Suicide Across Cultures

Oxford Cultural Psychiatry Series

Psychiatry of Intellectual Disability Across Cultures
Samuel Tromans, Regi Alexander, Satheesh Kumar Gangadharan, Chaya Kapugama, Sabyasachi Bhaumik

Homelessness and Mental Health
João Mauricio Castaldelli-Maia, Antonio Ventriglio, Dinesh Bhugra

Spirituality and Mental Health Across Cultures
Alexander Moreira-Almeida, Bruno Paz Mosqueiro, Dinesh Bhugra

Terrorism, Violent Radicalization, and Mental Health
Bhui, Dinesh Bhugra

Urban Mental Health
Dinesh Bhugra, Antonio Ventriglio, João Castaldelli-Maia, Layla McCay

Early Intervention in Psychiatric Disorders Across Cultures
Eric Y. H. Chen, Antonio Ventriglio, Dinesh Bhugra

Suicide Across Cultures

Edited by

Meryam Schouler-Ocak and
Murad M. Khan

Series editor

Dinesh Bhugra

OXFORD
UNIVERSITY PRESS

OXFORD
UNIVERSITY PRESS

Great Clarendon Street, Oxford, OX2 6DP,
United Kingdom

Oxford University Press is a department of the University of Oxford. It furthers the University's objective of excellence in research, scholarship, and education by publishing worldwide. Oxford is a registered trade mark of Oxford University Press in the UK and in certain other countries

Published in the United States of America by Oxford University Press
198 Madison Avenue, New York, NY 10016, United States of America

British Library Cataloguing in Publication Data

Data available

Library of Congress Control Number: 2024932761

ISBN 978–0–19–884340–5

DOI: 10.1093/med/9780198843405.001.0001

Printed and bound by
CPI Group (UK) Ltd, Croydon, CR0 4YY

Foreword

Suicide is a universal challenge that transcends geographical boundaries and cultural divides. Yet cultural influences profoundly impact individuals' and communities' attitudes toward suicide. In this complex landscape, there is a need to recognize the shared elements of human suffering and despair as well as to acknowledge the unique cultural nuances that shape individual responses to life's hardships and mental health problems.

By approaching the sensitive topic of suicide through the cultural lens, this important and insightful book guides us toward a more comprehensive understanding of the issue that goes beyond statistics and explores the intricate interplay of cultural norms, values, prejudices, and beliefs.

In many countries, mental health problems, including suicidal thoughts and behaviour, are stigmatized due to prevailing societal attitudes and misconceptions that equate them with weakness, personal failure, or even moral shortcomings. The limited awareness of mental health issues results in a lack of public health preventive efforts, a substantial misclassification or underreporting of suicide as a cause of death, and, ultimately, prevents individuals from seeking help.

'Suicide Across Cultures' encourages overcoming stigma and discrimination and offers a broader and more inclusive perspective on suicide that recognizes the inherent diversity of human experiences. Furthermore, by adopting an interdisciplinary approach, the book bridges the gaps between the genetic, psychological, and sociological viewpoints. Finally, it represents a call to action for researchers, clinicians, and policymakers to engage in suicide preventive interventions adapted to and respectful of the sociocultural context.

It is my sincere hope that this book sparks deep conversations and contributes to the ongoing global efforts to prevent suicide and promote global mental health.

Danuta Wasserman, MD, PhD
President, World Psychiatric Association (WPA)
Professor of Psychiatry and Suicidology, Karolinska Institutet (KI), Stockholm, Sweden
Head and Founder, National Centre for Suicide Research and Prevention of Mental Ill-Health (NASP) at KI
Director, WHO Collaborating Centre for Research, Methods Development, Training in Suicide Prevention

Contents

Part 5 **Prevention concepts and programs**

Contributors

Dahlia
Universitas Syiah Kuala,
School of Psychology, Banda Aceh,
Indonesia

Dana Alonza
Fordham University
Graduate School of Social Service
New York, NY, USA

Gregory Armstrong
Nossal Institute for Global Health
Melbourne School of Population
and Global Health The University of
Melbourne, Australia

Anil Arora
Graduate College of Social Work
University of Houston
Houston, TX, USA

Nargis Asad
Associate Professor, Clinical
Psychologist, Aga Khan University
Hospital, Karachi, Pakistan

Jason Bantjes
Faculty of Medicine and Health
Sciences,
Department of Global Health,
Department of Psychiatry and
Mental Health, University of Cape
Town,
Stellenbosch University,
Alcohol, Tobacco and Other Drug
Research Unit, South African
Medical Research Council,
Institute for Life Course Health
Research, South Africa

Isabella Berardelli
Research Fellow of Psychiatry
Department of Psychology,
Sapienza University of Rome
Rome, Italy

Dinesh Bhugra
Institute of Psychiatry,
Kings College London
London, UK

Eva Döring-Brandl
Alexianer Krankenhaus
Hedwigshöhe, Berlin, Germany

Elsie Breet
Faculty of Medicine and Health
Sciences,
Department of Global Health,
Institute for Life Course Health
Research,
Stellenbosch University, South Africa

Marcus Brown
PhD Student, Graduate College of
Social Work, University of Houston
Houston, TX, USA

Sean Burr
Graduate College of Social Work
University of Houston
Houston, TX, USA

Báltica Cabieses
Universidad del Desarrollo Chile
University of York, UK

Silvia Sara Canetto
Department of Psychology
Colorado State University
Fort Collins, CO, USA

Vladimir Carli
National Centre for Suicide Research and Prevention (NASP)
Karolinska Institutet
Stockholm, Sweden

Chan Lai Fong
National University of Malaysia (UKM), Malaysia

Chen Ying-Yeh
Taipei City Hospital
National Yang-Ming University, Taipei City, Taiwan

Mehmet Eskin
Department of Psychology
Koc University
Istanbul, Turkey

Özlem Eylem-van Bergeijk
Psychiatry Research Group
The Netherlands Manchester Global Foundation
Webster University Leiden Campus
Global Mental Health Cultural
Manchester, UK

Liza Fathiariani
Aceh Psychiatric Hospital
Banda Aceh, Indonesia

Francesco D. Fritz
Department of Psychiatry and Neurosciences Charité Campus Mitte
Berlin, Germany

Robin Edward Gearing
Center for Mental Health Research and Innovation in Treatment Engagement and Service (MH-RITES Research Center)
Graduate College of Social Work
University of Houston
Houston, TX, USA

Ina Giegling
Comprehensive Center for Clinical Neurosciences and Mental Health (C3NMH)
Medical University of Vienna, Austria

Stefan Gutwinski
Department of Psychiatry and Psychotherapy
University Medicine Charité Berlin, Germany

Sahar N. Hamid
Assistant Professor Institute of Business Administration
Cognitive and Perceptual Psychologist
Karachi, Pakistan

Annette M. Hartmann
Department of Psychiatry and Psychotherapy
Comprehensive Center for Clinical Neurosciences and Mental Health (C3NMH)
Medical University of Vienna, Austria

Nusrat Husain
Director Research Global Mental
University of Manchester, UK

Miriam Iosue
Karolinska Institutet
Stockholm, Sweden

Ashraf Kagee
Department of Psychology
Stellenbosch University South Africa

Murad M. Khan
Department of Psychiatry,
Aga Khan University,
Karachi, Pakistan

Marianne C. Kastrup
Specialist in Psychiatry former Treasurer World Association Social Psychiatry former Secretary General European Psychiatric Association former Member Executive Committee World Psychiatric Association
Hvidovre, Denmark

Sangina Khudododova
Graduate College of Social Work
University of Houston
Houston, TX, USA

Dorian A. Lamis
Associate Professor, Emory University School of Medicine, Atlanta, Georgia, US

Felicia Boma Lazaridou
Psychiatry and Psychotherapy Clinic
CCM Charité Univesitätsmedizin
Berlin, Germany

Ying Ma
PhD Student Graduate College of Social Work University of Houston
Houston, TX, USA

Fauzia Mahr
Associate Professor of Psychiatry and Pediatrics
Child and Adolescent Psychiatrist
Penn State Milton S Hershey Medical Center
Hershey, USA

José Manoel Bertolote
Department of Neurology, Psychology, and Psychiatry, Botucatu Medical School – UNESP, Botucatu, Brazil

Marthoenis Marthoenis
Department of Psychiatry and Mental Health Nursing, Universitas Syiah Kuala, Banda Aceh, Indonesia

Stephan Maul
Neurologist, Johann-Gottfried-Boltze-Straße, Salzatal, Germany

Sascha Milin
Department of Psychiatry and Psychotherapy
University Medical Center
Hamburg-Eppendorf
Germany

Adrian P. Mundt
Universidad Diego Portales y Universidad de Chile Santiago, Chile

Tania Nadeem
Aga Khan University Hospital

Maria Panagioti
University of Manchester, Manchester, UK

Maurizio Pompili
Department of Medical and Molecular Sciences
School of Health Sciences, Sapienza University of Rome
Rome, Italy

Aaron Poppleton
Keele University
Stoke-on-Trent, UK

Ajay Risal
Consultant Psychiatrist & Somatic Experiencing Practitioner (SEP)
Dhulikhel Hospital
Kathmandu University School of Medical Sciences (KUSMS)
Kathmandu University Hospital
Dhulikhel Kavre, Nepal

Elena Rogante
Department of Psychology, Sapienza University of Rome, Italy

Wulf Rössler
Professor of clinical psychiatry
Director of the Clinic for Social Psychiatry
General Psychiatry Zurich
Department of Psychiatry and Psychotherapy
University Medicine Charité
Berlin, Germany

Dan Rujescu
Department of Psychiatry and Psychotherapy Comprehensive Center for Clinical Neurosciences and Mental Health (C3NMH)
Medical University of Vienna, Austria

Nani Safuni
Department of Medical Surgical Nursing, Universitas Syiah Kuala
Banda Aceh, Indonesia

Pooja Saini
School of Psychology, Liverpool John Moores University, UK

Shahnaz Savani
Social Work
University of Houston-Downtown
Houston, TX, USA

Barbara Schneider
Abteilung Abhängigkeitserkrankungen, Psychiatrie und Psychotherapie
LVR-Klinik Köln

Meryam Schouler-Ocak
Psychiatric University Clinic of Charité
St. Hedwig Hospital Berlin
Berlin, Germany

Stefanie Schreiter
Department of Psychiatry and Psychotherapy University Medicine Charité, Berlin, Germany

Dan J. Stein
Faculty of Health Sciences
Department of Psychiatry and Mental Health
University of Cape Town
South Africa

Antonio Ventriglio
University of Foggia Foggia, Italy

Lakshmi Vijayakumar
Department of Psychiatry Voluntary Health Services
SNEHA Suicide Prevention Centre, Chennai, India

Danuta Wasserman
National Centre for Suicide Research and Prevention of Mental Ill-Health
Karolinska Institutet Stockholm, Sweden
World Psychiatric Association (WPA) - Section on Suicidology

Cameron Watson
Barts NHS Trust, London

Thomas Wenzel
World Psychiatric Association, Scientific Section on Psychological Aspects of Torture and Persecution, Switzerland

Manfred Wolfersdorf
Former Medical Director
Bezirkskrankenhaus Bayreuth
Germany

Anna Wong
The Education University of Hong Kong Pokfulam, Hong Kong

Chen Ying-Yeh
Taipei City Hospital
National Yang-Ming University,
Taipei City, Taiwan

Paul Yip
Faculty of Social Sciences
Department of Social Work and
Social Administration
University of Hong Kong Pokfulam,
Hong Kong

Melissa Yoong
University of Nottingham Malaysia
Selangor, Malaysia

Introduction

According to the World Health Organization (WHO), more than 700,000 people take their own lives every year globally, i.e. one death by suicide every 40 seconds.[1] Among teenagers and young adults, suicide is the second most common cause of death after road traffic accidents.[1] Overall, almost three times as many men than women die by suicide. The global age-standardized suicide rate was 9.0 per 100 000 population for 2019. Rates varied between countries from fewer than two deaths by suicide per 100 000 to over 80 per 100 000.[2] Thus, an incredibly large number of people die by suicide globally, every year.

Every death is a tragedy for family, friends and colleagues. Suicide is etiologically heterogeneous and occurs due to a convergence of a broad spectrum of individual and non-individual risk factors, with significant differences in its patterns across gender, age, culture, geographic location and personal history.

With respect to epidemiology, the impact of culture on the suicide rates across cultures are well established. Culture influences the psychopathology of suicidal behaviour. These aspects are of high relevance for the understanding and assessment of a suicidal crisis, since the suicidal person is influenced by deep rooted traditions of suicidal behaviour in his/her culture of origin. Thus, this book aims to generate a broader understanding of suicide across cultures, which, we hope, will contribute to the understanding of effective multicultural suicide prevention programs and treatment for those who are suffering from mental health issues. It offers the opportunity to expand knowledge beyond majority groups and to look further than the dominant frame in suicide research, treatment and prevention. With majority of global suicides taking place in non-Western societies as well as the increase of ethnic minorities and immigrants across the globe, and with immigrant and minority status conferring a risk of suicide, the manifestation of suicidal behaviour among minorities is an important area in suicide research.

Experts from different parts of the world were invited to contribute to this book covering different aspects of suicidal behaviors from a variety of perspectives.

As can be seen, we have included topics and regions that usually are not covered in texts on suicide and self-harm. Some of these include social minority group in Latin America, suicidal behavior in sub-Saharan Africa and countries such as Nepal and Indonesia, migrant populations in Hong Kong and Germany, influence of religion on euthanasia and physician assisted suicide, suicidality in Blacks and People of Colour communities etc. amongst others. These chapters are in addition to the more 'traditional' topics such as epidemiology of suicide and self-harm, genetics aspects of suicide and national suicide prevention strategies etc.

Schneider, Milin and Wolfersdorf explain the terminology of suicidal behaviours, particularly the meaning of suicide in different cultural backgrounds. They underline that the meanings of suicidal behaviour in all forms like death wishes, suicidal thoughts, suicide attempts, death by suicide, and self-destructive behaviours. These are all different, because they are based on different cultural traditions.

Watson and Bhugra give an overview of cultural factors in suicide and point out that cultures have different patterns and types of suicide and that cultural values can contribute to suicidal ideation and acts of deliberate self-harm across cultures.

In his chapter on 'The role of culture in suicidal process', Eskin outlines how culture might be involved in the suicidal process and highlights methodological considerations in surveys and scientific work on the relationship between religion, individualism-collectivism, and self-construal with suicidal behavior. He gives examples of three cultural manifestations that scientific work identified earlier as representing cross-cultural variations and ends with some conclusions and recommendations for future scientific work.

Rössler, Schreiter and Gutwinski focus on the 'Epidemiological aspects of Suicide and Suicidality'. Lifetime prevalence rates for suicidal ideation lie around 40–50% in the general population. The authors contend that looking from the burden of disease perspective, the impact of suicide is comparable to that of cardio-vascular disease.

Giegling, Maul, Hartmann, and Rujescu highlight the genetic aspects of suicide. Genes are implicated in suicidal behavior and partially overlapping genetic backgrounds are beginning to emerge as samples sizes increase in candidate gene and genome-wide association studies, and polygenic risk score predictions are conducted, though no conclusive results can be given at present.

Yoong, Chan and Chen share the result of a systematic review of empirical studies on gender inequality and suicide. They found that although some studies suggest that higher female labour force participation is associated with an increased suicide risk, this was not observed in latter investigations, which implies that the relationship between suicidal behaviour and gender equality may have changed over time. Other contextual factors such as the quality of a country's human capabilities may also affect suicidality as gender norms within the society shift.

Gearing, Alonza, Savani, Burr, Arora and Khudododova in their chapter 'Suicide and Religion: A Comparative Analysis of a Complex Relationship to Inform Practice', examine the complex relationship between suicide and religion across five dominant world religious groups, including Buddhism, Christianity, Hinduism, Islam, and Atheism/Agnosticism. The role of religious doctrine, degree of affiliation, and level of participation are explored for their association with suicide ideation and behavior to clarify the current state of evidence and inform suicide prevention and intervention efforts.

Wong and Yip discuss a case study suicide among Asian migrants in Hong Kong. They underline that the healthy migrant effect must be viewed together with risk and protective factors specific to each migrant group with the knowledge of both their native culture and the sociocultural context of the migration destination. Some tailor-made services should be made available in helping these migrants to cope with difficulties and to mitigate suicidal risks.

Bantjes, Breet, Kagee and Stein's chapter focusses on suicide prevention in sub-Saharan Africa, a region about which very little is known in the context of suicide. They explore common contextual and cultural factors which may have an important bearing on suicide prevention in the region. Opportunities for potential collaboration across the region to advance the research and practice of culturally informed suicide prevention are discussed.

Mundt, Fritz and Cabieses analyse suicide risk in social minority groups (international migrants, prison populations and sexual minorities) in Latin America. Prison populations has more than doubled in Latin America in the past two decades. In this vulnerable population, mental disorders, substance use problems and suicide risk are highly prevalent, while access to care is still poor. The authors could not find reliable estimates of suicide rates in migrants for Latin American countries.

Eylem-van Bergeijk and Eskin work on suicidal behaviour and social cultural factors among immigrants of Turkish origin in Germany. The chapter outlines risk and precipitating factors in the research on suicidal behaviours among Turkish populations in Europe and Turkey. Additionally, identified risk and precipitating factors that lead to suicidal behaviours are discussed in the context of religion and migration and customised to their needs and expectations, in preventing, caring and treating suicidal behaviours. Their findings apply to all immigrant populations around the world.

Poppleton, Saini, Panagioti and Husain in their chapter on 'Suicidal behaviour and sociocultural factors among South Asians in the UK' explore a range of factors predisposing and protecting British South Asian individuals from self-harm and suicide. include mental health stigma, cultural identity, religion, marriage and relationships, domestic violence and mental and physical health conditions. Training in cultural competence, and adaptation of psychological interventions and therapies to address interpersonal triggers for self-harm and suicide are needed.

Lazaridou and Schouler-Ocak in their chapter 'Suicidality in Black and People of Colour Communities' provide a theoretical and conceptual overview of suicidality in black and people of colour communities, a hitherto rather neglected vulnerable group that suffers particularly from the influence of racism, and other forms of discrimination: interpersonal, institutional and structural. The connection to centering the thwarted social belongingness of racism's structural exclusion as suicide risk is also discussed.

We also included a few chapters from settings about which relatively little is known on suicidal behaviors. Two such settings are Nepal and Indonesia, both South Asian developing countries. In their chapter on suicide in Nepal, Wenzel and Risal report that suicide rates, especially in women, are high, and might reflect discriminative practices against women in general. The complex multi-ethnic and multi-religious setting does not permit simplified conclusions as to the influence of these factors on suicide rates. Prevention strategies are possible but the resources and complex challenges in the country are limited.

Marthoenis, Safuni, Dahlia and Fathiariani in their chapter on 'Suicide in Indonesia' highlight that suicide has become a serious problem in Indonesia. Even though the estimated rate of suicidal behavior is increasing, the exact number remains unknown. As reasons, they mention that cultural beliefs, financial and familial issues, and the Islamic beliefs of the Indonesian population all play a role. Suicide prevention activities nationwide are also discussed.

In her chapter on 'Suicide scripts of the Nacirema' (American spelled backwards), Canetto uses an interesting satirical approach to challenge the dominant American view of suicide from the point of view of an imaginary outsider. Canetto argues that Nacirema/America suicide is a deeply cultural act and the necessity of a cultural perspective in suicide theory, research, and prevention. Kastrup in her chapter on 'Suicidality and Trauma MANUS' writes that PTSD has high comorbidity with pre-trauma depressive disorders and having a depressive diagnosis is associated with an increased risk of dying by suicide. Hence, adjusting for other psychiatric disorders, the association between the presence of post traumatic disorder and suicidal ideation is weakened.

Berardelli, Rogante, Lamis and Pompili in their chapter on 'Suicide and Psychiatric Disorders' shed light on the current knowledge of the relation between psychiatric disorders and suicide risk (suicide attempts and suicide ideation), focusing on bipolar disorder, major depressive disorder, schizophrenia, personality disorders, anxiety disorders, dissociative disorders and alcohol and substance abuse disorders.

In their chapter 'Bullying, Cyberbullying and Suicide', Nadeem, Hamid, Mahr & Asad discuss different forms of bullying and its association with suicide especially focusing on data from lower- and middle-income countries and the effect of culture in this paradigm. They explore the importance of preventive programs focusing on individuals, families, communities and schools.

Although books on suicide rarely include topics of euthanasia and/or physician assisted suicide, we decided to include these as they have important religious and cultural connotations. Savani, Arora, Brown, Ma and Gearing in their chapter on 'The Influence of Religion on Euthanasia and Physician Assisted Suicide' investigate the association and influence of religion on the perspectives and attitudes toward euthanasia and PAS across five of the dominant world religions, specifically Buddhism, Christianity, Hinduism, Islam, and Judaism.

Wasserman, Iosue and Carli in their chapter on 'Suicide during the COVID-19 pandemic in the world' underline that the majority of studies on suicidality during the COVID-19 pandemic comes from high- and middle-income countries. The research on this topic is particularly lacking in South America, African and East-Mediterranean Regions. According to the authors, efforts should be made to overcome the research and treatment gap in mental health that affect low- and middle-income countries and rural communities.

Bertolote in his chapter on 'National Strategies and Plans for the Prevention of Suicide: Why and Why Do Not Countries Have Them?' highlights despite majority of countries accepting that suicide is a major public health problem, less than forty countries have a national suicide prevention strategy as hundreds of thousands of lives continue to be unnecessarily lost every year around the world.

Armstrong and Vijayakumar in their chapter on 'Mass media and suicide in low and middle-income countries: learnings from India' share their findings from research into media and suicide in India, including the impact of culture and colonial legacies on media reporting, and the need to understand the broader ecosystem within which media reporting takes place. Their findings and recommendations apply equally well to all LMICs.

Brandl reviews ethnic aspects in pharmacological treatment of suicidality. Ethnopsychopharmacology is an important but frequently overlooked subject, more so in the pharmacological treatment of suicidality. In her chapter 'Ethnic aspects in pharmacological treatment of suicidality', Brandl addresses this important topic and summarizes current findings on ethnic factors influencing treatment response and/or occurrence of side effects.

We hope that these contributions would stimulate a perspective that is sensitive to the variation and complexity of the suicidal process across ethnicities and cultures, and underline the impact of the intersections of ethnicity, culture, gender, and age to suicide.

We would like to take this opportunity to thank all authors for their contributions.

We would also like to thank Dinesh Bhugra for providing the theme for the book.

We thank Adam Breivik for his continued very helpful support.

Last but not least, we thank Oxford University Press for making this publication possible.

The Editors

References

1. https://www.paho.org/en/topics/suicide-prevention_access 03.05.2023
2. **Suicide worldwide in 2019**: global health estimates. Geneva: World Health Organization; 2021.

Part 1

Influencing factors on suicide and suicidal behaviour

Chapter 1

Terminology of suicide and suicidal behaviour, and the meaning of suicide in different cultural backgrounds

Barbara Schneider, Sascha Milin, and Manfred Wolfersdorf

Introduction

It is obvious that societal suicide rates differ widely across nations of the world.[1] Lower suicide rates have been found in nations with less economic development and where Islam is the dominant religion. One possible explanation for the differences in national suicide rates is that different nations vary in their physiology. For example, there are clear differences in the frequency of genes in people from the different nations of Europe. Thus, different nations and cultures may differ in their genetic structure. Furthermore, for almost all nations, with only a few exceptions, male suicide rates are higher than those of female suicide. However, non-fatal suicidal behaviour appears to occur at a higher rate in women than in men and, as a result, it has come to be viewed as a 'feminine' behaviour.[2] In high-income countries, mental disorders are present in up to 90% of people who die by suicide; however, mental disorders seem to be less prevalent among those who die by suicide in some Asian countries, as shown in studies from China and India.[3,4] Furthermore, suicide patterns are different in Asia, as compared to those in Western countries.[5,6] Age distribution and male-to-female ratios are different—rates are highest in the elderly in Western countries, but highest in young people in Asia. In the former, the male-to-female ratio is greater at 3:1 (or higher), whereas in the latter, the ratio is lower at 2:1, with China showing higher suicide rates among women.

Terminology is a discipline that systematically studies the 'labelling or designating of concepts'. Terminology consists primarily of aspects such as analysing the concepts and concept structures used in a field or domain of activity and identifying the terms assigned to the concepts. Terminology science also concerns itself with the formation and development of concepts, as well as with the principles of exposing the existing relations between concepts and classifying concepts.

Meaning is defined as the interpretation evoked in a person by an object or event at a given time, and cultural meaning is defined as 'the typical (frequently recurring and widely shared aspects of the) interpretation of some type of object or event evoked in people as a result of their similar life experiences'(p. 6).[7] Meanings have to be placed in relation to the context,[8] because meaning is always something that exists in relation to, and cannot be separated from, the background context of human lives. The meaning of suicide must be differentiated from the definition of suicide.[9]

Definition and terms of suicidality in Western culture

In either Western or other cultures, there is no unique and universally valid definition of suicidality. Furthermore, there is no definition of suicidality that encompasses all aspects of this phenomenon, factoring in human thoughts, behaviour, and experience. The need for a standardized and shared nomenclature for suicidal ideation and behaviours has long been recognized. There has been an ongoing discussion for years regarding the effective provision of an acceptable basis for an internationally shared agreement on the use of a given nomenclature (available from: https://www.iasp.info/nomenclature.php). Even within Western countries, there are differing opinions on the interpretation and correct definition of each different form of suicidal (and non-suicidal) manifestations.[10]

The World Health Organization[3] pointed out in its report that different definitions may be useful for specific cases. For the purpose of its report, suicide was defined as an act of deliberately killing oneself. The term 'suicidal behaviour' describes a number of behaviours such as suicidal thoughts, plans, and attempts, and the act of suicide itself. Here too, the authors point out that the assignment of suicidal thoughts to the spectrum of suicidal behaviour is widely discussed academically and was chosen for pragmatic reasons. In German-speaking countries, there are also various definitions. One of the broadest definitions was conceived by Haenel and Pöldinger[11] who defined suicidality as 'the potential of all mental powers and functions, which tends towards self-destruction'.

According to Wolfersdorf, suicidality is the sum of all ways of thinking, behaving, and experiencing of people who strive for their own death in their thoughts, through active doing or passive omission, or through letting someone taking action, and who accept death as the possible result of an action.[12,13,14] Suicide is an available course of action for all people, but it often occurs in psychosocial crises and mental illness ('medical–psychosocial paradigm'). Suicide is a 'self-inflicted or self-induced self-damaging action with the aim of being dead and of achieving this goal with the knowledge, expectation, or belief, with the method applied; the outcome of the action is the death of the actor'.[15]

Psychodynamics of suicide

In Western culture, suicidality has been seen for centuries on the background of a primarily Christian sociocultural context, but also in the context of illness.[16] Burton treats suicide as the outcome of melancholy. A more recent definition from a psychodynamic point of view was developed by the Hamburg research group 'Suicidality and Psychotherapy':[17] Suicidality is understood as 'an expression of the escalation of a mental development in which people are hopeless and desperate and experience their situation as hopeless' (S. 20).[18] Suicidality is not understood in the sense of a specific illness, but rather as a developmental experience that is individually and differently pronounced, which can be updated in different (sub)cultural contexts and in different phases of life, with different illnesses and with gender-specific correspondence of varying intensity.[17] From a psychoanalytical, object–relations theoretical perspective, the triggers of suicidal experience (e.g. experiences of illness) that are mostly accessible to consciousness lead to destabilization of the previously functional defence. In particular, experiences of separation and—often conflictual—changes in interpersonal relationships, the loss of occupational identity, changes in the body and its functions, and one's own serious illnesses can trigger suicidal tendencies in the phase of life at an advanced age.

There still is no uniform model of aetiopathogenesis of suicidal tendencies. In Western culture, there are several models (e.g. 'development models', 'aetiopathogenetic models', and 'complex development models') of suicidality.[15] Development models describe the path from a triggering event to a suicidal action, independently of the respective aetiology. The two best-known clinically used development models of suicidal tendencies are:[15]

- The 'presuicidal syndrome' by Ringel[19]—which describes the mental state of a person with increasing loss of inner and outer degrees of freedom: increasing constriction (situational constriction, dynamic constriction, and constriction of interpersonal relationships), aggression congestion and aggression reversal (lack of aggression rebuttal and turnaround of aggression against one's own person), and suicidal fantasies (actively intended, passively pushing oneself forward);

- The model by Pöldinger,[20] describing the stages and dynamics of suicidal development: 'considering' phase (suicidal thoughts; preserved ability to distance and control, with hints and appeals), ambivalence phase (suicidal impulses; limited ability to distance and control with cries for help and announcements), and intention phase (suicidal action, suicide preparation: suspended ability to distance and control; resignation and deceptive calm [so-called 'calm before the storm']).

Aetiopathogenetic models of suicide

The aetiopathogenetic models claim to explain suicidal behaviour by psychodynamic, biological, or sociological causes. Complex development models[15] are based on psychobiosocial initial conditions, together with biographical development. This can result in a mental disorder with suicidal psychopathology on the one hand. On the other hand, it can result in a 'psychologically healthy personality' with self-destructive styles of conflict resolution, often combined with facts promoting suicidality and hopelessness, sometimes with a role model of suicide. Both paths lead from a narrowing of experience and behaviour to suicidality.

Meanings of suicidal behaviour in different cultures

Cultural aspects had been largely excluded in concepts of suicidal behaviour.[21] However, the ethnocultural context of suicidal behaviour is important.[22,23] Culture contributes to the nature and severity of the distress that people may suffer. It affects the development of psychopathology,[24] which, in turn, affects suicide rates. Culture can have effects on a person's choice of suicide over other possible solutions to their problems. Several authors[23,25,26] criticized the overboarding medical specially psychiatric view and the theoretical explanations of suicidal behaviour according to psychopathology and psychoanalytic psychodynamics. They recommend to study the different cultural and indigenous aspects, and concepts and meanings of suicidal behaviour to get a basis for culturally informed suicide prevention and suicide intervention efforts—besides concepts such as the interpersonal theory or cognitive models of suicidality or Shneidman's idea of an intolerable psychological pain or the 'escape' model.[27]

Already more than a century ago, Durkheim presented a complex sociological perspective, according to which suicide could not be fully explained by psychological factors, religious affiliations, geographical location, or climate.[28]

A major premise of his theory is that '[s]uicide varies inversely with the degree of integration of the social groups of which the individual forms a part' (p. 209).[29] Durkheim identified three forms of suicide in his analysis of this pattern: egoistic, altruistic, and anomic.

Durkheim[28] described in his famous book a sociological theory of suicide. He looked at social integration and different forms of suicidal behaviour: the so-called egoistic suicide, altruistic suicide, and anomic and fatalistic suicide. The Hungarian author Emil Szittya (1886–1964) edited a book called *Selbstmörder. Die erste Kulturgeschichte des Selbstmordes aller Zeiten und Völker*;[30] he had collected a large number of suicides and showed the relation with sociocultural factors in the persons' life. In 1990, Baumeister[27] focused on the 'escape model of suicide' as an attempt to die by suicide because of unbearable problems. Shneidman's theory of 'psychache'[31] was followed by Joiner's 'interpersonal theory of suicide'[32] describing the burden and feelings of social disconnection, and by Chandler's 'model of cultural continuity'[33] which tries to connect traditional past, contemporary context, and future events.[23]

Cultural meanings of suicidal behaviour

Culture affects the particular meaning attributed to suicidal behaviour. Suicide is viewed very differently by different cultural groups, and culture influences the form, meaning, and frequency of suicide.[34,35,36] It is not merely the cognitive meanings of suicide that very likely vary from one society to another and from one subsociety to another. Boldt[9] stated that meaning goes beyond the universal criteria for certifying and classifying self-destructive deaths to how suicide is conceptualized in terms of cultural normative values. There are different sociocultural concepts of suicide;[9] suicide can be seen as: (1) an unforgivable sin; (2) a psychotic act; (3) a human right; (4) a ritual obligation; and (5) an unthinkable act. Furthermore, suicide can be a symbolic act of rebellion and revenge.[37] However, a complete understanding of the meanings of suicide is very difficult.[9]

Examples for suicide cases in different cultures

Case: two sisters in Kabul, Afghanistan

Based on extensive ethnographic fieldwork in Afghanistan,[38] the communitive dimension of female suicide and suicide attempts can be analysed in the complex situation of contemporary and often contradictory Afghan culture, influenced by Islam, local traditions, war, and post-war experiences of migration and what is perceived as foreign and modern influences. Female suicides in Afghanistan are often conducted by means of self-immolation, which some

Afghans regard as foreign to local social practices, whereas others insist that self-immolation had a long tradition in Afghan society, even though Islam does not allow suicide. Kerosene, used for self-immolation, can be found easily in Afghan houses to light the kitchen fire and therefore could be attributed to the female realm, other than bullets or ropes, which are perceived as being more masculine as they are used in war activities or to tie up cattle. But there is more to this very specific way of dying by suicide. Such dramatic and painful performances do not totally contradict traditional Afghan ideas of the women's nature, which is by local beliefs associated with inherent emotional fragility and irrationality, even with the burden to endure pain and suffering. On the other hand, female suicidal behaviour seems to be one of the most powerful ways to express discontent, to rebel, and to achieve goals where there are no other means and no culturally accepted ways to communicate this verbally or by other means. It is subversive and powerful in nature, because it 'brings shame to men whose first responsibility is to ensure the well-being and respectability of their family', as Billaud[38] put it.

Billaud's[38] ethnographic observations focus on two sisters who live in the Girl's Dormitory at the University of Kabul, where women with very different social backgrounds regarding their rural heritages, financial situations, and migration histories are accommodated together. Girls there 'shared with a mixture of excitement, admiration and disapproval melodramatic stories of female suicide'.[38] This might be understood by the influence of modern and ancient tales and poetry, mainly influenced by the Persian version of romantic love tales, that have a strong emphasis on the dilutional nature of true love and its connection with madness on the men's side and the more honourable suffering of the girl.

The two sisters residing in this dormitory at the University of Kabul subsequently committed suicide attempts by swallowing overdoses of pills bought at the local bazaar. These attempts had happened after serious disputes with their father in the rural village from where they came. Even though they both fulfilled traditional duties and lived by Islamic values, their westernized behaviour in Kabul became more and more suspicious to their father, who blamed them for not following Islamic rules and for dishonouring the family. One of the sisters had studied music and engaged in popular music projects in Kabul, and the other sister had practised and taught kung fu in urban sport schools. Even long disputes and claims to live Islam in their own way did not help. It seemed to be very crucial to both girls to validate the rightfulness of their way. The older sister stated, 'if they cannot get this, then there is no point for me to live either.'

Subsequently, the social situation of the two sisters improved after they survived their suicide attempts. These actions deprived their father of any legitimate means to continue to disregard his daughters' voice. 'The threat of suicide acted as a gesture of protest against imposed roles, an assertion of other possible ways of being,' Billaud concluded. She argued that 'the performance of pain had brought an indisputable element of truth to (the) daughter's speech'.

Case: suicide of a young woman of the Ch'ol, an indigenous group in Mexico

An ethnographic study of the Ch'ol, an ethnic group native to Chiapas in southern Mexico,[39] demonstrated how both traditional belief systems and belief systems that have evolved from processes of cultural change contribute to the attribution of causes for suicidality. In this regard, the author sees traditional logic, which consists of a religious syncretism of Mayan beliefs and Catholicism introduced during the colonial period, as more likely to include ideas that causes are not subject to an individual's free will. These external causes can be of a supernatural nature such as magic, witchcraft, or divine destiny. However, they can also be inevitable, and thus also non-self-determined consequences of certain occurrences, usually as a result of excessive consumption of alcohol or marijuana.

On the other hand, however, there are also ideas that a suicidal act is based on a free decision. In this case, suicide is seen as a voluntarily chosen way out of subjectively unmanageable problems in life. This second idea of causal explanations seems to have been added rather later and seems to be related to the recent challenges for this ethnic group within the Mexican and global economy.

This interplay of assumed causes is illustrated by the example of a young woman from the Ch'ol group who died by suicide by hanging herself with a hammock in her parents' house. Her father's known alcohol dependency played a certain role in the perception of this suicide, which, on the part of some neighbours, is seen as a sign of inner family problems and thus comes into question as an indirect cause, whereas the girl's mother rejects this causal connection. She rather suspects, based on observed behavioural problems, that the girl's friends, who had taken jobs outside the village in the nearby city, were a bad influence on her and may have brought her into contact with alcohol or marijuana. Equally, however, explanations such as a divine plan or witchcraft have been considered and shamans and fortune tellers have been consulted. These had identified witchcraft as the cause. The signs were interpreted in such a way that, due to envy of the family that was very prestigious and financially well off in the village, a contracted sorcerer had manipulated the girl's spirit with evil intent. Finally, another external cause is thought to be that the physical peculiarity of the girl born as an albino and the limitations associated with it, such as not being able to work in the fields in bright sunlight, made it seem impossible for her to marry and take on the traditional role of a wife.

If one considers these different explanations, it will surprise a Western observer that these subjectively perceived causes stand side by side and can all appear equally plausible to the relatives of the suicide victim, as well as to the village community. In principle, an assumed harmful spell would be sufficient as a sole explanation. The fact that, at the same time, personal problems and a more or less free decision resulting from them are supposed to be causal, however, is not regarded by this group as a contradiction. In this, this ethnic group differs little from other non-Western societies. The high tolerance for accepting causes that can be attributed to a self-made decision due to 'problems' and, at the same time, explanations that do not see the causes in the individual themselves but in external interferences appear impressive regarding the understanding of suicidality.

Case: suicides of young male Inuits in Canada

Historically, suicidal behaviour dramatically increased among the Inuits in the 1950s and 1960s in Canada and Alaska.[23] Kral[40] suggested that this rise in suicides emerged because of changes partially resulting from actions of the Canadian government in the Arctic, which dramatically affected kin relationships, roles, and responsibilities, but also romantic relationships.

'Suicide is embedded in these relationships,' wrote Kral[40] and called it 'postcolonial suicides'. One of the author's own experience (M. W., 1987) with young male Inuits in Barrow's Top of the World in Northern Alaska at the ice showed that the loss of traditional roles as hunters on the one hand, and money from oil companies and the army on the other hand, as well as alcoholism, were significant reasons for the increase in suicide rates among young male Inuits.

Historically, suicidal behaviour among the Inuits has been known as 'altruistic', according to Durkheim's sociological concept of altruistic and anomic suicide motivations.

According to Kral,[40] nowadays suicide is seen in the context of political changes instigated by the Canadian government and leads to 'suicidal sadness' among the Inuits, who considered suicidality primarily in the absence of family, talking, and cultural values and practice. Belonging to the family groups was most important and romantic relationships were the most significant triggers for suicide among young male Inuits. The government initiated intervention programmes based on the concept of suicide as a mental health problem, but also began intervention programmes based on traditional cultural healing programmes with counsellors from inside the Inuit groups. Kral[40] studied the negative effects of such social changes, instigated by the government, on family, parenting, and romantic relationships in Inuit communities.

Conclusion

In the Western world, for many centuries till now, suicidal behaviour was mostly seen in the context of melancholia and depression. The meaning was 'suicide is a symptom of depression and a psychiatric problem'. Then the view changed—nowadays, we can find a tendency in the literature to focus more on (psycho) social and existential problems, as well as on psychodynamic factors in the development of suicidality, as described in the presuicidal syndrome by Ringel.[19]

In non-Western cultures, suicidal behaviour is seen in a complex scenery of different factors: situational, existential, religious and mystic factors, somatic health, duties in families, relationships, understanding one's own role, mental health, views of the future, and hope due to possible changes, etc. Such concepts of suicidality (e.g. crisis or disorder, psychopathology or personality, cultural accepted behaviour or disorder) are found in our cases from Mexico, Afghanistan, and Canada (the Inuits). Relationships, styles of living, consequences of governmental decisions about living styles, (female) role expectancies, traditional belief systems of witchcraft and magic powers, alcohol abuse, and altruistic ideas of not becoming a burden to others are all factors that are found in the understanding, interpretation, and cultural meanings of suicide in different parts of the world.

In conclusion, theories of suicidal behaviour in Western cultures are mainly based on psychophysiological and psychological concepts. Suicidality is understood as a symptom or behaviour of a mental disorder, mostly depression, alcoholism, or schizophrenia. Epidemiological research on risk factors for suicide provides evidence for this hypothesis. The role of psychiatric disorders or severe crisis situations is at the centre of understanding the meaning of suicidal behaviour and, as a consequence, the basis of suicide prevention strategies. Boldt[9] wrote in his paper *The meaning of suicide: implications for research*: '. . . no one who commits suicide does so without reference to the prevailing normative standards and attitudes of the cultural community.' Additionally, Colucci[22] quoted in *The cultural meaning of suicide*:[41] 'Individual live in a meaningful world: Culture may give us meaning in the world . . . This is true about suicidology . . . Suicide has different meanings for different cultures.'

So we have culturally seen different points of view or interpretations of suicidal behaviour: a medical–psychiatric view, a traditional meaning of altruistic suicidal behaviour of not to be a burden to the family, and a relationship-oriented psychodynamic view (see Box 1.1).

We identified many universal principal aspects in the suicidal context; these observed cross-cultural commonalities in the characteristics of individuals who die by suicide (such as depression, hopelessness, and relational problems) let us

Box 1.1 Common topics

According to all theories of suicidality, there are three common topics:

1. Suicidal behaviour is closely connected with mental disorders and substance abuse;
2. Relationships are an important factor in the psychodynamics of the development of suicidality; and
3. A range of cultural ideas and meanings from ideas of magic create suicide wishes, like in early Christian times (who kills oneself must be obsessed by the devil) up to modern role expectations which cannot be fulfilled.

The altruistic idea of killing oneself, and not to become a burden to the group, is again a subject of discussion according to the severe problem of (assisted) suicide (see Chu et al.),[42] particularly in the elderly, a recent discussion in different countries nowadays).

assume universality and invariance in cross-cultural meanings. However, the individual interpretation of suicidal behaviour must always include the cultural imprint, including gendered meanings, in order to meet the future challenges of suicide prevention, especially on the background of a rapid sociocultural transition. Therefore, we need specific suicide prevention and intervention programmes for different sociocultural settings. Only by differentiating as precisely as possible the ethnic-, culture-, and subculture-dependent meanings of suicide, and by systematically bringing these into research paradigms, can the development of valid theories of causation, prediction, and intervention and prevention programmes be supported.

References

1. **World Health Organization** (2021). Suicide worldwide in 2019: global health estimates. Available from: https://www.who.int/publications/i/item/9789240026643
2. **Linehan MM.** Suicide and attempted suicide: study of perceived sex differences. Perceptual and Motor Skills. 1973;**37**(1):31–4.
3. **World Health Organization** (2014). Suicide prevention: a global imperative. Available from: https://www.who.int/publications/i/item/9789241564779.
4. **Schneider B.** *Risikofaktoren für Suizid.* Regensburg: Roderer; 2003.
5. **Mayer P, Ziaian T.** Suicide, gender, and age variations in India. Are women in Indian society protected from suicide? Crisis. 2002;**23**(3):98–103.
6. **Vijayakumar L, John S, Pirkis J, Whiteford H.** Suicide in developing countries (2): risk factors. Crisis. 2005;**26**(3):112–19.

7. **Strauss C, Quinn N.** *A Cognitive Theory of Cultural Meaning.* New York, NY: Cambridge University Press; 1997.
8. **Bracken P.** Cultural syndromes and cognitive psychology. Transcultural Psychiatry. 2002;**39**:214–19.
9. **Boldt M.** The meaning of suicide: implications for research. Crisis. 1988;**9**(2):93–108.
10. **Schneider B, Müller RS, Sperling U.** Voluntarily stopping eating and drinking (VSED): a suicidological perspective. Journal of Gerontopsychology and Geriatric Psychiatry. 2020;**34**:1–10.
11. **Haenel T, Pöldinger W.** Erkennen und Beurteilen von Suizidalität. **In: Kisker KP, Lauter H, Meyer JE**, et al., editors. *Psychiatrie der Gegenwart* **II.** Berlin: Springer; 1986. pp. 107–32.
12. **Wolfersdorf M.** *Der suizidale Patient in Klinik und Praxis.* Stuttgart: Wissenschaftliche Verlagsgesellschaft; 2000.
13. **Wolfersdorf M.** *Suizid bei stationären psychiatrischen Patienten.* Regensburg: Roderer; 1989.
14. **Wolfersdorf M, Etzersdorfer E.** *Suizid und Suizidprävention* [*Suicide and Suicide Prevention*]. 2. Auflage, 2nd edition. Stuttgart: Kohlhammer; 2021.
15. **Wolfersdorf M.** Suizidalität [Suicidality]. Nervenarzt. 2008;**79**(11):1319–34.
16. **Burton R.** *Anatomie der Melancholie.* 1. Auflage Oxford. München: Artemis Verlag; 1621.
17. **Lindner R, Fiedler G, Götze P.** Diagnostik der Suizidalität. Deutsches Ärzteblatt. 2003;**100**(A):1004–7.
18. **Lindner R.** *Suizidale Männer in der psychoanalytisch orientierten Psychotherapie. Eine systematische qualitative Untersuchung.* Gießen: Psychosozial-Verlag; 2006.
19. **Ringel E.** *Der Selbstmord. Abschluss einer krankhaften psychischen Entwicklung.* Wien: Maudrich; 1953.
20. **Pöldinger W.** *Die Abschätzung der Suizidalität.* Bern, Stuttgart, Wien: Hans Huber Verlag; 1968.
21. **Colucci E.** Cultural meaning(s) of suicide: a cross-cultural study. In: **Colucci E, Lester D**, editors. *Suicide and Culture: Understanding the Context.* Göttingen: Hogrefe Publishing; 2013. pp. 93–195.
22. **Colucci E.** Cultural issues in suicide risk assessment. In: **Kumar U, Mandal MK**, editors. *Suicidal Behavior: Assessment of People at Risk.* Washington, DC: Sage; 2010. pp. 107–35.
23. **O'Keefe VM, Tucker RP, Cole AB, Hollingsworth DW, Wingate LR.** Understanding indigenous suicide through a theoretical lens: a review of general, culturally-based, and indigenous frameworks. Transcultural Psychiatry. 2018;**55**(6):775–99.
24. **Cohen Y, Spirito A, Apter A, Saini S.** A cross-cultural comparison of behavior disturbance and suicidal behavior among psychiatrically hospitalized adolescents in Israel and the United States. Child Psychiatry and Human Development. 1997;**28**(2):89–102.
25. **Kral MJ.** Book Review: **Honkasalo M-L** and **Tuominen M**, editors. *Culture, Suicide, and the Human Condition.* New York, NY: Berghahn. Transcultural Psychiatry. 2015;**52**(6):NPI14–15.
26. **Honkasalo ML, Tuominen M.** *Culture, Suicide, and the Human Condition.* New York, NY: Berghahn; 2015.

27. **Baumeister RF.** Suicide as escape from self. Psychological Review. 1990;**97**(1):90–113.
28. **Durkheim E.** *Le Suicide.* New York, NY: Free Press; 1897.
29. **Durkheim E.** *Suicide: A Study in Sociology* (English translation of original publication '*Le Suicide*', 1897). New York, NY: Free Press; 1951.
30. **Selbstmörder SM.** *Ein Beitrag zur Kulturgeschichte aller Zeiten und Völker.* 2. Auflage 2016, **Bucherverlag König, Greiz** ed. Leipzig: C. Weller & Co. Verlag; 1925.
31. **Shneidman ES.** Suicide as psychache. In: **Goldblatt M, Maltsberger T**, editors. *Essential Papers on Suicide.* New York, NY: New York University Press; 1996. pp. 633–8.
32. **Joiner TE.** *Why People Die by Suicide.* Cambridge, MA: Harvard University Press; 2005.
33. **Chandler MJ, Lalonder CE.** Cultural continuity as a hedge against suicide in Canada's First Nations. Transcultural Psychiatry. 1998;**35**(2):191–219.
34. **Maris RW.** *Pathways to Suicide: A Survey of Self-Destructive Behaviors.* Baltimore, MD: John Hopkins University Press; 1981.
35. **Hendin H.** *Suicide in Scandinavia.* New York, NY: Doubelday; 1965.
36. **Farberow NL.** *Suicide in Different Cultures.* Baltimore, MD: University Park Press; 1975.
37. **Meng H, Bilke O, Braun-Scharm H, Zarotti G, Burgin D.** [Indications for inpatient child and adolescent treatment]. Praxis der Kinderpsychologie und Kinderpsychiatrie. 2002;**51**(7):546–58.
38. **Billaud J.** Suicidal performances: voicing discontent in a girls' dormitory in Kabul. Culture, Medicine, and Psychiatry. 2012;**36**:264–85.
39. **Imberton G.** Chol understandings of suicide and human agency. Culture, Medicine, and Psychiatry. 2012;**36**:245–63.
40. **Kral MJ.** Postcolonial suicide among Inuit in Arctic Canada. Culture, Medicine, and Psychiatry. 2012;**36**(2):306–25.
41. **Leenaars AA, Anawak J, Brown C, Hill-Keddie T, Taparti L.** Genocide and suicide among indigenous people: the north meets the south. Canadian Journal of Native Studies. 1999;**19**:337–63.
42. **Chu C, Buchman-Schmitt JM, Stanley IH,** et al. The interpersonal theory of suicide: a systematic review and meta-analysis of a decade of cross-national research. Psychological Bulletin. 2017;**143**(12):1313–45.

Chapter 2

Cultural factors in suicide

Cameron Watson, Dinesh Bhugra, and Antonio Ventriglio

Introduction

Suicide is not an uncommon phenomenon and is seen in cultures around the world. The reasons for dying by suicide can be personal, social, cultural, psychiatric, or other. It is inevitable that cultural factors will influence all of these reasons—however, some more than others. It is well recognized that cultures mould personality and cognitive and social development. In addition, various social determinants, such as poverty, unemployment, economic downturn, and urbanization, including overcrowding, lack of green spaces, and poor transport, can contribute to poor mental health and thereby contribute to the risk of suicide.

Suicide has been reported from across countries and cultures and history. Rates of suicide vary across cultures and regions within the same country. However, in many countries around the world, suicidal acts remain illegal, which makes accurate data collection quite problematic. Cultural factors can be crucial to the aetiology, genesis, perpetuation, and outcome of many psychiatric disorders, which, in themselves, can lead to suicidal ideation and suicide. Not all individuals who have suicidal ideation go on to the suicidal act. Psychosocial and cultural perspectives of suicide are important and have to be understood in the context of an individual's culture and cultural background.

In this chapter, we aim to highlight some of the key cultural factors and the role they may play in contributing to the act of attempted or completed suicide, and we will illustrate these from both historical and current perspectives. We believe that cultural determinants of health play a major role in the genesis of psychiatric disorders.

Culture

The term 'culture' has been used in three ways at least, firstly to describe the medium within which bacteria may grow or cultivation of crops. It also reflects the medium within which an individual is born, grows up, undergoes schooling, works, plays, lives, and dies. Culture is something we are not born with, but born into. Culture influences our cognitive and social development, and helps to develop our worldview. It must be remembered that culture is an integral part of who we are and what makes us, and yet is dynamic. We change in response to culture and, in turn, we change the culture. Culture has been defined as the complex whole which includes knowledge, beliefs, arts, laws, morals, customs, and any other capabilities and habits acquired as a member of society (p. 1).[1] Culture has been described as refinement (as in a cultured individual) to cultural identity and lastly as a way of life, including morals, laws, etc.[2] It is clear that all aspects of culture are acquired and relate to habits of the group and society within which individuals live, work, play, and age.[3]. The relationship between an individual and culture is complex and multilayered. It is a relational matter linking human beings with their environment and this is a bidirectional matter.[4] It can be seen as a web[5] and as daily lived experience and activities, including communication and social relations (p. 16).[6] Culture gives us a sense of belonging, purpose, and identity. Within cultural factors occur a number of characteristics which influence the individual in multiple ways. Cultural factors can be seen at personal, family, and larger social/societal levels, and their learning and impact on the individual will vary.

Cultural factors and the self

Understanding the self is crucial, as suicide and deliberate self-harm both concern the self. It is critical to understand the cultural differences in one's concept of the self. The self can be individual, familial, or universal.[7] Furthermore, very often in European countries, the self is egocentric, whereas in many traditional societies, it is sociocentric. As Morris[8] identified, there is a clear distinction between the Eastern and Western concepts of the self. These are also likely to be modulated through social and cultural exchanges, and may evolve in response to the process of acculturation. Furthermore, the act of suicide itself will be influenced by the type of self. As outlined by Morris,[8] it is entirely likely that in traditional societies like India, the emphasis is on kinship and families and the individual identity is embedded in a group and what has been described as weness.[9] However, there are two caveats to this—firstly that cultures are dynamic and culture in many parts of India is in transition, so things are changing. And secondly, it needs to be recognized that not every individual in a sociocentric culture is likely to be sociocentric. Self can be identified as a sense of 'who am I?', and the purpose of self-enhancement is a desire for positive feedback about the self and is rooted in the desire to seek pleasure and avoid pain. Self-knowledge is important simply because the self keeps changing in a dynamic way in response to external stimuli and sociocultural circumstances. It is important to recognize and acknowledge that multilayered complex nature of the self which is relevant in identifying what we mean by deliberate self-harm, as harm to a sociocentric self is likely to be very different from that to an egocentric self. The mind–body interaction or the dichotomy seen in some cultures can lead to some further difficulties in identifying the self and managing it.

Giddens[10] noted that suicide is a social fact and has to be explained by other social facts. Durkheim observed that the rates of suicide varied across countries and religions; as he had described,[11] there are different types of suicide. After observing the suicide rate of a religious community, he noted that this was inversely related to the level of social integration of that community: the more strongly integrated the religious society was, the lower its rate of suicide (p. 44).[10] It has been demonstrated that rates of crime, violence, mental disorders, and suicide are higher in egocentric societies.[12] The roles of cultural values and societal structures are worth remembering when interpreting data on rates of suicide or attempted suicide. Another major factor that needs to be remembered when looking at death rates due to suicide is how the data are collected and the stigma associated with suicide which may affect reporting and recording of suicides.

Durkheim described three types of suicide which are worth noting, as they play a significant role in developing interventions and these varieties are of significance even now. These are: egoistic, anomic, and altruistic suicides. He also noted that low suicide rates in many traditional societies may be due to counterpoint to egoistic suicide because death may be seen as a welcome release and may be meaningful. This does play a role in many countries, even now. For example, although farmers in India have been known to die by suicide due to financial problems,[13] compensation for the suicide from the government helps the family to repay debts.[14] Therefore, this is likely to contribute to increased rates of suicide, as the individual may choose to sacrifice themselves as part of an altruistic act.

The self across religions

In this section, we propose to briefly describe some illustrative concepts of the self as related to various religions. This is not a comprehensive review of the state but simply serves to highlight some of the religious and cultural variations across the globe.

Hinduism

Hinduism is more of a philosophy than a religion. Polytheistic in form, it does not have a single leader. Four Vedas are the traditional source of tenets and rules related to the Hindu way of life. The Ayurveda is a system of medicine where there is clear communication between mind and body and diseases are caused by diet, the environment, and other multiple factors. The mind is said to have two purposes—atomic and invisible unity—and directs the senses and control of the self, along with reasoning and deliberation (which could be equated with cognition). Beyond the mind lies the intellect. An individual is composed of 24 elements: the mind, along with 10 organs (five each cognitive and conative), five sense objects, and eight *prakriti* or evolutes of nature.[15] For most Hindus, religion is all-pervading, but the individual is left to their own devices to decide what to follow and when to attend services, etc. The practice is largely internalized and human beings are the highest level in living beings, and therefore one step away from nirvana by doing the right things to avoid reincarnation. One's present state and status in life may be predestined due to actions (karma) from previous birth. Hindu attitudes to suicide are ambivalent. Hindu identity is in terms of kin relations and caste membership. Religious suicides have been described in Hindu religious texts.[16] In ancient India, suicide was often seen as an act which was not a result of medical or psychiatric conditions. Several incidents of suicide have been described in the two scriptures of Hinduism. Self-immolation and death by drowning are described, perhaps related to a function of 'purification'. People with incurable diseases or those too old to carry out their appointed religious duties and ascetics are allowed to die by suicide. Attitudes and practice changed in medieval times and subsequently following invasions and colonization.

Buddhism, Sikhism, and Jainism

Buddhism, Sikhism, and Jainism emerged from Hinduism as a response to the increasing rigidity of the Hindu caste system, which, over time, had also created tensions among groups. Buddha's primary insight into interdependence and impermanence of everything forms the concept of the Buddhist self. His teachings suggested that one should refrain from taking life, and yet Buddhist monks often kill themselves by self-immolation in public places occasionally for political reasons and political statements. Buddhism extols the value of human life, and one of its five precepts is to do with refraining from taking life. Buddha himself chided a monk for attempting suicide, but not seriously enough to expel the monk from the order. It can be argued that as both Buddhism and Hinduism believe in reincarnation, this may seem to give permission to some vulnerable individuals to die by suicide in search of a better life in the next incarnation. Sikhism is monotheistic and sees the self as sociocentric, with God being responsible for the world, but with the world itself being an illusion. Their Holy Book is the Guru Granth Sahib, and all the tenets and principles of Sikhism are written in that. Jainism too is monotheistic; however, it sees suicide as vulgar and evil. One of the tenets of the religion is that individuals should avoid the desire for death, although death by fasting in calamities, famines, extremes of old age, and incurable diseases is accepted, but not encouraged. Wherever an act of suicide is accepted, it is often for those who have lived their life to the fullest extent and acquired the highest ascetic powers.[17,18]

Islam

Islam, as a religion, took off from north-west Arabia in the seventh century and rapidly spread further north and west.[19] Its spread to the east to India and on to Indonesia occurred over the subsequent few centuries. The ethical dimensions of Islam lie in the weaving of bringing together a just and fair society under the guidance of God. Individuals are equal in the eyes of God, and kindness is to be cultivated and encouraged. In ancient Egypt, suicide was discouraged, as by doing so, the soul would lose its home. It was said that Cleopatra's suicide was accepted because she was Greek, not Egyptian. Historically, Islam provides a framework for social and cultural living. Islam proscribes suicide because it is felt that only God can take life. Islam advocates that life is to be preserved and suicide is 'haram' (forbidden).

Suicide as a leading cause of death is seventh in Europe and eighth in Western Pacific, but twenty-fifth in the Eastern Mediterranean region of the WHO.[20,21] It is likely that as in many countries in the region, suicidal acts are illegal, reporting may be less than perfect. However, there is no doubt that Muslim countries by and large show lower rates of suicide. In Algeria, the rates of suicide reported are low, but those aged between 15 and 22 years are at high risk and the rates become even lower in the month of Ramadan.[22] A similarly low rate has been reported from Saudi Arabia,[23,24] Iran,[25] and Jordan,[26] although with cultures in transition, these may be beginning to change. The religion moulds our worldview through a spiritually charged vision on the one hand and through rationalism on the other. Islam offers paradigms for the role of the individual and community functioning along with a vision of the self and self-realization, which not only differs from Western cultures and religious concepts, but also gets misinterpreted.

Culturally recognized suicide

Interpretations of various religious texts and their precepts and tenets can vary widely, depending upon a number of factors, but it is clear that irrespective of religious attitudes to suicide, suicide exists across all cultures and religions, and attitudes to these acts also vary a lot.

We shall now look towards more culturally nuanced suicide (e.g. *hara-kiri* and *shinju* in Japan, and *sati* and *jauhar* in India.

Japan

In Japan, *hara-kiri*, or *seppuku* (belly-cutting), was undertaken as an act of loyalty to a superior or to restore injured honour if revenge seemed impossible. Japanese viewed this type of suicide as voluntary and obligatory. The ceremony was often performed in a temple. The obligatory variety of suicide was seen as capital punishment. The other two types of suicide described in Japan are *shinju*, or *aitashi*, and *junshi*. Whereas *shinju* is noted as a joint suicide by unhappy lovers who wish to escape difficulties, *junshi*, on the other hand, is a type of suicide where after the master has died, the servant chooses to die by suicide. Suicide in ancient Japan was classified by motive. An additional type of suicide described was when an individual chose to appear to river gods and be buried in the foundation of a bridge under construction. Kamikaze pilots carried out similar actions and motives. *Funshi*, or *munerbara*, was based on resentment, hatred, and enmity. *Kashitsu-shi*, or *sokatsu-bara* (suicide for exploiting mistakes), and *kanshi*, or *kanganeshi* (suicide for remonstration), were other types (see Iga and Tatai[27] and Tatai[28] for further descriptions and clarification). Saving honour is often a well-recognized reason for an act of suicide in many cultures. This has also been reported from India.

India

The practice of a Hindu widow jumping onto the funeral pyre of her husband and killing herself is described as *sati*. The word represents many meanings and the most common use refers to the act of dying by suicide, which was fairly common in north India in particular, until the British rulers made it an illegal act. As the term also is reflected as devotion, the actual act may have been due to devotion or coercion partly because looking after widows may have been seen as a burden for the family.[29] A system similar to this was reported by Westermarck[30] from China, by Petrie[31] from Egypt, and by Weinberger-Thomas[32] from Bali. The voluntary death of a wife over the death of her husband may reflect their gender role, gender role expectations by the community or the society and perceived inferior status to men, but also them being seen as a potential financial burden. Further details of the context of *sati* can be seen in Bhugra[18] (see also Thakur[33] and Bhugra[34]).

In Moghul India in particular, *jauhar* was also an act of suicide again 'chosen' by women in Rajasthan in India, to avoid falling into the hands of the enemy after losing the battle in a war or following an invasion. Although rare, *jauhar* was carried out for the sake of defence of the territory and for purity of the royal lineage.[35] It is likely that *jauhar* itself could eliminate a tribe within hours. This practice too is non-existent now, although occasional instances of *sati* have emerged in modern India. There have also been reports of tribes and groups in Western India who would die by suicide if attacked.[32] In the past few decades, protest suicides by burning by students and Buddhist monks for political reasons have been reported in many countries including India.[36] These observations confirm that variations of Durkheim's classification of suicides do exist across cultures in altered forms but are clearly influenced by cultural factors. There are several ways in which cultures have been classified, and cultural dimensions identified. Here we will focus on Hofstede's classification.

Egocentric versus sociocentric cultures

In a global study of multinational organizations, Hofstede[9] described various dimensions of cultures. These included egocentric/sociocentric, masculine/feminine, long-term orientation, the degree of closeness to power, and uncertainty avoidance. It is theoretically possible that all these dimensions can be applied to the study of rates of suicide. It is obvious that in sociocentric societies, the definition of the self will differ and the intention to harm oneself may unconsciously or subconsciously focus on others belonging to the sociocentric self. Similarly, the notion of we-ness embedded in sociocentric cultures will ensure that the act is likely to be directed at others (i.e. harming other selves represented by family or kinship members). The long-term orientation of these cultures may allow individuals to be more patient and forward-looking, but if there is a dissonance between individual and social expectations, this may produce something akin to Durkheim's notion of anomie. It is well recognized that in times of economic downturn, no matter which part of the world, the rates of mental illnesses and suicide rise.[37] In a similar vein, if the culture has a short-term orientation, individuals may feel frustrated and angry at the pace of change. If they do not feel close to the centre of power (i.e. they feel disempowered and trapped), they may use suicide as a way out. These multiple dimensions and their interactions with each other and the relationship with attempted and completed suicide need further detailed exploration, especially if adequate and acceptable interventions to prevent suicide and deliberate self-harm are to be developed.

Masculine versus feminine cultures illustrate another important way of looking at characteristics of cultures, and it is predictable that rates of suicide will vary. As Hofstede[9] and Hofstede et al.[38] described, masculine cultures have more controlling, less equal, and different gender roles and gender role expectations, which will vary and influence cultural mores and expectations. Attitudes of these groups towards authority, child rearing, responsibilities, and so forth will vary. In feminine cultures, the dominant values are caring for others and preservation; people and warm relationships are important, and everybody is supposed to be modest. Both parents deal with children on an equal basis, and in schools, boys and girls study the same subjects.

There is no doubt that attitudes towards sexual orientation and same-sex behaviour vary across these cultures. It is well recognized that the rates of suicide are higher among lesbian and gay individuals, so these cultural values introduce yet another dimension into our understanding of patterns of suicide. In a similar vein, different cultures see different substances and their abuse in different ways, which will also contribute to rates of suicide. As mentioned earlier, Maercker,[12] in a secondary analysis of data of primary health care attendees in different countries, demonstrated that egocentric countries have higher rates of psychiatric disorders, crime, and divorce and the rates of suicide will be affected by all of these factors. It is important to recognize that although multiple cultural dimensions may exist, these are not either/or, or exclusive, and there will be a degree of overlap and consonance.

As mentioned earlier, in many countries around the world, the act of suicide remains illegal. So if an individual survives the act of suicide, in theory, they may well be arrested and charged, although in practice, this is rare. This makes accurate collection of data difficult. However, it is well established that in most countries, men are more likely to die by suicide, whereas women are more likely to attempt suicide. Furthermore, when men choose to die by suicide, they are much more likely to use violent means such as guns, jumping from high buildings, and hanging. Of course, availability and accessibility of means will influence the choice of method.

The means to die by suicide are dependent upon availability of sources for these acts. In farming communities in high-income countries, guns are likely to be used, whereas in low- and middle-income countries, farmers are more likely to use pesticides. In the Indian subcontinent, hanging from a ceiling fan is often employed in urban settings. Where tall buildings are accessible, people may choose to jump off them. In many settings car exhausts are used for dying by suicide. There have been interesting interventions to reduce the rates of suicide. For example, control of the amount of paracetamol that can be bought over the counter has contributed to a drop in the rates of suicide in the United Kingdom, and locking up of pesticides has reduced the number of deaths in some farming communities in South India. Evidence suggests that the choice of the means may be related to what is available and also acceptable culturally.[39]

Gender and religion are another two significant cultural factors which play a role in the rates of suicide. If we look at the prevalence of psychiatric disorders across genders and cultures, another potential variable begins to emerge. Cultural contexts are indeed important, but these are also only one variable. Suicide needs to be studied in a qualitative manner, with cultural, social, and political contexts clearly identified, so that its implications can be studied in detail. In many cultures, psychiatric disorders and their comorbidities with substance abuse will be the primary reason, whereas in others, it will be the religious, political, or civil context. On occasions, the act of suicide may be seen as brave, courageous, or heroic, whereas in others, it may be seen as a coward's way out. Within the ambit of culture and its impact, various factors such as racism, sexual and emotional abuse, domestic interpersonal violence, and discrimination may need to be understood and explored.

In an interesting study in America although somewhat old, Hendin[40] reported that the rates of suicide among young black men were low, but the rates of homicide were much higher. He identified homicide/suicide as the two sides where often black men left home thinking that 'I will kill or get killed', thus adding yet another dimension to the expression and act of suicide. When gay black individuals were attracted to white partners, they were less forgiving of their mothers and had a degree of self-hatred, and Hendin's psychodynamic explanations highlighted violence to the self and others. Hendin noted that suicidal patients often hold up an exaggerating mirror to the problems of their culture or social group. He saw suicide among young black people in the ghettos as the result of a struggle dealing with the conscious rage and conscious murderous impulses. Of course, underlying the psychodynamic principles will also vary widely across cultures, even if the act, the means, and the method are similar.

Comorbidities between physical and psychiatric disorders can increase the likelihood and possibility of dying by suicide. Furthermore, comorbidities of psychiatric disorders and substances, including alcohol, can add variable. It is well recognized that individuals with some psychiatric disorders, including substance abuse, are much more likely to die by suicide. These indicate a multi-complex set of systems which will be influenced by a range of sociodynamic factors contributing to suicide.

Suicide can be seen as a communication of escape, protest, and rebellion,[41] and it is not only the act per se, but the method which conveys the intent and message. Suicidal behaviour does not begin with the intent and end with the act, but reflects individual and collective (cultural) pasts and future.[42] Thus, in order to understand suicide, a whole life and cultural narratives are required to understand the existential angst which may push or pull someone towards the actual act of suicide. Although it is important to know the extent of rates of suicide in any society, it is important to understand the context, methods, and causes, so that suitable interventions and public health measures can be put in place. Relational and sociocultural factors make us human, and in order to understand suicide, these contexts need to be explored and understood. In order to develop any suicide prevention strategies, it is critical to detail the social, cultural, and political contexts at the macro-level and the personal and psychological contexts at a micro-level. Any suicide prevention strategy has to be joined up with religious leaders, educationalists, patients, families, employers, educators, policymakers, voluntary agencies, and so forth, so that everyone agrees with the strategies. Each culture needs more culturally appropriate and culturally sensitive interventions. One size does not fit all. It needs to be recognized and remembered that policy may be developed centrally, but delivery has to be at a local level with local buy-in.

Conclusion

Cultural factors are a basic key to our understanding of human beings' worldview, as well as social and cognitive development. It can be argued that various cultures show varying rates of the suicidal act and different means. Religious attitudes may well affect individual behaviour, as well as public policy. In order to understand the complexity of the act, along with the multifaceted nature of the impact of culture, qualitative narratives are needed. The act is not an end to suicidal ideation but may well reflect the messages people are keen to leave behind for their loved ones, families, and others. Perhaps cultural differences in attitudes to suicide may reflect differing notions—both historical and current—of suicide. The communication thus may be seen in sociocultural perspectives studying changing social (macro) and personal (micro) contexts. What is seen as culturally normal or deviant may well be embedded in broader political contexts. The relationship between deliberate self-harm and its repetition and its relationship with suicide need to be seen in the changing context of cultures in transition, increased globalization, and its impact which may lead to rapid industrialization and subsequently urbanization. It is critical to explore individual concepts of the self and the meaning of self-harm and suicide. The role of culture and micro-identities may help for people to develop sensitive prevention and intervention strategies.

References

1. **Taylor E.** *Primitive culture.* London: John Murray; 1871.
2. **Kirmayer L.** Cultural psychiatry: a historical perspective. In: **Bhugra D**, **Bhui K**, editors. *Textbook of Cultural Psychiatry.* Oxford: Oxford University Press; 2018. pp. 1–17.
3. **Boas F.** Summary of the work of the committee in British Columbia. In: **Stocking GW**, editor. *A Franz Boas Reader: The Shaping of American Anthropology.* Chicago, Illinois: University of Chicago Press; 1982. pp. 87–107.
4. **Kroeber A**, **Kluckhohn C.** *Culture: A Critical Review of Concepts and Definitions. Papers of the Peabody Museum of American Archaeology and Ethnology.* Cambridge, MA: Harvard University Museum; 1952.
5. **Geertz C.** *The Interpretation of Cultures.* NY: Basic Books; 1973.

6. **Kleinman A.** How is culture important for DSM-IV? In: **Mezzich J, Kleinman A, Fabrega H**, et al., editors. *Culture and Psychiatric Diagnosis*. Washington, DC: American Psychiatric Association Press; 1996. pp. 15–25.
7. **Roland A.** *In search of self in India and Japan: Towards a cross-cultural psychology*. Princeton, NJ: Princeton University Press; 1991.
8. **Morris B.** *Anthropology of the Self: The Individual in Cultural Perspective*. London: Pluto Press; 1994.
9. **Hofstede G.** *Culture's Consequences*. Beverly Hills, CA: Sage; 1980/2000.
10. **Giddens A.** *Durkheim*. London: Fontana/Collins; 1978.
11. **Durkheim E.** *Suicide: A Study in Sociology*. Trans. Spauling JA, Simpson G. London: Routledge, Kegan Paul; 1897/1951.
12. **Maercker A.** Association of cross-cultural differences in psychiatric morbidity with cultural values: a secondary data analysis. German Journal of Psychiatry. 2001;**4**:17–23.
13. **Behere P, Bhise M.** Farmers suicide across cultures. Indian Journal of Psychiatry. 2009;**51**:242–3.
14. **Behere P, Behere A.** Farmers' suicide in Vidarbha district of Maharashtra state: a myth or reality. Indian Journal of Psychiatry. 2008;**50**:124–7.
15. **Caraka Samhita**. Trans. Sharma PV. Varanasi: Chaukhamba Orientalia; 2005.
16. **Dubois AJ.** *Hindu Manners, Customs and Ceremonies*. Trans. Beauchamp HK. New York, NY: Cosimo Classic; 1906 based on 1815 manuscript.
17. **Bhugra D.** *Psychiatry and Religion: Context, Consensus and Controversies*. London: Routledge; 1997/2019.
18. **Bhugra D.** *Culture and Self-Harm*. Hove: Psychology Press; 2004.
19. **Okasha A, Okasha T. Suicide** and **Islam**. In: **Wasserman D**, editor. *Oxford Textbook of Suicidology and Suicide Prevention*, 2 edn. Oxford Textbooks in Psychiatry (Oxford, 2021; online edn, Oxford Academic, 1 Jan. 2021), https://doi.org/10.1093/med/9780198834441.003.0008, accessed 4 Mar. 2024.
20. **World Health Organization**. *Preventing Suicide: A Global Imperative*. Geneva: World Health Organization; 2014.
21. **Lester D.** Suicide and Islam. *Archives of Suicide Research*. 2006;**10**:77–97.
22. **Al-Issa I.** Culture and mental illness in Algeria. In: **Al-Issa I**, editor. *Al-Junoon: Mental Illness in the Islamic World*. New York, NY: International University Press; 2000. Pp101-121
23. **Mahgoub OM, Al-Freihi H, Al-Mohaya S, Al-Nahdi M.** Deliberate self-harm in the Eastern region of Saudi Arabia. Annals of Saudi Medicine. 1988;**8**:126–30.
24. **Malik G, Bilal A, Mekki T, Al-Kinany H.** Drug overdose in the Asir region of Saudi Arabia. Annals of Saudi Medicine. 1996;**16**:33–6.
25. **Yesemi M, Sanei N.** Epidemiological study on suicide cases in the province of Kashan. [Cited by **Mehrabi F**, et al.: *Mental Health in Iran*] In: **Al-Issa I**, editor. *Al-Junoon: Mental Illness in the Muslim World*. New York, NY: International University Press; 1994. pp. 139–61.
26. **Daradkeh T.** Suicide in Jordan 1980–1985. Acta Psychiatrica Scandinavica. 1989;**79**:241–4.
27. **Iga M, Tatai K.** Characteristics of suicide and attitudes towards suicide in Japan. In: **Farberow NL**, editor. *Suicide in Different Cultures*. Baltimore, MD: University Park Press; 1975. pp 255–80.

28. **Tatai K.** Japan. In: **Headley LA**, editor. *Suicide in Asia and the Near East*. Berkeley, CA: University of California Press; 1983. pp. 12–58.
29. **Figueira DM.** Die Flanbierte Frau: Sati in European culture. In: **Hawley JS**, editor. *Sati: The Blessing and the Curse*. New York, NY: Oxford University Press; 1994. pp. 55–71.
30. **Westermarck E.** *Suicide in China*. Cited in U. Thakur: History of Suicide in India Delhi: Munshiram Manoharlal; 1962.
31. **Petrie WMF.** *Religious life in ancient Egypt*. London: Constable; 1924.
32. **Weinberger-Thomas C.** *Atlas of Immortality: Widow Burning in India*. Chicago, IL: University of Chicago Press; 2000.
33. **Thakur U.** *History of Suicide in India*. Delhi: Munshiram Manoharhal; 1962.
34. **Bhugra D.** Sati: a non-psychiatric type of suicide. Crisis. 2005; **26**:73–7.
35. **Oldenburg VT.** Comment: the continuing inventions of the sati tradition. In: **Hawley JS**, editor. *Sati: The Blessing and the Curse*. New York, NY: Oxford University Press; 1994. pp. 159–74.
36. **Bhugra D.** Politically motivated suicides. British Journal of Psychiatry. 1991;**159**:594–5.
37. **Stuckler D, Basu S.** *The Body Economic: Why Austerity Kills*. London Allen Lane; 2013.
38. **Hofstede G, Arrindell W, Best D**, et al. *Masculinity and Femininity: The Taboo Dimension of National Cultures*. Thousand Oaks, CA: Sage; 1998.
39. **Canetto S.** Women and suicidal behaviour: a cultural analysis. American Journal of Orthopsychiatry. 2008;**78**:259–65.
40. **Hendin H.** *Suicide in America*. New York, NY: Norton; 1995.
41. **Canetto S.** Suicidal behaviours among Muslim women: patterns, pathways, meanings and prevention. Crisis. 2015;**36**:447–58.
42. **Staples J, Widger T.** Situating suicide as an anthropological problem: ethnographic approaches to understanding self-harm and self-inflicted death. Culture, Medicine, and Psychiatry. 2012;**36**:183–203.

Chapter 3

The role of culture in a suicidal process*

Mehmet Eskin

Introduction

Suicidal phenomena are a global public health concern and cause many premature deaths. Suicide is a personal and social tragedy for the afflicted person and their families, friends, neighbours, and society. According to the World Health Organization (WHO), more than 800,000 people die by suicide annually, and it is the second leading cause of death among 15- to 29-year olds.[1] Seventy-eight per cent of all global suicides occur in low- and middle-income countries, and data indicate that there are 20 attempts for every suicidal death.[1] This means that globally, 16,000,000 individuals make at least one attempt to kill themselves per annum. Suicidal phenomena therefore constitute a significant burden on national health care systems.[2] For instance, the annual cost of suicide and suicide attempts is estimated to be $93.5 billion in the United States.[3]

Suicide is not an end in itself, but a result of a process comprising various cognitive, affective, social, interpersonal, and behavioural acts or omissions. Suicidal behaviour is an umbrella term used to denote a range of actions related to self-annihilation, from ideation to self-killing. The following distinctions are essential to make. Suicidal ideation includes thoughts of engaging in behaviour intended to end one's life, whereas suicidal plans involve formulating a specific method through which one wants to die. Suicide attempts constitute potentially self-injurious behaviour with at least some intent to die. Finally, suicidal death is intentionally ending one's life.[4]

* This is a slightly modified version of a paper entitled 'Suicide and culture' published in *Beirut Arab University Journal: Health and Wellbeing*. 2018;1(1):33–50.

Characteristics of suicidal behaviour

Research in suicidology has so far delineated several features of suicidal behaviour. The first feature of suicidal behaviour is that it is a process that starts first with an idea.[5] Another feature is that suicidal behaviour results from psychological pain exceeding a person's tolerance threshold.[6,7] The pathways to suicidal behaviour are multifaceted and might include intrapersonal, interpersonal, social, biological, and genetic factors. There is therefore no fixed cause of suicidal behaviour. Although there is a substantial overlap between mental disorders and suicide, this does not imply causality, and some claim that suicide is not always a sign of psychopathology.[8] Another characteristic of suicidal behaviour is that it is a significant public health problem and constitutes a severe economic burden on national health care systems.[3] A further feature of suicidal behaviour is that its prevalence rates vary from one sociocultural context to another.

Intersocietal variation of suicide

Table 3.1 presents international variations in age-standardized suicide rates (per 100,000 population) reported by the Member States of WHO for 2015.[9] The table groups Member States into quartiles based on their age-standardized suicide rates. Quartile 1 contains those states with the lowest suicide rates, and quartile 4 includes those with the highest suicide rates. As seen in the table, suicide rates vary considerably from one country to another. Despite this variation, suicides are relatively statistically stable across nations or social groups,[10] although they remain individually unpredictable events,[11] a phenomenon/something known as the conundrum of suicide.

Why is this variation? What is the aetiology of this variation? Is it living standards, widespread poverty, the availability or quality of (mental) health care systems, or abuse of alcohol and use of illicit drugs? Is it social and personal traumas like war, disasters, robberies, rapes, and the like, or purely social factors such as unemployment, divorce, and violence? Is it the prevalence of psychological conditions like depression and anxiety? Or is this variation simply an artefact of misreporting and underreporting?

The author of this chapter compared mean gross domestic product (GDP) based on purchasing power parity per capita in US dollars,[12] depression and anxiety rates,[13] and mean unemployment rates recorded for the countries in the first and fourth quartiles by using *t*-tests. Countries in the first and fourth quartiles did not differ in GDP (first quartile M = 18413.5755, standard deviation (SD) = 16974.29786 vs fourth quartile M = 19360.7885, SD = 23420.2358,

Table 3.1 International variations in age-standardized suicide mortality rates for 2015 (World Health Organization)

Quartile 1		Quartile 2		Quartile 3		Quartile 4	
Country	**Rate**	**Country**	**Rate**	**Country**	**Rate**	**Country**	**Rate**
Antigua and Barbuda	0.0	Macedonia	6.4	Ghana	10.2	Cambodia	12.8
Barbados	0.3	Malaysia	6.5	Liberia	10.3	Ethiopia	12.8
Grenada	0.4	Saint Lucia	6.7	Turkmenistan	10.3	Mozambique	12.9
Brunei Darussalam	1.4	Bahrain	6.9	Australia	10.4	Burundi	13.0
Jamaica	1.4	Samoa	7.0	Canada	10.4	Eritrea	13.2
Bahamas	1.6	Vanuatu	7.0	Namibia	10.4	Trinidad and Tobago	13.2
Pakistan	2.5	Afghanistan	7.1	Cuba	10.5	Lesotho	13.6
Saint Vincent and the Grenadines	2.6	Nepal	7.2	Kenya	10.5	Argentina	13.9
Sao Tome and Principe	2.6	Vietnam	7.2	Mali	10.5	Laos	14.0
Guatemala	2.7	Costa Rica	7.3	Czechia	10.6	Chad	14.2
United Arab Emirates	2.8	Dominican Republic	7.3	Switzerland	10.7	Finland	14.2
Indonesia	3.0	United Kingdom and Northern Ireland	7.4	Djibouti	10.8	Kiribati	14.8
Algeria	3.1	Ecuador	7.6	Malawi	10.8	Estonia	14.9
Azerbaijan	3.1	Madagascar	8.0	El Salvador	11.0	Benin	15.0
Egypt	3.1	Kyrgyzstan	8.2	Maldives	11.0	Slovenia	15.0
Lebanon	3.1	Belize	8.3	Tanzania	11.0	Nigeria	15.1
Venezuela	3.1	China	8.5	Ireland	11.1	North Korea	15.2
Greece	3.2	Luxembourg	8.5	Bulgaria	11.2	Uruguay	15.2
Syria	3.2	Niger	8.5	Micronesia	11.2	Japan	15.4
Iran	3.6	Portugal	8.5	Zambia	11.2	Togo	15.4
Albania	3.8	Singapore	8.6	Guinea	11.4	Hungary	15.7
Philippines	3.8	Somalia	8.6	Sudan	11.4	India	16.0

(*continued*)

Table 3.1 Continued

Quartile 1		Quartile 2		Quartile 3		Quartile 4	
Country	**Rate**	**Country**	**Rate**	**Country**	**Rate**	**Country**	**Rate**
Cyprus	3.9	Türkiye	8.6	The Gambia	11.6	Belgium	16.1
Jordan	3.9	Montenegro	8.7	Austria	11.7	Burkina Faso	16.5
Saudi Arabia	3.9	Seychelles	8.7	Haiti	11.7	Ukraine	16.6
Tonga	4.1	Mauritius	8.8	Iceland	11.8	Latvia	17.4
Iraq	4.1	Fiji	8.9	Senegal	11.8	Cameroon	17.5
Kuwait	4.1	Chile	9.1	Cabo Verde	11.9	Eswatini	17.9
Honduras	4.2	Denmark	9.1	Congo	11.9	Russian Federation	17.9
Myanmar	4.5	Germany	9.1	Papua New Guinea	11.9	Zimbabwe	18.0
Oman	4.8	Romania	9.2	Bhutan	12.1	Poland	18.5
Tajikistan	4.9	Uzbekistan	9.2	Croatia	12.1	Belarus	19.1
Malta	5.0	Norway	9.3	Serbia	12.1	Central African Republic	19.6
Mexico	5.0	Netherlands	9.4	Congo	12.2	Bolivia	20.5
Morocco	5.2	Solomon Islands	9.4	Comoros	12.3	Sierra Leone	22.1
Georgia	5.3	Timor-Leste	9.4	France	12.3	South Korea	24.1
Israel	5.4	Yemen	9.4	New Zealand	12.3	Angola	25.9
Italy	5.4	Guinea-Bissau	9.5	South Africa	12.3	Lithuania	26.1
Tunisia	5.4	South Sudan	9.6	Gabon	12.5	Equatorial Guinea	26.6
Panama	5.6	Mauritania	9.8	Moldova	12.5	Suriname	26.9
Qatar	5.7	Nicaragua	9.8	Botswana	12.6	Ivory Coast	27.2
Bangladesh	6.0	Paraguay	9.9	Rwanda	12.6	Kazakhstan	27.5
Brazil	6.0	Slovakia	9.9	Uganda	12.6	Mongolia	28.1
Colombia	6.0			United States	12.6	Guyana	30.6
Libya	6.0			Sweden	12.7	Sri Lanka	34.6
Peru	6.0			Thailand	12.7		
Spain	6.0						

$t_{(90)} = 0.824$; $p > 0.05$), rates of depression (first quartile M = 4.408, *SD* = 0.681 vs fourth quartile M = 4.427, SD = 0.722, $t_{(92)} = 0.899$; $p > 0.05$), rates of anxiety (first quartile M = 4.145, SD = 1.253 vs fourth quartile M = 3.960, SD = 1.228, $t_{(92)} = 0.472$; $p > 0.05$), and unemployment rates (first quartile M = 10.335, SD = 7.404 vs fourth quartile *M* = 7.960, SD = 6.044, $t_{(89)} = 0.098$; $p > 0.05$). As these comparisons show, socio-economic indicators and the prevalence of mental disorders seem to be unrelated to intersocietal variations in suicide rates.

Thus, social, economic, and mental health conditions are/would appear insufficient when accounting for intersocietal variations in suicidal mortality. Indeed, suicide is a multifaceted phenomenon, including biological, genetic, social, cultural, philosophical, existential, spiritual, and religious factors. Scholars often refer to 'culture' to make sense of these observed intersocietal variations in suicide rates. But how can 'culture' be understood in this context, and how is it connected to suicide?

Culture

Unaware of its immediate presence, human beings are submerged by culture; it is only once they are out of 'water', so to speak, that its absence is realized. Like a fish out of water, humans cannot survive without culture, even though it is often taken for granted or not recognized in daily life pursuits.

Culture can be defined in many ways. Kroeber and Kluckhohn, for example, describe it as follows: 'Culture consists of patterns, explicit and implicit, of and for behavior acquired and transmitted by symbols, constituting the distinctive achievements of human groups, including their embodiment in artifacts; the essential core of culture consists of traditional (i.e., historically derived and selected) ideas and especially their attached values; culture systems may, on the one hand, be considered as products of action, on the other, as conditional elements of future action' (p. 181).[14] Culture is also defined as the collective programming of the mind which distinguishes members of one group or category of people from another.[15] In short, culture can be defined as the cognitive, behavioural, and affective characteristics of people living in a society or group.

Another way to conceptualize culture is to distinguish between different levels of social reality. For instance, by surveying the previous intellectual work on culture in various scientific disciplines, Buono et al. delineated two aspects of culture. The first is the integrative concept of custom, also called social culture. This aspect includes traditional or regularized ways of doing things. In regard to the second aspect, they make a distinction between objective and subjective cultures. Objective culture refers to artefacts and material products of a society, whereas subjective culture is a cultural group's usual way of perceiving the manufactured part of its environment.[16] Subjective culture includes cognition, values, beliefs, and behaviours.

For Oyserman et al., humans need other humans for survival, which requires cooperation called 'sticking together.' According to the authors' analysis, sticking together is vital and problematic. They argue that culture solves the problems that arise from sticking together: managing relations to avoid conflict; clarifying boundaries; and facilitating innovation. They designate culture as situated cognition.[17,18] According to this view, all knowledge is situated in activities embedded in social, cultural, and physical contexts.

Culture makes people similar, yet different

Culture provides people with some ready-made packages of codes, content, and timing for what, how, why, when, and where to think, like, eat, wear, behave, do things, and feel. The package contains complex scripts and descriptions for behavioural patterns related to the world, others, self, production, reproduction, consumption, life, death, and afterlife. Culture signals what behaviours are deemed acceptable and desirable in what situations and what others are considered unacceptable or undesirable.

As people are born into families, they cannot choose; likewise, people cannot choose the culture into which they are born. This imperative makes some people/groups resemble one another but differ from others. As stated above, culture provides people with ready-made packages containing complex scripts and descriptions to point directions for behavioural patterns. Thus, a person born into a culture reacts to situations and demands from the inner and outer world through scripts and descriptions made available in that culture.

Culture can be conceived as a within-person and a between-culture variable.[19,20] Thus, culture can account for variations in interindividual differences within a culture and between cultural groups. The relative frequencies of the scripts and descriptions in cultural groups render group members similar or different. That is to say, a person's adoption of which scripts and descriptions to follow while responding to those situations/demands makes them different from others sharing the same culture. But at the same time, scripts/descriptions being limited/finite makes them similar to others sharing the same culture.

Culture–person interplay

There is a reciprocal dynamic relationship between culture and the person. The nature of this mutual interaction renders both culture and the person capable of having an impact on each other. Human beings create culture, but once created, culture recreates human beings. Human beings are reflexive and abstract-thinking meaning-makers. As their nature requires, humans have a natural propensity for a regulated, meaningful existence. As part of this meaningful existence, human beings need others to forge collective meanings while maintaining autonomy to establish personal meaning.

Relevance of culture to suicidology

The observation that suicide rates vary across societies is often taken as an indication of cultural differences—many researchers in suicidology attribute intersocietal variation in suicidal behaviour to manifestations of culture. Societal suicide rates show consistent patterns over time.[21] Like most human behaviour, culture influences suicide.[22,23,24] Therefore, for a better understanding of suicidal phenomena, some suicidologists have called for the inclusion of culture in suicide research.[25,26,27] Inclusion of culture in suicide research raises three questions. The first is 'What do we mean by culture, and how do we conceptualize it to include it in suicide research?'. The conceptualization of culture relates to the issue of precision. The second question is 'What role does culture play in a suicidal process?'. The role of culture in the suicidal process relates to the issue of mechanisms or processes. The third question is 'Do we conceptualize culture at the group or individual level?'. Conceptualization of culture at the group or individual level relates to the level of measurement.

How is culture involved in a suicidal process?

Scientific research on suicidology often compares groups of participants from different nations, countries, or social groups, and attributes findings to cultural factors. Suicide is a process starting from its onset to its reporting and recording. The scientific work must specify how culture may affect suicide to achieve precision. To better appreciate the possible role of cultural factors in a suicidal process, it is essential to identify the likely influence of culture in a suicidal process. The following is a list of how culture may affect a suicidal process.

- Culture might direct or signal what reactions to emit under stressful life conditions: people may behave in various ways under stressful life circumstances. Cultural values and codes may point to or prepare individuals to respond during adverse life circumstances.
- Culture may prepare or signal the tolerance threshold for psychological pain: it usually assumes that people engage in suicidal behaviour when experiencing psychological pain that exceeds their tolerance threshold. For instance, while the psychological pain resulting from cause *A* for individual *X*

in culture *I* may not be a sufficient condition to trigger a suicidal process, it may be adequate in culture *II*.

- Culture may shape help-seeking behaviour under stressful life conditions: people frequently consider a suicidal act as personal freedom and choice.[28,29] Consistent with this, most suicidal individuals usually seek neither professional nor non-professional help.[30,31] The perceived stigma, embarrassment, and a preference for self-reliance are the most common barriers to seeking help in young people with suicide and mental health problems.[32,33,34]
- Culture may shape attitudes towards suicide: cultural values and codes may shape attitudes towards controversial topics such as suicide. People usually assume that prevailing cultural values form peoples' attitudes towards suicide and hence account for intersocietal variation in suicidal behaviour. For instance, research suggests that cultural approval of, or permissive cultural attitudes towards suicide are associated with an increased propensity for suicidal behaviour.[35,36,37]
- Culture may shape and determine the social reactions to suicidal persons: similar to other controversial topics, culture may influence the nature of social responses to persons engaging in controversial behaviours like suicidal behaviour—although, to varying degrees, all religious traditions forbid self-killing, which is a sin. Social stigma surrounds suicidal behaviour and suicidal individuals.
- Culture may shape attitudes and reactions towards persons bereaved by suicide: the death of a close and beloved one is a heavy emotional burden on the person.[38,39] If death is by suicide, the matter becomes even more complicated due to societal reactions. Social stigma places a unique stress on the bereavement process. Hence, research shows that persons bereaved by suicide are at greater risk of suicide.[38,40,41,42]
- Culture may influence reporting and recording of suicidal behaviour: cultural values may also impact the mere recording and reporting of suicidal phenomena. The stigmatized nature of suicide renders its reporting problematic in several ways. Stigma around suicide stems from different layers of society. In societies such as Islamic ones, where suicide is considered a major sin, persons who engage in suicidal behaviour may find it difficult to reveal this even to health professionals. Likewise, cultural values may also influence the recording of suicidal behaviour.[43] Therefore, many researchers question the validity of suicide statistics for good reasons. For instance, it is a well-known fact that some Muslim nations report and record meager suicide rates. Yet the rates of non-fatal suicidal behaviours among youth in some Muslim societies are comparable to, or even higher than, in communities

with high suicide rates.[44,45,46,47,48] Having similar rates of non-fatal suicidal behaviour in some Muslim communities raises doubt that suicide rates are not as low as officially reported in Muslim countries. Scientific evidence supports this view, especially for Middle Eastern Arab nations. For instance, research shows that most suicides are misclassified as 'other violent deaths' in Middle Eastern Muslim Arab nations, but not in European Muslim nations such as Albania, Bosnia-Herzegovina, or Turkey.[49]

- Cultural values may influence suicide research: the topic of suicide has a taboo nature in almost all social contexts; it causes uneasiness in talking about suicide. Due to its controversial characteristic, the subject of suicide touches upon life values such as freedom, restraint, holiness, happiness, human rights, rationality, and so on. Ethical presuppositions play a role in pursuing suicide research.[50] For some, 'ideology, politics, power, and vested interests among influential professionals (p. 1)' play a role in establishing the truth about the relationship between mental illness and suicide.[8]
- Cultural values and codes may create or specify conditions for social inclusion and exclusion, which in turn may turn out to be risk factors for suicide. For instance, gender nonbinary persons, people with same-sex sexual attractions, and people with different colours or outlooks may be socially excluded or even bullied or harassed. All these conditions are known to be fertile soil for suicidal behaviours.

Culture and suicide: methodological caveats

Almost every researcher acknowledges that culture plays a role in a suicidal process, but how culture impacts suicide is unclear. It is because the term culture is an all-encompassing, fuzzy one. If you are comparing groups of people, you do not know what you are comparing. Assume that a researcher in a cross-cultural study compared the rates of youthful suicidal behaviour in country A and country B and found young suicidal behaviour rates to be lower in country B than in country A. What does this finding mean? What does it say about the role of culture in suicide? In what ways can our researcher explain their result? To what shall the researcher attribute differences in suicide rates between the two countries? These and other questions remain unanswered in comparisons between countries or groups.

One way to overcome this issue is to compare countries or cultural groups with known cultural characteristics (i.e. suicide rates, individualism–collectivism, religion, or any other cultural features of interest). It is possible that what is considered a cultural characteristic of a given socio-geographical region may function as an individual difference variable. In this case, one should ensure that the samples taken from two countries differ in cultural characteristics of interest. Another approach might be comparing samples from the same country or culture with known cultural characteristics. One should know (however?) that findings from all these comparative research designs are prone to ecological fallacy. Therefore, it is difficult to ascribe a causal role to culture in a suicidal process. To claim a causal role for culture in suicide, one should use creative experimental or longitudinal research designs.

Three conditions should be fulfilled to ascribe a causal role for culture in suicide. First, one should delineate a cultural characteristic or dimension from among a group of ingredients or measurements of culture. Second, this dimension should be able to account for as much variance as possible in intersocietal variation. Third, this dimension should be related to suicidal phenomena and variation in suicide. In the following sections, I will survey some manifestations or characteristics of culture for their association with suicidal behaviour. In doing this, I will aim to provide evidence for or against the role of culture (if any) obtained from empirical scientific investigations.

Manifestations of culture

Religion

Religion is an important indicator of culture, accounting for the most significant observed cross-cultural differences.[51] Religion and religious values are assumed to be related to intersocietal variation in suicidal behaviour. Tarakeshwar and colleagues believe religion is an overlooked dimension in cross-cultural psychology research.[52] All religions have explicit or implicit sanctions against self-killing, with varying severity. Among the three Abrahamic religions, Islam has the most explicit sanctions against suicide. Hence, low suicide rates reported in Muslim countries are often attributed to the prohibitive attitude of Islam to suicide. Religious values therefore can be said to determine social attitudes towards self-annihilation.

Why and how does religion protect against suicide? The evolutionary perspective posits that religion as an integral cultural syndrome has evolved to reduce fitness costs and improve fitness benefits for their fellow members at individual and group levels, along with cultural evolution.[53,54,55] Religious systems help to increase adaptive capacities of their believers in a constant social, physical, psychological, and existential flux.[56] As self-reflecting agents, human beings are aware of their inevitable death, which is a source of existential anxiety. Research provides empirical support to the view that religious beliefs help people to cope with this existential anxiety.[57]

How does religion then help improve its believers' adaptive capacity? Given that suicide is an extreme form of desperation, how does faith protect its believers against such anguish? What are the mechanisms by which religion exercises its protective function against suicidal behaviour? Suicidology literature has identified three theoretical formulations about the link between religion and suicide.[58] The first is the social integration theory,[59] and the second is the network theory.[59] Both approaches argue that religion exercises its protective function against suicide by developing informal relationships and promoting communal ties that increase networking and feelings of integration. On the other hand, the religious commitment theory[60,61] assumes that core religious beliefs opposing suicide prevent individuals from considering suicide during personal crises.

Empirical evidence indicates that religion may protect against diminished psychological well-being.[62,63,64] Findings from a longitudinal study showed that religious service attendance reduces depressive symptoms significantly.[65] Reduced mental health is one of the most substantial risk factors for suicidal behaviour. As for theoretical positions about the link between religion and suicide, faith is the most potent deterrent against suicidal behaviour, and research provides empirical evidence for this assertion.[66,67,68,69,70,71,72,73,74,75,76] Further, acceptability of suicide is lower among religious than among non-religious people.[37,77,78,79] Higher levels of suicide acceptability, in turn, were found to be associated with contemplating, planning, and attempting suicide.[46,80,81,82] In a recent review, religious affiliation was found to be a protective factor against suicide attempts and suicide, but not against suicidal ideation.[83]

However, other lines of research indicate that the protective function of religiosity against suicide cannot be generalized to some geo-sociocultural settings and groups.[84,85,86,87,88] Findings from a study on depressed patients showed that suicide attempts were more common in patients with a religious affiliation. Further, the researchers found that suicidal ideation was more significant among depressed patients who considered religion to be more important and among those who attended religious services more often.[89] In a recent paper, Lester and Walker showed religiosity to be protective against suicidal ideation in European American students, but not in African American students.[90] As mentioned before, Islamic scripture prohibits suicide. A recent study involving 5572 students from 12 countries reported associations of religious affiliation to suicidal behaviour in a multinational/multireligious sample. Results showed that affiliation with Islam was associated with a reduced risk of suicidal ideation; however, affiliating with Orthodox Christianity and with no religion was related to an increased risk of suicidal ideation. While affiliating with

Buddhism, Catholicism, and with no religion was associated with a lowered risk of attempting suicide, affiliation with Islam was related to a heightened risk of suicide attempt.[91]

Alongside religious affiliation, belief, importance, and attendance, religiosity has also been conceptualized in motivational terms. For instance, Allport and Ross differentiated between intrinsic and extrinsic motivations for religious belief. Individuals with an intrinsic orientation towards religion were described as wholly committed to their religious beliefs, and religiosity was evident in every aspect of their life. On the other hand, those with an extrinsic orientation used religion to participate in powerful in-group protection, consolation, and social status.[92] Empirical evidence indicates that intrinsic motivations for religious belief, as opposed to extrinsic orientation, may be protective against suicidal behaviour.[86,93,94] Evidence also suggests that extrinsic religious orientation has a negative impact on psychological well-being.[95]

Still another line of research conceptualizes religiosity as coping.[96] Pargament defines religion as 'a process, a search for significance in ways related to the sacred' (p. 32) and religious coping as 'a search for significance in times of stress' (p. 90). Pargament conceptualized religious coping in two dimensions: positive and negative. Accordingly, positive religious coping involves a secure relationship with a transcendent force, a sense of spiritual connectedness with others, and a benevolent worldview. On the other hand, negative religious coping involves underlying spiritual tensions and struggles within oneself, with others, and with the divine.[97] Research indicates that positive religious coping is related to positive, whereas negative religious coping is related to negative, psychological adjustment to stress.[98] Similarly, positive spiritual coping methods—like looking to God for strength, comfort, and guidance—were protective against suicide attempts and suicidal ideation.[99]

In a study of 7427 university students affiliating with Islam from 11 Muslim nations, my colleagues and I investigated the associations of religiosity, religious coping, and suicide acceptance with suicidal ideation and suicide attempts. Neither positive nor negative religious coping was related to suicidal ideation, but negative religious coping was negatively associated with suicide attempts. Accepting attitudes towards suicide had the most robust relationship with suicidal ideation and suicide attempts. Religiosity, conceptualized as affiliation and strength of religious belief, was an indirect deterrent against suicidality via its effects on suicide acceptability.[100]

Individualism–collectivism

Cultural or cross-cultural psychology has identified individualism–collectivism as a meaningful dimension along which cultures or cultural groups can be compared.[15,101] Cultures that emphasize individualism value personal autonomy, self-reliance, uniqueness, and independence, whereas those that emphasize collectivism value person–other relatedness or interdependence and the person as part of a collective.[102] The scientific literature indicates that individualism and collectivism as two worldviews[103] influence an array of psychological variables such as self-concept, motivation, affect, cognition, cognitive processing style, attribution, emotion regulation, and social support provisions.[104,105,106,107,108,109]

The influence of individualism and collectivism on suicidal behaviour has long been debated in suicidology. For instance, the seminal work of Durkheim[110] situated the cause(s) of self-killing within the relationship between the person and the collective. Individualism and collectivism refer to the nature of the individual and collective relationship. Individualism emphasizes self-reliance, personal uniqueness, independence, and a priority on personal goals. In contrast, collectivism stresses interdependence, relatedness, and the importance of group goals.[102] Although the cultural dimension of individualism–collectivism provides a significant source of information about intersocietal and interindividual differences, research has not yet fully integrated these into the science of suicide.

Durkheim situated the causal mechanism for suicide within the interplay between the person and culture. Individualistic–collectivistic values relate to the relationship between the person and the collective. Being situated at a certain point on the individualism and collectivism continuum may involve advantages or disadvantages for both the collective and the person. Researchers seem to hold conflicting views about the benefits and harms of being situated on a specific point on the individualism–collectivism divide/continuum regarding mental health and well-being.

Some researchers think cultural factors such as materialism and individualism are health hazards for a population's health and well-being.[111] Still, for others, individualism exerts a positive effect on mental well-being via its potential to create a context for freedom and choice.[112,113] One should, however, note that these findings stem mainly from ecological studies. From a methodological point of view, results from ecological research designs are prone to various confounders. The third line of inquiry has argued that what matters for better mental health is the level of person-culture match or fit.[114] This line of reasoning assumes that people at the extreme ends of the individualism–collectivism dimension, when incompatible with societal values, have disadvantages for personal adaptation. The data seem to support this view.[115,116]

Eskin has argued that individualism and collectivism might be involved in the onset, maintenance, and aggravation of a suicidal process in two ways. First, individuals with individualistic value orientations may feel a personal responsibility for what happened and blame themselves when confronted with, or under the influence of, adverse life circumstances. Feeling personal responsibility for unfavourable life circumstances may further aggravate the feelings of anger, unhappiness, and hopelessness, which are the predominant affective states in suicide.[117] On the other hand, in a similar situation, individuals with collectivistic value orientations may attribute responsibility to others or circumstances, diminishing the impact of anger, unhappiness, and hopelessness on them.[118]

Second, values related to individualism-collectivism may impact the social attitudes towards suicide as a phenomenon and suicidal persons. The defining features of individualism include independence, freedom, choice, personal responsibility, and competition.[119] The act of self-killing is frequently seen as involving personal freedom and choice.[28,29] In line with this, most suicidal individuals usually seek neither professional nor non-professional help,[30,31] and the perceived stigma and embarrassment, along with a preference for self-reliance, are the most common barriers to seeking help in young people with suicidal and mental health problems.[32,33,34] Within such a value matrix, it is reasonable to assume that people with an individualistic worldview will see suicide as a regular act compatible with their worldview. Subsequently, such persons will show higher acceptance of suicide than those with a collectivistic worldview. Since individualistic values are associated with context-independent information processing,[106] persons with an individualistic mindset may see the causes for a suicidal act as situated within the person and blame them for what happened.

On the other hand, since collectivism is associated with a context-dependent information processing style,[106] persons with a collectivistic mindset may see the doer or agent of a suicidal act as a victim and blame the situation or others for what happened. Thus, persons who attempt suicide and live in social contexts where individualistic values prevail may not receive the help they cry for through their attempts. By contrast, persons who attempt suicide and live in social contexts where collectivistic values prevail may receive the support they need.[118]

Is there any empirical evidence supporting these anticipations? Research suggests that, for both societies and individuals, having individualistic values is associated with increased rates of completed suicide and suicidal behaviour. Some ecological (group-level or geographical) studies yielded positive associations between individualism and suicide mortality,[36,121,122] whereas others did not find such an association.[123,124,125]

Associations of individualistic and collectivistic values with suicidal thoughts and suicide attempts seem more complex than one can imagine. In a study of 5572 university students from 12 culturally diverse nations, my colleagues and

I found that intermediate levels of individualism were protective against suicide attempts across all nations. Higher levels of collectivism were associated with fewer suicidal thoughts in individualistic countries. Lower levels of individualism were a risk factor for suicidal ideation, specifically in Muslim collectivistic cultures. Still, higher levels of individualism were a risk factor for suicidal ideation in Asian collectivistic cultures. The findings further demonstrated that collectivistic values were related to less permissive attitudes towards suicide in all countries, but individualistic values were associated with a more stigmatized view of suicidal behaviour.[126]

Except for Lester's findings, results from individual-level studies seem to confirm group-level effects. One study identified individualism as a risk factor for suicidal ideation among second-generation immigrant adolescents in France.[127] A study conducted on Australian university students found participants with strong individualistic values (idiocentrism), as opposed to those with strong collectivistic values, to be less satisfied with, and less inclined to, seek social support, presenting with higher levels of hopelessness and suicidal ideation.[128] Another study on Turkish adolescents and young adults concluded that suicidal thoughts and suicide attempts were more common among individualistic participants than among those with collectivistic tendencies.[118] Still, another study with Chinese participants showed individualistic orientation to be associated with increased hopelessness and substance use, along with reverse associations with collectivistic values.[129] Another study with US and Chinese college students found that high levels of suicidal ideation correlated with more idiocentrism (individualism) in women only. Still, more allocentrism (collectivism) was related to less suicidal ideation in both US and Chinese students.[130]

Scholarly work on associations of individualistic and collectivistic cultural orientations with suicidal attitudes seems to support a relationship between individualistic values and permissive attitudes towards suicide and suicide-related phenomena. For instance, among US college students, individualistic value orientations were associated with approval of physician-assisted suicide.[131,132] Among young Turkish adults and adolescents, Eskin demonstrated that participants valuing individualistic values over collectivistic ones displayed more positive and permissive attitudes towards suicide; however, they were less accepting of a suicidal close friend than those with collectivistic tendencies.[118]

There seems to be an asymmetry in the relationship between cultural orientation and social attitudes towards suicidal persons. The reasons behind seemingly rejective attitudes of individuals with individualistic values, compared to those with collectivistic values, towards persons engaged in suicidal behaviour, or vice versa, look benevolent. In a study of 857 Turkish university students, my colleagues and I investigated whether person exclusion or phenomenon exclusion would be perceived as more effective in preventing suicide. Results showed that participants with an individualistic value orientation believed person exclusion is more effective in preventing suicide. Still, participants with a collectivistic value orientation thought phenomenon exclusion was more effective.[133]

Another line of evidence for the potential role of individualistic values in a suicide process comes from the gender distribution of suicidal behaviour. In suicidology, it is well known that more women think about, and attempt, suicide, but more men kill themselves.[134] Masculinity's characteristics include striving for power and dominance, aggressiveness, courage, independence, efficiency, rationality, competitiveness, success, activity, control, and invulnerability.[135,136,137] As one may note, the attributes of masculinity overlap mainly with the defining characteristics of the individualistic worldview. For Möller-Leimkühler, people with an individualistic worldview attribute adverse or unfavourable life changes, such as loss of work and long-term unemployment, to personal failure rather than viewing them as social problems resulting in identity crises, loss of control, helplessness, and depression. Accordingly, the author concludes, 'Males respond to this with maladaptive coping strategies, triggered by norms of traditional masculinity or confusion resulting from gender-role conflict: emotional inexpressiveness, lack of help-seeking, aggressiveness, risk-taking behavior, violence, alcohol, and drug abuse and suicide' (p. 7).[136]

Self-construal

Self-construal refers to how individuals define and make meaning of the self. In essence, self-construal is about to what extent people define themselves by incorporating others into their own 'selves'. People may express themselves on a scale ranging from completely incorporating others into their selves to an absolute exclusion of others. Hence, Markus and Kitayama coined the terms independent versus interdependent self-construals. Research indicates that independent and interdependent self-definitions influence basic psychological processes such as motivation, cognition, emotion, social support provisions, and the like.[104,138]

There is a close link between individualism and collectivism dimensions and self-construal. People in collectivistic societies define themselves by incorporating others into their self-concepts; hence, when enquired, they sample relational aspects of their selves. On the other hand, people in individualistic societies or cultural settings define themselves as autonomous entities disconnected from others; hence, when enquired, they sample independent aspects of their selves. In this way, interdependent versus independent self-construals are not static self-qualities, but dynamic self-processes. Thus, as with individualism–collectivism, self-construal can be thought of as a between-culture,[139] within-culture,[140] and within-person[141] variable. In this way, self-construal may account for cross-cultural, interpersonal, and intrapersonal variations as a cultural ingredient or syndrome.

Do we have empirical work relating self-construal to suicidal behaviour and mental well-being? Empirical evidence for a role of self-construal in these issues comes from research on self-construal and social support help-seeking processes, subjective well-being, and psychopathology. Compared to those with an independent self-construal, people with an interdependent self-construal perceive meaningful relationships as closer and more committed,[142] social support to be more important for their self-esteem,[143] and life satisfaction.[144] Further, interdependent self-construal was associated with socially oriented subjective well-being,[140,145] more help-seeking,[146] dependency-oriented support,[144] and lower levels of post-traumatic stress disorder.[147] However, in Asian American and African American college students, distress was positively related to interdependent self-construal and negatively associated with independent self-construal.[148] These findings, however, can also be accounted for by a culture clash perspective. Research also shows that interdependent self-construal mitigates the fear of death,[149] a crucial factor in the interpersonal psychological theory of suicide.[150,151] Still, this effect could not be replicated in an independent sample.[152]

From the findings above, one can deduce that self-construal may be a critical variable in a suicidal process. Since individualism–collectivism and self-construal cultural conceptualizations overlap, we can assume that the proposed mechanisms for individualistic–collectivistic values in a suicide process also apply to self-construal. Unfortunately, there is a shortage of empirical work investigating the role of self-construal in suicide.

The interpersonal psychological theory of suicide (IPTS) assumes that a sense of thwarted belongingness and perceived burdensomeness make suicide a desirable option. However, it does not translate into action, unless coupled with reduced fear of death and increased pain tolerance.[151] From an IPTS perspective, research has examined the relationships among self-construal, thwarted belongingness, perceived burdensomeness, and suicidal ideation in Asian American college students. One study found that interdependent self-construal and independent self-construal both weakened the link between perceived burdensomeness and suicidal ideation on the one hand, and between thwarted belongingness and suicidal ideation on the other hand.[153] It would therefore seem that independent and interdependent self-concepts have some beneficial effects that can counter suicidal desire in times of perceived burdensomeness and thwarted belongingness among Asian American college students.

One thesis research (conducted under the author's supervision) on Turkish high-school students investigated the relationships of self-construal with non-fatal suicidal behaviours and suicidal attitudes.[154] Results showed that high scores on autonomous self-construal characterized students with suicidal ideation and suicide attempts. In contrast, high scores on the relational self-construal scale characterized those without such behaviours. Results also revealed that while the autonomous self-construal scale scores were positively related to suicide acceptance, relational self-construal scale scores were negatively related to accepting attitudes towards suicide. Thus, the findings from this investigation converge with the results from others on the relationships between individualistic–collectivistic values and suicidal behaviour and attitudes.

Research has demonstrated that while adverse life events and permissive attitudes towards suicide constitute a significant risk of suicidality, social support is a protective factor against it. In a study conducted on 7427 university students from 11 Muslim nations affiliated with Islam, my colleagues and I investigated the associations of negative life events, suicide acceptability, social support, and self-construal with suicidal ideation and suicide attempts. We found that while adverse life events and suicide acceptance positively predicted suicidal ideation, social support did so negatively. Persons with interdependent self-construal were less accepting of suicide, and adverse life events were the strongest predictor of suicide attempts. Self-construal moderated the relationship between negative life events and suicide attempts. Hence, people with low interdependent (independent) self-construal who experienced many adverse life events were more likely to report attempting suicide than others. Thus, interdependent self-construal may mitigate the suicidogenic effects of negative life experiences.[155]

Suicide is a goal-directed behaviour embedded in a social–historical context; hence, people engage in suicidal behaviour for various reasons. The literature identifies two types of motives for suicidal behaviour: escape and communication. In escape motives for suicide, the person tries to escape a harmful situation or state. In communication motives for suicide, people try to convey to others their goal or aim through their suicidal act. In a study done on 392 university students from 10 Muslim nations who attempted suicide, my colleagues and I investigated to what extent self-construal, suicide attempt motives, suicide acceptability, and strength of intention to die were associated with personal and interpersonal post-suicide attempt well-being. We found that permissive attitudes towards suicide were related to escape motives. Escape motives for suicide were negatively associated with post-suicidal well-being, but communication motives were not. We found that having an interdependent self-construal might be beneficial for post-suicidal well-being, and others' interpretation of suicidal acts might be critical for post-suicidal well-being.[156]

Other cultural ingredients or dimensions

Researchers have investigated associations of other value dimensions with suicidal behaviour and attitudes. One study found that while intellectual autonomy and secular–rational values were associated with higher suicide rates, characteristics typical of post-modern societies, such as self-expression values and egalitarian commitment, were associated with lower suicide rates.[157] Another study showed that self-expression values were associated with greater suicide acceptance, but survival values with lower suicide acceptability.[158]

Scientific work has shown that approval for suicide and social acceptance of suicidal persons are inversely correlated, and societies differ on these attitudinal dimensions.[46,80,159,160] In one study on multinational samples of young adults from 12 countries,[82] it was found that participants with accepting attitudes towards suicide, but rejecting attitudes towards suicidal persons, reported more suicidal behaviour and psychological distress. They were more often from countries and samples with high suicide rates than their counterparts, suggesting that they are caught in a fatal trap in which the most predominant feelings of suicidality, such as hopelessness or helplessness, are likely to occur. Countries with high suicide rates are characterized by high suicide approval, but a stigmatized view of suicidal persons.

Conclusion and future directions

The survey of results from the empirical work presented here allows for some tentative conclusions. The conclusions drawn from this brief survey may be summarized as follows.

- Although many scholars acknowledge the role of culture in suicide, very few empirical studies have been conducted so far. Therefore, more scientific work on culture's role in a suicidal process is warranted.
- Scientific studies involving country or group comparisons of suicidal behaviour and attitudes reveal that countries, cultures, or groups differ from, or resemble, one another. However, there are methodological caveats in terms of uncontrolled confounding variables regarding these findings. Thus, results from these kinds of comparisons, whether aggregate or individual-level data, pose severe threats to validity.
- The survey reveals that some cultural ingredients or syndromes may be related to suicidal processes. Among those variables, religion and the person–collective interface are the most salient. Scholarly work indicates

that religion may be a protective factor against suicidal behaviour. However, its protective function is not generalizable to specific sociocultural contexts and groups. Some scientific work suggests that individualistic values may be a risk factor and collectivistic values may be a protective factor against suicidality. Still, these findings cannot be generalized to all sociocultural contexts and groups.

- More scholarly work with methodological vigour is needed to explore the possible role of cultural factors in suicide. For instance, future work may benefit from clarifying what culture means, and future research designs should define what culture is and develop a measuring approach accordingly. The definition and conceptualization of culture entail a strict operational definition of cultural variables of interest.
- All research findings relating culture to suicidal behaviour are correlational. As we know, correlation does not allow us to infer causation. There may be a bidirectional causality between culture and suicidal behaviour. People who once engaged in suicidal behaviour may endorse less religiosity, an individualistic worldview, independent self-definition, etc. Therefore, suicidology needs creative and vigorous research designs to test for causal effects.
- Future scientific investigations may also benefit from using research designs to uncover the conditions under which cultural constructs might be a risk for, a facilitator of, or a protective factor against suicidal behaviour.

References

1. **World Health Organization.** *Mental Health. Preventing Suicide: A Global Imperative.* Geneva: World Health Organization; 2014.
2. **Goldman-Mellor SJ, Caspi A, Harrington H,** et al. Suicide attempt in young people: a signal for long-term health care and social needs. JAMA Psychiatry. 2014;**71**(2):119.
3. **Shepard DS, Gurewich D, Lwin AK, Reed GA, Silverman MM.** Suicide and suicidal attempts in the United States: costs and policy implications. Suicide and Life-Threatening Behavior. 2016;**46**(3):352–62.
4. **Nock MK, Borges G, Bromet EJ, Cha CB, Kessler RC, Lee S.** Suicide and suicidal behavior. Epidemiologic Reviews. 2008;**30**:133–54.
5. **Kral MJ.** Suicide as social logic. Suicide and Life-Threatening Behavior. 1994;**24**:245–55.
6. **Verrocchio MC, Carrozzino D, Marchetti D, Andreasson K, Fulcheri M, Bech P.** Mental pain and suicide: a systematic review of the literature. Frontiers in Psychiatry. 2016;7:108.
7. **Shneidman ES.** Perspectives on suicidology. Further reflections on suicide and psychache. Suicide and Life-Threatening Behavior. 1998;**28**(3):245–50.
8. **Hjelmeland H, Knizek BL.** Suicide and mental disorders: a discourse of politics, power, and vested interests. Death Studies. 2017;**41**(8):481–92.

9. **World Health Organization** (2016). Suicide rate estimates, age-standardized estimates by country. Available from: http://apps.who.int/gho/data/node.main.MHSUICIDEASDR?lang=en
10. **Ritter K, Chaudhry HR, Idemudia E**, et al. Suicide motives and culture: degree of modernization, response behavior and acceptance. World Cultural Psychiatry Research Review. 2008;**3**:69–76.
11. **Ribeiro JD, Franklin JC, Fox KR**, et al. Self-injurious thoughts and behaviors as risk factors for future suicide ideation, attempts, and death: a meta-analysis of longitudinal studies. Psychological Medicine. 2016;**46**(02):225–36.
12. International Moneytary Fund (I.M.F.) Gross domestic product based on purchasing-power-parity (PPP) percapita GDP. Retrieved from World Economic Outlook Database; 2015. (Accessed on 10 March 2018).
13. **World Health Organization**. Depression and other common mental disorders: global health estimates. Geneva: World Health Organization; 2017.
14. **Kroeber AL, Kluckhohn C.** *Culture: A Critical Review of Concepts and Definitions.* Papers. Boston; Peabody Museum of Archaeology and Ethnology; 1952.
15. **Hofstede G, Hofstede GJ, Minkov M.** Cultures and organizations: software of the mind. Cultures and Organizations. 2010;3–576. New York: McGraw Hill.
16. **Buono AF, Bowditch JL, Lewis JW.** When cultures collide: the anatomy of a merger. Human Relations. 1985;**38**(5):477–500.
17. **Oyserman D, Novin S, Flinkenflögel N, Krabbendam L.** Integrating culture-as-situated-cognition and neuroscience prediction models. Culture and Brain. 2014;**2**(1):1–26.
18. **Oyserman D, Lee SWS.** A situated cognition perspective on culture. Effects of priming cultural syndromes on cognition and motivation. In: **Sorrentino RM, Yamaguchi S**, editors. *Handbook of Motivation and Cognition across Cultures.* San Diego, CA: Academic Press; 2008. pp. 237–65.
19. **Leung AKY, Cohen D.** Within- and between-culture variation: individual differences and the cultural logics of honor, face, and dignity cultures. Journal of Personality and Social Psychology. 2011;**100**(3):507–26.
20. **Moorman R, Blakely G.** Individualism–collectivism as an individual difference predictor of organizational citizenship behavior. Journal of Organizational Behavior. 1995;**16**:127–42.
21. **Hansen L, Pritchard C.** Consistency in suicide rates in twenty-two developed countries by gender over time 1874–78, 1974–76, and 1998–2000. Archives of Suicide Research. 2008;**12**(3):251–62.
22. **Kral MJ.** Suicide and the internalization of culture: three questions. Transcultural Psychiatry. 1998;**35**:221–33.
23. **Maharajh HD, Abdool PS.** Cultural aspects of suicide. The Scientific World Journal. 2005;**5**:736–46.
24. **Lester D.** Suicide and culture. World Cultural Psychiatry Research Review. 2008;**2008**:51–68.
25. **Chu JP, Goldblum P, Floyd R, Bongar B.** The cultural theory and model of suicide. Applied and Preventive Psychology. 2010;**14**:25–40.
26. **Akotia CS, Knizek BL, Kinyanda E, Hjelmeland H.** 'I have sinned': understanding the role of religion in the experiences of suicide attempters in Ghana. Mental Health, Religion, and Culture. 2014;**17**:437–48.

27. **Hjelmeland H.** Cultural research in suicidology: challenges and opportunities. Suicidology Online. 2010;**1**:34–52.
28. **Wexler LM, Gone JP.** Culturally responsive suicide prevention in indigenous communities: unexamined assumptions and new possibilities. American Journal of Public Health. 2012;**102**(5):800–6.
29. **Wiesenhutter E.** Suicide as an element of human freedom? Praxis der Psychotherapie. 1971;**16**(4):194–205.
30. **Bruffaerts R, Demyttenaere K, Hwang I**, et al. Treatment of suicidal people around the world. British Journal of Psychiatry. 2011;**199**(1):64–70.
31. **Husky MM, McGuire L, Flynn L, Chrostowski C, Olfson M.** Correlates of help-seeking behavior among at-risk adolescents. Child Psychiatry and Human Development. 2009;**40**(1):15–24.
32. **Clement S, Schauman O, Graham T**, et al. What is the impact of mental health-related stigma on help-seeking? A systematic review of quantitative and qualitative studies. Psychological Medicine. 2015;**45**:11–27.
33. **Curtis C.** Youth perceptions of suicide and help-seeking: 'they'd think I was weak or "mental"'. Journal of Youth Studies. 2010;**13**(6):699–715.
34. **Gulliver A, Griffiths KM, Christensen H.** Perceived barriers and facilitators to mental health help-seeking in young people: a systematic review. BMC Psychiatry. 2010;**10:113:1–9**.
35. **Jeon HJ, Park JH, Shim EJ.** Permissive attitude toward suicide and future intent in individuals with and without depression: results from a nationwide survey in Korea. Journal of Nervous and Mental Disease. 2013;**201**:286–91.
36. **Lenzi M, Colucci E, Minas H.** Suicide, culture, and society from a cross-national perspective. Cross-Cultural Research. 2012;**46**:50–71.
37. **Stack S, Kposowa AJ.** The association of suicide rates with individual-level suicide attitudes: a cross-national analysis. Social Science Quarterly. 2008;**89**:39–59.
38. **Peters K, Cunningham C, Murphy G, Jackson D.** 'People look down on you when you tell them how he died': qualitative insights into stigma as experienced by suicide survivors. International Journal of Mental Health Nursing. 2016;**25**(3):251–7.
39. **Cvinar JG.** Do suicide survivors suffer social stigma: a review of the literature. Perspectives in Psychiatric Care. 2005;**41**:14–21.
40. **Pitman A.** Addressing suicide risk in partners and relatives bereaved by suicide. British Journal of Psychiatry. 2018;**212**:197–8.
41. **Pitman AL, Osborn DPJ, Rantell K, King MB.** Bereavement by suicide as a risk factor for suicide attempt: a cross-sectional national UK-wide study of 3432 young bereaved adults. BMJ Open. 2016;**6**:e009948:1–11.
42. **Pitman AL, Stevenson F, Osborn DPJ, King MB.** The stigma associated with bereavement by suicide and other sudden deaths: a qualitative interview study. Social Science and Medicine. 2018;**198**:121–9.
43. **De Leo D.** Can we rely on suicide mortality data? Crisis. 2015;**36**(1):1–3.
44. **Eskin M.** Suicidal behavior as related to social support and assertiveness among Swedish and Turkish high school students: a cross-cultural investigation. Journal of Clinical Psychology. 1995;**51**(2):158–72.
45. **Eskin M.** Gençler Arasında İntihar Düşüncesi, Girişimi ve Tutumları. Türk Psikoloji Dergisi. 2017;**32**(80):93–111.

46. **Eskin M, Palova E, Krokavcova M.** Suicidal behavior and attitudes in Slovak and Turkish high school students: a cross-cultural investigation. Archives of Suicide Research. 2014;**18**(1):58–73.
47. **Eskin M, Sun JM, Abuidhail J**, et al. Suicidal behavior and psychological distress in university students: a 12-nation study. Archives of Suicide Research. 2016;**20**(3):369–88.
48. **Eskin M.** Gender and cultural differences in the 12-month prevalence of suicidal thoughts and attempts in Swedish and Turkish adolescents. Journal of Gender, Culture, and Health. 1999;**4**(3):187–200.
49. **Pritchard C, Amanullah S.** An analysis of suicide and undetermined deaths in 17 predominantly Islamic countries contrasted with the UK. Psychological Medicine. 2007;**37**:421–30.
50. **Mishara BL, Weisstub DN.** Ethical and legal issues in suicide research. International Journal of Law and Psychiatry. 2005;**28**(1):23–41.
51. **Saucier G, Kenner J, Iurino K**, et al. Cross-cultural differences in a global 'survey of world views'. Journal of Cross-Cultural Psychology. 2015;**46**(1):53–70.
52. **Tarakeshwar N, Stanton J, Pargament KI.** Religion: an overlooked dimension in cross-cultural psychology. Journal of Cross-Cultural Psychology. 2003;**34**:377–94.
53. **Boyer P, Bergstrom B.** Evolutionary perspectives on religion. Annual Review of Anthropology. 2008;**37**(1):111–30.
54. **Pyysiäinen I, Hauser M.** The origins of religion: evolved adaptation or by-product? Trends in Cognitive Sciences. 2010;**14**(3):104–9.
55. **Wilson DS.** Testing major evolutionary hypotheses about religion with a random sample. Human Nature. 2005;**16**(4):382–409.
56. **Purzycki BG, Haque OS, Sosis R.** Extending evolutionary accounts of religion beyond the mind: religions as adaptive systems. In: **Watts F, Turner LP**, editors. *Evolution, Religion, and Cognitive Science: Critical and Constructive Essays*. Oxford: Oxford University Press; 2014. pp. 74–91.
57. **Vail KE, Arndt J, Abdollahi A.** Exploring the existential function of religion and supernatural agent beliefs among Christians, Muslims, Atheists, and agnostics. Personality and Social Psychology Bulletin. 2012;**38**(10):1288–300.
58. **Colucci E, Martin G.** Religion and spirituality along the suicidal path. Suicide and Life-Threatening Behavior. 2008;**38**:229–44.
59. **Pescosolido BA.** The social context of religious integration and suicide: pursuing the network explanation. Sociological Quarterly. 1990;**31**(3):337–57.
60. **Stark R, Doyle DP, Rushing JL.** Beyond Durkheim: religion and suicide. Journal for the Scientific Study of Religion. 1983;**22**:120–31.
61. **Stack S.** The effect of religious commitment on suicide: a cross-national analysis. Journal of Health and Social Behavior. 1983;**24**:362–74.
62. **Kang PP, Romo LF.** The role of religious involvement on depression, risky behavior, and academic performance among Korean American adolescents. Journal of Adolescence. 2011;**34**(4):767–78.
63. **Moreira-Almeida A, Neto FL, Koenig HG.** Religiousness and mental health: a review. Revista Brasileira de Psiquiatria. 2006;**28**(3):242–50.
64. **Smith TB, McCullough ME, Poll J.** Religiousness and depression: evidence for a main effect and the moderating influence of stressful life events. Psychological Bulletin. 2003;**129**(4):614–36.

65. **Zou J, Huang Y, Maldonado L, Kasen S, Cohen P, Chen H.** The efficacy of religious service attendance in reducing depressive symptoms. Social Psychiatry and Psychiatric Epidemiology. 2014;**49**(6):911–18.
66. **Dervic K, Oquendo MA, Grunebaum MF**, et al. Religious affiliation and suicide attempt. American Journal of Psychiatry. 2004;**161**:2303–8.
67. **Gearing RE, Lizardi D.** Religion and suicide. Journal of Religion and Health. 2009;**48**:332–41.
68. **Lizardi D, Gearing RE.** Religion and suicide: Buddhism, Native American and African religions, atheism, and agnosticism. Journal of Religion and Health. 2010;**49**:377–84.
69. **Neeleman J, Lewis G.** Suicide, religion, and socioeconomic conditions. An ecological study in 26 countries, 1990. Journal of Epidemiology and Community Health. 1999;**53**:204–10.
70. **Wu A, Wang JY, Jia CX.** Religion and completed suicide: a meta-analysis. PLoS One. 2015;**10**(6):e0131715:1–14.
71. **Sisask M, Varnik A, Kolves K**, et al. Is religiosity a protective factor against attempted suicide: a cross-cultural case-control study. Archives of Suicide Research. 2010;**14**:44–55.
72. **Gearing RE, Alonzo D.** Religion and suicide: new findings. Journal of Religion and Health. 2018;**57**:2478–99.
73. **Norko MA, Freeman D, Phillips J, Hunter W, Lewis R, Viswanathan R.** Can religion protect against suicide? Journal of Nervous and Mental Disease. 2017;**205**(1):9–14.
74. **Stack S.** The relationship between culture and suicide: an analysis of African Americans. Transcultural Psychiatry. 1998;**35**(2):253–69.
75. **Stack S, Wasserman I.** The effect of religion on suicide ideology: an analysis of the networks perspective. Journal for the Scientific Study of Religion. 1992;**31**:457–66.
76. **Hsieh N.** A global perspective on religious participation and suicide. Journal of Health and Social Behavior. 2017;**58**(3):322–39.
77. **Boyd KA, Chung H.** Opinions toward suicide: cross-national evaluation of cultural and religious effects on individuals. Social Science Research. 2012;**41**(6):1565–80.
78. **Eskin M.** The effects of religious versus secular education on suicide ideation and suicidal attitudes in adolescents in Turkey. Social Psychiatry and Psychiatric Epidemiology. 2004;**39**:536–42.
79. **Stack S, Kposowa AJ.** Religion and suicide acceptability: a cross-national analysis. Journal for the Scientific Study of Religion. 2011;**50**:289–306.
80. **Eskin M, Voracek M, Stieger S, Altinyazar V.** A cross-cultural investigation of suicidal behavior and attitudes in Austrian and Turkish medical students. Social Psychiatry and Psychiatric Epidemiology. 2011;**46**(9):813–23.
81. **Joe S, Romer D, Jamieson PE.** Suicide acceptability is related to suicide planning in US adolescents and young adults. Suicide and Life-Threatening Behavior. 2007;**37**(2):165–78.
82. **Eskin M, Kujan O, Voracek M**, et al. Cross-national comparisons of attitudes towards suicide and suicidal persons in university students from 12 countries. Scandinavian Journal of Psychology. 2016;**57**(6):554–63.
83. **Lawrence RE, Oquendo MA, Stanley B.** Religion and suicide risk: a systematic review. Archives of Suicide Research. 2016;**20**(1):1–21.

84. **Young R, Riordan V, Stark C.** Perinatal and psychosocial circumstances associated with risk of attempted suicide, non-suicidal self-injury and psychiatric service use. A longitudinal study of young people. BMC Public Health. 2011;**11:875:1–11**.
85. **Zhang J, Jia S, Jiang C, Sun J.** Characteristics of Chinese suicide attempters: an emergency room study. Death Studies. 2006;**30**:259–68.
86. **Nonnemaker JM, McNeely CA, Blum RW.** Public and private domains of religiosity and adolescent health risk behaviors: evidence from the National Longitudinal Study of Adolescent Health. Social Science and Medicine. 2003;**57**(11):2049–54.
87. **Thanh HTT, Tran TN, Jiang GX, Leenaars A, Wasserman D.** Life time suicidal thoughts in an urban community in Hanoi, Vietnam. BMC Public Health. 2006;**6**(1):76.
88. **Birkholz G, Gibson JM, Clements PT.** Dying patients' thoughts of ending their lives: a pilot study of rural New Mexico. Journal of Psychosocial Nursing and Mental Health Services. 2004;**42**(8):34–44.
89. **Lawrence RE, Brent D, Mann JJ**, et al. Religion as a risk factor for suicide attempt and suicide ideation among depressed patients. Journal of Nervous and Mental Disease. 2016;**204**(11):845–50.
90. **Lester D, Walker RL.** Religiosity is a protective factor for suicidal ideation in European American students but not in African American students. Omega (Westport). 2017;**74**(3):295–303.
91. **Eskin M, Poyrazli S, Janghorbani M**, et al. The role of religion in suicidal behavior, attitudes and psychological distress among university students: a multinational study. Transcultural Psychiatry. 2019;**56**(5):853–77.
92. **Allport GW, Ross JM.** Personal religious orientation and prejudice. Journal of Personality and Social Psychology. 1967;**5**(4):432–43.
93. **Stroppa A, Moreira-Almeida A.** Religiosity, mood symptoms, and quality of life in bipolar disorder. Bipolar Disorders. 2013;**15**(4):385–93.
94. **Lew B, Huen J, Yuan L**, et al. Religious orientation and its relationship to suicidality: a study in one of the least religious countries. Religions. 2018;**9**(2):15.
95. **Doane MJ, Elliott M, Dyrenforth PS.** Extrinsic religious orientation and well-being: is their negative association real or spurious? Review of Religious Research. 2014;**56**(1):45–60.
96. **Pargament KI.** *The Psychology of Religion and Coping: Theory, Research, Practice*. New York, NY: The Guilford Press; 1997.
97. **Pargament K, Feuille M, Burdzy D.** The Brief RCOPE: current psychometric status of a short measure of religious coping. Religions. 2011;**2**(4):51–76.
98. **Ano GG, Vasconcelles EB.** Religious coping and psychological adjustment to stress: a meta-analysis. Journal of Clinical Psychology. 2005;**61**(4):461–80.
99. **Taylor RJ, Chatters LM, Joe S.** Religious involvement and suicidal behavior among African Americans and black Caribbeans. Journal of Nervous and Mental Disease. 2011;**199**(7):478–86.
100. **Eskin M, Baydar N, El-Nayal M**, et al. Associations of religiosity, attitudes towards suicide and religious coping with suicidal ideation and suicide attempts in 11 Muslim countries. Social Science and Medicine. 2020;**265:113390:1–11**.
101. **Kagitcibasi C, Berry J.** Cross-cultural psychology: current research and trends. Annual Review of Psychology. 1989;**40**:493–531.

102. **Triandis HC.** Individualism–collectivism and personality. Journal of Personality. 2001;**69**:907–24.
103. **Oyserman D.** The lens of personhood: viewing the self and others in a multicultural society. Journal of Personality and Social Psychology. 1993;**65**:993–1009.
104. **Cross SE, Hardin EE, Gercek-Swing B.** The what, how, why, and where of self-construal. Personality and Social Psychology Review. 2011;**15**:142–79.
105. **Kitayama S, Uskul AK.** Culture, mind, and the brain: current evidence and future directions. Annual Review of Psychology. 2011;**62**:419–49.
106. **Kühnen U, Oyserman D.** Thinking about the self influences thinking in general: cognitive consequences of salient self-concept. Journal of Experimental Social Psychology. 2002;**38**:492–9.
107. **Matsumoto D, Yoo SH, Nakagawa S.** Culture, emotion regulation, and adjustment. Journal of Personality and Social Psychology. 2008;**94**:925–37.
108. **Oyserman D, Coon HM, Kemmelmeier M.** Rethinking individualism and collectivism: evaluation of theoretical assumptions and meta-analyses. Psychological Bulletin. 2002;**128**:3–72.
109. **Oyserman D, Lee SWS.** Does culture influence what and how we think? Effects of priming individualism and collectivism. Psychological Bulletin. 2008;**134**:311–42.
110. **Durkheim E.** *Suicide: A Study in Sociology*, Vol. **3**. New York, NY: New York Free Press; 1951.
111. **Eckersley R.** Is modern Western culture a health hazard? International Journal of Epidemiology. 2006;**35**:252–8.
112. **Veenhoven R.** Quality-of-life in individualistic society. Social Indicators Research. 1999;**48**:157–86.
113. **Fischer R, Boer D.** What is more important for national well-being: money or autonomy? A meta-analysis of well-being, burnout, and anxiety across 63 societies. Journal of Personality and Social Psychology. 2011;**101**(1):164–84.
114. **Fulmer CA, Gelfand MJ, Kruglanski AW**, et al. On 'feeling right' in cultural contexts: how person–culture match affects self-esteem and subjective well-being. Psychological Science. 2010;**21**(11):1563–9.
115. **Ogihara Y, Uchida Y.** Does individualism bring happiness? Negative effects of individualism on interpersonal relationships and happiness. Frontiers in Psychology. 2014;**5**:**135**:**1–8**(MAR).
116. **Caldwell-Harris CL, Ayçiçegi A.** When personality and culture clash: the psychological distress of allocentrics in an individualist culture and idiocentrics in a collectivist culture. Transcultural Psychiatry. 2006;**43**(3):331–61.
117. **Ellis TE, Rutherford B.** Cognition and suicide: two decades of progress. International Journal of Cognitive Therapy. 2008;**1**(1):47–68.
118. **Eskin M.** The effects of individualistic–collectivistic value orientations on nonfatal suicidal behavior and attitudes in Turkish adolescents and young adults. Scandinavian Journal of Psychology. 2013;**54**(6):493–501.
119. **Bryerton W.** That 'every man for himself' thing: the rationales of individualism among the urban poor. Sociological Inquiry. 2016;**86**(1):79–102.
120. **Waterman AS.** Individualism and interdependence. American Psychologist. 1981;**36**:762–73.

121. **Eckersley R, Dear K.** Cultural correlates of youth suicide. Social Science and Medicine. 2002;**55**:1891–904.
122. **Rudmin FW, Ferrada-Noli M, Skolbekken JA.** Questions of culture, age and gender in the epidemiology of suicide. Scandinavian Journal of Psychology. 2003;**44**:373–81.
123. **Lester D.** Individualism and suicide. Psychological Reports. 2005;**97**:576.
124. **Lester D.** Nations' rated individualism and suicide and homicide rates. Psychological Reports. 2003;**92**:426.
125. **Lester D.** Individualism and suicide. Perceptual and Motor Skills. 2000;**91**(3 Part 1):826.
126. **Eskin M, Tran US, Carta MG, et al.** Is individualism suicidogenic? Findings from a multinational study of young adults from 12 countries. Frontiers in Psychiatry. 20203;11:259:1–16.
127. **Van Leeuwen N, Rodgers R, Régner I, Chabrol H.** The role of acculturation in suicidal ideation among second-generation immigrant adolescents in France. Transcultural Psychiatry. 2010;**47**:812–32.
128. **Scott G, Ciarrochi J, Deane FP.** Disadvantages of being an individualist in an individualistic culture: idiocentrism, emotional competence, stress, and mental health. Australian Psychologist. 2004;**39**:143–54.
129. **Du H, Li X, Lin D, Tam CC.** Hopelessness, individualism, collectivism, and substance use among young rural-to-urban migrants in China. Health Psychology and Behavioral Medicine. 2014;**2**(1):211–20.
130. **Zhang J, Norvilitis JM, Ingersoll TS.** Idiocentrism, allocentrism, psychological well being and suicidal ideation: a cross cultural study. Omega (Westport). 2007;**55**(2):131–44.
131. **Kemmelmeier M, Burnstein E, Peng K.** Individualism and authoritarianism shape attitudes toward physician-assisted suicide. Journal of Applied Social Psychology. 1999;**29**(12):2613–31.
132. **Kemmelmeier M, Wieczorkowska G, Erb HP, Burnstein E.** Individualism, authoritarianism, and attitudes toward assisted death: cross-cultural, cross-regional, and experimental evidence. Journal of Applied Social Psychology. 2002;**32**(1):60–85.
133. **Eskin M, Köskün T, Harlak H.** Beliefs about suicide prevention by excluding the phenomenon versus the person: the role of cultural orientation, attitudes towards suicide, and social reactions to suicidal persons in Turkish university students. Scandinavian Journal of Psychology. 2022;**63**(2):83–90.
134. **Schrijvers DL, Bollen J, Sabbe BGC.** The gender paradox in suicidal behavior and its impact on the suicidal process. Journal of Affective Disorders. 2012;**138**:19–26.
135. **Connell RW, Messerschmidt JW.** Hegemonic masculinity rethinking the concept. Gender and Society. 2005;**19**(6):829–59.
136. **Möller-Leimkühler AM.** The gender gap in suicide and premature death or: why are men so vulnerable? European Archives of Psychiatry and Clinical Neuroscience. 2003;**253**(1):1–8.
137. **Schippers M.** Recovering the feminine other: masculinity, femininity, and gender hegemony. Theory and Society. 2007;**36**(1):85–102.
138. **Markus HR, Kitayama S.** Culture and the self: implications for cognition, emotion, and motivation. Psychological Review. 1991;**98**(2):224–53.

139. **Oetzel JG, Ting-Toomey S.** Face concerns in interpersonal conflict: a cross-cultural empirical test of the face negotiation theory. Communication Research. 2003;**30**(6):599–624.
140. **Suh EM, Diener E, Updegraff JA.** From culture to priming conditions: self-construal influences on life satisfaction judgments. Journal of Cross-Cultural Psychology. 2008;**39**(1):3–15.
141. **Gardner WL, Gabriel S, Lee AY.** 'I' value freedom, but 'we' value relationships: self-construal priming mirrors cultural differences in judgment. Psychological Science. 1999;**10**(4):321–6.
142. **Cross SE, Bacon PL, Morris ML.** The relational-interdependent self-construal and relationships. Journal of Personality and Social Psychology. 2000;**78**(4):791–808.
143. **Cross SE, Vick NV.** The interdependent self-construal and social support: the case of persistence in engineering. Personality and Social Psychology Bulletin. 2001;**27**(7):820–32.
144. **Heintzelman SJ, Bacon PL.** Relational self-construal moderates the effect of social support on life satisfaction. Personality and Individual Differences. 2015;**73**:72–7.
145. **Yamaguchi A, Kim MS.** Effects of self-construal and its relationship with subjective well-being across cultures. Journal of Health Psychology. 2015;**20**(1):13–26.
146. **Shea M, Yeh CJ.** Asian American students' cultural values, stigma, and relational self-construal: correlates of attitudes toward professional help seeking. Journal of Mental Health Counseling. 2008;**30**(2):157.
147. **Mordeno IG, Nalipay MJN, Sy DJS, Luzano JGC.** PTSD factor structure and relationship with self-construal among internally displaced persons. Journal of Anxiety Disorders. 2016;**44**:102–10.
148. **Christopher MS, Skillman GD.** Exploring the link between self-construal and distress among African American and Asian American college students. Journal of College Counseling. 2009;**12**(1):44–56.
149. **Orehek E, Sasota JA, Kruglanski AW, Dechesne M, Ridgeway L.** Interdependent self-construals mitigate the fear of death and augment the willingness to become a martyr. Journal of Personality and Social Psychology. 2014;**107**(2):265–75.
150. **Joiner T.** *Why People Die by Suicide*. Cambridge Massachusetts: Harvard University Press; 2007.
151. **Van Orden KA, Witte TK, Cukrowicz KC, Braithwaite SR, Selby EA, Joiner** TE. The interpersonal theory of suicide. Psychological review. 2010;**117**:575–600.
152. **Lester D.** Self-construal and the fear of death. Psychological Reports. 2015;**117**(2):376–9.
153. **Wong YJ, Koo K, Tran KK, Chiu YC, Mok Y.** Asian American college students' suicide ideation: a mixed-methods study. Journal of Counseling Psychology. 2011;**58**(2):197–209.
154. **Yavuz Yaren Ö**. *Self-Construal, Suicide and Attitudes to Suicide* [unpublished MA thesis, in Turkish]. Adnan Menderes University; 2013. Aydın.
155. **Eskin M, Baydar N, Harlak H**, et al. Cultural and interpersonal risk factors for suicide ideation and suicide attempts among Muslim college students from 11 nations. Journal of Affective Disorders. 2021;**294**:366–74.
156. **Eskin M, Baydar N, Moosa Khan M**, et al. Are nonfatal suicide attempts instrumental in achieving personal and interpersonal goals? Behavior Therapy. 2022;**53**(4):725–37.

157. **Schwarzenthal MJ, Milfont TL.** Suicide and culture: exploring country-level relations between suicide rates and dimensions of cultural variability. In: **Roland-Lévy C, Denoux P, Voyer B, Boski P, Gabrenya Jr WK**, editors. *Unity, Diversity and Culture: Research and Scholarship*. Melbourne, Florida USA: International Association for Cross-Cultural Psychology; 2016. pp. 312–19.
158. **Stack S, Kposowa AJ.** The effect of survivalism-self-expressionism culture on black male suicide acceptability: a cross-national analysis. Social Science and Medicine. 2011;**72**:1211–18.
159. **Eskin M.** Adolescents' attitudes toward suicide, and a suicidal peer: a comparison between Swedish and Turkish high school students. Scandinavian Journal of Psychology. 1995;**36**(2):201–7.
160. **Eskin M.** Social reactions of Swedish and Turkish adolescents to a close friend's suicidal disclosure. Social Psychiatry and Psychiatric Epidemiology. 1999;**34**:492–7.

Chapter 4

Epidemiological aspects of suicide and suicidality

Wulf Rössler, Stefanie Schreiter, and Stefan Gutwinski

Introduction

Epidemiological research on suicide can be traced back almost 100 years. Despite a large number of empirical findings, our theoretical understanding of suicide is still limited. One of the best known conceptualizations of suicide is found in the monograph by Emile Durkheim,[1] who described suicide not from an individual, but from a psychosocial perspective.

To this date, we still try to find a common denominator for the causes of suicide. But as suicidal acts obviously represent a very complex behaviour, similarly the number of factors involved are large, with each factor contributing a small effect.

Our current understanding is based on two models. Model A is primarily a psychosocial model, that is various stress factors lead to mental illness and eventually result in suicidal acts (model A). The main connection here is the link between psychosocial stress factors and suicidal acts. Model B emphasizes the importance of mental disorders which also may lead to psychosocial stress, resulting in suicidal acts. However, in model B, the predominant pathway is between mental disorders and suicidal acts. Model A is the preferred model in sociology, whereas model B is favoured in psychiatry.[2]

There are some caveats regarding the empirical findings presented in this chapter. Registering of suicide data may be incomplete, as it is a sensitive issue. Some countries do not register the causes of death at all and, as such, also do not register suicides. In some countries, suicide is still illegal or at least associated with shame and stigma for the person concerned and their affected family members. Therefore, a large number of suicides could also be registered under other causes (e.g. as an accident).

The validity of registered suicide data is even more restricted in the case of suicide attempts. Most countries do not register suicide attempts at all. Thus, most empirical knowledge concerning suicide attempts is not based on comprehensive epidemiological data, but rather on sporadic local assessments or health utilization data.

General epidemiological information on suicidal acts

In 2012, approximately 800,000 suicides were registered worldwide. The average age-standardized suicide rate is about 11.4 per 100,000 population. The age-standardized rates are slightly higher in industrialized countries, compared to low- and middle-income countries (LMICs). However, there is a strong predominance in LMICs, with about 75.5% of all suicides, compared to 24.5% of suicides in industrialized countries. Iemmi et al.[3] reported in a systematic review a strong association on an individual level between poverty and suicidal behaviour in LMICs.

Global suicide rates have risen by approximately 60% in the past 45 years, although Western countries have experienced a significant decrease over the same time period. It can be assumed that the increase in suicide rates is due to various psychosocial stresses (e.g. wars, migration factors, economic crises). Reasons for the decrease in suicide rates in Western countries is mostly not well understood, but it could be assumed that it is related to better access to psychiatric and psychotherapeutic treatment.

Suicide attempts are at least approximately 10–20 times more frequent than completed suicides, and the lifetime prevalence rates for suicidal ideation lie at around 40–50% in the general population. A prior suicide attempt is the strongest predictor of a later completed suicide.[4] Concerning the burden of disease, the impact of suicide is comparable to that of cardiovascular disease.[5]

The differences in suicide rates become even more pronounced when we look at individual countries:[6]

- The lowest suicide rates of between 0.0 and 4.9 were found in Antigua and Barbuda, Barbados, Pakistan, Guatemala, Egypt, Syrian Arab Republic, United Arab Emirates, Indonesia, Iraq, Venezuela, Algeria, Jordan, Saudi Arabia, the Philippines, Iran, Kuwait, Greece, and Morocco.
- Suicide rates of between 5.0 and 9.9 are documented in Mexico, Somalia, Bangladesh, Panama, Afghanistan, Libya, Tunisia, Peru, Nepal, Bosnia and Herzegovina, Brazil, Zambia, Kenya, Ghana, United Republic of Tanzania, Uganda, Kyrgyzstan, Vietnam, Ecuador, Namibia, Italy, Macedonia, Ethiopia, Mozambique, Spain, the United Kingdom, Turkey, Congo, Nigeria, Chile, and Singapore.

- Rates of between 10.0 and 14.9 are registered in China, South Africa, Gabon, Norway, Ireland, Romania, Bhutan, Australia, Cambodia, Cameroon, the Netherlands, Denmark, Lao People's Democratic Republic, Canada, Slovakia, New Zealand, Iceland, Germany, Portugal, Czech Republic, Argentina, and the United States.
- The highest rates of over 15 are registered in Switzerland, Sierra Leone, Sweden, India, Democratic People's Republic of Korea (North), Bulgaria, Thailand, Finland, Austria, France, Serbia, Bolivia, Estonia, Japan, Russian Federation, Belgium, Slovenia, Hungary, Latvia, Poland, Kazakhstan, Mongolia, Republic of Korea (South), Lithuania, and Sri Lanka.

Taken together, we find particularly high rates in industrialized countries, but high rates are also found in South East Asia. On the other side, we find comparatively low rates in Latin America or the Western Pacific region. But even in countries with traditionally low suicide rates like Brazil, looking at the spatial distribution, there is a remarkably wide, mostly unexplained variation in rates in various parts of the country of between 1.0 and 80 suicides per 100,000 population.[7]

Increasing studies report a higher risk of mental illness in urban areas. Meta-analyses of studies on the prevalence of mental illness among individuals living in urban settings have shown that for psychiatric disorders in general, the prevalence is increased by 38%, with a lingering effect when controlling for confounding factors.[8] But interestingly, recent studies indicate a higher risk of completed suicide in rural areas possibly due to limited access to health care services and a higher availability of certain suicide methods in rural areas.[9,10,11,12]

Risk factors

Although a variety of risk factors for suicide have been described, it sometimes remains difficult to identify precisely those individuals who have a high suicide risk. The accuracy of such a prediction is reported to be close to zero.[13]

Age and gender seem to be the best researched risk factors due to the fact that these data are assessed regularly in all routine and administrative statistics.

Age

In almost all regions of the world, suicide rates are highest in persons aged 70 years and older for both men and women. In some countries, suicide rates are highest among the younger population, and globally suicide is the second leading cause of death in 15- to 29-year olds.[4] Suicide data on those below the age of 15 are rare. In statistics from the National Center for Injury Prevention and Control in the United States,[14] suicide takes third place among the leading causes of death in 10- to 14-year olds. However, the absolute number of suicides are low, as the number of deaths are generally low in this age group.

In general, absolute suicide numbers are high among the young, but calculated in rates per 100,000 population, the rates in the elderly are up to eight times higher.[15] Suicide in older men is often connected to bereavement and social isolation. Maladaptive personality traits seem to be a risk factor for suicide in old age, which also might be related to the inability to adapt to changes in late life.[16]

Gender

Globally, suicides account for 50% of all violent deaths in men and for 71% in women.[4] Roughly there are about twice as many men as women dying by suicide (15.0 for men and 8.0 for women per 100,000 population). However, in industrialized countries, three times more men die of suicide than women, but in LMICs, the male-to-female ratio is only 1.5 men to each woman or even 0.9 in the Pacific region.[4] Highest rates of suicides in women were found in China (11.5), Angola (11.6), Japan and Belgium (12.4), Sri Lanka (13.7), India (14.3), North Korea (15.4), and South Korea (16.4).[4]

There are many considerations for these varying male-to-female ratios (e.g. differences in socially acceptable suicide methods, that is more aggressive methods associated with higher risks of dying, differences in alcohol consumption, or differences in help-seeking behaviours).

Some risk factors for suicidality are gender-distinctive, whereas some are not.[17] Overall, suicidality among women seems to be more commonly associated with childhood environmental risk factors, in particular in situations of low social support, broken home, and sexual abuse, whereas in men, certain depressive and anxious personality traits predominated, particularly in suicidal ideation.[18] These findings suggest that the risk factors for suicidality should be separately analysed in men and women.

Mental disorders

As mentioned above, there is a strong belief in psychiatry that most suicides are related to mental disorders. As Bertolote and Fleischmann[15] stated, 'it is generally acknowledged that over 90% of those who died by suicide had a psychiatric diagnosis at the time of death'. Bertolote and Fleischmann[15] conducted a review of 31 papers between 1959 and 2001, which demonstrated that 98% of those who died by suicide had a diagnosable mental disorder, mostly an affective disorder, a diagnosis of schizophrenia, or a diagnosis of a personality disorder. About one-tenth suffered from a substance-related disorder.

A systematic review by Knipe et al.[19] suggested a possibly lower prevalence of mental disorders among those with suicidal behaviour in LMICs. In relevant studies, there was a wide variability in the proportion of mental disorders in fatal (30–80%) and non-fatal (3–86%) suicidal behaviour, but on average, 58% of those who died by suicide and 45% of those who engaged in non-fatal suicidal behaviour had a mental disorder. Comparably to Bertolote and Fleischmann's findings,[15] affective disorders were the most prevalent disorder identified in both fatal and non-fatal suicidal behaviour.

A more recent extensive review on the risks of suicide in mental disorders was conducted by Chesney et al.[20] They identified 407 reviews, including over 1.7 million patients and over a quarter of a million deaths. All disorders had an increased risk of all-cause mortality compared to the general population, and many had higher or similar mortality risks compared to heavy smoking. Substance use disorders and anorexia nervosa were associated with the highest all-cause mortality risk. Borderline personality disorder, anorexia nervosa, depression, and bipolar disorder showed the highest suicide risks.

A recent study applying a machine-learning approach to predict the suicide risk by using single-payer health care registry data from Denmark tested 1365 parameters based on 334 individual predictors and highlighted the importance of psychiatric disorders as risk factors for suicide.[21] The analyses simultaneously considered somatic and psychiatric disorders and a few socio-demographic factors. It reported that diagnoses, such as schizophrenia and adjustment disorders, and markers of psychiatric morbidity, such as antidepressants and antipsychotics, are strongly associated with suicide.

For decades, insomnia has been identified as a risk factor for mental illnesses, mainly depression. More recently, insomnia demonstrated to be an independent risk factor for suicide.[22] Not only severe insomnia, but also sleep disturbance have been described as risk factors for suicidality. There is a growing body of evidence from clinical, as well as community, samples that such disturbances are, in fact, associated with an elevated risk of suicidality.[23,24] Sleep disturbances are highly prevalent—in up to 25% among young and middle-aged adults—and as such, indeed sleep is an important topic in the public mental health arena, with a focus on preventive measures.

Suicide methods

National studies on suicide indicate that the preferred suicide method varies across countries. Based on World Health Organization (WHO) mortality data, we published a comprehensive overview on suicide methods worldwide.[25]

The differences in suicide methods used in different countries are considerable. Three methods—hanging, pesticide suicide, and firearm suicide—predominate country-specific suicide patterns. Jumping from a height and poisoning occasionally appear as alternative methods.

Hanging is the main suicide method when no other major method is available. However, the prevalence of hanging typically decreases as the prevalence of either pesticide suicides or firearm suicides increases in populations.

Pesticide suicide has been recognized as a major public health problem in some developing countries.

Pesticides account for an estimated one-third of the world's suicides. Suicide by intentional pesticide ingestion primarily occurs in rural areas of LMICs in Africa, Central America, South East Asia, and the Western Pacific.

Firearm suicide predominates in several countries in the Americas and in some European countries. Firearm suicide is frequent in countries where firearms are common in private households.[25]

Men and women seem to choose very similar methods. There is a much larger difference in suicide methods across countries than between genders. When a suicide method is particularly often performed in men in a population, often it will also be practised by women, and vice versa. In general, underlying suicide patterns tell us more about the availability and acceptability of suicide methods than about gender disparities, with the exception of Europe. In Europe, suicide by poisoning, mainly with drugs, among women has overtaken firearm suicide, which is more common among men.

Seasonality

In the nineteenth century, higher suicide rates were reported in spring and early summer, compared to autumn and winter, whereas the seasonal effects of suicide have decreased over the twentieth century. There has been a shift from hanging and drowning to use of firearms and poisoning (i.e. from methods with strong seasonality to those with weak or no seasonality) (all literature in this chapter to be found in Ajdacic-Gross et al.)[26]

The seasonality effects in suicide have been confirmed in many different countries and regions worldwide. Typically, seasonality in suicide is found in both genders. Seasonal effects in suicide are stronger in rural than in urban communities. Evidence for seasonal effects with respect to different psychiatric disorders is not very strong.

However, understanding of these empirical findings is still poor. Today, explanations are sought on many different levels, including biological, psychopathological, sociological, and psychological. Also, the term 'seasonality' has lost its specific connection with the seasons. Today, the term is used in a much more general way to denote any kind of periodic variation such as short-term fluctuations of monthly or daily dates or minor periodic effects such as holidays or birthdays.

A notable example of short-term fluctuations is analysis of the decrease of suicide rates during the Advent season at the end of year.[25] Suicide data were extracted from individual records of the Swiss mortality statistics, 1969–2003. The decrease in suicide frequencies occurs throughout the whole Advent season and is accentuated at Christmas. After the New Year, there is a sharp recovery in men's suicide rates, but not in women's. The reduction in the suicide rate during the last weeks of the year exceeds the well-recognized effect of reduced rates on major public holidays. It implies significant challenges in terms of suicide prevention such as timing of campaigns and enhancement of social networks.

The relationship between the day of death and the birthday has been a subject of discussions for many years and is a good example of daily fluctuations.[26] The presumed relationship concerns important events, such as holidays or birthdays, with the time of death. One hypothesis has been that death on birthdays is less frequent, because death could possibly be postponed. Specific studies investigated, for example, the postponement of suicides after birthdays. The alternative hypothesis is called 'anniversary reaction' or 'birthday blues'. This means that deaths, including suicides, occur more frequently on birthdays.

In our analysis, we included data on 2,380,997 deaths over a period of 40 years.[26] Over the entire time series, which included all deaths, the rate of excess mortality between the date of death and the date of birth was about 14%, and roughly the same for both genders. Thus, it seems that birthdays are more likely to end fatally than one would expect. This is mainly due to cardiovascular and cerebrovascular diseases where the effects are more severe in women than in men, but also due to suicides and accidents where the rate of excess mortality is only confirmed in men.

Religion

Religion is generally regarded as a protective factor with regard to suicide and is associated with cultural factors, religious homogeneity, and age, as demonstrated in a recent meta-analysis comprising nine studies.[27] However, this is not as clear as it might appear, as religion is at least as complex as suicide itself.[28] Many world religions offer stability, order, structure, and a common understanding of the world,[1] but at the same time, they also rigorously condemn suicide. In many religions, to suffer seems to be more acceptable than to kill oneself. For this reason, suicide is stigmatized and tabooed in many of the world religions. Due to stigmatization of killing oneself, many world religions also prevent people from seeking appropriate help in their times of need. In strictly organized religious societies, prohibition of suicide is also reflected in the legislation, with the result that many suicides are not recorded in these countries. Where religion is experienced as helpful, this often has to do with the fact that many religions also offer community and social support.[29] Many religions also prohibit alcohol, which is a risk factor for suicidal behaviour, which, in turn, could partially explain reduced suicide rates in religious people.

Economy and unemployment

For decades, there has been an interest in the effect of economic recession—reflected in unemployment rates—on suicide rates. In a systematic review of suicide in economic recession, Oyesanya et al.[30] identified 38 studies, of which 31 showed a hypothesized link between suicide and economic recession.

Interest in this association was also heightened during the world economic crisis of 2008. In line with previous evidence, data from Europe, the United States, and Asia suggested a similar association between increased suicides rates and rising unemployment rates during the 2008 crisis.[31] The study authors also found that in all world regions, the relative risk of suicide associated with unemployment was increased by about 20–30% during the study period of 2000–11. The coronavirus disease 2019 (COVID-19) pandemic might have a similar effect, as rising unemployment during the pandemic might also result in higher suicide rates.[32]

However, the impact of economic recession on suicidality remains controversial. It was suggested that the effect of socio-economic factors on suicide tends to be overestimated when the contribution of psychiatric disorders is not taken into account. Many studies also ignore the dynamic nature of unemployment (i.e. the duration of unemployment). Longer durations of unemployment affect all-cause mortality over time. Variations in the effect of unemployment duration have also been shown in studies of psychological well-being, which demonstrated marked adverse mental health consequences the longer a person is unemployed. Finally, the consequences of unemployment are also influenced by the social welfare systems.[33]

Studies on socially marginalized populations, such as homeless people, revealed substantially increased mortality in the homeless group due to suicide and other causes.[34] A recent meta-analysis demonstrated a remarkably higher prevalence of suicidal ideation and suicide attempt among homeless people, as compared to that reported in the general population—current and lifetime prevalences of suicidal ideation among homeless people were 17.83% and

41.60%, respectively, whereas current and lifetime prevalences of suicide attempt were 9.16% and 28.88%, respectively.[35]

Media reports

Suicides following media stories are known as the 'Werther effect'. The term is derived from Goethe's novel *The Sorrows of Young Werther* published in 1774, which triggered an increase in suicides, leading to its ban in many European countries.

Empirical research has clearly demonstrated that extensive newspaper coverage of suicide is associated with a significant increase in suicide rates. The magnitude of the increase is proportional to the amount, duration, and prominence of media coverage. While most of the studies found an excess of deaths following the appearance of suicide stories, other earlier studies found a decrease in deaths during periods of story cessation, as occurring during newspaper strikes.[36,37]

Inappropriate media reporting practices can sensationalize and glamourize suicide, and can increase the risk of suicides among vulnerable people. Therefore, media practice is usually inappropriate when they report on celebrity suicides or unusual suicides, show photographs or information on the method used, or normalize suicide as an acceptable response to a personal crisis.[38]

A recent 'Werther' debate also arose around the multi-episode fictional Netflix series *13 Reasons Why* about various struggles, including suicide, in the lives of high-school students in the United States. A recent study showed evidence of an increase in suicide rates in the United States following the release of season 1 of the series on 31 March 2017. In an observational analysis on a macro-level, Bridge and colleagues estimated that an additional 195 suicide deaths (95% confidence interval (CI) 168–222) among 10- to 17-year-old youths occurred between 1 April and 31 December 2017 following the release of the series.[39] Studies have also reported on the beneficial effects of suicide content in the media, known as the Papageno effect.[40] There might be a decrease in suicide rates after specific suicide reports (e.g. following a story about positively coping with a suicidal crisis). As it is unlikely that all consumers would respond to the same media content in the same way, the underlying patterns should be of interest. Some authors argue that the Werther effect is a net effect on a macro-level—the same media contents may have harmful and/or helpful effects on an individual level on suicide-related ideation/behaviour, depending on the interaction between the contents and the consumer characteristics, and may or may not translate on a macro-level to Werther/Papageno effects.[41]

References

1. **Durkheim E.** *Le Suicide: Étude de Sociologie.* Paris: Felix Alcan; 1897.
2. **Hegerl U.** Prevention of suicidal behavior. Dialogues in Clinical Neuroscience. 2016;**18**:183–90.
3. **Iemmi V, Bantjes J, Coast E**, et al. Suicide and poverty in low-income and middle-income countries: a systematic review. The Lancet Psychiatry. 2016;**3**(8):774–83.
4. **World Health Organization** (2019). Age-standardized suicide rates: male:female ratio (per 100 000). Available from: https://www.who.int/gho/mental_health/suicide_rates_male_female/en/ (last updated 2024).
5. **De Leo D, Milner A, Fleischmann A**, et al. The WHO START study: suicidal behaviors across different areas of the world. Crisis. 2013(34):156–63.
6. **Bachmann S.** Epidemiology of suicide and the psychiatric perspective. International Journal of Environmental Research and Public Health. 2018;**15**(7):1425.
7. **Dantas AP, de Azevedo UN, Nunes AD, Amador AE, Marques MV, Barbosa IR.** Analysis of suicide mortality in Brazil: spatial distribution and socioeconomic context. Brazilian Journal of Psychiatry. 2017;**40**:12–18.
8. **Peen J, Schoevers RA, Beekman AT, Dekker J.** The current status of urban–rural differences in psychiatric disorders. Acta Psychiatrica Scandinavica. 2010;**121**(2):84–93.
9. **San Sebastián M, Edin-Liljegren A, Jonsson F.** Rural–urban differences in suicide attempts and mortality among young people in northern Sweden, 1998–2017: a register-based study. Scandinavian Journal of Public Health. 2020;**48**(8):794–800.
10. **Singh GK, Azuine RE, Siahpush M, Kogan MD.** All-cause and cause-specific mortality among US youth: socioeconomic and rural–urban disparities and international patterns. Journal of Urban Health. 2013;**90**:388–405.
11. **Page A, Morrell S, Taylor R, Dudley M, Carter G.** Further increases in rural suicide in young Australian adults: secular trends, 1979–2003. Social Science and Medicine. 2007;**65**(3):442–53.
12. **Goldman-Mellor S, Allen K, Kaplan MS.** Rural/urban disparities in adolescent nonfatal suicidal ideation and suicide attempt: a population-based study. Suicide and Life-Threatening Behavior. 2018;**48**(6):709–19.
13. **Belsher BE, Smolenski DJ, Pruitt LD**, et al. Prediction models for suicide attempts and deaths: a systematic review and simulation. JAMA Psychiatry. 2019;**76**(6):642–51.
14. **Centers for Disease Control and Prevention.** Using WISQARS®: 10 leading causes of death by age group, United States—2016. Available from: https://www.cdc.gov/injury/wisqars/LeadingCauses.html (last updated 2020).
15. **Bertolote JM, Fleischmann A.** A global perspective in the epidemiology of suicide. Suicidologi. 2002;7(2):6–8.
16. **Szücs A, Szanto K, Aubry J-M, Dombrovski AY.** Personality and suicidal behavior in old age: a systematic literature review. Frontiers in Psychiatry. 2018;**9**:128.
17. **Epstein JA, Spirito A.** Gender-specific risk factors for suicidality among high school students. Archives of Suicide Research. 2010;**14**(3):193–205.
18. **Angst J, Hengartner MP, Rogers J**, et al. Suicidality in the prospective Zurich study: prevalence, risk factors and gender. European Archives of Psychiatry and Clinical Neuroscience. 2014;**264**:557–65.

19. **Knipe D, Williams AJ, Hannam-Swain S**, et al. Psychiatric morbidity and suicidal behaviour in low- and middle-income countries: a systematic review and meta-analysis. PLoS Medicine. 2019;**16**(10):e1002905.
20. **Chesney E, Goodwin GM, Fazel S.** Risks of all-cause and suicide mortality in mental disorders: a meta-review. World Psychiatry. 2014;**13**(2):153–60.
21. **Gradus JL, Rosellini AJ, Horváth-Puhó E**, et al. Prediction of sex-specific suicide risk using machine learning and single-payer health care registry data from Denmark. JAMA Psychiatry. 2020;**77**(1):25–34.
22. **McCall WV, Black CG.** The link between suicide and insomnia: theoretical mechanisms. Current Psychiatry Reports. 2013;**15**:1–9.
23. **Malik S, Kanwar A, Sim LA**, et al. The association between sleep disturbances and suicidal behaviors in patients with psychiatric diagnoses: a systematic review and meta-analysis. Systematic Reviews. 2014;**3**:1–9.
24. **Rössler W, Angst J, Ajdacic-Gross V**, et al. Sleep disturbances and suicidality: a longitudinal analysis from a representative community study over 30 years. Frontiers in Psychiatry. 2018;**9**:320.
25. **Ajdacic-Gross V, Lauber C, Bopp M**, et al. Reduction in the suicide rate during Advent—a time series analysis. Psychiatry Research. 2008;**157**(1–3):139–46.
26. **Ajdacic-Gross V, Knöpfli D, Landolt K**, et al. Death has a preference for birthdays—an analysis of death time series. Annals of Epidemiology. 2012;**22**(8):603–6.
27. **Wu A, Wang J-Y, Jia C-X.** Religion and completed suicide: a meta-analysis. PLoS One. 2015;**10**(6):e0131715.
28. **Lawrence RE, Oquendo MA, Stanley B.** Religion and suicide risk: a systematic review. Archives of Suicide Research. 2016;**20**(1):1–21.
29. **Kleiman EM, Liu RT.** Prospective prediction of suicide in a nationally representative sample: religious service attendance as a protective factor. British Journal of Psychiatry. 2014;**204**(4):262–6.
30. **Oyesanya M, Lopez-Morinigo J, Dutta R.** Systematic review of suicide in economic recession. World Psychiatry. 2015;**5**(2):243–54.
31. **Nordt C, Warnke I, Seifritz E, Kawohl W.** Modelling suicide and unemployment: a longitudinal analysis covering 63 countries, 2000–11. The Lancet Psychiatry. 2015;**2**(3):239–45.
32. **Kawohl W, Nordt C.** COVID-19, unemployment, and suicide. The Lancet Psychiatry. 2020;7(5):389–90.
33. **Milner A, Page A, LaMontagne AD.** Long-term unemployment and suicide: a systematic review and meta-analysis. PLoS One. 2013;**8**(1):e51333.
34. **Fazel S, Geddes JR, Kushel M.** The health of homeless people in high-income countries: descriptive epidemiology, health consequences, and clinical and policy recommendations. The Lancet. 2014;**384**(9953):1529–40.
35. **Ayano G, Tsegay L, Abraha M, Yohannes K.** Suicidal ideation and attempt among homeless people: a systematic review and meta-analysis. Psychiatric Quarterly. 2019;**90**:829–42.
36. **Stack S.** Media coverage as a risk factor in suicide. Journal of Epidemiology and Community Health. 2003;**57**(4):238–40.

37. **Gould MS.** Suicide and the media. Annals of the New York Academy of Sciences. 2001(932):200–24.
38. **Marchant A, Hawton K, Stewart A**, et al. A systematic review of the relationship between internet use, self-harm and suicidal behaviour in young people: the good, the bad and the unknown. PLoS One. 2017;**12**(8):e0181722.
39. **Bridge JA, Greenhouse JB, Ruch D**, et al. Association between the release of Netflix's *13 Reasons Why* and suicide rates in the United States: an interrupted time series analysis. Journal of the American Academy of Child and Adolescent Psychiatry. 2020;**59**(2):236–43.
40. **Niederkrotenthaler T, Voracek M, Herberth A**, et al. Papageno v Werther effect. BMJ. 2010;**341**:c5841.
41. **Arendt F, Romer D.** Problems posed by the Werther effect as a 'net effect': a comment on recent scholarly work on the effects of *13 Reasons Why*. British Journal of Psychiatry. 2020;**217**(6):665–6.

Chapter 5

Genetic aspects of suicide

Ina Giegling, Stephan Maul,
Annette M. Hartmann, and Dan Rujescu

Introduction

Risk of suicidal behaviour (SB) results from a complex interplay of genetic, epigenetic, and environmental factors, as well as regulatory dimensions in between. Modelling of this phenotype needs to consider the dimensional changes of various risk factors throughout the lifespan, beginning with genetic vulnerability, and epigenetic adaptations initiated by environmental events starting at the prenatal stage (although transgenerational effects may occur). In addition, adverse environmental experiences during the lifespan also contribute to an increased risk. Various risk factors for SB have been described, including social, socio-economic, medical, cognitive, and biological parameters (e.g. genetics, epigenetics) and personality, as well as stressful and traumatic life events. A classification regarding their causative relevance is still under debate.[1] In addition, the phenotype itself is a heterogeneous complex phenomenon. At present, it is still being discussed whether suicidal ideation, suicide attempts, and completed suicide display manifestations of varying degrees of severity or are distinct phenotypic entities. Furthermore, comorbidity with mental illness is present in more than 90% of individuals, without diagnosis-specific accumulation.[2] These considerations show a major influence on study designs and may be, in part, responsible for often inconsistent results.

Heritability of suicidal behaviour

Evidence for a genetic component contributing to the risk of SB has been collected by using family, twin, and adoption studies. In a large epidemiological study comprising 83,951 suicide completers as index cases, comparison of the relative suicide risk between the biological family and the general population revealed an increasing risk with a decreasing genetic distance (2-fold in children of index cases and up to 15-fold in monozygotic twins),[3] confirming observations from an earlier prospective study.[4] This risk increase was influenced by an early onset of the first suicide attempt.[5] In adoption studies, the suicide rate of biological relatives was shown to be 6-fold higher in adoptees with SB, compared to those without,[6] which was even more pronounced if index cases also suffered from mood disorders.[7] This was reflected by an increase in SB in biological offspring if parents were suffering from psychiatric diseases.[8] In a meta-analysis including 32 studies, heritability of SB was estimated to be 30–35%, with concordance rates of 13.7% in monozygotic twins and 1.4% in dizygotic twins.[9] In an all-female sample, heritability estimates reached up to 58%.[10] In addition, single nucleotide polymorphism (SNP)-based heritability (i.e. the proportion of phenotypic variance explained by additive contributions from SNPs in unrelated individuals) was calculated to be approximately 4% for suicide attempt in a sample of European ancestry.[11] The gap between SNP-based heritability measures and those derived from family-based studies is most probably influenced by insufficient power and restriction to single-base pair variants only, but also by inconsistent population stratifications and phenotype definitions.

Personality traits as risk factors for suicidal behaviour

Personality traits have long been considered to be mediating endophenotypes by promoting a maladaptive response to risk factors later in life, thereby increasing the risk of suicidal events.[12] Studies exploring these traits rely heavily on the type of measurement (e.g. self-reporting questionnaires, neurocognitive measures or assessments supplied by third parties such as relatives), limiting comparability of the results because of the heterogeneity of the underlying constructs.[13,14] Although themselves complex, consistent associations with SB were identified for the personality traits of impulsivity, aggression, anger, and neuroticism.[15] A link between impulsivity and SB was found in a variety of studies, with a meta-analysis revealing a rather small effect (for a review and meta-analysis, see Anestis et al.[13]), which might be, in part, due to inadequate characterization of impulsivity and its (sub-)phenotypes.[16] The traits of anger and aggression are closely related, and a link with SB was described for various psychiatric disorders such as depression[17] and post-traumatic stress disorder.[18,19] Neuroticism is a major trait in personality models that appears to increase vulnerability to SB and psychiatric disorders such as depression, anxiety, and personality disorders, which, in turn, are also associated with SB.[20,21] As personality traits are under genetic control,[22] a better understanding of the underlying mechanisms of the respective traits provides the opportunity to study the molecular background of SB.

Molecular genetics

Early research on genetic susceptibility to SB was based on clinical observations of low serotonin metabolite levels in the cerebrospinal fluid (CSF) of patients as an indicator of a presumed reduction in serotonin turnover. Also, serotonergic function was regarded as crucial to the regulation of proposed risk personality traits, and lower amounts of the serotonin metabolite 5-hydroxyindoleacetic acid (5-HIAA) in the CSF were found to correlate with higher levels of aggressive behaviour, leading to a vast number of studies focusing on genes involved in the regulation of serotonergic transmission.[23]

TPH1 and *TPH2*

Association studies of SB with the gene encoding tryptophan hydroxylase 1 (*TPH1*), one of two rate-limiting enzymes in serotonin synthesis, mostly focusing on the intronic variants A218C and A779C, remained inconclusive,[23] although probably independent of the population structure underlying the investigated Caucasian, Asian, and African–American populations,[24] but dependent on the concomitant disease.[25] The personality traits of anger and aggression were also shown to be associated with *TPH1* variants, implicating a genotype-specific reduced ability to control anger.[26] *TPH2*, the gene encoding the second isozyme, which is predominantly expressed in the brain, was associated with completed suicide in an early study.[27] Also, a meta-analysis on attempted and completed suicides showed consistent results for an increased risk in G-allele carriers of A709G (rs4570625).[28] In accordance with an increased risk of SB, the 709G allele was also associated with increased aggressive behaviour and maladaptive impulsivity in young male adults.[29] Furthermore, *Tph2*$^{-/-}$ mice were shown to exhibit an increase in aggressive and motoric impulsive behaviour, as well as depression-like symptoms,[30] strengthening the findings from human association studies.

MAOA and *MAOB*

Monoamine oxidase A and B are responsible for metabolism of monoamine neurotransmitters (e.g. serotonin). Most association studies on variants in the *MAOA* gene, especially on a variant number tandem repeat (VNTR) polymorphism in the promoter region with influence on the transcription rate, revealed no direct association with SB.[23] Increasing evidence points to a modulatory role of this variant in the context of childhood trauma, with the low-activity allele being associated with an increased risk of antisocial behaviour later in life,[31] which, in addition, is also under the influence of epigenetic modifications.[32]

Serotonin transporter

The serotonin transporter (5-HTT) is responsible for the reuptake of released serotonin from the synaptic cleft. An insertion/deletion polymorphism in the promoter region of the *SCL6A4* gene, with the insertion carrying another SNP, was shown to have an influence on transcription efficiency.[33] A meta-analysis including 15,341 subjects from 45 studies failed to detect an association between low-expressing variants (S, L_G) and SB, even after subdividing into ethnicity-specific populations (European and Asian descent). However, an increased risk of violent suicide attempt for low-expression allele carriers was detected,[34] emphasizing the need to include the severity of SB in analyses. When considering personality traits, studies resulted in inconsistent findings (e.g. including questionnaires measuring differing traits,[35] ethnicities with differences in local haplotypes,[36] and interactions between genes and environment).[37]

Serotonin receptors

The 5-hydroxytryptamine receptors (HTRs) are G-protein-coupled receptors leading to inhibition of the adenylyl cyclase cascade (*HTR1A*, *HTR1B*) or stimulation of the phosphoinositide cascade (*HTR2A*, *HTR2C*). Although an early study implicated a functional variant in the promoter region of *HTR1A* (C-1019G, rs6295) as a promising candidate for SB,[38] these results were not replicated,[39] but an influence on impulsive behaviour was observed.[40] For *HTR1B*, in an early study,[41] a variant (G861C, rs6296) was associated with suicide attempts in personality disorders, but this was not confirmed in further studies.[42] In addition, associations of *HTR1B* variants with anger and aggression,[43] as well as with impulsivity and inattention, have been described.[44,45] The most extensively investigated polymorphisms of the *HTR2A* gene are the A1438G (rs6313) and T102C (rs6311) variants, which are in high linkage disequilibrium (LD) across ethnicities (r2 >90%). While some studies reported associations of subphenotypes of SB with variations in the *HTR2A* gene, mostly no associations were found.[23] Taking into account the genetic differences of the accompanying comorbidities, Wang et al.[46] detected an increased risk of suicide attempt for the 102CC genotype specifically in patients with schizophrenia. Regarding personality traits, the 102CC risk genotype was associated with increased impulsivity,[47] anger, and aggression.[48] Contribution of *HTR2C* receptor variants, especially C23S (rs6318), to SB seems unlikely, given the mostly negative association results.[49]

Other genes

Further candidate gene studies on SB focusing on catecholamine catabolism, neurotrophins, stress, or the immune system[50] are rare and show heterogeneous results. For example, studies on tyrosine hydroxylase, the pacemaker enzyme of catecholamine biosynthesis or the Val158Met polymorphism of the *COMT* gene, which inactivates the catecholamines dopamine and noradrenaline, show differing or negative results.[51] Studies on the gene encoding the growth factor brain-derived neurotrophic factor (*BDNF*) involved in neuronal development and synaptic plasticity, containing another Val/Met polymorphism (rs6265, 196G>A), was shown to be associated with suicide attempts in a meta-analysis including 3352 individuals,[52] but these could not be replicated in a larger sample.[53] In part, this could be based on underlying differences in the individuals studied, as this variation was shown to moderate the effect of adverse childhood experiences on impulsive aggression in patients with borderline personality disorder.[54]

Although associations of candidate genes with SB or related personality traits seem inconclusive, deeper knowledge might occur, including gene × gene and gene × environment interactions and epigenetic mechanisms.

Genome-wide association studies

As a result of ongoing technical development, the determination of about 1 million genetic variations and subsequent estimation of more than 20 million variants, based on the LD structure of the genome, are now standard in genome-wide association study (GWAS) approaches. In addition to genome-wide-associated single hits, data collected in the framework of GWAS also offer the possibility to perform gene-based evaluations and identify rare structural variants (copy number variations (CNVs)), and can be used to estimate the risk burden for a phenotype (polygenic risk score (PRS)).

Suicidal behaviour

The first GWAS on SB failed to identify significant signals.[23] This changed in more recent studies including significantly larger samples. In a gene-based analysis, three genes (*RETREG1*, *GSN*, and *CACNA1D*) were found to be significantly associated with severe suicide attempts. In addition, an over-representation of genes involved in synaptic function and brain development was detected.[55] By adjusting for comorbid psychiatric conditions, the first genome-wide-associated (p<10E-08) single variants were identified in a region on chromosome 20 between a non-coding ribonucleic acid (ncRNA) (*LOC105372646*) and the *PREX1* gene.[56] While taking into account the severity of SB, Levey et al.[57] revealed signals near the *LDHB* (European) and *FAH* (African) genes, as well as a significant overlap with the diagnosis of major depression. A GWAS using data from the UK Biobank revealed three new genome-wide significant loci (on chromosomes 9, 11, and 13), as well as a moderate-to-strong correlation between SB and psychiatric diagnoses, which was most pronounced for depression.[58] Another large GWAS on suicide attempt (SA) included individuals with major depression (1622 with SA, 8786 without), bipolar disorder (3264 with SA, 5500 without), and schizophrenia (1683 with SA, 2946 without). Genome-wide associations with SB were identified within the major depression (*ARL5B*) and bipolar disorder (ncRNA *LOC105374524*) subgroups. This locus and the *IWS1/MYO7B* region were also found to be significant in a meta-analysis on both disorders, but the findings were not replicated in two independent samples. PRS analysis showed that a genetic risk burden for major depression can predict an increased risk of SB not only in depression, but also in bipolar disorder and schizophrenia, suggesting an increased risk of SB across diagnoses, depending on the genetic burden for major depression.[59] Studies investigating genetic susceptibility to SB as a potential additive risk factor for treatment-emergent suicidal ideation (TESI) remained inconclusive (e.g. see Perroud et al.),[60] probably due to small sample sizes. In contrast, studies investigating the association of CNVs with SB produced no significant results, implicating a minor role in this phenotype.[61]

Aggression and anger

GWAS of aggression and anger have mainly been conducted in correlated phenotypes, including conduct disorder (CD), antisocial personality disorder (ASD), violent offending, aggressive behaviour, anger, and hostility,[62,63] with many of these studies performed in children or adolescents. In early studies on CD and antisocial behaviour, no genome-wide significant hits were detected due to insufficient statistical power.[63] In a sample of 3963 mixed-ancestry subjects with substance dependence, four variants in three independent regions (*C1QTNF7*, *LINC00331*, and *EEF1A2*—pseudogene *LOC642791*) were genome-wide-associated with CD symptom count, although this was abolished in ancestry-specific subsets[64] and could not be replicated in association with antisocial behaviour.[65] A meta-analysis of five population-based cohorts and three target samples on a broader phenotype of ASD, consisting of a considerably larger sample of 25,781 participants, revealed three genome-wide significant hits by using a sex-specific evaluation (females: *LHX4*, *NXPE2*; males:

intergenic variant). PRS extracted from the ASD GWAS showed predictive properties for antisocial phenotypes and conduct problems, but not for CD in independent samples, implicating a shared aetiology.[66] By comparing cohorts of Finnish criminal offenders with ASD to the general population, suggestive associations were obtained in the human leucocyte antigen (HLA) region in two clusters (6p21.2, 6p21.32). Follow-up by imputation of HLA alleles resulted in an independent nominal association with *DRB1**01:01 allele, and by replication and meta-analysis of the 6p21.2 region in a genome-wide significant association with rs4714329 (near *LINC00951*).[67] In addition, physical aggression in the context of cannabis abuse was genome-wide significantly associated with variants in the *HTR2B*/*PSMD1* locus in Americans of African, but not European, ancestry.[68] In a study of 18,988 children of North European ancestry, which also focused on aggressive behaviour, a near genome-wide-associated variant within an intergenic region on chromosome 2 (rs11126630; $p = 5.30 \times 10^{-8}$) was detected.[69] Finally, the NEO-PI-R neuroticism facet of angry hostility was genome-wide significantly associated with a variant in the *MIR548H3* gene in a cohort of 5584 Koreans.[70] While the functional significance of those associations remains to be investigated, the gene loci implicated in aggression and anger traits suggest an involvement of the immune- and neuroendocrine-related pathways, intracellular protein metabolism, and neuronal development.

Impulsivity

The heterogeneity of the construct of impulsivity is reflected in the numerous phenotypes studied in GWAS in this context, including inattention/hyperactivity–impulsivity,[71] emotional and mood instability,[72,73] addictions (for a review, see Hancock et al.),[74] and related personality traits such as extraversion[75] Klicken oder tippen Sie hier, um Text einzugeben. and excitement seeking.[76] A GWAS by Ehlers et al.[77] Klicken oder tippen Sie hier, um Text einzugeben. on impulsivity in an American Indian sample identified significant associations with two independent loci (*REG* gene cluster and ncRNA *LOC105377557*). In evaluating the genetic background of impulsive choice measured as delayed reward discounting,[78] a GWAS which included a small discovery sample of 986 young adults of European ancestry revealed an association with a gene desert locus on chromosome 2, which failed to be replicated in the 23andMe cohort.[79] Using this considerably larger sample which included 23,217 adults of European ancestry, a genome-wide association of a variant localized in the *GPM6B* gene was detected.[80] Attention-deficit/hyperactivity disorder (ADHD) is accompanied by a frequent display of hyperactive–impulsive behaviour in affected individuals,[71] with a considerable genetic overlap with bipolar disorder,[81] one of the main comorbidities found in patients with SB.

Using a GWAS on emotional instability in a highly traumatized sample of 2600 African–American adults, a male-specific genome-wide hit in the *IL2RA* locus was identified, as well as an enrichment of genes involved in calcium signalling.[72] Terracciano et al.[76] found another genome-wide significant association for a variation in the *CTNNA2* gene in a meta-analysis of six European samples ($n = 7860$) with the trait of excitement seeking, but which failed in the replication step. Genome-wide significance of mood instability, based on a single item of the Eysenck Personality Questionnaire, in 53,525 patients with psychiatric disorders, compared to 60,443 controls, was observed for four chromosomal regions: *CLDN23/MFHAS1* locus, *PTPRD*, a region on chromosome 14 containing 10 coding genes, and DCC.[73] Another GWAS analysis derived from a UK Biobank sample that included 328,339 participants of white British ancestry also identified 10 genome-wide significant loci associated with self-reported risk-taking. In a follow-up of the lead SNPs in four samples of different ethnic backgrounds, nominal significance was detected for variations in *CADM2*, *FOXP2*, and *CYP7B1* in the white, non-British group, and in *SOX2* and *FOXP2* in South Asians. In a meta-analysis across all ethnicities, seven loci remained genome-wide significant.[82] Investigating risk tolerance and risky behaviour, a GWAS conducted in a discovery sample of approximately 1 million participants from the UK Biobank and 23andMe identified 124 index SNPs located in 99 independent regions. By including six further samples, 444 distinct loci were found spread across all seven GWAS and (sub-)phenotypes. General risk-taking behaviour was associated with 94 regions, including a long-range LD region on chromosome 3, with the most significant SNP for this phenotype (rs993137; $p = 2.14 \times 10^{-40}$) localized in the *CADM2* gene. Pathway and gene network analyses separately point to a role for glutamatergic and GABAergic neurotransmission.[83] Interestingly, another variation in the *CADM2* gene was also associated with sensation-seeking in a cohort of 22,861 participants of European ancestry.[84]

Although replications of the GWAS results in independent samples are pending, recent evidence suggests that calcium metabolism, neuroendocrine signalling, and genes involved in cell–cell interactions may play a role in impulsive behaviour.

Neuroticism

Initial GWAS investigating neuroticism were not successful, mainly due to the small sample size.[22] The first study to identify a genome-wide significant association with neuroticism was a meta-analysis including over 70,000 participants which identified a variant in the *MAGI1* gene. Although replication failed, the PRS obtained from this meta-analysis successfully predicted neuroticism and major depression in independent cohorts.[85] Further GWAS were drawing data from large biobanks and commercial companies to significantly increase the sample size. Thus, 11 variants were significantly associated with neuroticism in a cohort of 170,911 subjects, two of which were located within inversion polymorphisms on chromosomes 8p23.1 and 17q21.3.[86] The locus on chromosome 8 was replicated in another meta-analysis on neuroticism that included approximately 200,000 subjects.[87] In the latter study, a missense variant in the *L3MBTL2* schizophrenia risk gene was associated. Interestingly, a PRS derived from the sample of Okbay et al.[86] Klicken oder tippen Sie hier, um Text einzugeben. successfully predicted neuroticism and major depression in a Han Chinese sample, indicating a trans-ancestral genetic overlap for these phenotypes.[88] Luciano et al.[89] Klicken oder tippen Sie hier, um Text einzugeben. conducted another GWAS on 329,821 participants from the UK Biobank and identified 116 independent loci associated with neuroticism, confirming most of the previously discovered variants and a substantial overlap with major depression. In the largest GWAS to date including 449,484 participants, a total of 136 independent loci were identified, with functional analyses indicating involvement of specific cell types, including dopaminergic neuroblasts, medium spiny neurons, and serotonergic neurons, and gene set analyses demonstrating enrichment within neurogenesis, behavioural response to cocaine processes, and the axon compartment.[90]

Thus, it is increasingly possible to identify genes, signalling pathways, and cellular structures that are relevant to complex traits, in order to uncover the biological background of neuroticism.

Conclusion and outlook

Although the genetic basis of suicidal behaviour is far from resolved, several results from the last years of research can be drawn. Suicidal behaviour itself is a complex trait, with several categories of severity. Whether these conduct separate entities or a continuous trait is still under discussion and needs to be considered in future studies. Furthermore, environmental influences, such as early stressful life events which can manifest as epigenetic changes, as well as gene × gene and gene × environment interactions, need to be considered. As sample sizes increase and genotyping techniques improve, it becomes more and more apparent that most past studies were underpowered, and hypothesis-driven candidate gene studies were too narrow in design. Taken together, genetic studies have led to interesting results, particularly in regard to phenotypic boundaries between suicidal behaviour, mental disorders, and allocated endophenotypes, as well as to their modes of inheritance, with implications for diagnostics and genetic counselling.

References

1. **Martin-Carrasco M, Evans-Lacko S, Dom G**, et al. EPA guidance on mental health and economic crises in Europe. Eur Arch Psychiatry Clin Neurosci. 2016;**266**(2):89–124.
2. **Nock MK, Hwang I, Sampson N**, et al. Cross-national analysis of the associations among mental disorders and suicidal behavior: findings from the WHO World Mental Health Surveys. PLoS Med. 2009;**6**(8):e1000123.
3. **Tidemalm D, Runeson B, Waern M**, et al. Familial clustering of suicide risk: a total population study of 11.4 million individuals. Psychol Med. 2011;**41**(12):2527–34.
4. **Brent DA, Melhem NM, Oquendo M**, et al. Familial pathways to early-onset suicide attempt: a 5.6-year prospective study. JAMA Psychiatry. 2015;**72**(2):160–8.
5. **Kenneally LB, Szűcs A, Szántó K, Dombrovski AY.** Familial and social transmission of suicidal behavior in older adults. J Affect Disord. 2019;**245**:589–96.
6. **Schulsinger F.** A family study of suicide. In: **Schou M, Stromgren E**, editors. *Origin, Prevention and Treatment of Affective Disorders*. New York, NY: Academic Press; 1979. pp. 277–87.
7. **Wender PH, Kety SS, Rosenthal D, Schulsinger F, Ortmann J, Lunde I.** Psychiatric disorders in the biological and adoptive families of adopted individuals with affective disorders. Arch Gen Psychiatry. 1986;**43**(10):923–9.
8. **Von Borczyskowski A, Lindblad F, Vinnerljung B, Reintjes R, Hjern A.** Familial factors and suicide: an adoption study in a Swedish National Cohort. Psychol Med. 2011;**41**(4):749–58.
9. **Voracek M, Loibl LM.** Genetics of suicide: a systematic review of twin studies. Wien Klin Wochenschr. 2007;**119**(15–16):463–75.
10. **Thornton LM, Welch E, Munn-Chernoff MA, Lichtenstein P, Bulik CM.** Anorexia nervosa, major depression, and suicide attempts: shared genetic factors. Suicide Life Threat Behav. 2016;**46**(5):525–34.
11. **Ruderfer DM, Walsh CG, Aguirre MW**, et al. Significant shared heritability underlies suicide attempt and clinically predicted probability of attempting suicide. Mol Psychiatry. 2020;25(10):2422–30.
12. **Turecki G, Brent DA, Gunnell D**, et al. Suicide and suicide risk. Nat Rev Dis Primers. 2019;**5**(1):74.
13. **Anestis MD, Soberay KA, Gutierrez PM, Hernández TD, Joiner TE.** Reconsidering the link between impulsivity and suicidal behavior. Pers Soc Psychol Rev. 2014;**18**(4):366–86.
14. **McHugh CM, Chun Lee RS, Hermens DF, Corderoy A, Large M, Hickie IB.** Impulsivity in the self-harm and suicidal behavior of young people: a systematic review and meta-analysis. J Psychiatr Res. 2019;**116**:51–60.
15. **Gvion Y, Horesh N, Levi-Belz Y, Apter A.** A proposed model of the development of suicidal ideations. Compr Psychiatry. 2015;**56**:93–102.
16. **Yen S, Shea MT, Sanislow CA**, et al. Personality traits as prospective predictors of suicide attempts. Acta Psychiatr Scand. 2009;**120**(3):222–9.
17. **Lewitzka U, Spirling S, Ritter D**, et al. Suicidal ideation vs suicide attempts: clinical and psychosocial profile differences among depressed patients: a study on personality traits, psychopathological variables, and sociodemographic factors in 228 patients. J Nerv Ment Dis. 2017;**205**(5):361–71.

18. **Fanning JR, Lee R, Coccaro EF.** Comorbid intermittent explosive disorder and posttraumatic stress disorder: clinical correlates and relationship to suicidal behavior. Compr Psychiatry. 2016;**70**:125–33.
19. **Dillon KH, van Voorhees EE, Dennis PA,** et al. Anger mediates the relationship between posttraumatic stress disorder and suicidal ideation in veterans. J Affect Disord. 2020;**269**:117–24.
20. **Draper B, Kõlves K, de Leo D, Snowdon J.** A controlled study of suicide in middle-aged and older people: personality traits, age, and psychiatric disorders. Suicide Life Threat Behav. 2014;**44**(2):130–8.
21. **Kotov R, Gamez W, Schmidt F, Watson D.** Linking 'big' personality traits to anxiety, depressive, and substance use disorders: a meta-analysis. Psychol Bull. 2010;**136**(5):768–821.
22. **Sanchez-Roige S, Gray JC, MacKillop J, Chen C-H, Palmer AA.** The genetics of human personality. Genes Brain Behav. 2018;**17**(3):e12439.
23. **Mirkovic B, Laurent C, Podlipski M-A, Frebourg T, Cohen D, Gerardin P.** Genetic association studies of suicidal behavior: a review of the past 10 years, progress, limitations, and future directions. Front Psychiatry. 2016;**7**:158.
24. **Li D, He L.** Further clarification of the contribution of the tryptophan hydroxylase (*TPH*) gene to suicidal behavior using systematic allelic and genotypic meta-analyses. Hum Genet. 2006;**119**(3):233–40.
25. **Saetre P, Lundmark P, Wang A,** et al. The tryptophan hydroxylase 1 (*TPH1*) gene, schizophrenia susceptibility, and suicidal behavior: a multi-centre case-control study and meta-analysis. Am J Med Genet B Neuropsychiatr Genet. 2010;**153B**(2):387–96.
26. **Baud P.** Personality traits as intermediary phenotypes in suicidal behavior: genetic issues. Am J Med Genet C Semin Med Genet. 2005;**133C**(1):34–42.
27. **Zill P, Büttner A, Eisenmenger W, Möller H-J, Bondy B, Ackenheil M.** Single nucleotide polymorphism and haplotype analysis of a novel tryptophan hydroxylase isoform (*TPH2*) gene in suicide victims. Biol Psychiatry. 2004;**56**(8):581–6.
28. **Ottenhof KW, Sild M, Lévesque ML, Ruhé HG, Booij L.** *TPH2* polymorphisms across the spectrum of psychiatric morbidity: a systematic review and meta-analysis. Neurosci Biobehav Rev. 2018;**92**:29–42.
29. **Laas K, Kiive E, Mäestu J, Vaht M, Veidebaum T, Harro J.** Nice guys: homozygozity for the TPH2-703G/T (rs4570625) minor allele promotes low aggressiveness and low anxiety. J Affect Disord. 2017;**215**:230–6.
30. **Kulikova EA, Kulikov AV.** Tryptophan hydroxylase 2 as a therapeutic target for psychiatric disorders: focus on animal models. Expert Opin Ther Targets. 2019;**23**(8):655–67.
31. **Balestri M, Calati R, Serretti A,** et al. Maoa and Maob polymorphisms and personality traits in suicide attempters and healthy controls: a preliminary study. Psychiatry Res. 2017;**249**:212–17.
32. **Checknita D, Bendre M, Ekström TJ,** et al. Monoamine oxidase A genotype and methylation moderate the association of maltreatment and aggressive behaviour. Behav Brain Res. 2020;**382**:112476.
33. **Lesch KP, Bengel D, Heils A,** et al. Association of anxiety-related traits with a polymorphism in the serotonin transporter gene regulatory region. Science. 1996;**274**(5292):1527–31.

34. **Fanelli G, Serretti A.** The influence of the serotonin transporter gene *5-HTTLPR* polymorphism on suicidal behaviors: a meta-analysis. Prog Neuropsychopharmacol Biol Psychiatry. 2019;**88**:375–87.
35. **Munafò MR, Freimer NB, Ng W**, et al. *5-HTTLPR* genotype and anxiety-related personality traits: a meta-analysis and new data. Am J Med Genet B Neuropsychiatr Genet. 2009;**150B**(2):271–81.
36. **Hemmings SMJ, Xulu K, Sommer J**, et al. Appetitive and reactive aggression are differentially associated with the STin2 genetic variant in the serotonin transporter gene. Sci Rep. 2018;**8**(1):6714.
37. **Waltes R, Chiocchetti AG, Freitag CM.** The neurobiological basis of human aggression: a review on genetic and epigenetic mechanisms. Am J Med Genet B Neuropsychiatr Genet. 2016;**171**(5):650–75.
38. **Lemonde S, Turecki G, Bakish D**, et al. Impaired repression at a 5-hydroxytryptamine 1A receptor gene polymorphism associated with major depression and suicide. J Neurosci. 2003;**23**(25):8788–99.
39. **Höfer P, Schosser A, Calati R**, et al. The impact of serotonin receptor 1A and 2A gene polymorphisms and interactions on suicide attempt and suicide risk in depressed patients with insufficient response to treatment: a European multicentre study. Int Clin Psychopharmacol. 2016;**31**(1):1–7.
40. **Benko A, Lazary J, Molnar E**, et al. Significant association between the C(-1019)G functional polymorphism of the *HTR1A* gene and impulsivity. Am J Med Genet B Neuropsychiatr Genet. 2010;**153B**(2):592–9.
41. **New AS, Gelernter J, Goodman M**, et al. Suicide, impulsive aggression, and *HTR1B* genotype. Biol Psychiatry. 2001;**50**(1):62–5.
42. **Sadkowski M, Dennis B, Clayden RC**, et al. The role of the serotonergic system in suicidal behavior. Neuropsychiatr Dis Treat. 2013;**9**:1699–716.
43. **Conner TS, Jensen KP, Tennen H, Furneaux HM, Kranzler HR, Covault J.** Functional polymorphisms in the serotonin 1B receptor gene (*HTR1B*) predict self-reported anger and hostility among young men. Am J Med Genet B Neuropsychiatr Genet. 2010;**153B**(1):67–78.
44. **Stoltenberg SF, Christ CC, Highland KB.** Serotonin system gene polymorphisms are associated with impulsivity in a context dependent manner. Prog Neuropsychopharmacol Biol Psychiatry. 2012;**39**(1):182–91.
45. **Bidwell LC, Gray JC, Weafer J, Palmer AA, de Wit H, MacKillop J.** Genetic influences on ADHD symptom dimensions: examination of a priori candidates, gene-based tests, genome-wide variation, and SNP heritability. Am J Med Genet B Neuropsychiatr Genet. 2017;**174**(4):458–66.
46. **Wang J-Y, Jia C-X, Lian Y, Sun S-H, Lyu M, Wu A.** Association of the HTR2A 102T/C polymorphism with attempted suicide: a meta-analysis. Psychiatr Genet. 2015;**25**(4):168–77.
47. **Gray JC, MacKillop J, Weafer J**, et al. Genetic analysis of impulsive personality traits: examination of a priori candidates and genome-wide variation. Psychiatry Res. 2018;**259**:398–404.
48. **Giegling I, Hartmann AM, Möller H-J, Rujescu D.** Anger- and aggression-related traits are associated with polymorphisms in the *5-HT-2A* gene. J Affect Disord. 2006;**96**(1–2):75–81.

49. **González-Castro TB, Hernandez-Diaz Y, Juárez-Rojop IE**, et al. The role of the Cys23Ser (rs6318) polymorphism of the *HTR2C* gene in suicidal behavior: systematic review and meta-analysis. Psychiatr Genet. 2017;**27**(6):199–209.
50. **Lengvenyte A, Conejero I, Courtet P, Olié E.** Biological bases of suicidal behaviours: a narrative review. Eur J Neurosci. 2021 Jan;**53**(1):330–51.
51. **González-Castro TB, Hernández-Díaz Y, Juárez-Rojop IE**, et al. The role of *COMT* gene Val108/158Met polymorphism in suicidal behavior: systematic review and updated meta-analysis. Neuropsychiatr Dis Treat. 2018;**14**:2485–96.
52. **Zai CC, Manchia M, de Luca V**, et al. The brain-derived neurotrophic factor gene in suicidal behaviour: a meta-analysis. Int J Neuropsychopharmacol. 2012;**15**(8):1037–42.
53. **Sadeghiyeh T, Hosseini Biouki F, Mazaheri M, Zare-Shehneh M, Neamatzadeh H, Poursharif Z.** Association between catechol-*O*-methyltransferase Val158Met (158G/A) polymorphism and suicide susceptibility: a meta-analysis. J Res Health Sci. 2017;**17**(2):e00383.
54. **Wagner S, Baskaya O, Dahmen N, Lieb K, Tadić A.** Modulatory role of the brain-derived neurotrophic factor Val66Met polymorphism on the effects of serious life events on impulsive aggression in borderline personality disorder. Genes Brain Behav. 2010;**9**(1):97–102.
55. **Sokolowski M, Wasserman J, Wasserman D.** Gene-level associations in suicide attempter families show overrepresentation of synaptic genes and genes differentially expressed in brain development. Am J Med Genet B Neuropsychiatr Genet. 2018;**177**(8):774–84.
56. **Erlangsen A, Appadurai V, Wang Y**, et al. Genetics of suicide attempts in individuals with and without mental disorders: a population-based genome-wide association study. Mol Psychiatry. 2020 Oct;**25**(10):2410–21.
57. **Levey DF, Polimanti R, Cheng Z**, et al. Genetic associations with suicide attempt severity and genetic overlap with major depression. Transl Psychiatry. 2019;**9**(1):22.
58. **Strawbridge RJ, Ward J, Ferguson A**, et al. Identification of novel genome-wide associations for suicidality in UK Biobank, genetic correlation with psychiatric disorders and polygenic association with completed suicide. EBioMedicine. 2019;**41**:517–25.
59. **Mullins N, Bigdeli TB, Børglum AD**, et al. GWAS of suicide attempt in psychiatric disorders and association with major depression polygenic risk scores. Am J Psychiatry. 2019;**176**(8):651–60.
60. **Perroud N, Uher R, Ng MYM**, et al. Genome-wide association study of increasing suicidal ideation during antidepressant treatment in the GENDEP project. Pharmacogenomics J. 2012;**12**(1):68–77.
61. **Gross JA, Bureau A, Croteau J**, et al. A genome-wide copy number variant study of suicidal behavior. PLoS One. 2015;**10**(5):e0128369.
62. **Salvatore JE, Dick DM.** Genetic influences on conduct disorder. Neurosci Biobehav Rev. 2018;**91**:91–101.
63. **Odintsova VV, Roetman PJ, Ip HF**, et al. Genomics of human aggression: current state of genome-wide studies and an automated systematic review tool. Psychiatr Genet. 2019;**29**(5):170–90.
64. **Dick DM, Aliev F, Krueger RF**, et al. Genome-wide association study of conduct disorder symptomatology. Mol Psychiatry. 2011;**16**(8):800–8.

65. **Tielbeek JJ, Medland SE, Benyamin B,** et al. Unraveling the genetic etiology of adult antisocial behavior: a genome-wide association study. PLoS One. 2012;**7**(10):e45086.
66. **Tielbeek JJ, Johansson A, Polderman TJC,** et al. Genome-wide association studies of a broad spectrum of antisocial behavior. JAMA Psychiatry. 2017;**74**(12):1242–50.
67. **Rautiainen M-R, Paunio T, Repo-Tiihonen E,** et al. Genome-wide association study of antisocial personality disorder. Transl Psychiatry. 2016;**6**(9):e883.
68. **Montalvo-Ortiz JL, Zhou H, D'Andrea I,** et al. Translational studies support a role for serotonin 2B receptor (*HTR2B*) gene in aggression-related cannabis response. Mol Psychiatry. 2018;**23**(12):2277–86.
69. **Pappa I, St Pourcain B, Benke K,** et al. A genome-wide approach to children's aggressive behavior: the EAGLE consortium. Am J Med Genet B Neuropsychiatr Genet. 2016;**171**(5):562–72.
70. **Kim SE, Kim H-N, Yun Y-J,** et al. Meta-analysis of genome-wide SNP- and pathway-based associations for facets of neuroticism. J Hum Genet. 2017;**62**(10):903–9.
71. **Palladino VS, McNeill R, Reif A, Kittel-Schneider S.** Genetic risk factors and gene–environment interactions in adult and childhood attention-deficit/hyperactivity disorder. Psychiatr Genet. 2019;**29**(3):63–78.
72. **Powers A, Almli L, Smith A,** et al. A genome-wide association study of emotion dysregulation: evidence for interleukin 2 receptor alpha. J Psychiatr Res. 2016;**83**:195–202.
73. **Ward J, Strawbridge RJ, Bailey MES,** et al. Genome-wide analysis in UK Biobank identifies four loci associated with mood instability and genetic correlation with major depressive disorder, anxiety disorder and schizophrenia. Transl Psychiatry. 2017;**7**(11):1264.
74. **Hancock DB, Markunas CA, Bierut LJ, Johnson EO.** Human genetics of addiction: new insights and future directions. Curr Psychiatry Rep. 2018;**20**(2):8.
75. **Van den Berg SM, de Moor MHM, Verweij KJH,** et al. Meta-analysis of genome-wide association studies for extraversion: findings from the Genetics of Personality Consortium. Behav Genet. 2016;**46**(2):170–82.
76. **Terracciano A, Esko T, Sutin AR,** et al. Meta-analysis of genome-wide association studies identifies common variants in *CTNNA2* associated with excitement-seeking. Transl Psychiatry. 2011;**1**:e49.
77. **Ehlers CL, Gizer IR, Bizon C,** et al. Single nucleotide polymorphisms in the REG-CTNNA2 region of chromosome 2 and NEIL3 associated with impulsivity in a native American sample. Genes Brain Behav. 2016;**15**(6):568–77.
78. **Gray JC, Sanchez-Roige S, de Wit H, MacKillop J, Palmer AA.** Genomic basis of delayed reward discounting. Behav Processes. 2019;**162**:157–61.
79. **MacKillop J, Amlung MT, Few LR, Ray LA, Sweet LH, Munafò MR.** Delayed reward discounting and addictive behavior: a meta-analysis. Psychopharmacology (Berl). 2011;**216**(3):305–21.
80. **Sanchez-Roige S, Fontanillas P, Elson SL,** et al. Genome-wide association study of delay discounting in 23,217 adult research participants of European ancestry. Nat Neurosci. 2018;**21**(1):16–18.
81. **O'Connell KS, Shadrin A, Bahrami S,** et al. Identification of genetic overlap and novel risk loci for attention-deficit/hyperactivity disorder and bipolar disorder. Mol Psychiatry. 2021 Aug;**26**(8):4055–65.

82. **Strawbridge RJ, Ward J, Lyall LM,** et al. Genetics of self-reported risk-taking behaviour, trans-ethnic consistency and relevance to brain gene expression. Transl Psychiatry. 2018;**8**(1):178.
83. **Linnér RK, Biroli P, Kong E,** et al. Genome-wide association analyses of risk tolerance and risky behaviors in over 1 million individuals identify hundreds of loci and shared genetic influences. Nat Genet. 2019;**51**(2):245–57.
84. **Sanchez-Roige S, Fontanillas P, Elson SL,** et al. Genome-wide association studies of impulsive personality traits (BIS-11 and UPPS-P) and drug experimentation in up to 22,861 adult research participants identify loci in the *CACNA1I* and *CADM2* genes. J Neurosci. 2019;**39**(13):2562–72.
85. **De Moor MHM, van den Berg SM, Verweij KJH,** et al. Genome-wide association study identifies novel locus for neuroticism and shows polygenic association with major depressive disorder. JAMA Psychiatry. 2015;**72**(7):642–50.
86. **Okbay A, Baselmans BML, de Neve J-E,** et al. Genetic variants associated with subjective well-being, depressive symptoms and neuroticism identified through genome-wide analyses. Nat Genet. 2016;**48**(6):624–33.
87. **Lo M-T, Hinds DA, Tung JY,** et al. Genome-wide analyses for personality traits identify six genomic loci and show correlations with psychiatric disorders. Nat Genet. 2017;**49**(1):152–6.
88. **Docherty AR, Moscati A, Peterson R,** et al. SNP-based heritability estimates of the personality dimensions and polygenic prediction of both neuroticism and major depression: findings from CONVERGE. Transl Psychiatry. 2016;**6**(10):e926.
89. **Luciano M, Hagenaars SP, Davies G,** et al. Association analysis in over 329,000 individuals identifies 116 independent variants influencing neuroticism. Nat Genet. 2018;**50**(1):6–11.
90. **Nagel M, Jansen PR, Stringer S,** et al. Meta-analysis of genome-wide association studies for neuroticism in 449,484 individuals identifies novel genetic loci and pathways. Nat Genet. 2018;**50**(7):920–7.

Chapter 6

Gender inequality and suicide: A systematic review of empirical studies

Melissa Yoong, Chan Lai Fong, and Chen Ying-Yeh

Introduction

It is well known that suicide rates in men are higher than in women in most parts of the world.[1] There is also a long tradition of theorizing in dominant suicidology which argues that women are protected from suicide. For example, Durkheim, one of the most prominent suicidologists, proposed that women are protected from suicide because they presumably are not as socialized and civilized as men and are tucked in the 'safety' of the domestic sphere.[2,3] Durkheim also believed that women specialized in 'affective functions', as opposed to 'intellectual functions', which he assumed belonged to men and proposed was an important factor in suicide contemplation and action.[2 (p. 60),4,5] Hence, according to Durkheim, suicide rates in women would rise if they became 'more like men' such as through their increased participation in the labour force, social groups, and political decision-making. Men's suicide rates too would grow if women stepped into men's public realm, as such social change would disrupt domestic integration.[6] Overall, based on Durkheim's theory, egalitarian gender norms would result in increased suicide rates in both men and women.

Paradoxically, women's lower social status is thought to be an important determining factor for the high female suicide rates in many Asian countries (e.g. China and India).[7,8] Marriage, which signifies domestic integration, is not a protective factor against suicide in Asia; it is a suicide risk factor in the region.[9] The dominance of extended family systems and the family-centred culture in Asia place young married women at the lowest rank in some Asian contexts.[10] Stuck in choiceless and hopeless family situations (e.g. domestic violence, bullying by in-laws), many young wives often consider suicide as a way out of an unbearable position. Hence, how women's status and gender equality affect suicide risk in men and women is intriguing. However, information from the Global South and dominant Western-based suicidology are contradictory, whereas no previous research has systematically reviewed the available evidence. The current chapter aims to review existing empirical studies on gender (in)equality and suicide to further our understanding about the impact of egalitarian gender norms on suicide risk.

Method

Using PubMed and the American Psychological Association's PsycInfo, we performed a search for the keywords 'suicide' and 'gender inequality', 'suicide' and 'gender equality', 'suicide' and 'egalitarian gender norms', and 'suicide' and 'women's status' in the titles and abstracts of English-language journal articles published from 1 January 1960 to 19 December 2022. We also scanned the reference lists of these publications to identify other relevant research papers. Figure 6.1 presents the steps taken in the search and selection process. A final total of 28 empirical studies were retrieved and reviewed.

Results

Table 6.1 summarizes information on the empirical studies, including the geographical setting, time period, and key findings of each study. Nine articles were published in the 1980s and 1990s, whereas 18 were published between 2000 and 2021. Overall, female labour force participation rate (FLPR) was the most commonly used indicator of gender equality in scholarship published before 2000 (7 out of 9 studies). The majority of studies during this period focused on the United States; the research design was mostly longitudinal time series analysis that explored the association between gender inequality (e.g. FLPR) and suicide rates over time.

As Table 6.1 shows, save for a few exceptions,[11,13,16,22] most of the studies found that egalitarian gender norms have no impact or are even beneficial for both women and men, particularly in times of economic crisis.[32,38] Notably, research conducted after the year 2000 used more delicate indicators of gender equality (or inequality) such as the Gender Empowerment Measure[22] and the Gender Inequality Index[36] developed by the United Nations Development Programme (UNDP).[42] Rather than solely talking about trends in suicide rates as women become 'more like men', studies have started to examine how men's involvement in activities that are traditionally regarded as 'women's work' (e.g. care work) can benefit both genders.[35,39]

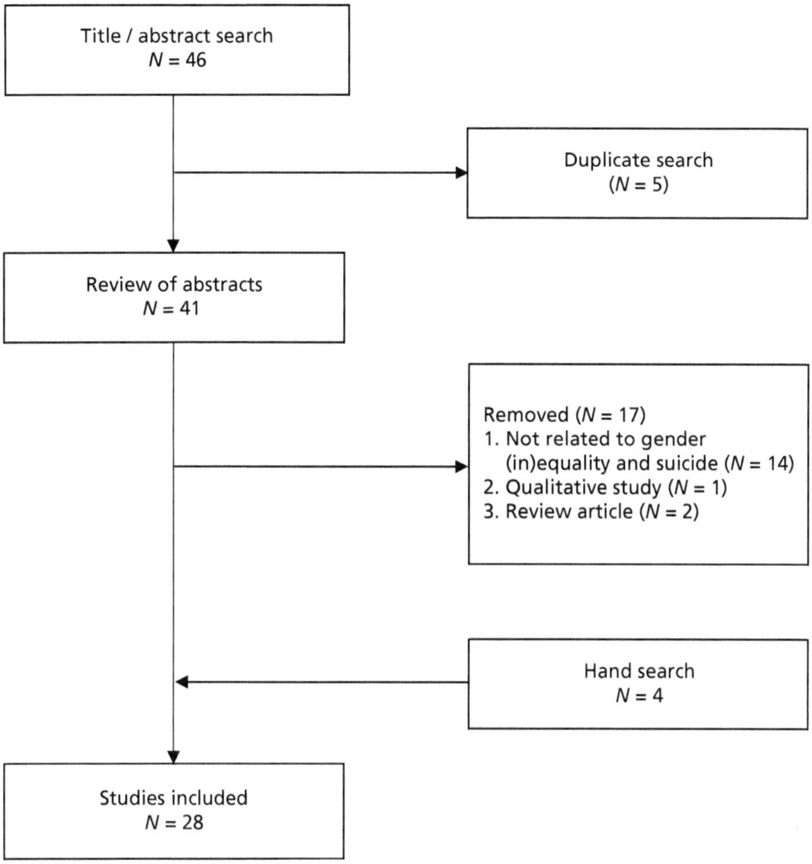

Figure 6.1 Selection process of empirical studies on gender inequality and suicide.

Discussion

Cultural and contextual effects

Our systematic review of empirical studies refutes theories from dominant suicidology that suggest gender equality to be a risk factor for suicides. On the contrary, our review indicates that egalitarian gender norms are associated with lower suicide risk for both men and women. This is particularly evident in the more recent studies that we reviewed (i.e. those published after 2000).

Apparently, Durkheim's theory is dated. His sociological analysis interpreted gender differences in suicide rates through an essentialist lens and overlooked cultural diversity. Canetto, a more recent theorist on gender and suicide,

Table 6.1 Summary of empirical studies on gender (in)equality and suicide

Authors (year)	Study setting	Study period	Research design	Indicator of gender (in)equality	Main findings
Davis (1981)[11]	USA	1950–69	Longitudinal time-series study	FLPR	FLPR was associated with higher female suicide rates, but lower male suicide rates NB this study did not control for potential covariates
Lester and Yang (1991)[12]	Australia USA	1946–84	Longitudinal time-series study	FLPR	After considering time trend, unemployment rates, and divorce rates, FLPR was associated with lower suicide rates in women, but not with male suicide rates, in Australia and the USA
Austin et al. (1992)[13]	USA	1950–69, 1970–84	Longitudinal time-series study	FLPR Educational attainment	Higher FLPR and educational attainment were associated with higher female-to-male suicide ratio in middle-aged women NB this study did not control for potential covariates
Lester (1992)[14]	USA	1980	Cross-sectional ecological study	Indicators of gender equality based on 24 indicators[15]	Gender equality was not associated with suicide rates
Lester et al. (1992)[16]	Japan USA	1953–82	Longitudinal time-series study	FLPR	In the USA, FLPR was not associated with suicide rates in the covariate-adjusted model In Japan, FLPR was associated with increased suicide rates in both women and men
Yang et al. (1992)[17]	Taiwan USA	1952–84	Longitudinal time-series study	FLPR	In both the USA and Taiwan, increased FLPR was associated with lower suicide rates in both men and women

Lester (1994)[18]	23 countries	1985	Cross-sectional ecological study	Gender equality indicator designed by Charles[19]	Gender equality was not associated with suicide rates in both women and men
Chuang and Huang (1996)[20]	Taiwan USA	1952–92	Longitudinal time-series study	FLPR	In both the USA and Taiwan, increased FLPR was associated with lower suicide rates in both men and women
Burr et al. (1997)[21]	USA	1970, 1980	Cross-sectional ecological study	FLPR	In 1970, FLPR was associated with male suicide rates, but not with female suicide rates In 1980, FLPR was associated with lower suicide rates in both women and men
Mayer (2000)[22]	26 countries	1996	Cross-sectional ecological study	Gender Empowerment Measure Gender-related development index	Higher levels of Gender Empowerment Measure were associated with higher suicide rates in both men and women Gender-related development index was not associated with suicide rates in either gender NB this study only used correlation matrix, with no adjustment for covariates
Lucey et al. (2005)[23]	Ireland	1968–2000	Longitudinal time-series study	FLPR	FLPR was not associated with gender-specific and overall suicide rates
Zhang et al. (2006)[24]	Dalian province, China	2003	Cross-sectional interview-based study	Perceived gender inequality	Perceived gender inequality was associated with higher suicide intent
Zhang and Xu (2007)[25]					NB Zhang et al. (2006) and Zhang and Xu (2007) used the same source population. The latter supplied additional information on suicide methods used

(continued)

Table 6.1 Continued

Authors (year)	Study setting	Study period	Research design	Indicator of gender (in)equality	Main findings
Shah (2008)[26]	69 countries	1991–2003	Cross-sectional ecological study	Gender Empowerment Measure Gender-related development index	No association between gender-related measures and suicide rates
Aliverdinia and Pridemore (2009)[27]	Iran	1997–2000	Cross-sectional ecological study	FLPR Educational attainment	Increased gender equality was associated with lower female suicide rates
Ying and Chang (2009)[28]	G7 countries: Canada, France, Germany, Italy, Japan, UK, USA	1982–2002	Longitudinal time-series across seven countries	FLPR	FLPR was associated with lower female suicide rates, but with higher male suicide rates
Barth et al. (2011)[29]	18 countries	1983–2007	Longitudinal time-series study across 18 countries	FLPR	Increasing FLPR was associated with lower female suicide rates
Phillips and Nugent (2014)[30]	USA	1997–2010	Longitudinal time-series study across 50 US states	FLPR	FLPR was not associated with overall and gender-specific suicide rates, but in states with high FLPR, the associations between unemployment rates and suicide rates were stronger

Nowotny et al. (2015)[31]	USA	1996	Cross-sectional survey, utilizing multilevel data (state-level data and individual-level survey)	16 questions on restricted gender norms	Youth, particularly female, in rigidly gendered contexts had a higher risk of suicidal ideation
Reeves and Stuckler (2016)[32]	20 European Union countries	1991–2011	Longitudinal time-series study across 20 European countries	Gender Equality Index	No association between gender equality and suicide rates in both women and men; however, gender equality buffers the association between unemployment rates and suicide rates
Chen et al. (2017)[33]	70 countries	2012	Cross-sectional ecological study across 70 countries	FLPR	The association between FLPR and suicide rates was context-dependent. In countries where human capabilities are strong, higher levels of FLPR were beneficial (particularly for women). However, the advantages of FLPR may reach a plateau in countries where the Human Development Index is at the very top. In countries where human capabilities are relatively less advanced, FLPR were positively associated with suicide rates
Assarsson et al. (2018)[34]	37 countries	2003–14	Cross-sectional ecological study across 37 countries	Gender Inequality Index	Gender inequality was associated with higher levels of suicidal ideation, especially for boys. In other words, conservative forms of masculinity may affect suicidality
Lee et al. (2018)[35]	Korea	2012, 2014	Cross-sectional survey	Satisfaction with husbands' participation in housework	Satisfaction with husbands' participation in housework was associated with lower risks of suicidal ideation in married working women in South Korea

(continued)

Table 6.1 Continued

Authors (year)	Study setting	Study period	Research design	Indicator of gender (in)equality	Main findings
Chang et al. (2019)[36]	174 countries	2012	Cross-sectional ecological study across 174 countries	Gender Inequality Index Sex ratios at birth	Male-to-female suicide rate ratios were higher in countries with more egalitarian gender norms, whereas lower suicide gender ratios were generally observed in countries with higher levels of gender inequality. Culture-based indicator of gender inequality (i.e. natality inequality/son preference) was more sensitive than economic-based indicator (i.e. the Gender Inequality Index)
Milner et al. (2020)[37]	87 countries	2006–16	Cross-sectional ecological study across 87 countries	Gender Gap Index	Increase in gender equality was associated with reduction in suicide rates in women
Chen et al. (2021)[38]	20 countries	2012	Cross-sectional ecological study across 20 countries	Male-to-female ratio of time spent on family care work	Men's higher involvement in care work was associated with lower suicide rates. Men's care work involvement buffers the association between unemployment rates and suicide rates
Cai et al. (2021)[39]	176 countries	2017	Cross-sectional ecological study across 176 countries	Laws discriminating against women	Legislative discrimination against women in low- and middle-income countries was found to be associated with smaller male-to-female suicide rate ratios (i.e. higher female suicide rates) in these countries
Navarro-Mantas et al. (2021)[40]	El Salvador	2013–14	Cross-sectional survey	Intimate partner violence against women	Women who experienced intimate partner violence had significantly poorer mental health and more suicidal ideation

proposes the 'cultural scripts theory' to explain gender differences in suicidal behaviours across different sociocultural contexts.[42] She posits that 'suicidal behavior is socially scripted and socially regulated in all cultures of the world'. In every community and nation, there exists 'collective, implicit beliefs about the meaning and permissibility of suicidal behavior. These scripts likely influence individual suicidal behavior, including when suicidal behavior becomes a possibility as well as the forms it takes' (p. 264).[42] Based on Canetto's cultural scripts theory, individuals draw on cultural scripts to initiate, contemplate, and conduct their suicidal behaviours; thus, suicidal acts have culture-specific meanings and significance. For example, in China and India, young married women's suicidal behaviours signify outcries of their oppressive experiences. The highly lethal methods that they adopt (e.g. pesticide, self-immolation) are also socially scripted. In the United States and many developed European countries, on the other hand, suicide is often portrayed as a masculine behaviour; once you decide to do it, you have to make it a 'success'. This might be the reason why, in earlier suicide research,[43] suicides that led to deaths were termed 'successful suicides' (i.e. a masculine act), whereas survived suicidal acts were characterized as 'failed suicide attempts' (i.e. feminine behaviour). These cultural scripts shape individual behaviours and guide communities' interpretations and responses to suicide.[44]

Our empirical observations also suggest that context matters. Gender relations evolve over time. The passage to gender equality may initially disrupt and unsettle traditional norms and values, but institutions will adjust, policies can be improved, and new norms will subsequently be created and operationalized.[45,46] Increased FLPR was reported to be associated with a higher suicide risk in some of the studies published before 2000, but this was not observed in any of the later research published after 2000 (see Table 6.1). Furthermore, suicidal behaviours also appear predicated on the quality of a nation's human capabilities. An international study across 70 countries using world mortality data from 2012 found that among countries equipped with better human capabilities, higher FLPRs were associated with a lower suicide risk. The reverse was observed in countries with lower human capabilities where higher FLPRs were associated with a higher risk.[33] Overall, the interplay between gender (in)equality and suicide risk is context-dependent; it varies over time and differs across cultural environments and national boundaries.

Research gaps and limitations of gender equality indicators

The majority of empirical studies were longitudinal time-series analysis or cross-sectional ecological studies; very few studies utilized information collected at individual level. In fact, only one study combined individual-level data and contextual-level (US states) information to assess the impact of restricted gender norms on the occurrence of suicidal ideation.[31] Nevertheless, this study is cross-sectional. At present, longitudinal multilevel studies assessing the relationships between gender (in)equality and suicide risk over time and across spaces are still lacking.

Half of the studies reviewed employed FLPR as a measure of national gender equality. However, it is crucial to go beyond the binary nature of this indicator and consider the gendered employment outcomes for working women and their exposure to occupational psychosocial risks that could affect their physical and psychological well-being. Even in countries that are close to parity in economic participation, 'the quality of employment and opportunities for better jobs continue to be unequally distributed between men and women' (p. 8).[48] Working women in many Global South nations tend to earn less than men and engage in low-productivity jobs, unpaid family work, and other forms of vulnerable work that do not enhance their economic empowerment or social position. In low-income nations, whether a woman works may be driven more by poverty than by choice or any widening of their educational and employment prospects. For example, the FLPR in Nepal is almost 80%, but women there mostly work in subsistence agriculture.[47] And while Bangladesh has experienced a rapid increase in FLPR, this growth has been fuelled by the garment manufacturing industry where the threat of sexual violence, low pay, and repetitive strain from physically demanding work make women vulnerable.[48] These poor work conditions have led to depression and its associated risk factors.[49,50] Hence, the impact of women's labour market involvement on suicide rates must be contextualized within the circumstances under which women enter and remain in the workforce, including their access to decent, secure, stable, and productive jobs.

It is equally important to examine the consequences of regressions in women's fragile workplace gains. Progress in women's economic inclusion is not linear, as the coronavirus disease 2019 (COVID-19) 'she-cession'[51] has shown. Historically, men, in particular those of working age, were at higher risk of suicide, compared to women, during periods of economic crisis.[52] However, emerging data seem to suggest that the pandemic may be exacerbating pre-existing gender inequalities that compound the socio-economic drivers of suicide in women. McKinsey Global Institute reported that from 2019 to 2020, women were at higher risk of job insecurity, compared to men, as employment in female-dominated service sectors has been the most negatively affected during the COVID-19 pandemic.[53] Similarly, UN Women's Rapid Gender Assessments in Asia Pacific have demonstrated that women are more prone to loss in paid work hours, in addition to shouldering greater unpaid domestic and care work, than men during lockdown. What is more, women are disproportionately at risk with regard to the mental health sequelae of the pandemic.[54] Taking Japan as a case in point, the country witnessed a rise in its suicide rate during the second wave of the pandemic after an initial decrease during the first wave.[55,56] Notably, the increase in suicide mortality was almost five times higher in women than in men. In particular, the younger age groups (below 49 years for women and below 30 years for men) were at higher suicide risk, compared to the elderly population.[56] Given that in Japan, women and younger adults comprise the majority of workers in hard-hit service industries (e.g. food and beverage, tourism, retail),[54,55] their elevated suicide risk could be associated with financial stress and unemployment. Domestic abuse is another potential factor contributing to the increased risk of suicide in women in Japan. The country reported an upsurge in domestic violence during the pandemic, with victims being predominantly female (exceeding 95%).[56] In South Korea where women are overrepresented in the informal economy and are vulnerable to poverty and violence, the female suicide rate increased by 1.4% between January and August 2020 despite an overall decrease in the total number of suicide deaths compared to the preceding year.[57] Reporting on low- and middle-income countries, Moussié and Staab described how many informal women workers have been forced to face gendered health and safety stresses such as traversing unsafe public spaces during lockdowns due to inadequacies in social protection measures.[58] The COVID-19 pandemic is expected to have long-lasting effects on gender equality in global labour markets. Hence, longitudinal data from countries of all levels of development are much needed to elucidate the mechanisms of a possible gender differential impact of the pandemic and its accompanying changes in occupational status and activities on suicidal behaviour.

Two studies reviewed[13,27] have taken educational attainment into account, alongside FLPR. Education is a significant factor that affects the type of employment women enter and their potential earnings. Nevertheless, Psaki et al.'s analysis of Demographic and Health Survey data from 43 countries showed that parity in attainment does not automatically translate into parity in school quality and learning, with female disadvantages more common than male disadvantages.[59] Thus, while a case can certainly be made for using female educational attainment to gauge changes in gender (in)equality, it is not a fine measure of the ability of girls and women to live healthy, satisfied lives following a good education.

Studies published after the year 2000 employed indicator(s) (e.g. Gender Inequality Index, Gender Gap Index) systematically collected by international organizations (e.g. the United Nations); these indicators may be better able to capture multiple dimensions of gender equality (e.g. women's political representation, reproductive rights, gender-equal legislation) over and above labour force participation. Nevertheless, these systematically collected composite indices are unable to grasp implicit or explicit gender inequality deeply rooted in a culture, such as gendered family norms, patrilocality, sexual bullying (e.g. slut-shaming, revenge porn, sextortion), child marriage, internalization of the female thin ideal, and son preference. One recent study explored the impact of the Gender Inequality Index and male-to-female ratio at birth (a measure of son preference), and found that the cultural-based measure was a more potent determinant of suicide risk than the political- and economic-based gender (in) equality index.[36] Furthermore, issues disadvantaging more men than women 'are not heavily weighted (if at all) in widely used measures of gender inequality, such as the highly cited Global Gender Gap Index' (p. 1).[60] In fact, most of the current gender (in)equality indicators treat men as the gold standard and examine how women can be more like men, rather than the other way around. Only two studies used men's care work involvement as an indicator of gender equality.[35,38] The advantages for men to participate in what has long been perceived as 'women's work' (e.g. childcare) have been less well researched. Additionally, with a few exceptions like the Gender Equality Index, the indices largely treat women and men as homogenous groups, failing to capture the disparate social impacts of intersectional discrimination.

Relatedly, even though the studies reviewed use keywords pertaining to *gender* equality, they appear to focus on equality between *cisgender* men and women, and overlook the particular set of equality issues for transgender and gender-non-conforming persons. Individuals who identify as transgender or gender-non-conforming are at increased risk of suicide as a result of sociocultural prejudice, family rejection, internalized anti-trans attitudes, fear of anti-trans stigma, and a lack of gender-appropriate spaces.[61,62,63] However, because gender identity is not always recorded on death certificates, precise suicide rates are difficult to establish.[64] When interpreting the findings in Table 6.1, it is important to bear in mind the existence of gender diversity hidden by the binary categories of men and women, and to recognize that transgender and gender-non-conforming persons may face many more specific suicide risk factors,[62] which are not adequately addressed through traditional efforts to promote equality such as mobilizing women into the workplace and political arena.

Conclusion

This study conducted a systematic review of empirical research on gender (in) equality and suicide published in the last four decades (1981 to 2022), to establish a clearer understanding of the effects of egalitarian gender norms on suicide risk. The general trend across the 28 studies disproves Durkheim's theory that suicidal behaviour would rise as more women join the 'male' public sphere. The findings indicate that suicide rates in both men and women tend to decrease as gender barriers collapse or, in some cases, are not associated with these changes. Additionally, although a handful of studies published in the previous millennium suggested that women's engagement in the workforce is closely correlated with an increased suicide risk, this was no longer observed in later investigations, which implies that the relationship between suicidal behaviour and transformations in gendered systems of power is not static but evolves over time. Suicide rates in women and men are also influenced by other contextual factors such as the quality of their country's human capabilities. As the first study to undertake a systematic review of empirical research on gender equality and suicide, the present work provides a much-needed overview of how structural change can benefit men and women. Nevertheless, given that many economically developing countries do not have the resources to systematically collect suicide-related data, information in certain regions may be only informed by small-scale qualitative studies. Hence, reviews of pertinent qualitative literature would enrich our understanding of gender equality and suicidal behaviour.

References

1. **World Health Organization** (2019). Global Health Observatory (GHO) data: suicide mortality rates (per 100 000 population). Available from: https://www.who.int/gho/mental_health/suicide_rates_male_female/en/
2. **Durkheim E.** *The Division of Labor in Society*. New York, NY: Free Press; 1893/1933.
3. **Durkheim E.** *Suicide: A Study in Sociology*. New York, NY: Free Press; 1897/1951.
4. **Canetto SS.** Gender and suicide in the elderly. Suicide and Life-Threatening Behaviour. 1992;**22**(1):80–97.
5. **Lehmann JM.** *Durkheim and Women*. Lincoln, NE: University of Nebraska Press; 1994.
6. **Fernquist RM, Cutright P.** Societal integration and age-standardized suicide rates in 21 developed countries, 1955–1989. Social Science Research. 1998;**27**(2):109–27.
7. **Yip PSF, Liu KY.** The ecological fallacy and the gender ratio of suicide in China. British Journal of Psychiatry. 2006;**189**:465–6.
8. **Wu KCC, Chen YY, Yip PSF.** Suicide methods in Asia: implications in suicide prevention. International Journal of Environmental Research and Public Health. 2012;**9**(4):1135–58.
9. **Yip PSF, Chen YY, Yousuf S**, et al. Towards a reassessment of the role of divorce in suicide outcomes: evidence from five Pacific Rim populations. Social Science and Medicine. 2012;**75**(2):358–66.
10. **Chen YY, Wu KCC, Yousuf S, Yip PSF.** Suicide in Asia: opportunities and challenges. Epidemiologic Reviews. 2012;**34**(1):129–44.

11. **Davis RA.** Female labor force participation, status integration and suicide, 1950–1969. Suicide and Life-Threatening Behaviour. 1981;**11**(2):111–23.
12. **Lester D, Yang B.** The relationship between divorce, unemployment and female participation in the labour force and suicide rates in Australia and America. Australia and New Zealand Journal of Psychiatry. 1991;**25**(4):519–23.
13. **Austin RL, Bologna M, Dodge HH.** Sex-role change, anomie and female suicide: a test of alternative Durkheimian explanations. Suicide and Life-Threatening Behaviour. 1992;**22**(2):197–225.
14. **Lester D.** Gender equality, legitimization of violence, social disorganization and rates of personal violence (suicide and homicide) in America. Psychological Reports. 1992;**71**(2):626.
15. **Baron L, Straus MA.** Four theories of rape: a macrosociological analysis. Social Problems. 1987;**34**(5):467–89.
16. **Lester D, Motohashi Y, Yang B.** The impact of the economy on suicide and homicide rates in Japan and the United States. International Journal of Social Psychiatry. 1992;**38**(4):314–17.
17. **Yang B, Lester D, Yang CH.** Sociological and economic theories of suicide: a comparison of the U.S.A. and Taiwan. Social Science and Medicine. 1992;**34**(3):333–4.
18. **Lester D.** Gender equality and the sex differential in suicide rates. Psychological Reports. 1994;**75**(3 Pt 1):1162.
19. **Charles M.** Cross-national variation in occupational sex segregation. American Sociological Review. 1992;**57**(4):483–502.
20. **Chuang HL, Huang WC.** A reexamination of 'sociological and economic theories of suicide: a comparison of the U.S.A. and Taiwan'. Social Science and Medicine. 1996;**43**(3):421–3.
21. **Burr JA, McCall PL, Powell-Griner E.** Female labor force participation and suicide. Social Science and Medicine. 1997;**44**(12):1847–59.
22. **Mayer P.** Development, gender equality, and suicide rates. Psychological Reports. 2000;**87**(2):367–72.
23. **Lucey S, Corcoran P, Keeley HS, Brophy J, Arensman E, Perry IJ.** Socioeconomic change and suicide: a time-series study from the Republic of Ireland. Crisis. 2005;**26**(2):90–4.
24. **Zhang J, Jia S, Jiang C, Sun J.** Characteristics of Chinese suicide attempters: an emergency room study. Death Studies. 2006;**30**(3):259–68.
25. **Zhang J, Xu H.** The effects of religion, superstition, and perceived gender inequality on the degree of suicide intent: a study of serious attempters in China. Omega (Westport). 2007;**55**(3):185–97.
26. **Shah A.** Association of suicide rates for elderly age bands with gender equality. Psychological Reports. 2008;**102**(3):887–92.
27. **Aliverdinia A, Pridemore WA.** Women's fatalistic suicide in Iran: a partial test of Durkheim in an Islamic Republic. Violence Against Women. 2009;**15**(3):307–20.
28. **Ying YH, Chang K.** A study of suicide and socioeconomic factors. Suicide and Life-Threatening Behaviour. 2009;**39**(2):214–26.
29. **Barth A, Sogner L, Gnambs T, Kundi M, Reiner A, Winker R.** Socioeconomic factors and suicide: an analysis of 18 industrialized countries for the years 1983 through 2007. Journal of Occupational and Environmental Medicine. 2011;**53**(3):313–17.

30. **Phillips JA, Nugent CN.** Suicide and the Great Recession of 2007–2009: the role of economic factors in the 50 U.S. states. Social Science and Medicine. 2014;**116**:22–31.
31. **Nowotny KM, Peterson RL, Boardman JD.** Gendered contexts: variation in suicidal ideation by female and male youth across U.S. states. Journal of Health and Social Behavior. 2015;**56**(1):114–30.
32. **Reeves A, Stuckler D.** Suicidality, economic shocks, and egalitarian gender norms. European Sociological Review. 2016;**32**(1):39–53.
33. **Chen YY, Chen M, Lui CSM, Yip PSF.** Female labour force participation and suicide rates in the world. Social Science and Medicine. 2017;**195**:61–7.
34. **Assarsson R, Petersen S, Hogberg B, Strandh M, Johansson K.** Gender inequality and adolescent suicide ideation across Africa, Asia, the South Pacific and Latin America: a cross-sectional study based on the Global School Health Survey (GSHS). Global Health Action. 2018;**11**(sup3):1663619.
35. **Lee SA, Park EC, Ju YJ, Han KT, Yoon HJ, Kim TH.** The association between satisfaction with husband's participation in housework and suicidal ideation among married working women in Korea. Psychiatry Research. 2018;**261**:541–6.
36. **Chang Q, Yip PSF, Chen YY.** Gender inequality and suicide gender ratios in the world. Journal of Affective Disorders. 2019;**243**:297–304.
37. **Milner A, Scovelle AJ, Hewitt B, Maheen H, Ruppanner L, King TL.** Shifts in gender equality and suicide: a panel study of changes over time in 87 countries. Journal of Affective Disorders. 2020;**276**:495–500.
38. **Chen YY, Cai Z, Chang Q, Canetto SS, Yip PSF.** Caregiving as suicide-prevention: an ecological 20-country study of the association between men's family carework, unemployment, and suicide. Social Psychiatry and Psychiatric Epidemiology. 2021;56(12):2185–98. doi:10.1007/s00127-021-02095-9
39. **Cai Z, Canetto SS, Chang Q, Yip PSF.** Women's suicide in low-, middle-, and high-income countries: do laws discriminating against women matter? Social Science and Medicine. 2021;**282**:114035.
40. **Navarro-Mantas L, de Lemus S, Megías JL.** Mental health consequences of intimate partner violence against women in El Salvador. Violence Against Women. 2021;**27**(15–16):2927–44.
41. **United Nations Development Programme** (2017). Gender Inequality Index (GII). Available from: http://hdr.undp.org/en/content/gender-inequality-index-gii
42. **Canetto SS.** Women and suicidal behavior: a cultural analysis. American Journal of Orthopsychiatry. 2008;**78**(2):259–66.
43. **Kushner HI.** Women and suicide behavior: epidemiology, gender and lethality in historical perspective. In: **Canetto SS, Lester D**, editors. Women and Suicide Behavior. New York, NY: Springer; 1995. Pp. 11–34.
44. **Canetto SS, Lester D.** Gender, culture, and suicidal behavior. Transcultural Psychiatry. 1998;**35**(2):163–90.
45. **Stack S.** The effect of female participation in the labor force on suicide: a time series analysis, 1948–1980. Sociological Forum. 1987;**2**(2):257–77.
46. **Pampel FC.** National context, social change, and sex differences in suicide rates. American Sociological Review. 1998;**63**(5):744–58.
47. **Verick S.** Female labor force participation in developing countries. IZA World of Labor. 2014;**2014**(87):1–10.

48. **Kabir H, Maple M, Usher K, Islam MS.** Health vulnerabilities of readymade garment (RMG) workers: a systematic review. BMC Public Health. 2019;**19**(1):70.
49. **Akhter S, Rutherford S, Akhter Kumkum F**, et al. Work, gender roles, and health: neglected mental health issues among female workers in the ready-made garment industry in Bangladesh. International Journal of Women's Health. 2017;**9**:571–9.
50. **Fitch TJ, Moran J, Villanueva G, Sagiraju HKR, Quadir MM, Alamgir H.** Prevalence and risk factors of depression among garment workers in Bangladesh. International Journal of Social Psychiatry. 2017;**63**(3):244–54.
51. **Bluedorn J, Caselli F, Hansen N, Shibata I, Tavares MM** (2021). Gender and employment in the COVID-19 recession: evidence on 'she-cessions'. Available from: https://www.imf.org/en/Publications/WP/Issues/2021/03/31/Gender-and-Employment-in-the-COVID-19-Recession-Evidence-on-She-cessions-50316
52. **Gunnell D, Chang SS.** Economic recession, unemployment, and suicide. In: **Connor RCO, Pirkis J**, editors. *The International Handbook of Suicide Prevention*. Chicester: Wiley-Blackwell; 2016. pp. 284–300.
53. **McKinsey Global Institute** (2020). COVID-19 and gender equality: countering the regressive effects. Available from: https://www.mckinsey.com/featured-insights/future-of-work/covid-19-and-gender-equality-countering-the-regressive-effects
54. **Seck PA, Encarnacion JO, Tinonin C, Duerto-Valero S.** Gendered impacts of COVID-19 in Asia and the Pacific: early evidence on deepening socioeconomic inequalities in paid and unpaid work. Feminist Economics. 2021;**27**(1–2):117–32.
55. **Sakamoto H, Ishikane M, Ghaznavi C, Ueda P.** Assessment of suicide in Japan during the COVID-19 pandemic vs previous years. JAMA Network Open. 2021;**4**(2):e2037378.
56. **Tanaka T, Okamoto S.** Increase in suicide following an initial decline during the COVID-19 pandemic in Japan. Nature Human Behaviour. 2021;**5**(2):229–38.
57. **Kim AM.** The short-term impact of the COVID-19 outbreak on suicides in Korea. Psychiatry Research. 2021;**295**:113632.
58. **Moussié R, Staab S; UN Women** (2020). Three ways to contain COVID-19's impact on informal women workers. Available from: https://data.unwomen.org/features/three-ways-contain-covid-19s-impact-informal-women-workers
59. **Psaki SR, McCarthy KJ, Mensch BS.** Measuring gender equality in education: lessons from trends in 43 countries. Population and Development Review. 2018;**44**(1):117–42.
60. **Stoet G, Geary DC.** A simplified approach to measuring national gender inequality. PLoS One. 2019;**14**(1):e0205349.
61. **Narang P, Sarai SK, Aldrin S, Lippman S.** Suicide among transgender and gender-nonconforming people. Primary Care Companion for CNS Disorders. 2018;**20**(3):18nr02273.
62. **Wolford-Clevenger C, Cannon CJ, Flores LY, Smith PN, Stuart GL.** Suicide risk among transgender people: a prevalent problem in critical need of empirical and theoretical research. Violence and Gender. 2017;**4**(3):69–72.
63. **Tebbe EA, Moradi B.** Suicide risk in trans populations: an application of minority stress theory. Journal of Counseling Psychology. 2016;**63**(5):520–33.
64. **Centre for Suicide Prevention** (2019). Transgender people and suicide. Available from: https://www.suicideinfo.ca/resource/transgender-people-suicide/

Chapter 7

Suicide and religion: A comparative analysis of a complex relationship to inform practice

Robin Edward Gearing, Dana Alonza, Shahnaz Savani, Sean Burr, Anil Arora, and Sangina Khudododova

Introduction

Research examining the relationship between religion and mental health dates back well over 100 years. Emile Durkheim,[1] as early as 1897, proposed that spiritual commitment and religious connections contribute to emotional well-being, as they provide a source of meaning and order in the world. Yet, this relationship is complex, and efforts to identify how much religiosity and through which denomination the greatest effects are derived have failed to provide a consistent answer. This may be, in part, due to the fact that in the literature, the terms religiosity/religion are used inconsistently and, at times, interchangeably with the terms spiritual/spirituality. For the purposes of our discussion, we use spirituality to refer to personal views or beliefs of the presence or existence of something greater than the self, and religion to refer to a specific religious denomination.

Understanding the influence of religion is even more complex when applied to an equally complex concept such as suicide. Religious beliefs and expectations play a key role in how individuals experience and manage suicidal thoughts and feelings. Research consistently indicates that the rate of suicide varies across religions. Most religions hold specific conceptualizations about death and dying in general, and about suicide in particular. The degree of one's religious affiliation and commitment, as well as the specific doctrine of a given religion as it relates to concepts of life and death, exerts influence on the factors that will serve to increase the risk of suicide and protect against suicide, and on the expectations individuals may have regarding suicidal behaviour. Although it is now generally accepted that religion largely serves as a protective factor against suicide across religious denominations, there are aspects of religiosity that are also recognized as contributing to an increased suicide risk for some adherents that require understanding and consideration.

Given the association between religion and suicidal thoughts and behaviours, an understanding of the role of religion in one's life is essential to determining an accurate estimation of suicide risk. Further, an effective assessment of a client's religiosity can serve to identify potential areas that treatment could target and to enhance life-affirming beliefs and expectations.

This chapter provides an analysis of the current state of knowledge regarding the relationship between religion and suicide across the five dominant world religions of Buddhism, Christianity, Hinduism, Islam, and atheism/agnosticism, with the recognition that these religions are not homogenous groups but comprise a multitude of sects and subgroups, each with some shared central tenets, but also with distinct interpretations and unique and differing religious customs.

Six dimensions are presented for each religion, including doctrine, affiliation, participation, ideation and behaviour (planning, attempt, completion), risk factors, and protective factors.

Method

A search for peer-reviewed published articles on religion and suicide was conducted by using PsycINFO, MEDLINE, and PubMed databases. The search was limited to English language journals, and there were no restrictions to the search period. The Boolean search strategy and keywords included the religious terms: Christianity; Christian; Protestant; Catholic; Judaism; Jewish; Buddhism; Buddhist; Buddhists; Hinduism; Hindu; Islam; Muslim; Islamic; atheism; agnosticism; and, the suicide terms: suicide; suicide attempt; or suicidal. Searches of the three databases yielded 1673 articles. A total of 613 duplicate articles were removed, which resulted in 1060 remaining articles. An additional 53 articles were added to the review after also reviewing the reference sections of these articles for other relevant articles, to a total of 1113 articles. Three authors reviewed the abstracts and content of the remaining articles and excluded 904 articles, including letters to the editor, editorials, book reviews, and articles that were not a research study or not focused on one of the identified aspects of the relationship between suicide and religion (e.g. not focused on risk factors, affiliation, etc., and on the identified religions). A final total of 209 articles were included in this review on the relationship between suicide and the religions of Buddhism, Christianity, Hinduism, Islam, Judaism, and non-religious affiliations, specifically atheism and agnosticism (see Figure 7.1).

The articles included in this review were assessed and coded by the research team, including three PhD-level professors and three doctoral students. Each

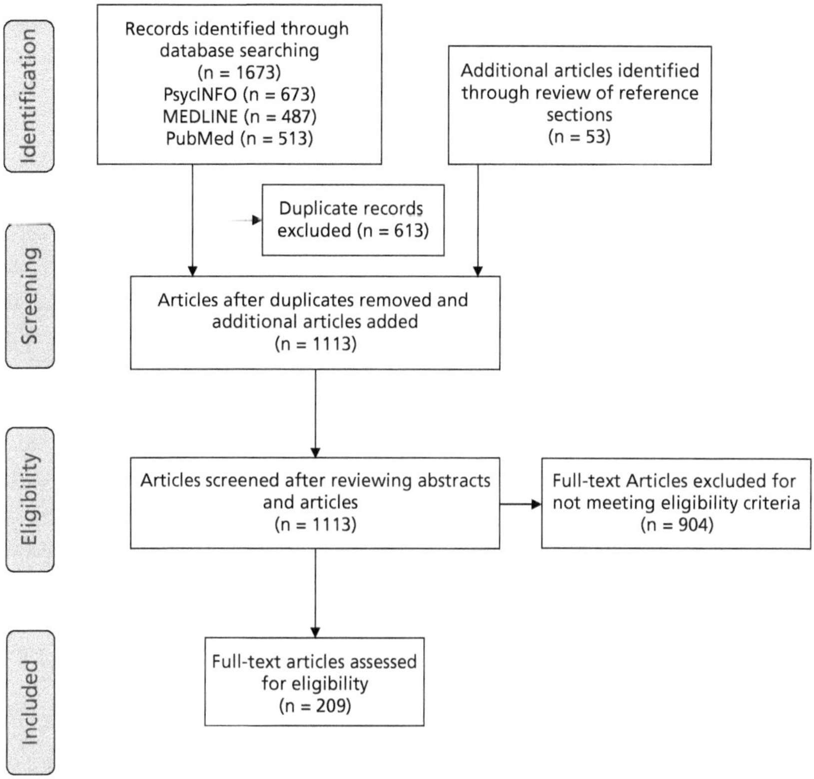

Figure 7.1 Flow diagram.

eligible article was coded by two members of the research team by using a data abstraction form developed to synthesize findings from all eligible peer-reviewed published studies. Each study was coded for religious doctrine, affiliation, participation, suicidal ideation, suicide planning, suicide attempts, and completed suicide. Research studies and review articles focused on the relationship between suicide and religion in terms of doctrine, affiliation, participation, suicidality (suicidal ideation, planning, suicide attempts, and completed suicide), and risk and protective factors were included in this review.

Buddhism

Systematic search

Of the 22 articles identified specifically focusing on Buddhism, seven articles referenced Buddhist doctrines regarding suicide, whereas 13 articles investigated affiliation with Buddhism. Only six articles discussed suicidal ideation among those identifying as Buddhist, and 13 articles explored the actual risk and protective factors for suicide among Buddhists. None of the identified articles differentiated between suicidal ideation, suicide attempt, and suicide completion.

Doctrine

According to the World Religion Database, there are approximately 500 million individuals who adhere to Buddhism worldwide, making it the fourth largest religion in the world.[2] Buddhism comprises three major schools: Theravada, Mahayana, and Vajrayana. These three branches span from India, Sri Lanka, Thailand, Cambodia, Myanmar, Laos, China, Japan, Taiwan, Tibet, Nepal, Mongolia, Korea, and Vietnam.[3] Data collection on the incidence and prevalence of suicide among those who identify as Buddhists are limited.[3] Buddhist doctrine can be interpreted in many ways, leading to a range of perspectives on suicide.[4]

To understand Buddhism's stance on suicide, it is necessary to explore the religion's views on life and death in general. Buddhism's teachings emphasize cultivating respect for life and avoiding all actions that result in suffering to oneself or others.[4,5] This is reflected in *Ahimsa*, the Buddhist principle that focuses on not harming or killing any living beings.[4,6,7]

The Four Noble Truths serve as the foundation of Buddhist philosophy. They are considered to reflect the realization that led the Buddha to enlightenment and teach that all stages of life are full of suffering and dissatisfaction. At all developmental stages, individuals are consumed by want and desire, manifested in *unskilful* mental states, which serve as the foundation for this suffering and dissatisfaction.[4,8,9] Suicide is considered just one of many forms of suffering. In some Buddhist texts, suicide is characterized as the result of *moha*, or delusion, as it reflects failure by the individual to realize that death is the ultimate suffering.[10,11]

Buddhists do not see death as the end of life, but rather as a transition to another life.[12] Suicide is not considered an escape from that cycle.[12] Rather, Buddhist teachings explain that suicidal behaviour competes with the cycles of reincarnation leading to further suffering in one's next life and causing suffering, or *dukkha*, to others.[4,9,13,14] As such, suicide may actually serve to perpetuate one's suffering, as those who attempt to take their own lives through suicide are motivated by anger or aggression and are bound to reincarnation in hell (*Niraya*).[8]

How then can one stop this cycle of suffering? According to Buddhist doctrine, the cycle of life and death is continuous and cannot be stopped by any means other than by reaching nirvana, a state characterized by no longer experiencing desire and suffering, while achieving bliss and peace.[3,8] It is a teaching across all traditions of Buddhism that enlightenment can only be obtained while in the state of a human body; hence, one's physical form must be treated with great respect. Buddhist teachings generally view suicide as disrespect against the human body.[10]

In order to reach nirvana, the Noble Eightfold Path must be followed. It serves as the path to liberation from suffering through *skilful* actions and mind states grounded in contentment. The Noble Eightfold Path comprises three overarching domains, including moral/ethical conduct (*sila*), mental discipline (*samadhi*), and wisdom (*panna*), to be practised simultaneously, rather than hierarchically. They specifically include: (1) Right Understanding (*Samma ditthi*); (2) Right Thought (*Samma sankappa*); (3) Right Speech (*Samma vaca*); (4) Right Action (*Samma kammanta*); (5) Right Livelihood (*Samma ajiva*); (6) Right Effort (*Samma vayama*); (7) Right Mindfulness (*Samma sati*); and (8) Right Concentration (*Samma samadhi*).

Within the doctrine of the Noble Eightfold Path, the Buddha promotes *Right Livelihood*, through which he teaches that there are five kinds of trade that are unacceptable (weapons, meat, human beings, liquor, and poison).[8] These teachings also include abstaining from bringing harm to other beings. This can be connected to prevention of suicide, as trade of weapons, poison, or substances that could be used to engage in suicidal behaviour is prohibited.[8]

Religious monks are duty-bound to instil a respect for life and the virtues of the Noble Eightfold Path, and to provide guidance not only through Buddhist doctrine, but also from their own experiences with suffering and to support those who experience mental health challenges.[8] Monks strive to protect Dharma (universal Buddhist teachings) and encourage individuals to care for their own body, as it is essential for spreading the Buddhist doctrine.[4,12] Some literature explicitly states that the Buddha warned monks that assisting in suicide would lead to them being banished from the spiritual community (Sangha).[5,11]

In accordance with the Noble Eightfold Path, adherents to the religion follow five precepts of conduct, including: (1) to abstain from taking life; (2) to abstain from taking what is not given; (3) to abstain from sensuous misconduct; (4) to abstain from false speech; and (5) to abstain from intoxicants as they tend to cloud the mind. The first of these precepts can be seen as prohibiting suicide, as it promotes abstinence from killing all living beings, including intentionally taking one's own life by one's own hand.[9,11,15]

Yet Buddhist teachings emphasize the importance of examining and understanding intention, often more so than the action itself. The precepts of Buddhism are not considered absolutes or global rules, but rather are intended to be applied on a situational basis.[10] For example, certain Buddhist texts present suicide as an admirable sacrifice motivated by compassion as opposed to by despair.[4] A Bodhisattva (a person who is on the right path) may be able to sacrifice their life to end suffering for others and to bring happiness and peace to themselves.[4,12] Other instances where the motivation of suicide can be seen as altruistic is when a Bodhisattva is seen as repaying kindness to their parents.[12] Further, research has found that Buddhist priests teach that what matters when determining the acceptability of suicide is the individual's attitude at the moment of death.[16,17,18,19] For example, a suicide resulting from a mind still attached to worldly desires or consumed by hatred or anger would suffer the consequence of the negative karmic chain and negative rebirths.[17]

To this extent, Buddhist doctrine relating to suicide makes a distinction regarding whether it is acceptable or will lead to reincarnation in hell, based on the motivation for the behaviour. When driven by self-sacrifice, it is seen as acceptable and merits compassion; when motivated by a desire to escape suffering, it is seen as fruitless, counterproductive, and unacceptable.[20,21]

Affiliation

Buddhism, like other religions, offers perspectives on suicide through doctrine. Affiliation to the religion must also be assessed to understand the influence of religion on suicide risk. Affiliation may provide some degree of protection through connection to the community. However, affiliation to a minority religious group may also cause feelings of isolation.[22] Research has found that in East Asia, suicide rates range from 18 to 27 per 100,000 individuals, which is higher than the global average.[6,23] Research has also found that the rates of suicide are higher among women in Buddhist countries.[6,24] In the same study, findings indicated that countries with large populations of Buddhist-identifying individuals have relatively high suicide rates.[6,25] By contrast, others have found that in Thailand, where over 90% of the population identify as Buddhist, the suicide rate is 8 per 100,000.[6,8]

In another study, university students in 12 countries who self-reported as Buddhist were the least accepting of suicide.[26] The same study found that affiliation with Buddhism was associated with a lower risk of attempting suicide.[26] Conversely, in another study in China examining methadone maintenance therapy, results indicated that suicide risk was significantly higher among those who were affiliated with the Buddhist religion in comparison to non-religious believers.[9]

Overall, research examining the degree of religious affiliation with Buddhist doctrine and suicide risk is quite sparse and inconsistent. Further research is needed to better understand this relationship and provide a more accurate picture that can inform assessment and intervention.

Participation

The rates of suicide in East Asian countries are the highest in the world, but individuals' level of religious participation remains low in these countries.[6] A recent study in East Asia found that a 1% percent increase in religious participation was associated with a 1% increase in suicide rates.[6,27] Conversely, another study found participating in organized religious activities had a moderating effect on depression and suicidal ideation among those who identify as Buddhist.[28,29] Research on participation and suicide is limited and even contradictory, and further research is recommended to better understand the relationship between religious participation and suicide.

Suicide dimensions: ideation, planning, rehearsals, attempts, and suicide

Overall, only a few studies have examined the relationship between Buddhism and the various dimensions of suicidal behaviour. One qualitative study found that Buddhism lowered the risk of suicidal ideation among individuals due to the religious views influencing individuals to not attempt suicide.[30] Consistent with these findings, another study in Vietnam found that Buddhist beliefs were associated with a lower risk of suicidal ideation.[26,31] This study further identified that Buddhist beliefs were associated with a lower risk of suicide attempts among university students.

Fang et al.[32] examined the relationship between suicidal ideation and suicide attempts among participants belonging to Buddhist, Catholic, Taoist, and Christian groups in Taiwan. This study had a total of 4000 participants, with 1000 participants from the four target religious groups. In the sample of individuals identifying as Buddhist, the average age was 41 years and 62% were female. Results indicated that there was an association between those who identified with religious faith and experiences and previous suicide attempts or suicidal ideation. The study also revealed that religious leaders could support suicide prevention through educating members, as well as offering empathy and care for new members. Through these interactions, it is possible to decrease suicidal ideation and suicide attempts.

Saiz and colleagues[33] conducted a study with 82,898 participants from 60 countries and examined their attitudes towards suicide while considering subjective religiosity and religious practices. Results demonstrated that the attitude towards suicide among those who identified as Buddhist did not depend on whether the person was perceived as religious, non-religious, or atheistic. For

Buddhists in this sample, their attitude towards suicide was equal or greater, the more the person values God or gods. Overall, Buddhists who prayed several times a day also had a favourable attitude towards suicide in comparison to those who prayed once a year or less. Similarly, Huang et al.[9] found a positive association between Buddhist belief and increased suicide risk.

Risk factors

Lew et al.[34] collected data from undergraduate students from six different provinces in China from 2017 to 2018, and found that religious denomination could be both a risk factor for, and a protective factor against, suicidality. Findings from the study revealed that risk factors for suicide, such as hopelessness, were significantly higher across all religions (including Buddhism), in comparison to no religion.[34] Other risk factors that were significant among those who identified as Buddhist were depression and distress. Zhang et al.[35] explained that in China, those who grapple between Western and Chinese religious practices may perceive that Buddhist incarnation encourages suicide as it glorifies the ending of one's life.

Disayavanish et al.[8] described that in Thailand, mental health organizations have developed Buddhist suicide prevention measures to empower and encourage groups and individuals to work together. The authors listed nine ways in which Buddhists should approach suicide prevention: (1) Buddhist attitude towards suicide; (2) faith and confidence in life after death; (3) providing monks with general knowledge and understanding about suicide and life after death; (4) early identification of mental disorders and persons at risk of suicide, and prompt referral to appropriate mental health professionals; (5) control of access to instruments of suicide; (6) control of alcohol and drug abuse; (7) prevention of HIV infection; (8) responsible media reporting; and (9) practice of meditation.

Protective factors

Lew and colleagues[34] investigated both risk and protective factors for suicide among undergraduate students, comparing Buddhists to all other religious groups. They found fewer protective factors against suicidal thoughts and behaviours, specifically in terms of self-esteem, social support, and purpose in life.[34] Other studies examined the moderating effect of religion on the relationship between depression and suicidal ideation among older adults. Findings indicated that having limited organized religious activity for those who identify as Buddhist could explain the small number of protective factors against suicide among adherents to this religion.[29] Lawrence et al.[22] conducted a systematic review exploring religion as a protective factor against suicide, which showed inconsistencies, and this area needs to be further investigated. This assertion appears particularly relevant for Buddhism, given the very sparse research specifically examining suicide risk among its adherents.

Buddhism and suicide: implications

A central tenet within Buddhism is respect for life and limiting harm to other living beings.[4,5,6] On the surface, suicide is in contradiction with these, as well as with other key teachings within Buddhism (e.g. non-violence, reincarnation, Right Livelihood).[4,6,7,8,13] However, when explored more deeply, it becomes clear that there are exceptions to this position such as when suicide is motivated by compassion or altruistic purposes. Such instances of suicide appear to be permissible and reframed as self-sacrifice.[4,12,20] Across the different dimensions of suicide, a belief in Buddhism has been shown to reduce the risk of suicidal ideation and suicide risk in some studies, whereas other research has shown an increased risk.[9,26,30,31] In terms of broader affiliation, countries in East Asia that have higher proportions of individuals who are Buddhist demonstrate higher rates of suicide compared to other major religions.[6,25] Nevertheless, a low level of religious participation is seen in these countries, which may provide some explanation for these higher rates. Some research demonstrates the protective role of increased religious participation in any religion against suicide.[6,28,29] This finding is complicated by other research that shows that an increase in religious involvement may be associated with increased suicide rates among Buddhists and research demonstrating that affiliation with Buddhism has limited associations with attitudes towards suicide.[6,27,33]

These mixed and contradictory findings relating to affiliation and participation indicate the need for further research to determine how participation may contribute to the high suicide rates seen in countries that have high numbers of Buddhists. Given the generally prohibitive stance of Buddhist doctrine towards suicide, it remains unclear as to why the relative rates in these countries are elevated. Further, the relatively high rates of suicide among women in these countries also indicate that the intersection of gender, Buddhism, social factors, and suicide risk must also be further investigated.[6,24]

The extant literature on risk and protective factors indicates that Buddhists possess fewer protective factors against suicidality, whereas psychiatric disorders relating to alcohol and drug abuse appear to increase the risk of suicide among adherents.[8,34] Positive outcomes have also been demonstrated in training religious leaders to provide mental health, addiction, and suicide prevention education and activities.[32,34] Although preliminary, given the high rates of suicide in East Asian countries, any interventions that decrease suicidality for this population should be further developed and tested.

Christianity

In comparison to all other religions, there is more research available on Christianity and suicide. Extensive research has been conducted on risk and protective factors and suicide, and the extent to which individuals participate in, and affiliate with, Christianity. A systematic search for the literature on Christianity and suicide produced 44 relevant articles. Of the 44 articles identified, only five articles commented on Christian doctrines regarding suicide, whereas 27 articles investigated affiliation with Christianity. Nine of the articles investigating religious affiliation also examined religious participation and its relationship to suicide. Sixteen articles examined suicidal ideation among individuals identifying as Christian. Fourteen articles discussed protective factors against suicide, and 18 articles discussed risk factors for suicide among Christians.

Doctrine

In Christianity, as in other monotheistic religions, attempting suicide is condemned.[29,36] Christianity's perspective towards suicide has remained firm since the fifth century,[37] when St Augustine proposed that suicide is a violation of the sixth commandment (Thou shall not kill).[37,38,39,40] St Thomas Aquinas expanded on this conceptualization and described suicide as a sin against self, neighbour, and God.[37,38,41] Within Christianity, suicide is equated with other sins resulting in the taking of life such as murder and abortion.[39,42,43] Further, according to Christian doctrine, when an individual dies, s/he faces judgement by God and only God can decide if the individual will enter heaven or go to hell or purgatory. It is argued that the act of suicide because of everyday challenges and turmoil would be considered a *breach of trust*, the trust that God has bestowed upon human beings by granting the gift of life.[44] Moreover, it is believed that God would never abandon his believers at any given time; thus, suicide is not an option for avoiding life challenges.[45] Hence, it is believed that harming yourself is considered an offence to God, as the Holy Bible states that, 'I have authority to lay it down and authority to take in up again. This command I received from my Father' (p. 840).[46] Therefore, suicide is generally viewed as an interference in God's will.[44,46] Although several suicides are reported in the Old Testament, the characters are not exemplary.[44]

It has also been argued that belief in the existence of life after death could lead believers to not be afraid of death.[46] Such an understanding could make suicide more likely for believers. However, there remains a caveat. According to the Catechism of the Catholic Church,[47] individuals have to be mentally competent in order for the act in which they partake to be considered a sin. Therefore, if suicide is interpreted as an act demonstrative of mental illness, it may serve to mitigate the equation of the act with sin.[41] One study illustrates this concept by describing that across various Christian denominations, clergy who attributed suicide to mental illness endorsed a compassionate, rather than a punitive, response.[48] Along these lines, in 1983, the Roman Catholic Church removed suicide from the list of mortal sins, proposing the belief that suicide is often the result of untreated depression, pain, or other mental suffering.

Affiliation

Among the dominant Christian denominations (Catholics, Baptists, and Protestants), the highest suicide rates are found among Protestants, and the lowest rates of suicide among Catholics and evangelical Baptists.[49,50] On a national level, Catholic countries report an overall lower rate of suicide than Protestant countries. Further, in Protestant countries, within areas where there is a higher population of Catholics, suicide rates are lower.[41,51] Moreover, within Christianity, orthodox and more radical denominations most strongly condemn suicide.[29,52] Lastly, research indicates that there are significantly higher suicide rates among men and the elderly in Catholic and Christian orthodox countries, as compared to rates among those groups in non-Catholic and orthodox countries.[53,54]

Within Christianity, Catholics are stricter in their condemnation of suicide, as compared to Protestants.[36,55,56] Catholics believe that *life is a gift from God* and only God can decide when life should start or end; therefore, suicide would be going against the wish of the Lord (p. 338).[57] However, the research is rather inconsistent. In comparison to Protestants, some research has found that suicide is more prevalent among Catholics,[36] whereas other studies have found that Catholics have a lower rate of suicide than Protestants.[49,55] Thus, affiliation with any Christian religious denomination does not always denote suicide risk.[36,55,56] However, studies in this area are general and vague, and thus present different views and findings. For example, Eskin et al.[26] stated that religious affiliation in general is associated with low suicidal ideation, and yet the same article posited that religious affiliation might be too general a concept to determine its effect on suicidal ideation. Further, in comparison to all religions, Christianity (Catholics) was found to be associated with less suicidal ideation and attempts than other faith groups.[59] Research by Eskin et al.[26] showed that being affiliated with Christianity, specifically with Catholicism, is usually associated with better mental health, which clearly indicates that there is definitively a low risk of suicidal ideation with being affiliated with Christianity and with religion in general.[36] Considering all this, a study by Panczak et al.[49] suggested that it is important for public health practitioners to come up with strong interventions for those who do not affiliate with any religion, as they have a higher risk of suicide attempts and suicidal ideation.

Participation

Research indicates that not merely religious affiliation, but also actual participation in religion and religious ceremonies associated with Christianity affect attitudes towards suicide.[55] For example, studies demonstrated an increased frequency of prayer, church attendance, and religious ceremonies was associated with lower suicidal ideation and psychiatric hospitalizations.[33,55,59]

Research has demonstrated that Catholics and Baptists have higher levels of religious participation and are more likely to be actively involved in church activities.[50] As a result, they may benefit more from the expanded social support networks offered by being an active member of the church community.[50] Others have found lower rates of suicide among Catholics, as compared to Protestants, even after controlling for quantity and quality of social and religious networks.[55] Still others have proposed that the lower rates of suicide found among conservative Catholics may be due to their lower rates of alcohol consumption and engagement in other risk behaviours rather than due to higher level of participation in religious-related activities.[60]

The rate of suicide among Protestants seems to be higher than among Catholics. Some researchers have suggested that Catholics promote higher involvement in religious activities and church attendance, compared to Protestants, and that this higher degree of participation may account for the lower rates of suicide.[55] Also, community support mechanisms in religious communities can be very strong, leading to higher social and emotional support, and consequently to lower suicide risk.[55,62] Research involving more than 20,000 participants found that those attending church 24 times or more in a year had lower suicidal ideation compared to those who never attended church.[52] Overall, participation in Christianity is positively associated with a lower level of suicidal ideation and behaviour.

In a prospective study examining suicide risk by Christian religious affiliation, approximately 1,106,104 individuals aged 16–74 years in the United Kingdom were followed for nine years, and their level of religious activity and degree of commitment tracked. It was hypothesized that if church attendance was the most important determinant of suicide risk, the risk would be lowest among Roman Catholics, and highest among those with no religion. Conversely, if religiosity was the most important determinant, then *conservative* Christians would present as being at lowest risk. Results indicated that Roman Catholics, Protestants, and those professing to having no religion recorded similar risks. However, the risk associated with conservative Christians was lower than that with Catholics.[60]

Interestingly, research has found that suicide rates decrease in December when Christmas is approaching, only to return to normal levels again at the start of the New Year.[61] This may speak to the importance of religious participation rather than the degree of adherence to religious doctrine, as Christmas is a widely practised holiday across different levels of religiously committed individuals.

Suicide dimensions: ideation, planning, rehearsals, attempts, and suicide

Historically, the rate of suicide before the Renaissance was much lower than during the Renaissance.[36,49] Researchers suggested that this difference in the rate of suicide was because before the Renaissance, religion was more powerful and the secular philosophy of the Renaissance made religion weaker by challenging the ideology of Christianity.[36] As a result, suicidal ideation, the number of suicide attempts, and deaths by suicide increased.[36,49]

Research on suicide (the participants of which were both Christians and Muslims) indicated that ongoing stressful events in life, exposure to challenges, and the absence of support led to suicidal ideation among individuals.[46] Jung et al.[29] suggested that religious variables could reduce the impact of life challenges on suicidal ideation. However, Eskin et al.[26] found that religious affiliation worked as a protective factor against suicide and suicide attempts, but less against suicidal ideation, which was equally relevant to various communities.

Current research shows that within Christianity, suicidal ideation and suicide planning and attempts are mostly observed among people who identify themselves as belonging to a sexual and gender minority.[62] Reconciling sexual orientation with religious and spiritual beliefs can be challenging for individuals who identify as Christian, as many Christian churches continue to teach that non-heterosexual behaviour is a sin. The effects of this conflict have been found to include alienation, depression, guilt, anxiety, and suicidal ideation.[63]

While many studies have found that Catholics have a lower rate of suicidal ideation than other denominations, not all studies revealed the same findings. For example, Kelleher et al.[36] found that comparing between Catholics and Protestants, Catholics have higher reports of suicidal behaviour and ideation. Some research suggested that among Christians, the type of God representation held by the individual predicts the severity of suicidal ideation. A positive–supportive God representation is negatively correlated with suicidal ideation, whereas a passive–distressing God representation has a positive correlation with suicidal ideation.[52]

Protective factors

Much research indicates that religion usually acts as a support system for individuals and is considered as a source of hope and empowerment, making it a protective factor for suicide.[29,36,52,55,59,64,65] Christian religiosity motivates church attendance, and church attendance is considered as one of the ways in which people usually meet and form cycles of support and community.[29,46,52] Together, the teachings of Christianity that promote supporting one another, enhanced community belongingness, and the improved networking created from church attendance make Christianity a protective factor against suicide and suicidal ideation.[26,29,46,52,62] Research further suggests the belief that prayer can protect against the experience of adversity also reduces suicide risk.[55] Furthermore, Christians believe that God always watches over them and provides protection and care, instilling hope and reducing suicide risk.[55] Suicide prevention is also encouraged in religious teachings and the religion's condemnation of suicide.[46,55]

Risk factors

While a majority of the studies indicate that Christianity serves as a protective factor against suicide and suicidal ideation, there are several studies that have found Christianity to be a risk factor for suicide.[29,59] This research has found that for sexual and gender minority (SGM) young populations, religion can serve as a risk factor for suicide.[62,65,66] Except for cisgender and heterosexual individuals, SGM children's identity is usually not accepted by parents and people who are religious.[62] Additionally, most religious ideologies do not acknowledge the identity of the minority genders and sexual groups. Anderson et al.[62] found that due to such unacceptability and negative attitudes and relationships of religious family members with Christian SGM children, suicidal ideation, suicide attempts, and suicides are high among these youth.

Research by Waitz-Kudla and colleagues[59] indicated that people who often attend church and religious ceremonies usually prefer to reach out to clergy for emotional support while facing mental health issues. However, seeking help from mental health professionals and going through treatment and rehabilitation contribute towards the reduction of suicide and suicidal ideation.[29] The preference for reaching out to clergy for help not only limits receiving care from professional mental health practitioners who are actually trained in this field, but also generally reduces the help-seeking ability among Christians.[59] One of the reasons why individuals struggling with suicidal thoughts and behaviours prefer to seek help from clergy is that reaching out to the Church involves less stigma than going to mental health practitioners.[59,67]

Christianity and suicide: implications

Christian doctrine strongly prohibits suicide.[29,36,45] A central belief is that life is a gift from God and suicide is a transgression of God's will.[44,46] In terms of religious affiliation and suicide, although several articles were identified, the results are contradictory or limited. Nevertheless, the literature does provide sufficient information to determine that Christian affiliation is associated with less suicidality when compared to other faith groups.[68] Interdenominational investigations have compared Catholic and Protestant affiliations, and although Protestants typically demonstrated higher rates of suicide, the results were mixed.[36,55,56] Further research into suicidality and these two denominations is recommended. Further research into non-denominational Christians is very limited and is needed to fully understand this group's relationship to suicide.

Research into religious participation indicates that greater participation in Christian religious activities appears to reduce suicidality. The literature identifies higher incidences of prayer, church attendance, and involvement in religious ceremonies as associated with lowered suicidality.[33,55,59] Evidence for church attendance is particularly strong, as increased attendance is associated with lower levels of suicidal ideation.[52] The benefit of increased participation is not well differentiated across different demographic groups, and further research is needed across diverse samples such as SGM youth.

Another important implication relates to help-seeking and mental health. Research indicates that Christians with regular church involvement often prefer to connect with faith leaders or clergy for mental health support.[59] Although potentially motivated by a desire to avoid the stigma associated with accessing formal mental health care, this preference can increase the risk of suicide as appropriate mental health interventions are not accessed.[59,67] Practice implications include development and implementation of programmes that train faith leaders and clergy in mental health assessment and referral, as well as collaborations with community mental health agencies. Broader research implications include investigating how to reduce stigma relating to accessing mental health care services for this population.

Hinduism

A systematic search for literature on Hinduism and suicide yielded 30 relevant articles. Scanning of the bibliographies of these articles yielded an additional 20 articles that met criteria for inclusion. There were approximately 12 articles for each category, including, affiliation, suicidal ideation and behaviour, and risk factors. Additionally, there were eight articles related to protective factors, five articles related to doctrine, and two articles related to participation. India is the most populous Hindu country in the world, and much of the research on Hinduism and suicide comes from India. It is important to note that 20% of the population of India does not identify as Hindu. However, most of the data on suicide and Hinduism are not sufficiently nuanced to address.

Doctrine

Compared to the more defined doctrinal positions taken by the other world religions, Hinduism's stance regarding suicide has been described as ambiguous.[42,69,70] As the oldest of the major religions, Hinduism is more of a way of life when compared to the defined doctrines of the other major religions.[70] Hinduism's religious texts, namely the Vedas and Upanishads, alongside several epics, such as the Mahabharata, provide Hinduism's philosophical and moral positions.[70] An examination of these texts for Hinduism's stance on suicide reveals conflicting viewpoints. Several scholars have described these contrasting positions by distinguishing between Hinduism's stance on general suicides and its stance towards religious suicides.[69,70]

In the Upanishads, suicide is categorically condemned.[70] According to the *Dharmashastra* (the book of code, conduct, and ethics), suicide and attempted suicide are considerable sins.[70] A part of the Mahabharata describes that those who die by suicide cannot enter heavenly worlds, and the *Garuda-purana* (a religious text in Hinduism) declares that those who die violently, including by suicide, may become ghosts.[69] The *Arthasastra* and *Manu-smriti* (Laws of Manu) bar cremation rites for those who die by suicide and prohibit ritualistic offerings to the deceased,[70] and the *Yama-smriti* (another religious text) states that the bodies of those who die by suicide ought to be dishonoured.[69,70] It is suggested that underlying much of this prohibitive stance to suicide is Hinduism's tenet of reincarnation.[42,69]

Hinduism believes that all beings contain an *atman*, or a soul. The atman goes through cycles of death and rebirth, based on its karmas (translated into deeds or acts), until it reaches *moksha* (liberation) and the ultimate reality, known as Braham, is realized.[70] As this process can take more than one lifetime, how a Hindu dies (which is related to how they live through the principle of karma) is preparatory for their spiritual progress into the next reincarnation. Given this emphasis on death, suicide (which, in Sanskrit, is *Pranatyaga* or *Atmahatya* and means abandoning life force) can be seen as not ideal for pursing spiritual progress in the next life.[42,69] It is also noted that the tenet of karma may also be protective in that it encourages Hindus to tolerate worldly suffering as it is considered a part of their given fate.[70,71]

However, there are exceptions to this understanding, as Hinduism allows for several types of religious suicides. Within these practices, suicide is redefined as a process by which a person can progress further along their spiritual path. For example, the *Dharmashastra* contains a section entitled *allowable suicides*.[70] As these books are the ancient law books for religious conduct (900–700 BC), they provide insight into the cultural and theological factors underpinning allowable suicides.

For example, translated as the *Great Journey*, Mahaparasthana was a sanctioned practice whereby a person walks in a north-east direction towards Mount Kailash—a holy site—without food until they die.[69,70] Certain rivers and their confluence (e.g. Prayag, the area near the Ganges, Yamuna, and Saraswathi rivers) also hold religious significance.[70] It is described that if a person dies at one of these sites, they can be relieved of the cycle of reincarnation. During the annual wheeling out of the deity at the Jagannath Temple (in the city of Puri), people threw themselves under the wheels, killing themselves, with the belief they could attain *moksha*, until a ban was placed on the practice in 1802.[72] Additionally, in rare contexts, euthanasia was permitted in Hindu communities, but only through fasting and in accordance with community rules. Ascetics were also permitted to die by fasting according to Laws of Manu.[69]

As another example, the practice of Sati, or self-immolation of women, has existed in Hinduism from ancient times. The first recorded historical instance occurred in 316 BC.[70] Connected to the mythology of the goddess Sati, the practice involves the widow ascending the funeral pyre of her husband or resolving to die by her own funeral pyre following the cremation of her husband.[69] Although illegal in modern times, Sati continues to be practised in parts of the Indian subcontinent. However, scholars suggest that in the modern context, the motivation no longer appears to be religious, but rather sociocultural relating to the lowered status of women and other patriarchal values.[70,73]

Affiliation

Hinduism has an estimated 1.1 billion followers, and is behind Christianity and Islam in terms of percentage of the world's population (Christianity 31.5%, Islam 23.2%, Hinduism 15–16%).[42,74,75] India is the most populous Hindu country, with 79.8% of its population identifying as Hindu.[76] Compared to the other major religions, India's rate of suicide is higher than both Christian and Muslim countries, but lower than Buddhist and atheist countries.[68]

According to the World Health Organization,[68] India's suicide rate is significantly higher than the global average of 11.4 deaths per 100,000, with roughly 21 deaths per 100,000. The suicide rate for Indian males in 2012 was estimated at 19.98 per 100,000, and 9.74 for Indian females.[68] From 2005 to 2015, the suicide rate in India increased only marginally (from 10.3% to 10.6%) and the male-to-female ratio of suicides remained at 2:1.[70]

As most of India's population are religiously affiliated with Hinduism, the extant literature often uses suicide data from India as being representative of Hinduism's relationship to suicide. It is important to note that India also comprises individuals religiously affiliated with Islam (14.2%), Christianity (2.3%), Sikhism (1.7%), Buddhism (0.7%), and Jainism (0.4%).[76] This trend is also seen in studies on suicidality within the Indian diaspora or among immigrants of Indian background. Hindu affiliation is considered the majority affiliation among participants, and as such, suicidality is interpreted in the context of the sociocultural influences of Hinduism.[13,77,78] Our findings are presented in the context of these limitations.

Participation

The high rates of suicide in Hindu countries could lead to the false assumption that greater participation in Hinduism may increase suicide risk. A case-control study in Bengaluru, the capital city of Karnataka, India looked at risk factors for suicide.[80] Psychological autopsies were conducted with 269 families of individuals who had suicided in the preceding three months compared to 269 controls. Lack of religious belief was found to be a risk factor for suicide (odds ratio (OR) 19.18, confidence interval (CI) 4.17–30.37).[79] Another population-based case-control study with psychological autopsies of individuals who suicided in Chennai, the capital city of Tamil Nadu, India produced similar findings.[80] For those who suicided in Chennai, lack of belief in God was associated with an OR of 6.83 (CI 2.88–19.69). This study also found that among those who suicided and were regular worshippers, 11% lost their faith in the three months prior.[80] It is important to note that neither of these studies identified the religious affiliation of their samples, and so despite the high rates of Hinduism in the states of Karnataka and Tamil Nadu (84% and 88%, respectively), these study results and how they pertain to participation in Hinduism must be interpreted with caution.[76]

Suicide dimensions: ideation, planning, rehearsals, attempts, and suicide

Limited research exists across the different suicide dimensions. India's National Crime Records Bureau (NCRB)[81] reported on suicide methods and frequency of use for 2013. Data on suicide methods inform an understanding of planning and rehearsals in this population when considering research that indicates method substitution for suicide is less common.[82,83] Additionally, the choice of suicide method has an association with suicide attempts.[84] According to the NCRB, in 2014, suicide by hanging and poisoning (39.8%) were the most prevalent, followed by burning (7.4%) and lastly drowning (5.7%).[69,81] Gururaj et al.[79]

conducted a case-control study of completed suicides in Bangalore, India and similarly found the three most common methods to be hanging, poisoning, and self-immolation. Regarding poisoning, analysis of data from 2001 to 2005 showed 68% of fatal episodes of self-poisoning were due to ingestion of pesticides.[85] Due to these high rates of poisoning by pesticides, it has been recommended that India places a comprehensive national ban on the most hazardous pesticides.[86]

Self-immolation, or Sati, is highly lethal and unlike many other methods of suicide, the ratio of attempters-to-completers is 1:25.[70,87] It is also the only suicide method for which women outnumber men (61% vs 39%).[70,88] Contemporary reasons for its persistence as a method of suicide is partially attributable to the ease with which kerosene is available and the frequency of its use in homes for cooking.[70] This trend in self-immolation among women also occurs outside India. A study by Raleigh et al.[78] found that even among female immigrants of Indian ethnic origin in England and Wales, self-immolation was a common method of suicide. Women also appear to be more vulnerable to suicide pacts relative to men.[70,89] Like the practice of Sati, it is suggested that this also may be linked to the patriarchal cultural pressures placed upon women in India.[70]

A minimal amount of research exists pertaining to suicidal ideation and Hinduism. A recent study by Blosnich et al.[66] examined how suicidal ideation (in the past 12 months) varied by sexual orientation among college students (aged 18–29 years) of different religious affiliations. Compared to heterosexual Hindu students, Hindu students who identified as belonging to a sexual minority (i.e. bisexual, gay/lesbian, questioning) were more likely to report recent suicidal ideation (OR 9.22, 95% CI 3.32–25.64).

Risk factors

Given the high proportion of adherents to Hinduism in India, examination of suicide data from the country revealed important information relating to risk factors. Patel et al.[90] completed a nationally representative study on suicide mortality in India. Data from the 1991 census were used to direct field-surveyor visits to every home where a death had been recorded from 2001 to 2003. The authors[90] found a bimodal age pattern for male suicides, with peaks at the age of 30–44 years and of 70 years and above. For females, the age pattern was downsloping, peaking at the age of 15–29 years.[90,91] The age-standardized suicide rate for males aged 15 years and older was 26.3 per 100,000 for men, and 17.5 for women. Other suicide rate figures confirmed that for Indian women, childbearing age and older age are key risk periods, and for men, young adulthood and older age are periods of high risk.[73,91]

In broad terms, Agoramoorthy et al.[69] described men as choosing suicide due to socio-economic problems, whereas women choose suicide due to emotional and personal reasons. A study on the trends and socio-economic determinants of suicide in India from 2001 to 2013 examined the different rates and patterns of suicide across states and territories. States with more economic development had suicide rates 3–4 times higher than those that are less economically developed.[91,92] The authors noted that this may be because more developed states report deaths by suicide more accurately.[91,92] Further key findings were that states with higher literacy rates, higher levels of male unemployment, and more agricultural employment were at higher risk of suicide.[92] The Maharashtra state recorded the highest suicide rate (12.3%), and also has a history of mass suicides by farmers.[69,92]

In 2015, India's NCRB[88] identified causes of suicide for all women aged 18–29 years. Family problems (32%), dowry-related issues (8%), other marriage-related issues (7%), and love affairs (6%) were described as the causes of most suicides for women in this age group.[88] For women in India, unlike in many other countries, marriage is less protective against suicide.[73,91] It has been suggested that this is due to the patriarchal system that is present in India, with factors including early and arranged marriages, domestic violence, economic dependence, and young motherhood.[73,91] It has also been suggested that the lower status of women at an early age results in lower self-esteem and poor coping skills, further contributing to the high rates of suicide during this period.[70]

The elevated suicide risk among older persons stands in stark contrast to data from Eastern and Western countries. From 1990 to 2016, suicide rates among elderly males and females in India saw a significant increase, whereas late-life suicide rates declined in places such as the United States, China, Japan, and the United Kingdom.[91] Data from 2013 of four Indian states (Tamil Nadu, Kerala, Maharashtra, and Andhra Pradesh) exposed the severity of this vulnerability where roughly 55% of suicides in these states were among citizens aged 60 years or older.[69] Cited causes of suicidal ideation in this group include functional disability, perceived burdensomeness on family, social isolation, and depression.[73,91]

Another risk factor for suicide among followers of Hinduism may be membership within the Indian diaspora. As a result of colonization, many persons from India settled in other Asian, Caribbean, and Western countries such as the United States.[70] Several studies have shown that in these various countries, Indians demonstrated a comparatively higher rate of suicide relative to other groups, which certain authors have suggested is due to religious and cultural factors relating to Hinduism.[70,93,94,95,96]

There are mixed results as to the extent that mental health disorders are risk factors for suicide. A study by Manoranjitham et al.[97] utilized a matched case-control and psychological autopsy design to examine risk factors for suicide in rural South India. Their findings suggested that, as opposed to psychiatric disorders, psychosocial stress and social isolation are risk factors for suicide in rural South India. However, another matched case-control study that utilized psychological autopsies from the State of Karnataka found contrary results.[79] Although they did not use any diagnostic instruments, Gururaj et al.[79] observed suicide risk increased 10-fold with the presence of an unclassified mental health disorder. This result aligns with the finding from Vijaykumar et al.'s[80] case-control study in India where the presence of Axis I disorders (mood disorders, substance use disorders, and psychotic disorders) increased the risk of suicide by 20 times. Further research needs to be conducted into the role that mental health and psychosocial stress have on suicide risk among adherents of Hinduism. More broadly, further research is recommended into risk factors for suicide and Hinduism uses samples comprising religious Hindus as opposed to only nationals of India.

Protective factors

Compared to the literature on risk factors for suicide, the literature on Hinduism and protective factors is sparse. Overall, it is suggested that the Hinduism tenet of karma allows for Hindus to better tolerate adversity and hardship, and thereby functions as a protective factor against suicide.[70]

Part of the case-control study conducted by Gururaj and colleagues[79] looked at the role and association of several protective factors in the State of Karnataka. Results indicated that 80% or more of cases that suicided did not have a positive outlook on life, had consistent difficulties in coping with problems, described a lack of faith in religious beliefs and activities, and had an inability to solve problems and low satisfaction with their lives. Other protective factors that were absent included non-availability of help in crises (69%), and absence of proper communication skills (73%) and social support (65%).[79] The authors[79] conducted a stepwise logistic regression analysis and found that not having access to resources in crisis situations (OR 11.47, CI 4.56–28.82) and absence of social support (OR 3.1, CI 1.09–8.48) emerged as significant. The role of faith and involvement in religious activities as protective factors was also found in the study by Vijayakumar et al.[80] Along these lines, Agoramoorthy et al.[69] recommended encouraging greater 'devotion, prayers, and visiting temples' (p. 810) as a way for at-risk farmers to avoid suicidal thoughts. In their recommendations for suicide prevention, Manoranjitham et al.[97] advocated for macro-level interventions that address poverty, economic inequality, and social justice for reducing suicide rates at the population level in India and other low- and middle-income countries. Although helpful in the short term, these authors did not view psychiatric or counselling services capable of making population-based changes regarding suicide.[97]

Hinduism and suicide: implications

Hindu doctrine in relation to suicide is complex. The Vedas, Upanishads, and epics contain significant material relating to death and dying, as well as suicide. In interpreting these texts, scholars appear to distinguish between general suicides, which are prohibited, and religious suicides that have historically been permitted.[69,70] In modern times, although certain practices such as Sati persist, it is difficult to define them as religiously motivated in the context of other sociocultural factors in India (the most populous Hindu country).[70,73]

Hindus die by suicide at a rate significantly higher than the global average, and only Buddhist and atheist countries have higher rates.[68] Only a few studies were identified relating to religious participation, but results indicate that greater belief and participation in religion lessen suicide risk.[79,80] These results demonstrate the need for further studies to replicate these findings and to further investigate the mechanisms involved in the association between participation and suicidality. If greater participation does reduce suicidality, it may be a possible way to intervene in relation to the high rates of suicide in this population. There already exist recommendations that certain high-risk groups, such as farmers, may be encouraged to participate more actively in religious activities as a means of suicide prevention.[69]

Self-immolation is a highly lethal method of suicide and is the only method where women outnumber men.[70,87,88] Compared to data on suicide, research into Hinduism and its relationship to suicidal ideation and suicide attempts is very limited. Further research will be necessary into these other domains to better understand how the various aspects of suicidality manifest among adherents.

Regarding risk factors for suicide, both sexes appear to have an increased risk during youth and young adulthood (females, aged 15–29 years; males, aged 30–40 years) and again in older adult years.[73,90,91] Consequences of the patriarchal system in India (family violence, early marriages, economic dependence) and related family and marriage issues seem to drive suicide among females.[73,91] Among males, socio-economic problems appear to be central drivers for suicide.[69] Increased risk of suicide among older adults (aged 60 years and older) appears to be related to social isolation, burdensomeness on the family, and functional disability.[73,91] Addressing the various drivers associated with an increased risk across genders and age cohorts is complex, which is why advocates assert the need for macro-level interventions focused on addressing broader root causes of suicide that cause psychosocial stress such as poverty and social inequities. This stated, there is sufficient support in the literature that indicates developing population-specific interventions for these groups (males, females, and the elderly).

Although Manoranjitham et al.[97] did not find psychiatric disorders as a prominent risk factor for suicide in rural South India, other investigations found mental health disorders to be associated with a significant increase in suicide risk in other states.[79,80] As India is a diverse and populous country, research into suicide and risk factors within Hindu communities needs to attend carefully to contextual factors. Relatively little research has been conducted on protective factors against suicide. In this review, one study that focused on protective factors found that access to resources in crisis situations and to social support were particularly significant variables.[79] More attention to protective factors is indicated, and like risk factors, contextual factors will need to be considered carefully.

One important limitation on the existing research regarding suicide in this population is the confounding of Indian with Hindu. While it is true that the majority of the population in India practise Hinduism, research in this area does not present socio-demographic data regarding religious group affiliations, limiting understanding of whether there are differences based on Hindu affiliation versus other group religions in India. Further research is needed that specifically addresses this gap.

Islam

A systematic search for the literature on Islam and suicide yielded a total of 43 pertinent articles. Of those, 10 articles commented on Muslim doctrine regarding suicide, whereas 33 articles investigated affiliation with Islam. Only 11 articles discussed participation within the Islamic religion in relation to suicide, and 17 articles discussed the four dimensions. Finally, 38 articles mentioned some aspect of risk factors for, and protective factors against, suicide among those who follow Islamic practices.

Doctrine

Islam condemns the taking of one's life, as it interferes with the work of God (Allah) and results in exclusion from heaven.[42,98,99] Multiple verses of the Quran directly address suicide. Low suicide rates in persons affiliating with Islam and in nations with predominantly Muslim populations are attributed either to the explicit condemnation of suicide by Islamic scriptures[100,101] or to under-reporting.[53,102]

Suicide is considered a sin and is a crime under Islamic law, and suicide attempts can lead to prosecution in some countries. On the severity scale, suicide ranks high, and people are not allowed to offer funeral prayers for a suicide death.[103] However, in modern times, Muslims may be more willing to accord funeral rites to suicides.[104]

According to Islamic law, suicide is regarded as homicide and, as such, is forbidden. Life and death are considered God's will, and therefore, suicide is sin and shameful. The Quran (4:29) states: '... You shall not kill yourself. God is merciful towards you'.[105] Suicide is seen as shameful within families, and there is reluctance to report or seek help for suicidal thoughts and feelings. Due to the collective familial culture within Muslim families, suicide can also impact the families of the victim who may face social sanctions, and possibly exclusion, within their communities.[106]

Other verses of the Quran relevant to suicide state, 'Nor take life—which God has made sacred—except for just cause' (Al-Israa' 17:33), and 'If anyone killed a person not in retaliation for murder (without just cause), or to spread mischief in the land, it would be as if he killed all mankind, and if anyone saved a life, it would be as if he saved all mankind' (Al-Ma'idah 5:32).[105] An individual who prevents a person from suicide is a hero. Within Muslim doctrine, God gives and takes life. The Quran states: 'Have you not turned your gaze to one who disputed with Abraham about his Lord because God granted him power?' Abraham said, 'My Lord is He who gives life and death' (Al-Baqarah 2:258).[105]

According to Islam, life is given by God to each person for a purpose, and adherents are here on earth to fulfil that purpose. Adherents are therefore not free to decide when their purpose is complete and when they should die. If a Muslim takes or attempts to take their own life, they are believed to be performing a function that belongs to God. The Quran states: 'Nor kill nor destroy yourselves, for surely God has been to you Most Merciful' (An-Nisaa' 4:29).[105] According to prophetic tradition (Hadith), a person who attempts suicide will be tormented. The Prophet said: 'He who commits suicide by throttling shall keep on throttling himself in the Hellfire (forever), and he who commits suicide by stabbing himself shall keep on stabbing himself in the Hellfire' (Al-Bukhari Volume 2, Book 23, Number 446).[105] Thabit bin Ad-Dahhak narrated: 'The Prophet said, "... whoever commits suicide with piece of a iron will be punished with the same piece of iron in the Hellfire," and, "A man was inflicted with wounds and he committed suicide, and so Allah said: My slave has caused death on himself hurriedly, so I forbid Paradise for him" '

(Al-Bukhari Volume 2, Book 23, Number 445).[98] Among all major world religions, Islam offers the strongest prohibition for suicide in the scripture and sayings of the Prophet.

Suicide remains a criminal offence in 25 countries around the world,[107] most of which are Muslim-majority counties.[108,109,110] However, there is some historical evidence of liberal and humane non-judgemental responses to mental illness within Islam. For example, Muslim doctors, such as the great Avicenna and Elrazi, positively influenced their more primitive medieval European contemporaries to view mental illness with compassion.[111,112,113]

Affiliation

Eskin et al.[26] conducted a study with 8417 university students from 12 Muslim-majority countries and found that affiliation with Islam increases suicide attempts and the level of psychological distress, but reduces the odds for suicidal ideation. A study conducted by Shaheen Al Ahwal et al. in 2016 on a sample of Muslim cancer patients explored the role of religiosity as a predictor of depression and suicidal ideation. Those with greater religious affiliation showed less suicidal ideation and fewer depressive symptoms.[42,114]

Other studies have looked into the prevalence of suicide, suicide attempts, and suicidal ideation among Arab and Jewish individuals in Israel. Although Arabs have a lower prevalence of completed suicide, compared to Jews,[98,115] they have a higher prevalence of suicidal ideation and higher rates of suicide attempts.[115,116] It should also be noted that although not all Arabs are Muslim, the majority of Arabs in Israel are Muslim.

The lower prevalence of completed suicide among Arabs has been attributed to stronger social ties and collectivist values characterizing the Arab society, in addition to leading an overall more religious way of life, compared to the Jewish population.[98] Religiosity and stronger social ties are known to serve as protective factors against suicide.[46]

Participation

As a result of strict prohibition around suicide, few Muslim countries report on suicide and very few Islamic countries record suicides or report suicide rates.[53,110] Taboo and stigma associated with, and criminalization of, suicide have made it harder to collect accurate data on participation.[42,53,109,110,117] Stack et al.[118] conducted a cross-national analysis filling in the gaps, mentioning that Islam lends itself to a more religiously based lifestyle leading to lower suicide acceptability and low prevalence rates. Undetermined deaths are classified by the World Health Organization (WHO) as Other Violent Deaths (OVD) in International Classification of Diseases, Ninth Revision (ICD-9), or as Other External Causes

(OEC) in International Classification of Diseases, Tenth Revision (ICD-10). To avoid under-reporting of suicides, both formal suicide verdicts and OVD need to be considered together because OVD may contain *hidden* suicides.[53] Social stigma may also contribute to under-reporting of suicide, as research points to rates of Muslim suicide as not being so low.[41,118,119]

Suicide dimensions: ideation, planning, rehearsals, attempts, and suicide

Suicidal ideation

In a study conducted by Benatov and colleagues,[120] 3554 students studying in high schools completed a self-report survey evaluating serious suicidal ideation, suicide attempts, depression, anxiety, somatization, self-efficacy, sense of belonging, and socio demographic variables. Results from the study found that students from minority backgrounds, including Arab Muslim, Bedouin Arab Muslim, and Druze, were more likely to have considered attempting suicide and have suicidal ideations in comparison to their Jewish counterparts.[121] Among the reasons for this are higher levels of depression among Bedouin Arab Muslim students. However, the overall rate of suicidal ideation and suicide attempts among vocational education students was lower, compared to students in the regular educational system, for both Jews and Arabs. This finding is in line with the study by Tandon et al.,[121] suggesting that the pressure they experience may be lower compared to students in the regular education system. The vocational education high school system in Israel, characterized by small class size, high student–personnel ratio, and availability of in-school psychological services, may serve as a protective factor against suicidal ideation and suicide attempts among its students.[120,121] Similarly, a study by Khokher et al.[122] found that suicidal ideation among college students in Pakistan (a Muslim-majority country) was high for both men and women.[41]

Suicide attempts

Sharia (Islamic law) is ingrained in the legal system in multiple Middle Eastern countries, leading to suicide attempts remaining as a criminal offence.[42,108,110,119,123] Specifically, in Iran, women who experience social regulation or those who hold traditional beliefs experience higher rates of suicide.[42,124] Another study raised awareness to the issue of increasing suicide rates among young females in Islamic Middle Eastern countries.[42,125] One study identified Islamic intrinsic religiosity to be a protective factor against suicide attempts.[42,126]

Klomek et al.[116] completed a study examining suicide and suicide attempts among four Arab groups defined by religious affiliation in Israel—Bedouins, Muslims (other than Bedouins), Christians, and Druzes—by using national databases of suicide (1999–2011) and suicide attempts (2004–2012). Age-specific and age-adjusted rates and ratios of suicides-to suicidal behaviour were calculated and compared to the total Israeli population rates. Age-adjusted suicide rates were lowest among non-Bedouin Muslims (2.5 per 100,000 population), followed, in ascending order, by Bedouins (3.2 per 100,000 population) and Christian Arabs (3.3 per 100,000 population). The highest rate was found among Druzes (8.7 per 100,000 population), particularly among young males. Rates among Arab groups were lower than among the total Israeli population (7.9 per 100,000 population), except for Druzes.[116]

Age-adjusted suicide attempt rate over the period of 2004 and 2012 in this study was highest among Muslims (84.8 per 100,000 population), compared to 72.4 among Bedouins, 64.9 among Druzes, and 58.6 among Christian Arabs, all per 100,000 population.[116] All rates were slightly lower than the rate for the total Israeli population (89.8 per 100,000 population), and the rate ratios of the Arab groups, compared to the total Israeli population, were between 0.7 and 0.9. The age range of 15–24 years was seen as the highest rate of suicide across all groups and genders. Among females, the highest rates at this age were among Muslims (270.7 per 100,000 population), followed by Bedouins (235.7 per 100,000 population), both being higher than the total Israeli population rate (229.8 per 100,000 population). Among males, a particularly high rate was found at this age among Druzes (285.9 per 100,000 population). This rate is almost three times higher than the female Druze rate of 108.4 per 100,000 population, which was the lowest of all Arab female groups.[116]

Completed suicide

The same study[116] found that suicide rates, however, were lowest among Muslims, with an age-adjusted rate of 2.5 per 100,000 population for total suicide, compared to 3.2 among Bedouins, 3.3 among Christian Arabs, and 8.7 (highest) among Druzes (all per 100,000 population). The difference between the rate of the groups and the total population was even higher among males, where the Muslim rate was 4.1 per 100,000 population, about a third of the total population rate, whereas the age-adjusted rate among male Druzes was 15.6 per 100,000 population, a rate ratio of 1.2 compared to the total population. Suicide rates were highest at ages of 15–24 years for all Arab groups other than Muslims. Muslims had slightly higher rates at 3.1 and 2.6 per 100,000 population at ages of 25–44 years and 45–64 years, respectively, compared to 2.4 per 100,000 population at ages of 15–24 years. Rates for the total Israeli population, however, increased with age. In all Arab groups, suicides at ages of 65 years and older were rare.[116]

Risk factors

Based on several studies in Muslim countries, including Egypt, Iran, Pakistan, Saudi Arabia, and Turkey,[110,123,127,128,129] it is clear that suicides are under-reported in official national statistics and suicide remains a largely taboo subject.[53,110,123,129]

Depression and unemployment have been found to be risk factors for suicide in this population. In 2014, unemployment rates were 5.7%, 8.1%, 6.1%, and 7.3% among Jews, Arab Muslims, Christians, and Druzes, respectively.[120] Although unemployment rates among minority groups in Israel are not high compared to some Arab countries in the region, such as Egypt (13.1%) or Jordan (11.55%), relative to the majority group of Jews in Israel, they remain higher. Employment prospects are also highly related to education. Although the percentage of minority youth attending higher education has been rising in recent years, Arab minority students are still under-represented in higher educational institutions in Israel. These gaps between minorities and the majority group may serve as contributing factors to the higher prevalence of suicidal ideation reported among minority youth. Arab Israelis have a suicide rate that is higher compared to residents of Arab countries in the region.[120]

Protective factors

Little information was found on protective factors in the existing research. Kamal et al.[99] looked at suicidal beliefs and behaviour among young Muslims and Hindus in the United Kingdom. Results indicated that Muslims endorsed high moral values, which included religious reasons for living, as well as survival and coping beliefs. Another study conducted in six Asian countries found a significant relationship between Islam and suicidality as Islam forbids suicide and contributes to low suicide rates.[130,131,132] There is some evidence that religious beliefs are protective against suicide, but there is little consensus as to how. While reviewing the evidence, Sarfraz et al.[119] noted the reasons for difficulties in obtaining accurate statistics on suicide in Islam. These include historical context, negative associations between religion and suicide, lack of research in Muslim countries or data not sent to the WHO, different cultural understandings of death in the West in comparison to Eastern Countries, different religious beliefs, and not studying suicide at an individual level for those who identify as Muslim.[119]

Islam and suicide: implications

Islamic doctrine categorically prohibits suicide. The Quran, Islam's holy book, contains multiple verses that explicitly condemn suicide, viewing it as a crime and a sin analogous to homicide. Accordingly, Islamic countries have some of the lowest rates of suicide relative to countries from the other major religions.[68] Islam's strong prohibitory stance to suicide is a possible explanation for the low rates of suicide seen among Muslims and nations that have large Muslim populations.[100,101] Another explanation for the lower suicide rates is under-reporting of suicide data from Muslim countries.[53,102] Due to the taboo around suicide, countries may misclassify deaths by suicide (e.g. as OVD) or simply not share their data with organizations that gather and report on suicide globally (e.g. the WHO).[53,119] Regardless of the cause, affiliation with Islam appears to be associated with a reduced risk of suicide, despite the problems with under-reporting.

Overall, research into religious participation within Islam and suicide is limited. This may also be related to the strong condemnation of suicide in countries with Muslim-majority populations, some of which have criminalized suicide. Research on suicide at an individual level is limited.[108,109,110,119] There is a considerable gap in the literature, which emphasizes the importance of multinational research collaborations with institutions and universities in Muslim countries. Additionally, suicide prohibitions and criminal exposure of individuals in Muslim countries significantly limit researchers working with Muslim populations, requiring them to exhibit cultural awareness. For example, cultural brokers and translators for research and clinical practice need to be considered when working with Muslim communities in the area of suicide research.

However, some important findings should be recognized. There are higher rates of Muslim women attempting suicide than men, and the age group of 15–24 years appears to be at particularly high risk.[116] Research conducted in Israel, where there is a significant minority of Arab Muslim population, indicates that the rate of female Muslims attempting suicide is higher than that of the total population, which includes Jewish and Christian groups. A large multinational study that included Muslim countries similarly found a heightened risk of Muslims attempting suicide compared to Hindus, Buddhists, Orthodox Christians, and Catholics, as well as to those with other religions and no religion.[26] These findings, which are in contradiction to broad narratives of Muslims being at low risk of suicide, are significant and need to be further investigated. Understanding the relationship between high rates of suicide attempts and low completed suicide rates in this population may help inform interventions for this population, as well as guide possible learnings for other religious groups.

The literature focusing specifically on suicidal ideation among Muslims is limited. A multinational study that included Muslim countries found identification with Islam to be associated with a reduced risk of suicidal ideation.[26] Another study on vocational education students in Israel found significantly greater incidences of suicidal ideation among Arab Muslims and Bedouin Arab Muslims compared to Jewish students.[133]

Similarly, research into risk and protective factors among Muslims is limited and the effect sizes are small. Initial findings for protective factors among high-school students indicated that higher levels of self-efficacy and sense of belonging were negatively associated with experiences of suicidal ideation and behaviour. Higher levels of depression, anxiety, and somatization were found to be positively associated with suicidal ideation and behavior.[133] This study also indicated that high levels of depression might increase the risk of serious suicidal ideation and suicide attempt relative to Jewish students. These results on suicidal ideation and protective and risk factors are limited by several factors (diversity of samples, demographics, small number of studies, and inadequate statistical power), and further research is warranted in these domains.

Challenges associated with data collection and research conducted within Muslim populations on suicide due to religious and cultural factors pose a significant barrier to furthering understanding of this phenomenon within this group. Cross-country collaborations and sharing of resources may help to build research infrastructure in these countries and to develop means to address such structural barriers.

Judaism

A systematic search for the literature on Judaism and suicide yielded 19 relevant articles. By scanning the bibliographies of these articles, an additional 14 articles were also found to meet the criteria for inclusion. Across the six categories searched (doctrine, affiliation, participation, four dimensions, risk factors, and protective factors), articles focusing on risk factors and affiliation were most common (more than 25 articles), and those focusing on doctrine, participation, and four dimensions were less common (less than 15 articles).

Doctrine

Suicide is present in the Torah, as well as in the written version of Jewish oral law known as the Talmud, and in other early rabbinical writings. In Judaism, humans are created in God's image and life is considered to be a gift from God. One's life belongs to God and an individual is responsible for it for a fixed time.[134,135] God is the ultimate judge of who gives and takes life, so the act of suicide is seen as superseding God's role.[136] Although recognizing the right to self-determination, the emphasis in the Jewish religious tradition is on the duties human beings have to others and to God.[137,138] Theologically, humans are meant to co-partner with God, with the aim of recreating another Garden of

Eden on earth, and therefore, suicide is seen as disrupting this central purpose for a Jewish life.[136]

In Judaism, murder is a cardinal sin and is one of the few commandments that cannot be violated, even in the case of permitting the loss of another life.[135] Talmudic sages extend the commandment prohibiting murder from the book of Exodus (20:13) to suicide and interpret it as a form of murder. Suicide is seen as more reprehensible than homicide, as the one who commits murder still can repent, whereas this is not possible with suicide.[136] The Torah does not differentiate murder according to reason or motive, and so euthanasia, like suicide, is prohibited. Adding to the stance against euthanasia, as the body belongs to God, Judaism believes human beings have an obligation to heal.[134]

Gvion and colleagues[135] stated that the story of Noah from the book of Genesis (9:15) is the earliest example of Judaism's disapproval of suicide. The Talmud interprets God saying to Noah that He will demand the blood of every man's life as meaning that a person cannot wound or take one's own life (B. Bava Kama 90b).[135] In addition, Kaplan et al.[136] suggested Judaism's opposition to suicide is based on the core tenet of *tzibbur*, or the broader community, and the ethical expectations a Jewish person has to this community. According to these authors,[136] Jews should live as Jewish persons despite the difficulties they may face in the world as well as within themselves. There is an emphasis on commitment to the community over the individual.[136]

Regarding the burial of those who suicided, the Halakhah, which is the set of Torah commandments, Jewish practices, and rabbinic law, does not permit Jews who die by suicide to receive a full burial.[135] For Jews who die by suicide, rites such as reciting of the Kaddish, the mourner's prayer, or sitting Shiva, the period of mourning for relatives, are contentious.[135] It is important to distinguish that Judaism's focus and condemnation are on the act of suicide itself, as opposed to the person.[136] Therefore, considerable attention goes into defining whether the death was or was not a suicide. The forgoing of traditional burial rituals is only done if the individual who suicided is deemed to have killed themselves *lada-at*, or wittingly.

As Kaplan et al. described,[136] if any indications of pathological behaviour are shown by the individual prior to their suicide, the label of *shoteh* can be given that refers to a person displaying abnormal behaviour. The individual and their act are then removed from the suicide category. Examples of individuals who can fall within this category are those under the influence of drugs and alcohol or minors as they are too young to understand the severity of their actions.[136] In modern Israel, in practice, the assumption is that the person who suicides is not in a normal state of mind and the event is most often treated as a normal death.[135]

Gvion et al.[135] noted there are scriptural instances where suicide is permitted. Suicide is permittable to avoid betraying one's faith such as when King Saul killed himself out of fear that he would be forced to worship other gods by his enemies (Ben Avraham Ishbili, 1959, Torah commentary, fourteenth century).[135] Heroic suicide is also a typology in Judaism. This typology is most prominently seen in Samson felling a house where his captors were residing alongside himself (Judges 16: 25-30).[135,139] The Battle of Masada, which resulted in the collective suicide of Jews to avoid enslavement by the Romans and during the Holocaust where individual and mass suicides occurred as an attempt to resist the prescribed Nazi deaths further exemplify the heroic suicide typology that exists in Judaism.[42,135,139,140]

Relating to end of life and sickness, Jews are allowed to pray to God for death to come, as there are several prayers in the Talmud on the subject.[134] Generally, Judaism does not permit anything to quicken death, but it also does not suggest the dying process should be prolonged. Most Jewish denominations, including those that are Orthodox, permit Jews to enter hospices for end-of-life care. Comfort, as opposed to cure, is deemed as an acceptable goal in these situations.[134]

Affiliation

In 2019, the Jewish population worldwide was estimated at 14,707,400.[141] Israel and the United States accounted for over 84% of this total population. Suicide rates among Jewish populations in these two countries have historically been low.[42] A study by Bailey et al.[142] in the United States analysed the Jewish population and suicide rates for each state. A negative association ($r = -0.26$; $p = 0.03$, one-tailed test) was found, indicating that states with larger Jewish populations had lower rates of suicide.[142] Jewish suicide rates in Israel have been lower than in the United States, but there have been significant fluctuations since Israel gained its independence in 1948.[42,139,143]

Suicide rates in Israel in the 1950s were approximately 18 per 100,000 and decreased to 11–14 per 100,000 in the 1960s and 1970s.[139] The beginning of the 1980s saw suicide rates of 8.1–8.5 per 100,000, which then rose to 10.8–11.2 per 100,000 in the mid 1980s until the mid 1990s.[139] From 1995 to 2009, the rate ranged approximately from 6.3 to 9.4 per 100,000.[139] Recently, according to the WHO's report 'Suicide worldwide in 2019: global health estimates',[144] Israel had an age-standardized suicide rate of 5.1 for all ages per 100,000. As most of the adherents to Judaism live in Israel, an understanding of the country's context, including suicide rates and possible socio-demographic processes, need to be considered when investigating Judaism's relationship with suicide. For example, the high suicide rates seen in the 1950s could be due to the sociopolitical instability Israel was facing at the time as a new nation, and the rise in suicides beginning in the mid 1980s may be due to the influx of immigration that Israel experienced during this period.[139,143,145]

Comparatively, suicide rates in Israel have been consistently lower than rates in most European and North American countries, but higher than those in Muslim countries located in Asia or North Africa.[139] Interreligious comparisons showed Jews having higher rates of suicide than Muslims,[42,146] and consistently lower rates compared to Protestants as well as Catholics in most cases.[139,143]

Participation

Minimal research has been conducted on how factors such as greater religious commitment and religious attendance may impact suicidality for adherents to Judaism.[139] There appears to be only one study that examined the relationship between religiosity and suicidal behaviour in an adult Jewish Israeli population,[147] and two studies that focused on this relationship among Jewish adolescents.[148,149]

Burshstein et al.[147] used cross-sectional data from an epidemiological study of mental disorders among adults in Israel in the 1980s and longitudinally examined self-reported data on religiosity and completed suicides 25 years later. In the Jewish sample of nearly 5000 subjects, Burshstein et al.[147] examined suicidal behaviour (ideation, attempts, completed suicide) by the religious subjects (secular, partially observant, religious). Results indicated that suicidal ideation among subjects who identified as religious, partially religious, and secular was 6.2%, 6.7%, and 9.4%, respectively.[147] Rates of suicide attempts among religious, partially observant, and secular subjects were 0.4%, 2.5%, and 2.4%, respectively. Confounding demographic (e.g. marital status) and clinical variables (e.g. substance use) for both suicidal ideation and suicide attempts were controlled for in determining these associations. For completed suicides, a follow-up was conducted 25 years after the baseline assessment, which found eight people from the original cohort had died by suicide (equivalent to a rate of 6.7 per 100,000 per year). Analysing religiosity among these subjects who had died by suicide, none were religious, one was partially observant, and seven were secular. Although these findings were not significant, the authors suggested this is most likely due to power considerations. Subjects who were secular were 8.5 times more likely to complete suicide as compared to those who were partially observant.[147]

Amit and colleagues[148] investigated the association between self-injurious thoughts and behaviours and religiosity in 620 Jewish adolescents. Their analysis demonstrated that after adjusting for depression and socio-demographic factors, adolescents who were religious (ultra-orthodox and observant) had a decreased likelihood of self-injurious thoughts and behaviours by 55% compared to non-religious (non-observant) adolescents.[148] An earlier study by Stein et al.[149] assessed the attitudes of 525 Israeli adolescents towards suicide and suicidal ideation. Greater Jewish religious affiliation was found to be significantly associated with decreased suicidal ideation and decreased tolerance of suicide.[149]

Results of these studies demonstrate that, in general, greater participation in Judaism is associated with lessened suicidal thoughts and suicide attempts. Further research is required to understand the role of religiosity more fully in completed suicides. The study by Burshstein et al.[147] provides preliminary evidence that greater religiosity is associated with fewer suicides, but there are limitations to this finding given the small sample size.

Additionally, further studies examining religiosity and suicidality in Jewish populations outside Israel is necessary. A study by Rasic et al.[150] examined longitudinal relationships of religiosity and suicidality in north-eastern United States, but under 1% of its sample were adherents to Judaism. Given that the United States has the second largest population of Jewish adherents,[141] and there are several cultural, political, and economic differences between Israel and the United States, further research into Jewish religiosity and suicidality in the United States is necessary.

Suicide dimensions: ideation, planning, rehearsals, attempts, and suicide

Suicidal ideation

Gal et al.[116] used data from the Israel National Health Survey from 2003 to 2004, and found that the estimated lifetime prevalence rate of suicidal ideation among Jewish Israelis was 5.5% and the lifetime prevalence rate for planning was 1.9%. A sample of 525 Israeli adolescents were assessed in terms of attitudes to suicide and suicidal ideation.[149] The authors found that adolescent attitudes towards suicide were significant predictors of suicidal ideation, and religious involvement was highly associated with four attitudinal conceptual factors. The identified factors related to attitudes towards the ability of society to prevent suicide, whether suicide is a symptom of mental illness, the right of the individual to talk openly about suicide, and the seriousness with which suicidal behaviour is viewed. Non-religious subjects were found to display a more approving attitude towards suicide than those who considered themselves as religious.[149]

There is less information about suicidal ideation within Jewish populations at higher risk of suicide, but some research does exist. In a national community survey of recent Jewish immigrants to Israel from the former Soviet Union, 15.1% of the sample were found to have suicidal ideation compared to 6.6% in an indigenous sample of Jews in Russia.[151] Among Jewish male soldiers, a high-risk population, a post-mortem study of 43 suicides found that suicidal ideation was not communicated to significant others and professional help-seeking was avoided.[139,152] For Jewish sexual minority populations, Blosnich et al.[66] examined how recent suicidal ideation (past 12 months) varied by sexual orientation among college students (aged 18–29 years) of different religious affiliations. For heterosexuals, Jewish affiliation was associated with significantly lower odds of suicidal ideation in the previous 12 months compared to atheist/agnostic/secular-identifying heterosexuals. Notably, compared to heterosexual Jewish students ($n = 1017$), Jewish students who identified as belonging to a sexual minority group (i.e. bisexual, gay/lesbian, questioning) ($n = 76$) were more likely to report recent suicidal ideation.[66] This finding is particularly striking as it contradicts the assumption that all types of affiliation with Judaism are associated with low levels of suicidality.

A thematic qualitative analysis of religiosity, coping, and suicidality among a religious Zionist community (associated with the modern Orthodox sector of Judaism) found that of the participants who experienced suicidal thoughts, the majority failed to connect the subject of suicide to their religious belief or faith.[153] The authors suggested that this apparent dissonance is perhaps emblematic of the tension the modern Orthodox sector of Judaism must hold between modernity and religious tradition. To manage this, the authors[153] suggested that a degree of compartmentalization occurs through which certain areas are categorized as being of either secular or religious importance. Accordingly, the phenomenon of suicidal thoughts may be subsumed under a secular understanding (i.e. mental health).[153]

Suicide attempts

A study analysing the socio-demographic factors associated with suicide in two Israeli cities during an 8-year span found that a greater distribution of the 2150 suicide attempts examined were among Israelis born in the Americas and Europe, which the authors suggested were most likely Jews of Ashkenazi descent.[154] A higher prevalence of repeated suicide attempts was found among Israelis born in Africa and Asia, which the authors[154] suggested were most likely Jews of non-Ashkenazi descent. This difference in suicide attempts and repeated suicide attempts between these two groups has been found in other studies.[139,143,154,155] Higher religiosity found among Jews of non-Ashkenazi descent is often attributed to the lower rates of suicide in their country of origin (Asia and Africa), compared to the higher rates found in the country of origin (Europe and America) of Ashkenazi Jews.[154] It is postulated that higher rates of repeated attempts among Jews of Asian and African origins may be reflective of the greater expression of frustrations and other emotions externally through behavioural or psychosomatic means.[154] In addition, Shoval et al.[156] emphasized the stress involved in acculturation to the Israeli society, given the vast differences in culture and technology, compared to Ethiopia, when they examined the higher risk of suicide among Ethiopian immigrants (Jews of non-Ashkenazi descent) in Israel. Overall, in the two Israeli cities analysed by Stein et al.,[154] the attempted suicide rate showed an almost constant decrease over the 8-year period from 1990 to 1998.

These authors[154] also examined gender and age with regard to suicide attempts. For males, two peaks were observed; the highest rates were between the ages of 25 and 28 years (121.4 per 100,000), and a second smaller peak for suicide attempts was found after the age of 65 years. For females, the highest rate of attempts was seen between the ages of 15 of 19 years (411 per 100,000). Apart from the age group of 65–74 years, female participants had consistently higher rates of suicide attempts relative to male participants. The mean ratio of female-to-male suicide attempts for all age groups in the study was 1.8.[154]

Gal et al.[115] conducted a comparative study comparing suicidal behaviour between Muslims and Jews in Israel. In the period of 2003–2007, the rate of attempted suicides among Jewish men was higher compared to Muslim men. For the same period, Jewish and Muslim women aged between 15 and 44 years showed no differences in attempted suicide rates. According to Israel National Health Survey data from 2003 to 2004, self-reported lifetime suicide attempts were significantly higher among Muslims compared to Jews (2.8% vs 1.2%, respectively). Although it was a small sample size, adjusted logistic regression analysis showed a significant association between religion and attempted suicide for Muslims compared to Jews.[115]

Completed Suicide

Gal et al.[115] found that in Israel, based on 1843 suicides recorded between 2003 and 2007, the completed suicide rate for Jewish Israelis was 8.2 per 100,000. This rate was comparatively higher than that found for Muslim Israelis of 3.0 per 100,000 during the same period. In terms of gender, a study completed by Stein et al.[154] found the suicide rate for both male and female residents of two Israeli cities increased with age. The male-to-female suicide ratio for the population of the two cities was 2:1 during the 5-year period of 1990–1995.[154] An epidemiological study of suicide that examined suicide rate trends in Israel from 1984 to 1994 found males to be particularly vulnerable.[146] Jewish males were found to have the highest suicide rate of any subgroup, as well as a pattern of increasing rates, during the study time periods. The authors found that the Jewish male group suicided at a rate of 11 per 100,000 in 1984–5 to a rate of 15.9

per 100,000 in 1992–4. The age cohort at greatest risk within this subgroup were males aged 18–21 years, who saw a significant increase in suicide rates of over fourfold from 3.9 to 18.2.[146]

A study by Lubin and colleagues[146] examined six suicide methods in a specific high-risk population of Jewish men aged 18–21 years. According to death certificates, the following means of suicide were used: firearms; poisoning; hanging; jumping; unspecified; and other suicides (not already specified). There was a dramatic change in the method employed to complete suicide. In 1984–5, the primary methods of suicide were jumping followed by hanging. Poisoning and firearms were the least common means. In 1992–4, the percentage of suicides by firearms rose to 77%, up from 11% in 1984–5, and became the primary method of suicide for Jewish men in this age group of 18–21 years. The authors[146] noted this trend relating to firearms was also present for females, but given that the actual number of female suicides was so minimal, it did not impact the overall figures. The authors[146] suggested that this particularly striking increase may be related to the influx of immigrants at this time from the former Soviet Union, which had extremely high suicide rates. In addition to issues associated with immigration, stresses related to compulsory military service and widespread access to firearms while in the army also may have contributed to this sharp increase in suicides as well as in the use of firearms. Looking at another vulnerable subgroup, a psychological autopsy of suicides of Ethiopian Jewish immigrants occurring between 1991 and 1992 found only two methods of suicide, both of which had the same distribution for males and females.[157] Hanging accounted for 62% of the deaths, and jumping off high places accounted for 38% of the remaining cases. According to Witztum et al.,[139] the use of violent methods has been replicated in other studies of Ethiopian suicides, as well as the use of more violent means of suicide by both genders.

Risk factors

Immigration appears to be a particularly salient risk factor for suicide in Jewish persons. A third of all suicides in Israel from 2000 to 2009 were among immigrants, a percentage that greatly exceeded the proportion of suicides among the larger population.[139] As noted above, one Jewish population that is at particularly high risk of suicide are Jewish immigrants from the former Soviet Union or those of Russian descent. Ponizovsky et al.[151] completed a national community survey examining suicidality in a sample of 788 Russian-born and recent Jewish immigrants, and an indigenous sample of Jews in Russia ($n = 411$). Suicidal ideation among the immigrant sample was found to be significantly higher than in Russian controls (15.1% vs 6.6%, respectively). Additionally, 5.5% of immigrants had made a suicide attempt at some point in their lives compared to only 0.5% of Russian controls. Several risk factors were identified, the strongest of which were higher levels of psychological distress and symptoms, including hostility, depression, and paranoid ideation. A study on attempted suicide in Israel looked at emergency services used in the cities of Holon and Bat Yam ($n = 1774$) for the period between 1990 and 1998.[154] The authors noted that the two cities selected were representative of the urban population in the centre of Israel. During the study period, there was an almost constant decrease in the rate of attempted suicides, except for the period of 1990–2, which saw higher rates. The authors suggested that this increase was associated with approximately 400,000 Jews from the former Soviet Union immigrating to Israel during the period of 1988–90.[154] Within this group of immigrants from the former Soviet Union, youth aged 15–24 years had the highest suicide rate.[139] Immigration may be a particularly salient risk factor for adolescents of Russian origin due to loss of familial support, identity crisis, and lack of integration in the new country.[158]

Immigration also appears to increase the risk of suicide for non-Ashkenazi Jews from North Africa and Middle Eastern countries, and specifically Jews from Ethiopia.[139] Up until the mid 1980s, Jews from these countries showed a lower rate of suicide, which has been attributed to the higher religiosity found among Jews of non-Ashkenazi descent.[139,154] A shift occurred in the mid 1990s, as the suicide rates among Jews from these countries reached rates similar to those among European and American-born Jews, and again in 2000 where the highest rates of suicide were among Israelis born of non-Ashkenazi descent.[139] Ethiopian Jewish immigrants were found to be particularly vulnerable within this group and have therefore been the topic of multiple studies.[139,156,157,159]

A particularly vulnerable group for suicides among Ethiopian immigrants are males aged 15–24 years.[135,139,159] A psychological autopsy was conducted surveying Ethiopian suicide victims ($n = 44$) who had immigrated to Israel.[157] The proportion of suicide victims who were male was higher than the proportion of males in the entire Ethiopian community by a ratio of almost 2:1, and the proportion of victims aged 20–39 years was also higher than the similar age group for the entire community (48.6% vs 29.1%, respectively).[157] From 2000 to 2004, young Ethiopian males had 7.4 times higher suicide rates compared to non-immigrant Israeli Jews, and this trend continued from 2007 to 2009, but to a lesser extent.[139] It has been suggested that the acculturation process for Ethiopian male immigrants disrupts traditional gender roles of male dominance within the family structure, and loss of this role can lead to distress and frustration, contributing to the higher rates of suicide among this population.[135,137] Results also indicated that the ratio of male-to-female suicides among Ethiopian immigrants was twice that of the general Israeli population.[139,157] It has been suggested that the immigration process also creates a vulnerability for Ethiopian Jewish women in that they lose critical social supports when faced with domestic violence and therefore see suicide as a last resort.[157]

Another serious risk factor for young Israeli Jews appears to be military service. Kohn et al.[155] examined socio-demographic correlates and temporal trends in suicide among Israeli youth between 1975 and 1989. Suicide rates were examined by variables that included gender and national/religious affiliation (Jews, Moslem Arabs, Christian Arabs, and Druzes). Results demonstrated that Jewish males in the army age group (age range 18–20 years) had a marked increase in their risk of suicide (OR 3.8, 95% CI 2.6–5.5) when compared to the younger adolescent age group (age range 15–17 years). Jewish males in the army age group also had a higher risk of suicide, combined with undetermined causes of death, when compared to the next older age group of individuals who had completed military service (age range 21–29 years) (OR 1.6, 95% CI 1.4–1.8). When undetermined causes of death were removed, Jewish males in the army age group had a suicide risk equal to that of the completed military service group (OR 1.0). Gender differences were also found in the army age group, with a greater frequency of males dying by suicide than females (OR 3.2, 95% CI 2.2–4.6).[155]

There are several suspected causes for the increased risk of suicide among males during the compulsory three years of military service. Psychosocial stress and demands of entering military service, loss of previous social support that was present during recruitment, and availability of firearms have been suggested as possible causes.[139,155] A clinical post-mortem study of 43 Israeli male suicides that occurred during compulsory military service (age range 18–21 years) was conducted.[152] A major finding of the study was the seemingly high degree of general functioning and low levels of diagnosable or significant psychopathological disorders at induction of duty. The authors noted that the absence of antisocial behaviour and substance abuse in the sample was strongly contrasted by what was seen in post-mortem studies of military suicides in a similar-age cohort from the United States and Scandinavia.[152]

Another risk factor for increased suicidality is survival of the Holocaust.[139,160] Medical records of 921 older adult suicidal patients who had been admitted to a psychiatric hospital during a 5-year period in Israel were retrospectively evaluated and compared to patients who had not attempted suicide.[160] The authors aimed to investigate whether ageing in this population with possible reactivation of traumatic syndromes, physical disorders, and psychological distress might increase suicide risk. Results indicated that the risk of attempted suicide among Holocaust survivors was significantly increased (OR 3.53, 95% CI

1.8–5.4) and therefore emphasized the importance of preventive strategies for this population.[160]

Protective factors

The pattern of suicide among the Jewish population in the Middle East seems to follow that in Western countries. At the aggregate level, low levels of suicide tolerance and high levels of religious beliefs were associated with low suicide rates.[162] From 1981 to 2009, the average suicide rate in Israel, which is home to the largest number of adherents to Judaism, was 9 per 100,000.[139] Over this 30-year period, this was one of the lowest suicide rates in the Western world. Judaism's strong negative perspective towards suicide has contributed to a relatively consistent low suicide rate among Israeli Jews. While there are certain groups that are at higher risk of suicide and suicidal behaviour (immigrants, Holocaust survivors, and male soldiers), affiliation and participation in Judaism act as protective factors against suicide.[139]

Although limited, several studies have demonstrated the direct independent protective effect of religiosity in Judaism against suicidality.[147,148,149] Amit et al.,[148] in their study of 620 Jewish Israeli adolescents, found that religiosity in Judaism decreased the likelihood of self-injurious thoughts and behaviours by 55% for the adolescents. This finding is consistent with an investigation by Stein et al.[149] who found that attitudes towards suicide were significant predictors of suicidal ideation and individuals who identified as religious were less accepting of suicide. Religious involvement was one of the most influential psychosocial parameters associated with all four of the identified attitude factors.[149] Further, Burshstein et al.,[147] in a large sample of adult Jewish Israeli adults ($n = 4914$), found that religious Jews were less likely to act on their suicidal ideation compared to secular Jews.

A thematic qualitative analysis of religiosity, coping, and suicidality among a group of young participants (age range 18–24 years) from a religious Zionist community found that the degree of religiosity had a relatively low impact on coping during times of acute stress and trauma.[153] Many of the study participants described having difficulties accessing their reserves of religious strength in response to harsh life situations. The authors[153] suggested that although research has often found religion to be a protective buffer against suicide, the rise of individualism in Israel due to its rapid modernization may impact the level of support traditionally provided by its religious communities that are characterized as possessing a high degree of cohesion. This analysis by Band et al.[153] relates to what another research has highlighted about modern-day Israel.[135,139] As a relatively young nation, Israel remains in transition through ongoing demographic shifts and sociocultural changes that will continue to shape the country, and therefore Judaism's relationship to suicide.

Judaism and suicide: implications

Judaism prohibits suicide as a Jewish person's life is believed to ultimately belong to God.[136] Jews are duty-bound to use the gift of life they have been given to contribute to others, the community, and God.[134,135] Instances of suicide exist in the Torah, and there are references to it in the Talmud and other rabbinical writings.[135] Although a heroic suicide typology exists in Jewish scriptures and history (e.g. Battle of Masada, Holocaust), there is no contemporary religious practices that relate, or offer any flexibility pertaining, to suicide being permittable. This doctrinal stance presumably contributes to the consistently low suicide rates observed in Israel where the majority of Jewish adherents reside.[139] The Jewish population in the United States also historically demonstrates a low suicide rate.[42,142] It is important to note that most studies relating to Jewish affiliation and suicide are based on Israeli and American Jewish populations. As culture and religion overlap considerably, research focusing on Jewish communities outside these two countries could add further understanding of this religion's relationship to suicide.

Existing research on how religious participation influences suicidality indicates that greater participation in Judaism is associated with a reduction in suicidal thoughts and suicide attempts.[147,148] Limited information exists relating to participation in Judaism and suicide, but preliminary findings have suggested that greater religiosity may be associated with fewer suicides.[147]

For the four dimensions of suicide, an examination of suicidal ideation and Judaism produced some key findings from the literature. Estimated lifetime prevalence of suicidal ideation for Jewish Israelis has been found to be low,[115] although certain Jewish populations appeared to be at higher risk of suicidal ideation, including former Jewish immigrants to Israel from the former Soviet Union,[151] Jewish male soldiers,[139,152] and Jewish sexual minorities.[66] A thematic qualitative analysis found that respondents who experienced suicidal thoughts failed to make the connection between their suicidality and religious belief or faith.[153] Although limited to a small sample of religious Zionists (associated with the modern Orthodox sector of Judaism), these results could indicate that respondents relegated their suicidal experiences to a secular domain (e.g. mental health) as opposed to considering their experiences through a religious lens.[153] A disconnect between suicidality and religious belief could have several implications, and further research into the experience of contemporary Jews with suicide is indicated.

The identified studies relating to suicide attempts and Judaism found the highest rates among males aged between 25 and 28 years and among females aged 15–19 years.[149] Jewish females were found to have consistently higher states of suicide attempts compared to Jewish males. The literature also identified a difference in suicide attempts between Jews of Ashkenazi descent and those of non-Ashkenazi descent.[139,143,154,155] Generally, it appeared that Israelis born in America and Europe (of Ashkenazi descent) were more likely to attempt suicide, whereas Israelis born in Africa and Asian (of non-Ashkenazi descent) were found to be more likely to have repeated suicide attempts.[154] It is suspected this difference corresponds to the levels of religiosity in each group's respective country of origin (e.g. low religiosity in Europe and America contributing to higher levels of suicidality compared to high religiosity in Africa and Asia contributing to lower levels of suicidality).[154] It is suggested that Jews of Asian and African origins may be more apt to externalize emotions and frustrations behaviourally (suicide attempts) in relation to acculturative stress generated by the challenges of adapting to life in Israel.[156] Several implications for policy and practice for Jewish immigrants of Asian and African origin are associated with these findings. These include targeting immigrants from these backgrounds for programming aimed at reducing acculturative stressors, and focused suicide prevention counselling among attempters in the population to reduce their heightened risk of future attempts.

Pertaining to Judaism and completed suicides, the literature shows Jewish males as particularly vulnerable to suicide and a male-to-female suicide ratio of 2:1.[115,146] Examination of the suicide method in the most at-risk age cohort of Jewish men (age range 18–21 years) found firearms to be the primary method of suicide.[146] This coincides with the period when young Israeli Jews are required to serve in the military and so there is widespread access to firearms.[155] Implications from these findings indicate the need for stricter gun safety measures in place for this population. Male and female Ethiopian Jewish immigrants appear to use primarily two methods (hanging and jumping from high places) for suicide, a finding that has been replicated.[139,157]

The literature identified several risk factors for suicide among Jewish persons. Immigration to Israel from the former Soviet Union, North Africa, and the Middle East appears to increase suicide risk.[139,154,158] Several studies demonstrated that young Ethiopian males seemed to be particularly vulnerable to immigration.[135,139,157,159] Military service is also a serious risk factor for young Israeli Jews. Jewish males in the army age group (age range 18–21 years) were found to be at comparatively high risk of suicide relative to Israelis of other religious affiliations or gender.[155] Survival of the Holocaust has also been identified as a risk factor for older Jewish adults.[16] Suicide prevention efforts and interventions should be implemented that target the known risk factors related to these specific populations.

Evidence supports that religiosity, and particularly increased religious involvement and less tolerant attitudes towards suicide, acts as a protective factor against suicidality among Jewish adherents.[135,147,148,149] As some authors noted, modern-day Israel is changing at a rapid pace and this will have an impact on how Judaism is practised at individual and community levels.[135,139,153] Therefore, ongoing research is required to better understand Judaism's relationship to suicide.

Atheism and agnosticism

Very limited research was identified that focused on atheist and agnostic affiliation and suicide. We found only four articles, with three having a loose association with non-religious groups. Due to limited available data, this section comments on the six dimensions of suicide and religion highlighted for the previous religious groups; however, we could not comment on each of these dimensions separately but rather merged them accordingly.

In the United States, 13.2% of the population view themselves as non-religious, whereas only 3.1% of the population consider themselves atheist and 4% agnostic.[3,6,42]

It is important to define the terms atheists and agnostics in order to discuss their beliefs in relation to suicide. Atheists are individuals who do not believe in the existence of God or a supreme power, and therefore focus their beliefs on logical answers to their questions. In comparison to the dominant religions, atheists and agnostics neither endorse the existence of God or a supreme power nor reject this belief, suggesting this knowledge is unknowable.[3,6]

Doctrine, affiliation, and participation

In the absence of specific religious doctrine and a religious framework for conceptualizing death, atheist and agnostic cultural worldview (which may or may not include religion) serves as a source of coping and provides a guide for achieving meaning and purpose in life.[162] As such, atheist and agnostic perceptions and attitudes towards suicide are more likely to reflect or align with the values and attitudes of their cultural affiliation and worldview rather than with any direct religious precepts or teachings.

Further, it has been suggested that atheism is, in and of itself, a worldview and should be considered as meaningful of a sociocultural variable in mental health research as religiosity of any other specific religious affiliation.[163] Research in support of this view has found that those individuals with higher belief certainty in either direction, who are confidently religious or firmly atheist, have greater well-being as compared to individuals with low certainty (i.e. religiously unsure or agnostic). This lends support to the idea that well-being may be related to a clearer, more confident worldview rather than to belief in a specific religious doctrine.[164]

The literature on the relationship between suicide and atheists and agnostics is quite limited. However, some research has addressed perceptions of life and death among these groups. Wulff,[165] for example, proposed a model for conceptualizing degrees of religiosity that may further lend to an understanding of how atheists and agnostics approach death, dying, and suicide.

This model proposes four basic attitudes, including: (1) literal inclusion; (2) literal exclusion; (3) symbolic inclusion; and (4) symbolic exclusion. Literal inclusion refers to individuals who define themselves as religious and who interpret religious contents in a rigid, close-minded, and dogmatic manner. They strictly adhere to religious content as taught by a particular religious tradition. Symbolic inclusion refers to individuals who define themselves as religious, yet tend to process religious content in a more open and tolerant manner. They acknowledge that varied interpretations of religious content are possible and try to find an interpretation that is personally meaningful. Literal exclusion refers to individuals who reject entirely the possibility of a religious reality based on strict, literal arguments (i.e. the lack of scientific evidence for the miraculous stories in the Bible). Lastly, symbolic exclusion refers to individuals who define themselves as non-religious, yet are generally more tolerant of, and less judgemental towards, religiosity compared to those endorsing literal exclusion. Individuals who report high symbolic exclusion consider religion as one way of giving meaning to life, among many other possible methods. They respect other's choices to adhere to a particular religion, yet do not themselves need religion to find personal meaning in life.[165]

Overall, atheists and non-believers are less social, less conformist, and more individualistic than individuals who identify as religious, regardless of denomination.[166] Although there are exceptionally limited data on the relationship between atheism, agnosticism, and suicide, the few studies that do exist demonstrate a relationship between these schools of belief and life and death attitudes and decisions.[118,167] Some research has examined religious beliefs versus non-believers. One study found that participants identifying as religiously unaffiliated had significantly more lifetime suicide attempts and more first-degree relatives who died by suicide than those who endorsed a religious affiliation. Unaffiliated participants were younger, more often single and without children, and reported less contact with family members, representing groups that are at high risk of suicide. Further, participants identifying as having no religious affiliation reported fewer reasons for living, particularly fewer moral objections to suicide, and greater lifetime impulsivity and aggression, and were more likely to report prior history of substance use disorder, all of which are risk factors for suicide.[168]

Ideation, risk factors, and protective factors

Only one study could be identified that specifically examined suicidal thoughts among atheists and agnostics.[169] This study compared atheists and agnostics with individuals endorsing a belief in spiritism (often called Kardecism, or the belief that God is the creator, the Supreme Intelligence, and the primary cause of all things, the immortality of the soul, and communication with spirits)[170] on key clinical and socio-demographic variables, acute life weariness (tiredness of life), and suicidal thoughts. The main findings of the study showed that atheism and agnosticism were associated with lower rates of life weariness and suicidal thoughts than spiritism.[169]

Despite being limited, research examining risk factors for, and protective factors against, suicide among atheists and agnostics has identified notable findings. For example, life weariness, or losing interest in life, has been shown to serve as a risk factor for suicide among atheists and agnostics.[6,169] A higher rate of suicide has been observed among those who do not ascribe to any religion or who consider themselves atheists.[33] If atheists do not find meaning in life, they are more likely to consider suicide instead of looking for ways to restore their interest in life.[6]

Research examining death and religion using Wulff's[165] model has found that those individuals endorsing a symbolic exclusion attitude attempt to find meaning in life itself without relying on a religious, transcendent reality, and as such, they also consider death a natural part of life.[171] This indicates that among atheists and agnostics, those who struggle with finding meaning in life have a more accepting attitude towards, or are more likely to consider, suicide as an option.

This research also demonstrated that individuals endorsing rigid, literal scientific explanations reflective of an attitude of literal exclusion may well be judgemental towards religious individuals due to their own anxiety about death and dying.[171] Another possible interpretation of the relationship between atheism and agnosticism and attitudes towards, and acceptance of, suicide, is that specifically their fear of, and anxiety and uncertainty regarding, death and dying may make them less likely to consider suicide as an option and to engage in suicidal behaviour.

One study examined the association between moral and religious beliefs and suicidality among individuals diagnosed with bipolar disorder. Findings indicated that religiously affiliated participants reported fewer past suicide attempts, had fewer suicides among first-degree relatives, and were older at the time of the first suicide attempt than participants who identified as religiously unaffiliated.[167]

Other studies have suggested atheism and non-religion could also serve as protective factors against suicide and suicidal ideation for the sexual minority population.[66] It is proposed that given that most religions/religious populations condemn SGMs, SGM individuals who identify as religious or belong to families that adhere to those religions experience social and psychological pressure, isolation, stigma, and rejection, which results in mental health problems and increased suicide risk.[62,66] However, for non-religious and atheist SGM individuals, the lack of religious affiliation and identification with stigmatizing doctrine may serve as a protective factor against suicide and suicidal ideation.[62,66]

Other studies have examined dimensions of religiosity and their relationship to suicidality. Findings of this research indicated that within communities that were highly religious, even those who identified as non-religious or religiously unaffiliated experienced a protective effect and reported lower levels of suicide attempts.[118,172]

Non-religion (atheism and agnosticism) and suicide: implications

Atheists and agnostics collectively comprise a significant number of individuals in the United States, albeit in relatively small populations. Data on suicide prevalence, as well as on the relationship between atheist and agnostic affiliation and suicide, are extremely limited. This research did not confirm that atheists and individuals who identify as having no religion are at increased risk of suicide.[33] Several scholars have postulated possible ways in which these populations may be at greater or lesser risk of suicide.[6] One population in whom atheism and non-religious affiliation may be protective against suicide is that of SGMs.[62,66] This is an important line of inquiry that deserves further attention, considering the increased risk of suicide associated with other major religious groups.[66] Overall, further research is required to begin to understand these populations' relationships with suicide.

Recommendations and clinical implications

Despite the widely accepted role of religiosity in relation to suicidal ideation and behaviour, and the fact that most mental health disciplines have formally acknowledged the importance of religion and spirituality in training,[173] formalized evidence-based religious competencies and methods to assess them remain undeveloped.[174]

Some have suggested that the same criteria applied to multicultural competencies in clinical practice should be extended to cultural differences involving religion and spirituality,[175] often referred to as *spiritual competence*.[176] Multicultural and spiritual competence is characterized by a dynamic process comprising three interrelated parts: (1) awareness of one's personal worldview, along with its associated assumptions, limitations, and biases; (2) an empathic, strength-based understanding of the client's spiritual worldview; and (3) the ability to develop and utilize intervention approaches that are sensitive to the client's spiritual worldview.[175,176]

Moreira-Almeida and colleagues[173] have recommended the following general principles for mental health clinicians to consider, including: (1) maintaining ethical boundaries and recognizing that incorporating religion into treatment should be patient-centred and not prescribing, imposing, or proselytizing; (2) maintaining a person-centred approach; (3) being attentive to countertransference, acknowledging that the clinician's own values, beliefs, and history may raise important issues and influence practice (i.e. having a strong reaction to religious topics, avoiding religious issues, or stressing upon them too much); (4) remaining open-minded while expressing genuine interest in, and respect for, the patient's beliefs, values, and experiences; and (5) avoiding self-disclosure of one's own religious beliefs as it may lead to disagreement, conflict, or avoidance.[173]

A more targeted set of clinical guidelines for effectively integrating religiosity into suicide risk assessment has also now been clearly established.[6,177] For a comprehensive and effective suicide risk assessment, this set of guidelines recommend that clinicians incorporate a discussion of the following 10 key areas:

1. The importance of religion to the client: clinicians should include questions such as: what the client's degree of religious affiliation is; how often they attend services; whether they engage in religious rites like prayer or reading of religious texts; and whether they socialize with members of their religious community.
2. The importance of religion to the client's family/significant others: given that social support networks often exert significant influence on health, mental health, help-seeking behaviours, and treatment engagement and utilization, clinicians should include questions such as: how important religion is in the lives of the client's family members, partner(s), and friends; how supportive the client's significant others are of the client's religious beliefs; and how this may facilitate or limit support and treatment.
3. The importance of religion to the client's identity: given the relationship between suicide risk and religious affiliation, clinicians should include

questions such as: how strongly the client identifies with their religion's tenets; whether the degree of their religious commitment has recently changed; and how this aspect of the client's identity interconnects with their ideas of suicide or mental illness.

4. How suicide is conceptualized and perceived in the client's religion: given the relationship between attitudes towards suicide and suicide risk, clinicians should include questions such as: whether the client's religion has sanctions against suicide; whether there are circumstances when it may be an acceptable act; whether there are varying interpretations of suicidality within the religion; whether this perspective represents a conflict with the client's personal beliefs; and if so, how they address this conflict and its impact on their faith.
5. The role of religiosity during previous times of stress and difficulties: as previous coping skills are associated with current suicide risk, clinicians should include questions such as: whether the client's religiosity has served as a source of comfort or as a coping mechanism in past difficulties or whether it has contributed to her/his level of distress; whether the client's religiosity has served to neither positively nor negatively influence his/her level of distress during times of crisis; if religion has been utilized, how so (e.g. relying on religious figures as sources of guidance and support; increasing involvement in religious activities such as attendance at, and participation in, religious rituals); and if religion has not been utilized, why not.
6. The value of strengthening the client's religiosity and participation in their religion: for some clients, focusing at least some part of treatment on increasing their religiosity may serve as a relevant way to increase the client's protective factors against suicide. As such, clinicians should include questions such as: which elements of the client's religiosity provide protection; how the client can find ways to maximize the support they receive from their religiosity. In contrast, if religion has been a source of distress or difficulty, it is important to examine: which elements of the client's religiosity have added to her or his distress; and how the client can find ways to minimize these harmful effects.
7. Belief in an afterlife: as several of the religions have specific views concerning the nature of what happens when one's body is declared dead, and this directly relates to attitudes towards suicide, clinicians should include questions such as: what the client's beliefs are regarding life after death; whether the client believes in the possibility of redemption in another life; whether the client believes he/she will have a chance to do things over/better/more successfully in an afterlife; and whether the client believes one

would be subject to an afterlife of pain and suffering as a result of taking his/her own life.

8. Meaning in life: given the research indicating that religion serves as a basis for finding meaning in life and that having meaning in life is an important protective factor against suicidality, clinicians should include questions such as: whether the client reports having a meaning in life; in what ways the client finds meaning in life; whether the client feels as though life is purposeless; whether the client thinks it is possible to find meaning in life; and whether the client is hopeless.
9. Strength of conviction: as research has demonstrated a greater risk of suicide among those who report strong belief in either direction, the existence of God or that there is no higher power, clinicians should include questions such as: how strongly the client believes that a higher power exists/does not exist; whether there are times when the client has doubts in their conviction; what those times are like; and when the last time was.
10. The role of traditional folk leaders/figures, spiritual healers/guides, and gurus: research has demonstrated the important role that traditional folk and spiritual figures/leaders/guides can play in reducing risk of, and serving as a protective factor against, suicide. As such, clinicians should include questions such as: who the client considers to be their spiritual and/or religious leader; whether the client considers this person a source of support; whether the client has access to this person; and whether the client is currently consulting with them for guidance.

Conclusion

The relationship between religion and suicide is complex. Although it is now generally accepted that religion most often serves as a protective factor against suicide across religious denominations, there is growing acknowledgement that certain aspects of religion may also represent risk factors for suicide among some followers. Further research is warranted in the area of religion and suicidality to better understand the relationship between religiosity and gender, age, sexual orientation, culture, and ethnicity.

The significant lack of consistent data for many of the dominant religious groups regarding the relationship between religious affiliation and participation and suicide risk serves as a barrier to developing targeted prevention and intervention efforts. It is important to recognize that affiliation with a religious denomination and actual participation in religious activity are conceptually different notions. Individuals might affiliate with a religion but not be an active participant in its activities. The influence of religious affiliation versus various levels of active participation on suicide needs to be studied distinctly to gather a more nuanced understanding of its association with suicide.

We recommend that future research considers the following key factors that we propose will significantly impact the role of religion as both a risk factor for, and a protective factor against, suicide moving forward. Secularization and its impact on the traditionally protective effects of religion on suicide need to be considered. Initial research has demonstrated that even in secular zones where there has been a significant decline in religious influence, such as in certain European nations, religiousness is associated with lower suicide rates.[179] Further explorations into secularization and suicide in different cultural and religious contexts are necessary. Another key consideration is the role of technology. It is predicted that factors such as expansion of mobile networks and more affordable handsets will continue to increase the use of technology globally.[180] To improve accessibility to mental health and suicide prevention interventions, several mobile applications have been developed. Further research is required into the efficacy of these interventions, but preliminary results showed they can reduce suicide-specific outcomes such as suicidal ideation.[181] As the evidence base for these mobile health interventions increases, and they are disseminated more widely, their influence on traditional protective factors such as religion needs to be considered. Additionally, there may also be opportunities for these new interventions methods to incorporate and reinforce established protective components of religion (e.g. encouraging attendance at religious ceremonies).

Lastly, while suicide is taboo in most cultures and religions, criminalization of suicide, in addition to such stigma, serves as a critical barrier to fully understanding the risk of suicide in Muslim populations. Within Muslim countries, where suicide is viewed as a sin and those who attempt suicide face a real risk of criminal exposure, data collection on any of the suicide dimensions is very difficult. Further, suicide is seen to bring shame to families, and therefore, suicide attempts are largely hidden and not reported. This leads to misreporting and under-reporting. While under-reporting is the norm, in instances where suicides are reported, there is a risk of prosecution, harassment, and extortion by the authorities. High levels of stigma, low levels of help-seeking behaviour, and fear and risk of prosecution add to the barriers to collecting accurate data among Muslim populations. Nuanced research into at-risk subgroups within Muslim populations, such as youth, women, and sexual minorities, is needed to understand specific vulnerabilities associated with these groups. Efforts to address this structural barrier and enhance psychoeducation will be key to improving research in these communities to more accurately identify rates of suicide and related risk and protective factors.

References

1. **Durkheim E.** *Suicide: A Study in Sociology*. London: Routledge; 2005.
2. **Borup J.** Who are these Buddhists and how many of them are there? Theoretical and methodological challenges in counting immigrant Buddhists: s Danish case study. Journal of Contemporary Religion. 2016;**31**(1):85–100.
3. **Lizardi D, Gearing RE.** Religion and suicide: Buddhism, Native American and African religions, atheism, and agnosticism. Journal of Religion and Health. 2010;**49**(3):377–84.
4. **Kelly BD.** Self-immolation, suicide and self-harm in Buddhist and Western traditions. Transcultural Psychiatry. 2011;**48**(3):299–317.
5. **Harvey P.** *An Introduction to Buddhist Ethics: Foundations, Values and Issues*. Cambridge: Cambridge University Press; 2000.
6. **Alonzo D, Gearing RE.** Suicide across Buddhism, American Indian–Alaskan Native, and African traditional religions, atheism and agnosticism: an updated systematic review. Journal of Religion and Health. 2021;**60**(4):2527–46. doi: 10.1007/s10943-021-01202-z
7. **Sangharakshita.** *The Ten Pillars of Buddhism*. United Kingdom: Windhorse Publications; 1996.
8. **Chamlong Disayavanish M, Primprao Disayavanish M, Tala Thammaroj M, Surut Jianmongkol M, Kimaporn Kamanarong M, Somjit Prueksaritanond M.** A Buddhist approach to suicide prevention. Journal of the Medical Association of Thailand. 2007;**90**(8):1680–8.
9. **Huang JX, Xu YM, Zhong BL.** Relationship between Buddhist belief and suicide risk in Chinese persons undergoing methadone maintenance therapy for heroin dependence. Frontiers in Psychiatry. 2020;**11**:414.
10. **Gouin M.** Self-immolation and martyrdom in Tibet. Mortality. 2014;**19**(2):176–83.
11. **Keown D.** Suicide, assisted suicide and euthanasia: a Buddhist perspective. Journal of Law and Religion. 1998;**13**(2):385–405.
12. **Shih HC.** *The Sutra on Upāsaka Precepts*. BDK English Tripiṭaka; 1994.
13. **Kok LP, Aw SC.** Suicide and parasuicide. Medicine, Science, Law. 1990;**30**:225–33.
14. **Harvey P.** *An Introduction to Buddhist Ethics: Foundations, Values and Issues*. Cambridge: Cambridge University Press; 2000.
15. **Kalra S, Priya G, Grewal E**, et al. Diabetes management and the buddhist philosophy: toward holistic care. Indian Journal of Endocrinology and Metabolism. 2018;**22**(6):806.
16. **Corcoran JJ.** *Selflessness or Sinfulness? How the Peoples of the East and West Differ in Their Views on Suicide* [Doctoral dissertation, University of Marquette]. Available from:http://academic.mu.edu/meissnerd/corcoran.html
17. **Picone M.** Suicide and the afterlife: popular religion and the standardisation of 'culture' in Japan. Culture, Medicine, and Psychiatry. 2012;**36**(2):391–408.
18. **Sisask M, Värnik A, Kolves K**, et al. Is religiosity a protective factor against attempted suicide: a cross-cultural case-control study. Archives of Suicide Research. 2010;**14**(1):44–55.
19. **Wu A, Wang JY, Jia CX.** Religion and completed suicide: a meta-analysis. PLoS One. 2015;**10**(6):e0131715.
20. **Bendall C, Rouse WH**, editors. *Śikṣā Samuccaya: A Compendium of Buddhist Doctrine*. India: Motilal Banarsidass Publisher; 1981.

21. **Ohnuma R, Kitts M.** To extract the essence from this essenceless body: self-sacrifice and self-immolation in Indian Buddhism. In: *Martyrdom, Self-Sacrifice, and Self-Immolation: Religious Perspectives on Suicide*. United States: Oxford University Press; 2018. pp. 241–65.
22. **Lawrence RE, Oquendo MA, Stanley B.** Religion and suicide risk: a systematic review. Archives of Suicide Research. 2016;**20**(1):1–21.
23. **Bertolote JM, Fleischmann A.** A global perspective in the epidemiology of suicide. Suicidologi. 2002;7(2):6–8.
24. **Ritter K, Zitterl W, Stompe T.** Religion and suicide-part 2: confessions, religiousness, secularisation and national suicide rates. Neuropsychiatrie. 2011;**25**(3):127–34.
25. **Vijayakumar L, Pirkis J, Huong TT, Yip P, Seneviratne RD, Hendin H.** Socio-economic, cultural and religious factors affecting suicide prevention in Asia. Suicide and Suicide Prevention in Asia. 2008;**2008**:19–30.
26. **Eskin M, Poyrazli S, Janghorbani M**, et al. The role of religion in suicidal behavior, attitudes and psychological distress among university students: a multinational study. Transcultural Psychiatry. 2019;**56**(5):853–77.
27. **Hsieh N.** A global perspective on religious participation and suicide. Journal of Health and Social Behavior. 2017;**58**(3):322–39.
28. **Nisbet PA, Duberstein PR, Conwell Y, Seidlitz L.** The effect of participation in religious activities on suicide versus natural death in adults 50 and older. Journal of Nervous and Mental Disease. 2000;**188**(8):543–6.
29. **Jung J, Roh D, Moon YS, Kim DH.** The moderating effect of religion on the relationship between depression and suicidal ideation in the elderly. Journal of Nervous and Mental Disease. 2017;**205**(8):605–10.
30. **Jo KH, An GJ, Sohn KC.** Qualitative content analysis of suicidal ideation in Korean college students. Collegian. 2011;**18**(2):87–92.
31. **Thanh HT, Tran TN, Jiang GX, Leenaars A, Wasserman D.** Life time suicidal thoughts in an urban community in Hanoi, Vietnam. BMC Public Health. 2006;**6**(1):1–8.
32. **Fang CK, Lu HC, Liu SI, Sun YW.** Religious beliefs along the suicidal path in northern Taiwan. Omega (Westport). 2011;**63**(3):255–69.
33. **Saiz J, Ayllón-Alonso E, Sánchez-Iglesias I, Chopra D, Mills PJ.** Religiosity and suicide: a large-scale international and individual analysis considering the effects of different religious beliefs. Journal of Religion and Health. 2021;**60**(4):2503–26. https://doi.org/10.1007/s10943-020-01137-x
34. **Lew B, Kõlves K, Zhang J**, et al. Religious affiliation and suicidality among college students in China: a cross-sectional study across six provinces. PLoS One. 2021;**16**(5):e0251698.
35. **Zhang J, Wieczorek WF, Conwell Y, Tu XM.** Psychological strains and youth suicide in rural China. Social Science and Medicine. 2011;**72**(12):2003–10.
36. **Kelleher MJ, Chambers D, Corcoran P, Williamson E, Keeley HS.** Religious sanctions and rates of suicide worldwide. Crisis. 1998;**19**(2):78–86.
37. **Phipps W.** Christian perspectives on suicide. The Christian Century. 1985;**30**:970–2.
38. **Kennedy TD.** Suicide and the silence of scripture. Christianity Today. 2000;**26**:2008.
39. **Maris RW, Berman AL, Silverman MM.** *Comprehensive Textbook of Suicidology*. New York: Guilford Press; 2000.

40. **Retterstøl N.** *Suicide: A European Perspective*. Cambridge: Cambridge University Press; 1993.
41. **Gearing RE, Lizardi D.** Religion and suicide. Journal of Religion and Health. 2009;**48**(3):332–41.
42. **Gearing RE, Alonzo D.** Religion and suicide: new findings. Journal of Religion and Health. 2018;**57**(6):2478–99.
43. **Wogaman PJ.** *Ethical Perspectives for the Community*. England: Westminster/John Knox Press; 1990.
44. **Amundsen DW.** Suffering and the sovereignty of God: one Evangelical's perspective on doctor-assisted suicide. Christian Bioethics. 1995;**1**(3):285–313.
45. **Kaplan KJ, Schwartz MB.** *A Psychology of Hope: A Biblical Response to Tragedy and Suicide*. Grand Rapids, Michigan, USA: Wm. B. Eerdmans Publishing; 2008.
46. **Kakounda Muallem H, Israelashvilli M.** Religiosity as a buffer against suicidal ideation: a comparison between Christian and Muslim-Arab adolescents. Mental Health, Religion and Culture. 2015**18**(10):838–49.
47. **XVI PB, von Schönborn C.** *Introduction to the Catechism of the Catholic Church*. San Francisco: Ignatius Press; 1994.
48. **Leavey G, Rondon J, McBride P.** Between compassion and condemnation: a qualitative study of clergy views on suicide in Northern Ireland. Mental Health, Religion and Culture. 2011;**14**(1):65–74.
49. **Panczak R, Spoerri A, Zwahlen M, Bopp M, Gutzwiller F, Egger M.** Religion and suicide in patients with mental illness or cancer. Suicide and Life-Threatening Behavior. 2013;**43**(2):213–22.
50. **Pescosolido BA, Georgianna S.** Durkheim, suicide, and religion: toward a network theory of suicide. American Sociological Review. 1989;**54**(1):33–48.
51. **Hood-Williams J.** Studying suicide. Health and Place. 1996;**2**(3):167–77.
52. **Jongkind M, van den Brink B, Schaap-Jonker H, van der Velde N, Braam AW.** Dimensions of religion associated with suicide attempt and suicide ideation in depressed, religiously affiliated patients. Suicide and Life-Threatening Behavior. 2019;**49**(2):505–19.
53. **Pritchard C, Amanullah S.** An analysis of suicide and undetermined deaths in 17 predominantly Islamic countries contrasted with the UK. Psychological Medicine. 2007;**37**(3):421–30.
54. **Spoerri A, Zwahlen M, Bopp M, Gutzwiller F, Egger M.** Religion and assisted and non-assisted suicide in Switzerland: national cohort study. International Journal of Epidemiology. 2010;**39**(6):1486–94.
55. **Torgler B, Schaltegger C.** Suicide and religion: new evidence on the differences between Protestantism and Catholicism. Journal for the Scientific Study of Religion. 2014;**53**(2):316–40.
56. **Moksony F, Hegedűs R.** Religion and suicide: how culture modifies the effect of social integration. Archives of Suicide Research. 2019;**23**(1):151–62.
57. **Mason K, Kim E, Blake Martin W, Gober R.** The moral deliberations of 15 clergy on suicide and assisted death: a qualitative study. Pastoral Psychology. 20171;**66**(3):335–51.
58. **Moreno-Montoya J, Palacios-Espinosa X, Gracia-Ruiz J.** Association between religion and suicidal behaviors in cancer patients. Revista Colombiana de Psiquiatria. 2017;**46**(4):209–14.

59. **Waitz-Kudla SN, Daruwala SE, Houtsma C, Anestis MD.** Help-seeking behavior in socially conservative and Christian suicide decedents. Suicide and Life-Threatening Behavior. 2019;**49**(6):1513–22.
60. **O'Reilly D, Rosato M.** Religion and the risk of suicide: longitudinal study of over 1 million people. British Journal of Psychiatry. 2015;**206**(6):466–70.
61. **Plöderl M, Fartacek C, Kunrath S,** et al. Nothing like Christmas—suicides during Christmas and other holidays in Austria. European Journal of Public Health. 2015;**25**(3):410–13.
62. **Anderson SO, Lough BJ.** Sexual and gender minoritized youth in Christian home schools: perceptions of climate and support. Journal of LGBT Youth. 2021;**18**(4):438–58.
63. **Subhi N, Geelan D.** When Christianity and homosexuality collide: understanding the potential intrapersonal conflict. Journal of Homosexuality. 2012;**59**(10):1382–402.
64. **Barranco RE.** Suicide, religion, and Latinos: a macrolevel study of US Latino suicide rates. The Sociological Quarterly. 2016;**57**(2):256–81.
65. **Berry D, Bass CP, Shimp-Fassler C, Succop P.** Risk, religiosity, and emerging adulthood: description of Christian, Jewish, and Muslim university students at entering the freshman year. Mental Health, Religion and Culture. 2013**16**(7):695–710.
66. **Blosnich JR, De Luca S, Lytle MC, Brownson C.** Questions of faith: religious affiliations and suicidal ideation among sexual minority young adults. Suicide and Life-Threatening Behavior. 2020;**50**(6):1158–66.
67. **Toussaint L, Wilson CM, Wilson LC, Williams DR.** Religiousness and suicide in a nationally representative sample of Trinidad and Tobago adolescents and young adults. Social Psychiatry and Psychiatric Epidemiology. 2015;**50**(9):1441–50.
68. **World Health Organization.** *Preventing Suicide: A Global Imperative.* Geneva: World Health Organization; 2014.
69. **Agoramoorthy G, Hsu MJ.** The suicide paradigm: insights from ancient Hindu scriptures. Journal of Religion and Health. 2017;**56**(3):807–16.
70. **Vijayakumar L, John S.** Is Hinduism ambivalent about suicide? International Journal of Social Psychiatry. 2018;**64**(5):443–9.
71. **Vijayakumar L.** 13 psychosocial risk factors for suicide in India. In: **Lakshmi Vijayakumar,** editor. *Suicide Prevention: Meeting the Challenge Together.* India: Orient Blackswan; 2003. p. 149.
72. **Leenaars A, Connolly J, Cantor C,** et al. Suicide, assisted suicide and euthanasia: international perspectives. Irish Journal of Psychological Medicine. 2001;**18**(1):33–7.
73. **Dandona R, Kumar GA, Dhaliwal RS,** et al. Gender differentials and state variations in suicide deaths in India: the Global Burden of Disease Study 1990–2016. The Lancet Public Health. 2018;**3**(10):e478–89.
74. **Hackett C, McClendon D.** *Christians Remain World's Largest Religious Group, but They Are Declining in Europe.* Pew Research Center; 2017. https://www.pewresearch.org/short-reads/2017/04/05/christians-remain-worlds-largest-religious-group-but-they-are-declining-in-europe/
75. **Pew Research Center** (2012). Religious composition by country. Available from: chrome-extension://efaidnbmnnnibpcajpcglclefindmkaj/https://assets.pewresearch.org/wp-content/uploads/sites/11/2012/12/globalReligion-tables.pdf

76. **Kramer S** (2021). Key findings about the religious composition of India. Pew Research Center. Available from: https://www.pewresearch.org/fact-tank/2021/09/21/key-findings-about-the-religious-composition-of-india/
77. **Morris P, Maniam T.** Ethnicity and suicidal behaviour in Malaysia: a review of the literature. Transcultural Psychiatry. 2001;**38**(1):51–63.
78. **Raleigh VS, Bulusu L, Balarajan R.** Suicides among immigrants from the Indian subcontinent. British Journal of Psychiatry. 1990;**156**(1):46–50.
79. **Gururaj G, Isaac MK, Subbakrishna DK, Ranjani R.** Risk factors for completed suicides: a case-control study from Bangalore, India. Injury Control and Safety Promotion. 2004;**11**(3):183–91.
80. **Vijayakumar L, Rajkumar S.** Are risk factors for suicide universal? A case-control study in India. Acta Psychiatrica Scandinavica. 1999;**99**(6):407–11.
81. **National Crimes Records Bureau.** *Accidental Deaths and Suicides in India*. New Delhi: Ministry of Home Affairs, Government of India; 2014.
82. **De Leo D, Dwyer J, Firman D, Neulinger K.** Trends in hanging and firearm suicide rates in Australia: substitution of method? Suicide and Life-Threatening Behavior. 2003;**33**(2):151–64.
83. **Van Orden KA, Witte TK, Cukrowicz KC, Braithwaite SR, Selby EA, Joiner Jr TE.** The interpersonal theory of suicide. Psychological Review. 2010;**117**(2):575.
84. **Giner L, Jaussent I, Olié E**, et al. Violent and serious suicide attempters: one step closer to suicide? Journal of Clinical Psychiatry. 2014;**75**(3):e191–7.
85. **Alex R, Prasad J, Kuruvilla A, Jacob KS.** Self-poisoning with pesticides in India. British Journal of Psychiatry. 2007;**190**(3):274–5.
86. **Bonvoisin T, Utyasheva L, Knipe D, Gunnell D, Eddleston M.** Suicide by pesticide poisoning in India: a review of pesticide regulations and their impact on suicide trends. BMC Public Health. 2020;**20**(1):1–6.
87. **Rao AV, Mahendran N, Gopalakrishnan C**, et al. One hundred female burns cases: a study in suicidology. Indian Journal of Psychiatry. 1989;**31**(1):43.
88. **National Crimes Records Bureau.** *Accidental Deaths and Suicides in India*. New Delhi: Ministry of Home Affairs, Government of India; 2015.
89. **Vijayakumar L, Thilothammal N.** Suicide pacts. Crisis. 1993:43–6.
90. **Patel V, Ramasundarahettige C, Vijayakumar L**, et al.; **Million Death Study Collaborators.** Suicide mortality in India: a nationally representative survey. The Lancet. 2012;**379**(9834):2343–51.
91. **Snowdon J.** Indian suicide data: what do they mean? Indian Journal of Medical Research. 2019;**150**(4):315.
92. **Arya V, Page A, Dandona R, Vijayakumar L, Mayer P, Armstrong G.** The geographic heterogeneity of suicide rates in India by religion, caste, tribe, and other backward classes. Crisis. 2019:370–4.
93. **Haynes RH.** Suicide and social response in Fiji: a historical survey. British Journal of Psychiatry. 1987;**151**(1):21–6.
94. **Hutchinson G, Daisley H, Simeon D, Simmonds V, Shetty M, Lynn D.** High rates of paraquat-induced suicide in southern Trinidad. Suicide and Life-Threatening Behavior. 1999;**29**(2):186–91.
95. **Maharajh HD.** Transgenerational cultural conflicts and suicide among Hindu girls. Caribbean Medical Journal. 1998;**60**(1):16–18.

96. **Maniam T.** Suicide and parasuicide in a hill resort in Malaysia. British Journal of Psychiatry. 1988;**153**(2):222–5.
97. **Manoranjitham SD, Rajkumar AP, Thangadurai P, Prasad J, Jayakaran R, Jacob KS.** Risk factors for suicide in rural south India. British Journal of Psychiatry. 2010;**196**(1):26–30.
98. **Morad M, Merrick E, Schwarz A, Merrick J.** A review of suicide behavior among Arab adolescents. Scientific World Journal. 2005;**5**:674–9.
99. **Kamal Z, Loewenthal KM.** Suicide beliefs and behaviour among young Muslims and Hindus in the UK. Mental Health, Religion and Culture. 2002;**5**(2):111–18.
100. **Lester D.** Suicide and islam. Archives of Suicide Research. 2006;**10**(1):77–97.
101. **Shah A, Chandia M.** The relationship between suicide and Islam: a cross-national study. Journal of Injury and Violence Research. 2010;**2**(2):93.
102. **Nelson G, Hanna R, Houri A,** Klimes-**Dougan B.** Protective functions of religious traditions for suicide risk. Suicidology Online. 2012;**3**(1):59–71.
103. **Jahangir F, ur Rehman H, Jan T.** Degree of religiosity and vulnerability to suicidal attempt/plans in depressive patients among Afghan refugees. International Journal for the Psychology of Religion. 1998;**8**(4):265–9.
104. **Ineichen B.** The influence of religion on the suicide rate: Islam and Hinduism compared. Mental Health, Religion and Culture. 1998;**1**(1):31–6.
105. Haleem AMAS, translator. *The Qur'an: English Translation and Parallel Arabic Text*. Oxford: Oxford University Press; 2010.
106. **Savani S, Gearing RE, Frantuz Y, Sozinova M.** Suicide in Central Asia. Suicidology Online. 2020;**11**(1):1–12.
107. **Mishara BL, Weisstub DN.** The legal status of suicide: a global review. International Journal of Law and Psychiatry. 2016;**44**:54–74.
108. **Suleiman MA, Moussa MA,** El-**Islam MF.** The profile of parasuicide repeaters in Kuwait. International Journal of Social Psychiatry. 1989;**35**(2):146–55.
109. **Khan MM.** Suicide and attempted suicide in Pakistan. Crisis. 1998;**19**(4):172–6.
110. **Khan MM, Hyder AA.** Suicides in the developing world: case study from Pakistan. Suicide and Life-Threatening Behavior. 2006;**36**(1):76–81.
111. **Sarhill N, LeGrand S, Islambouli R, Davis MP, Walsh D.** The terminally ill Muslim: death and dying from the Muslim perspective. American Journal of Hospice and Palliative Medicine. 2001;**18**(4):251–5.
112. **Ruthven M, Hourani A.** *A History of the Arab Peoples*. London, UK: Faber & Faber; 2002.
113. **Okasha A.** Mental health in Egypt. Israel Journal of Psychiatry. 2005;**42**(2):116.
114. **Shaheen Al Ahwal M, Al Zaben F, Sehlo MG, Khalifa DA, Koenig HG.** Religious beliefs, practices, and health in colorectal cancer patients in Saudi Arabia. Psycho-oncology. 2016;**25**(3):292–9.
115. **Gal G, Goldberger N, Kabaha A,** et al. Suicidal behavior among Muslim Arabs in Israel. Social Psychiatry and Psychiatric Epidemiology. 2012;**47**(1):11–17.
116. **Klomek AB, Nakash O, Goldberger N,** et al. Completed suicide and suicide attempts in the Arab population in Israel. Social Psychiatry and Psychiatric Epidemiology. 2016;**51**(6):869–76.
117. **Al-Harrasi A, Al Maqbali M, Al-Sinawi H.** Surviving a suicide attempt. Oman Medical Journal. 2016;**31**(5):378.

118. **Stack S, Kposowa AJ.** Religion and suicide acceptability: a cross-national analysis. Journal for the Scientific Study of Religion. 2011;**50**(2):289–306.
119. **Sarfraz MA, Castle D.** A Muslim suicide. Australasian Psychiatry. 200;**10**(1):48–50.
120. **Benatov J, Nakash O, Chen-Gal S, Brunstein Klomek A.** The association between gender, ethnicity, and suicidality among vocational students in Israel. Suicide and Life-Threatening Behavior. 2017;**47**(6):647–59.
121. **Tandon SD, Marshall B, Templeman AJ, Sonenstein FL.** Health access and status of adolescents and young adults using youth employment and training programs in an urban environment. Journal of Adolescent Health. 2008;**43**(1):30–7.
122. **Khokher S, Khan MM.** Suicidal ideation in Pakistani college students. Crisis. 2005;**26**(3):125–7.
123. **Al-Jahdali H, Al-Johani A, Al-Hakawi A**, et al. Pattern and risk factors for intentional drug overdose in Saudi Arabia. Canadian Journal of Psychiatry. 2004;**49**(5):331–4.
124. **Aliverdinia A, Pridemore WA.** Women's fatalistic suicide in Iran: a partial test of Durkheim in an Islamic Republic. Violence against Women. 2009;**15**(3):307–20.
125. **Rezaeian M.** Suicide among young Middle Eastern Muslim females. Crisis. 2010:36–42.
126. **Akbari M, Haghdoost AA, Nakhaee N, Bahram NA, Baneshi MR, Zolala F.** Risk and protective factor for suicide attempt in Iran: a matched case-control study. Archives of Iranian Medicine. 2015;**18**(11):747–52.
127. **Coşar B, Kocal N, Arikan Z, Işik E.** Suicide attempts among Turkish psychiatric patients. Canadian Journal of Psychiatry. 1997;**42**(10):1072–5.
128. **Khan MM, Reza H.** Gender differences in nonfatal suicidal behavior in Pakistan: significance of sociocultural factors. Suicide and Life-Threatening Behavior. 1998;**28**(1):62–8.
129. **Moghadamnia AA, Abdollahi M.** An epidemiological study of poisoning in northern Islamic Republic of Iran. Eastern Mediterranean Health Journal. 2002;**8**(1):88–94.
130. **Lim AY, Lee AR, Hatim A**, et al. Clinical and sociodemographic correlates of suicidality in patients with major depressive disorder from six Asian countries. BMC Psychiatry. 2014;**14**(1):1–8.
131. **Chen YY, Chien-Chang Wu K, Yousuf S, Yip PS.** Suicide in Asia: opportunities and challenges. Epidemiologic Reviews. 2012;**34**(1):129–44.
132. **Hendin H; World Health Organization**. *Suicide and Suicide Prevention in Asia*. Geneva: World Health Organization; 2008.
133. **Benatov J, Nakash O.** Religious-ethnic differences in prevalence and correlates of suicidal ideation and attempts among Israeli vocational education students. Israel Journal of Psychiatry and Related Sciences. 2016;**53**(3):40–6.
134. **Dorff EN.** End-of-life: Jewish perspectives. The Lancet. 2005;**366**(9488):862–5.
135. **Gvion Y, Levi-Belz Y, Apter A.** Suicide: the Jewish perspective. Crisis. 2014;**35**(3):141–4.
136. **Kaplan SJ, Schoeneberg LA.** Defining suicide: importance and implications for Judaism. Journal of Religion and Health. 1988;**27**(2):154–6.
137. **Baeke G, Wils JP, Broeckaert B.** 'We are (not) the master of our body': elderly Jewish women's attitudes towards euthanasia and assisted suicide. Ethnicity and Health. 2011;**16**(3):259–78.
138. **Jotkowitz AB, Glick S.** The Israeli terminally ill patient law of 2005. Journal of Palliative Care. 2009;**25**(4):284–8.

139. **Witztum E, Stein D.** Suicide in Judaism with a special emphasis on modern Israel. Religions. 2012;**3**(3):725–38.

140. **Ryn Z.** Suicides in the Nazi concentration camps. Suicide and Life-Threatening Behavior. 1986;**16**(4):419–33.

141. **DellaPergola S.** World Jewish population. In: **Arnold Dashefsky**, editor. *American Jewish Year Book 2019–2020*. University of Connecticut, Storrs, CT, USA, Ira M. Sheskin, University of Miami, Coral Gables, FL, USA, Cham: Springer; 2019. pp. 263–353.

142. **Bailey WT, Stein LB.** Jewish affiliation in relation to suicide rates. Psychological Reports. 1995;**76**(2):561–2.

143. **Levav I, Aisenberg E.** Suicide in Israel: crossnational comparisons. Acta Psychiatrica Scandinavica. 1989;**79**(5):468–73.

144. **World Health Organization**. *Suicide Worldwide in 2019: Global Health Estimates*. Geneva: World Health Organization; 2021.

145. **Nachman R, Yanai O, Goldin L, Swartz M, Barak Y, Hiss J.** Suicide in Israel: 1985–1997. Journal of Psychiatry and Neuroscience. 2002;**27**(6):423.

146. **Lubin G, Glasser S, Boyko V, Barell V.** Epidemiology of suicide in Israel: a nationwide population study. Social Psychiatry and Psychiatric Epidemiology. 2001;**36**(3):123–7.

147. **Burshtein S, Dohrenwend BP, Levav I, Werbeloff N, Davidson M, Weiser M.** Religiosity as a protective factor against suicidal behaviour. Acta Psychiatrica Scandinavica. 2016;**133**(6):481–8.

148. **Amit BH, Krivoy A, Mansbach-Kleinfeld I**, et al. Religiosity is a protective factor against self-injurious thoughts and behaviors in Jewish adolescents: findings from a nationally representative survey. European Psychiatry. 2014;**29**(8):509–13.

149. **Stein D, Brom D, Elizur A, Witztum E.** The association between attitudes toward suicide and suicidal ideation in adolescents. Acta Psychiatrica Scandinavica. 2007;**97**(3):195–201.

150. **Rasic D, Robinson JA, Bolton J, Bienvenu OJ, Sareen J.** Longitudinal relationships of religious worship attendance and spirituality with major depression, anxiety disorders, and suicidal ideation and attempts: findings from the Baltimore epidemiologic catchment area study. Journal of Psychiatric Research. 2011;**45**(6):848–54.

151. **Ponizovsky AM, Ritsner MS.** Suicide ideation among recent immigrants to Israel from the former Soviet Union: an epidemiological survey of prevalence and risk factors. Suicide and Life-Threatening Behavior. 1999;**29**(4):376–92.

152. **Apter A, Bleich A, King RA**, et al. Death without warning?: a clinical postmortem study of suicide in 43 Israeli adolescent males. Archives of General Psychiatry. 1993;**50**(2):138–42.

153. **Band M, Dein S, Loewenthal KM.** Religiosity, coping, and suicidality within the religious Zionist community of Israela thematic qualitative analysis. Mental Health, Religion and Culture. 2011;**14**(10):1031–47.

154. **Stein D, Asherov J, Lublinsky E**, et al. Sociodemographic factors associated with attempted suicide in two Israeli cities between 1990 and 1998. Journal of Nervous and Mental Disease. 2002;**190**(2):115–18.

155. **Kohn R, Levav I, Chang B, Halperin B, Zadka P.** Epidemiology of youth suicide in Israel. Journal of the American Academy of Child and Adolescent Psychiatry. 1997;**36**(11):1537–42.

156. **Shoval G, Schoen G, Vardi N, Zalsman G.** Suicide in Ethiopian immigrants in Israel: a case for study of the genetic-environmental relation in suicide. Archives of Suicide Research. 2007;**11**(3):247–53.
157. **Arieli A, Gilat I, Aycheh S.** Suicide among Ethiopian Jews: a survey conducted by means of a psychological autopsy. Journal of Nervous and Mental Disease. 1996;184(5):317–19.
158. **Ponizovsky A, Safro S, Ginath Y, Ritsner M.** Suicide ideation among recent immigrants: an epidemiological study. Israel Journal of Psychiatry and Related Sciences. 1997;**34**(2):139–48.
159. **Ratzoni G, Apter A, Blumensohn R, Tyano S.** Psychopathology and management of hospitalized Ethiopian immigrant adolescents in Israel. Journal of Adolescence. 1988;**11**(3):231–6.
160. **Barak Y, Aizenberg D, Szor H, Swartz M, Maor R, Knobler HY.** Increased suicidal risk amongst aging holocaust survivors. Annals of General Hospital Psychiatry. 2003;**2**(1):1.
161. **Neeleman J, Halpern D, Leon D, Lewis G.** Tolerance of suicide, religion and suicide rates: an ecological and individual study in 19 Western countries. Psychological Medicine. 1997;**27**(5):1165–71.
162. **Beck R.** Defensive versus existential religion: is religious defensiveness predictive of worldview defense? Journal of Psychology and Theology. 2006;**34**(2):142–52.
163. Whitley **Jr BE.** Religiosity and attitudes toward lesbians and gay men: a meta-analysis. International Journal for the Psychology of Religion. 2009;**19**(1):21–38.
164. **Galen LW, Kloet JD.** Mental well-being in the religious and the non-religious: evidence for a curvilinear relationship. Mental Health, Religion and Culture. 2011;**14**(7):673–89.
165. **Wulff DM.** *Psychology of Religion: Classic and Contemporary*, 2nd edition. Hamilton: Hamilton Printing; 1997.
166. **Caldwell-Harris CL.** Understanding atheism/non-belief as an expected individual-differences variable. Religion, Brain and Behavior. 2012;**2**(1):4–23.
167. **Dervic K, Carballo JJ, Baca-Garcia** E, et al. Moral or religious objections to suicide may protect against suicidal behavior in bipolar disorder. Journal of Clinical Psychiatry. 2011;**72**(10):1390–6.
168. **Dervic K, Oquendo MA, Grunebaum MF, Ellis S, Burke AK, Mann JJ.** Religious affiliation and suicide attempt. American Journal of Psychiatry. 2004;**161**(12):2303–8.
169. **Brunoni AR, Nunes MA, Lotufo PA, Benseñor IM.** Acute suicidal ideation in middle-aged adults from Brazil: results from the baseline data of the Brazilian Longitudinal Study of Adult Health (ELSA-Brasil). Psychiatry Research. 2015;**225**(3):556–62.
170. Cavalcanti MLV, Romera EJ. Life and death in Kardecist Spiritism. Religion and Society. 2006;**1**:1–15.
171. **Dezutter J, Soenens B, Luyckx K**, et al. The role of religion in death attitudes: distinguishing between religious belief and style of processing religious contents. Death Studies. 2008;**33**(1):73–92.
172. **Van Tubergen F, Te Grotenhuis M, Ultee W.** Denomination, religious context, and suicide: neo-Durkheimian multilevel explanations tested with individual and contextual data. American Journal of Sociology. 2005;**111**(3):797–823.

173. Moreira-**Almeida A, Koenig HG, Lucchetti G.** Clinical implications of spirituality to mental health: review of evidence and practical guidelines. Brazilian Journal of Psychiatry. 2014;**36**:176–82.

174. **Schafer RM, Handal PJ, Brawer PA, Ubinger M.** Training and education in religion/spirituality within APA-accredited clinical psychology programs: 8 years later. Journal of Religion and Health. 2011;**50**(2):232–9.

175. **Vieten C, Scammell S, Pilato R, Ammondson I, Pargament KI, Lukoff D.** Spiritual and religious competencies for psychologists. Psychology of Religion and Spirituality. 2013;**5**(3):129.

176. **Hodge DR.** Spirituality and people with mental illness: developing spiritual competency in assessment and intervention. Families in Society. 2004;**85**(1):36–44.

177. **Alonzo D, Gearing RE.** *Suicide Assessment and Treatment: Empirical and Evidence-Based Practices.* New York: Springer Publishing Company; 2017.

178. **Stack S, Laubepin F.** Religiousness as a predictor of suicide: an analysis of 162 European regions. Suicide and Life-Threatening Behavior. 2019;**49**(2):371–81.

179. **International Data Corporation** (2021). Smartphone shipments to grow 5.5% in 2021 driven by strong 5G push and pent-up demand.

180. **Torok M, Han J, Baker S,** et al. Suicide prevention using self-guided digital interventions: a systematic review and meta-analysis of randomised controlled trials. The Lancet Digital Health. 2020;**2**(1):e25–36.

181. **Goodman M, Tomas IA, Temes CM, Fitzmaurice GM, Aguirre BA, Zanarini MC.** Suicide attempts and self-injurious behaviours in adolescent and adult patients with borderline personality disorder. Personality and Mental Health. 2017;**11**(3):157–63.

182. **Hovey JD.** Acculturative stress, depression, and suicidal ideation in Mexican immigrants. Cultural Diversity and Ethnic Minority Psychology. 2000;**6**(2):134.

183. **Lijtmaer RM.** Splitting and nostalgia in recent immigrants: psychodynamic considerations. Journal of the American Academy of Psychoanalysis and Dynamic Psychiatry. 2001;**29**(3):427–38.

184. **Perreira KM, Ornelas I.** Painful passages: traumatic experiences and post-traumatic stress among US immigrant Latino adolescents and their primary caregivers. International Migration Review. 2013;**47**(4):976–1005.

185. Polanco-**Roman L, Miranda R.** Culturally related stress, hopelessness, and vulnerability to depressive symptoms and suicidal ideation in emerging adulthood. Behavioral Therapy. 2013;**44**(1):75–87.

186. **Revollo HW, Qureshi A, Collazos F, Valero S, Casas M.** Acculturative stress as a risk factor of depression and anxiety in the Latin American immigrant population. International Review of Psychiatry. 2011;**23**(1):84–92.

187. **Lara M, Gamboa C, Kahramanian MI, Morales LS, Hayes Bautista DE.** Acculturation and Latino health in the United States: a review of the literature and its sociopolitical context. Annual Review of Public Health. 2005;**26**:367–97.

188. **Finch BK, Vega WA.** Acculturation stress, social support, and self-rated health among Latinos in California. Journal of Immigrant Health. 2003;**5**(3):109–17.

189. **Yoo HC, Gee GC, Takeuchi D.** Discrimination and health among Asian American immigrants: disentangling racial from language discrimination. Social Science and Medicine. 2009;**68**(4):726–32.

Part 2

Suicidality, migrants and ethnic minorities

Chapter 8

Suicide among Asian migrants in Hong Kong: A case study

Anna Wong and Paul Yip

Introduction

Background

Asia both exports and hosts the highest number of international labour migrants, which are one of the fastest growing migrant populations in the world.[1] Migration is linked directly or indirectly to the quest for decent work opportunities.[2] For employment opportunities, international migration generally involves movement of people from low-income to high-income countries.[3] Asia will continue to play a major role in global migration patterns, with some variation in the short term. Evidence showed that more migrant women than non-migrant women (67% as compared to 50.8%, respectively) participate in the labour force, whereas for men, migrant and non-migrant rates are similar.[2] Also, they have experienced large increases in remittance flows in recent years.[4] Nowadays temporary labour migration has become a way of life in many outflow labour migration countries such as the Philippines and Indonesia. Much evidence showed that remittances did help improve the quality of life of labour migrants and their families, with a huge percentage going towards child education—essential for human capital formation. The emphasis is on economic contribution; however, the mental wellness of migrants has always been overlooked. Particularly, the suicide patterns and behaviour of the growing population of Asian migrants are not well understood.

This chapter examines the hypothesis that Asians who migrate and subsequently identify as ethnic minorities or migrants are at increased risk of suicide. The underlying assumption is that the challenges often experienced by ethnic minorities and migrants in the migration destination, together with the stigma rooted in the culture of their original country, make them more vulnerable to the risk of suicide. At the same time, there are studies providing evidence that migrants experience better health compared to people remaining in their country of origin. These contradictory findings have been attributed to a complex relationship between migration and migrant health, which is influenced by factors from population to individual levels.

Research and theories on migrants' well-being and suicide

Numerous international studies have been conducted and theories developed to explore and capture the complexity of the relationship between migration and migrants' well-being. However, due to lack of research conducted on suicides of Asian migrants, there is insufficient understanding to inform suicide prevention strategies for this group. To address this gap, this study draws on theories of migration and health, together with identification of risk and protective factors during migration and acculturation, to examine the case of suicide among Asian migrants in Hong Kong.

A widely recognized theory of migration and health is known as the healthy migrant effect, which proposes that a selection bias at migration favours healthier individuals, resulting in better health in migrants compared to the natives.[5,6] Further, since those who succeed in moving from one country to another tend to be the ones with stronger resilience and better resources to begin with, it follows that they would have greater ability to cope with the stress brought about by the migration process itself and life after migration. Although the healthy migrant effect has found support in some studies on migration in North American countries,[7,8] a systematic review of publications on European countries found that ethnic minority groups and migrants had poorer self-perceived health, even after controlling for age, gender, and socio-economic factors.[9] Further research on African, Asian, and European countries revealed mixed findings, with a more complex picture.[10,11,12] It is important to understand the complexity in order to develop more effective programmes to promote mental wellness among migrants.

These research studies looked beyond migration selection as the only influential health determinant and identified additional risk and protective factors in the place of destination that influenced physical health, mental health, and suicide risk among ethnic minorities and migrants. At the country level, several influential conditions have been identified as determinants of health gaps between ethnic minorities and migrants and the natives or majority population. These included the respective health status of the populations in the original and destination countries, as well as the destination country's health care system, inequalities in access to care, and social capital and social cohesion.[12] At the individual level, health determinants included language proficiency, living and working conditions, and the degree of integration and assimilation as reflected by the duration of stay and living outside an immigrant ethnic enclave.[13] Although these migration studies focused on physical health, research has found positive associations between physical illnesses and suicide risk.[14,15,16,17]

Mental disorder is another significant predictor of suicide.[18] Studies examining migrants' mental health have shown that migrants typically experience stress due to disconnection from the place of origin and acculturation in the destination country.[19] For migrants who become a socially and economically disadvantaged minority in the destination country, the stress can be all the more difficult to cope with. As with migration and physical health, the relationship between migration and mental health is also complex and varies according to a range of factors such as pre-migration planning and preparation,[20] financial and employment difficulties,[21,22] working conditions,[11] duration of residence,[23] degree of acculturation,[24] perceived discrimination,[25] and social isolation.[26] These are potential risk factors that threaten migrants' mental health and their capability to cope with the stress of migration, ultimately leading to a greater risk of suicide.

At the same time, migration can enhance migrants' mental health through improvement in certain life domains that motivated their move in the first place.[27,28] In addition, research studies have identified protective factors that moderate effects of migration stress on migrants' mental health. These beneficial conditions range from a better quality of life in the migration destination[29] and perceived social support from family, peers, and the neighbourhood[25,30,31] to individual factors such as success in goal-striving,[11] fulfilment of migration purpose,[21] social competence,[32] personal resilience, and family resilience.[33]

Many of these studies are based on existing theories and knowledge about suicide presented as part of a Westernized medical or mental health model. In contrast, cultural perspectives on suicide are equally important, if overlooked, in development of the field,[34] engaging a context-sensitive and in-depth approach to studying suicidal individuals in their specific cultural contexts. This approach offers new and crucial insight into suicidal patterns and behaviours of less studied populations and subgroups, while contributing to the overall study of suicide. A valuable contribution can be made by bringing in cultural perspectives to generate new knowledge about suicide among ethnic minorities and migrants in Asia.

In the current study, these conceptualizations and approaches to studying migration and its benefits and harms on individuals will be applied to lend insight into observed patterns of migrant suicides.

Hong Kong as a case study

Hong Kong, with a population of 7.3 million and a special administrative region (SAR) of China since 1997, as well as a former British colony, offers a unique case study for examining suicide of economically active immigrants from Asian countries as well as of internal migrants from mainland China. Although its population is predominantly Chinese, there has been a long history of non-Chinese and mainland-born Chinese migrants in Hong Kong. The proportion of non-Chinese migrants in Hong Kong has seen a steady rise from 5% (343,950) in 2001 to 8% (593,483) in 2016, whereas the total number of one-way permits granted to mainland-born Chinese for permanent settlement in Hong Kong has grown to beyond 1 million from 1997 to 2018.[35] One-way permit is an arrangement for migrants from the mainland who are usually the spouse and children of Hong Kong residents; a daily quota of 150 are allowed to enter Hong Kong, based on a quota system which was mutually agreed between Hong Kong SAR and the mainland government.[36] In the past two decades, the number of marriages between mainland and Hong Kong residents (mainly mainland brides and Hong Kong bridegrooms) have been increasing, accounting for nearly 40% of marriages registered in Hong Kong.[37] They represent the majority of one-way permit holders. Also, of non-Chinese migrants in Hong Kong, a vast majority come from the Philippines and Indonesia and are employed as foreign domestic workers (also known as domestic helpers). In contrast, mainland-born Chinese migrants are demographically more heterogeneous, taking on varied roles in the society. Foreign domestic helpers have played a significant role in Hong Kong community, especially in providing assistance to childcare and older adult support and housework for many Hong Kong families. It is estimated one in six households in Hong Kong has a foreign domestic helper. In 2020, there were nearly 400,000 foreign domestic helpers across 2.4 million households. Mainland-born Chinese migrants, despite being ethnically Chinese, are usually considered to be a socioculturally separate group from local-born Chinese.[22,38,39]

Foreign domestic workers and mainland-born Chinese migrants occupy unique positions in Hong Kong and Asia; yet there is currently a lack of research studies on their suicide patterns and behaviours. Therefore, an examination of suicide victims from these two migrant groups, including their characteristics and unique issues they face, is warranted.

This study

Taking Asian migrants in Hong Kong as a case study, suicide data were examined in detail to determine whether or not Asian migrants are at increased risk of suicide, and why. Firstly, the suicide rates of Filipino, Indonesian, and mainland-born Chinese migrants were compared to the general population in their host countries. Secondly, the economic, social, and mental health characteristics of migrant suicides were also presented. These findings were examined by using existing concepts of migration, mental health, and suicide, noting cultural particulars and deviations that emerged from the analysis to generate further insight into suicides among ethnic minorities and migrants in Asia beyond what was already known.

Methods

Data collection

This study utilized data compiled from the Hong Kong Coroner's Court Report on 15,534 suicide death records in 2002–17, 4498 (29.0%) of which were identified as Filipino, Indonesian, and mainland-born Chinese.[i] The study also drew on statistical data from the Hong Kong Government's population census and special reports, suicide statistics compiled by the World Health Organization (WHO), reports and news articles on issues faced by the migrant groups in question, and research findings from academic literature.

Characteristics of migrant groups

Filipino and Indonesian domestic workers

Filipino and Indonesian domestic workers make up more than half of ethnic minorities in Hong Kong. According to the population by-census published in 2016,[42] Filipinos and Indonesians constituted 31.5% and 26.2%, respectively, of the ethnic minority population, 99% of whom were female. Their numbers also saw a significant increase from 2006 by 71,628 to 184,081 among Filipinos, and from 65,459 to 153,299 among Indonesians.

A recent survey[43] estimated the economic contribution of the 385,000 foreign domestic workers in Hong Kong to be around USD12.6 billion in 2018, which was 3.6% of the gross domestic product (GDP). Their economic contribution has been calculated from care work for children, the elderly, and the disabled; domestic tasks such as cleaning, cooking, and washing; and enabling more mothers to join the labour force.

In sum, Filipino and Indonesian migrants are predominantly economic migrants who are female, of working age, and employed in the elementary occupation of domestic work. However, there are crucial differences between the two groups that have a significant impact on their respective suicide risks. Their similarities and differences would be explored in more detail.

---

[i] Of the 4498 suicides, six Filipino and three Indonesian male migrants were excluded from analysis and discussion.

Mainland-born Chinese migrants

Most mainland-born Chinese migrants living in Hong Kong today are no longer 'new arrivals', as they were once commonly called. The largest subgroup consists of those who have resided in Hong Kong for over 10 years. Yet, there is still a prevalent attitude towards mainland-born Chinese that is driven not only by differences in sociocultural values and practices between locals and migrants, but also by the locals' dissatisfaction and resentment of the way Hong Kong has been governed since becoming a part of mainland China after the handover of its sovereignty in 1997. A recent study showed that many Chinese migrants are still experiencing neighbourhood discrimination in the forms of social distance and avoidance.[22] Further, mainland-born Chinese migrants are often perceived as increasing strains on the society and competing for essential resources such as schooling, housing, and health care.[38,39]

Mainland-born Chinese migrants can apply for permanent residence in Hong Kong through several means. The most common is through the one-way permit scheme, which primarily grants spouses in a cross-border marriage or members of a cross-border family permanent residence in Hong Kong for the purpose of family reunion. The average waiting time to entering into Hong Kong is about three years and it was much longer a decade ago. Due to the unique nature of the scheme, female migrants far outnumber male migrants. Female and male migrants differ in their characteristics and suicide risks, therefore warranting examination as two separate groups.

Results

Comparison of suicide rates of Filipino, Indonesian, and mainland-born Chinese migrants in Hong Kong to suicide rates in countries of origin

According to age-standardized estimates provided by WHO,[43] China has the highest suicide rate of the three countries, at 8.0 suicides per 100,000 persons. Suicide rates are lower in the Philippines and Indonesia, both at 3.7 per 100,000. Comparing these figures to age-standardized suicide rates of the three ethnic groups in Hong Kong (per 100,000 person-years, across 2002–17) (see Figure 8.1), suicide rates among both mainland-born Chinese and Filipinos are lower in Hong Kong than in their countries of origin. In other words, Chinese and Filipino migrants have lower suicide rates than Chinese and Filipino natives who did not migrate to Hong Kong. Conversely, suicide rates among Indonesian migrants are higher than among the natives in Indonesia. Table 8.1 presents a breakdown of age-standardized suicide rates among migrant groups and local populations according to sex.

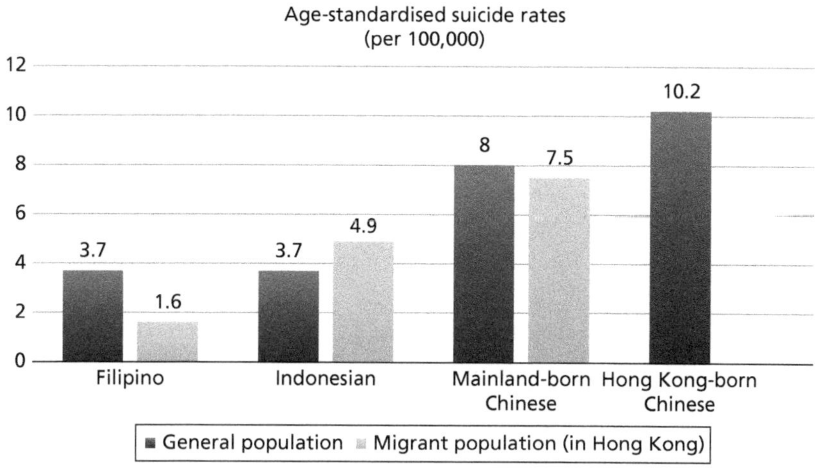

Figure 8.1 Estimated age-standardized suicide rates among Filipino, Indonesian, and mainland-born Chinese in the general population in their respective place of origin compared to migrant populations in Hong Kong.

Table 8.1 Estimated age-standardized suicide rates per 100,000 person-years according to sex in Filipino, Indonesian, mainland-born Chinese, and Hong Kong-born Chinese

Ethnicity	Sex	Age-standardized suicide rate in place of origin, 2016^	Age-standardized suicide rate[ii] (and number) in Hong Kong, 2002–17*	Difference from place of origin
Filipino	Female	2.3	1.6 (44)	–32%
Indonesian	Female	2.2	4.9 (51)	121%
Mainland-born Chinese	Female	8.3	5.6 (1762)	–33%
	Male	7.9	9.8 (2632)	25%
Hong Kong-born Chinese	Female	n/a	7.0 (2580)	n/a
	Male	n/a	13.5 (4922)	n/a

^ Figures extracted from WHO (2018).[43]

* Population sizes by age group and ethnicity are from HK Census 2001, 2006, 2011, and 2016. Linear interpolation is used to calculate values for missing years between 2001 and 2016; 2017 figures are estimated by fitting a linear trend to 2011 and 2016 figures.

ii Age-standardized rates are calculated by multiplying the age-specific crude rates by the age-specific WHO weights, divided by the sum of all weights.

As mentioned, Filipino and Indonesian migrants in Hong Kong are predominantly working-age females employed as domestic workers, whereas mainland-born Chinese migrants are a more heterogeneous group. Comparing Filipino and Indonesian females in the countries of origin with female migrants in Hong Kong, both the decrease (32%) and increase (121%) in suicide rates among Filipinos and Indonesians, respectively, are notable and worth examining for their underlying reasons. The breakdown also shows that female Chinese migrants in Hong Kong, in fact, had a 33% lower suicide rate than females in mainland China. However, the suicide rate of male Chinese migrants was 25% higher than that of males in the general population back home. This gender difference, in addition to effects that migration has on both male and female migrants, also warrants further examination.

Discussion

Initial findings partially support the healthy migrant effect theory. Filipino and mainland-born Chinese women seemingly have better chances of survival against suicide as migrants in Hong Kong, lending support to the theory. However, Indonesian women and mainland-born Chinese men both appear more vulnerable to suicide as migrants, thus representing a contradiction to the theory of healthy migrant effect. This reinforces the notion of one size does not fit all. To gain more insight into their differing patterns, further examination of migration-related risk and protective conditions, together with cultural perspectives on suicide of these subgroups, was conducted.

Female domestic workers from the Philippines

Prior to obtaining a contract and work visa in Hong Kong, domestic helpers are required to submit a valid medical certificate to demonstrate that they are physically and psychologically fit for employment as a domestic worker.[35] This requirement provides support for a positive selection bias, according to the healthy migrant theory. There is also evidence that they generally maintain a healthy lifestyle in Hong Kong, as characterized by a satisfactory diet and low rates of alcohol, nicotine, and coffee consumption. However, once living and working in Hong Kong, domestic helpers encounter various conditions that may adversely or positively affect their mental health. An early study by Bagley *et al.* identified two types of Filipino domestic workers who had particularly poor mental health. One group had employment-related issues, whereas the other group was confronted with debt and family issues.

Despite having a stable income, work conditions for a domestic worker can nevertheless be challenging. Long working hours and having nowhere to escape are common features of their compulsory lived-in arrangement.[43] Accounts of conflict and abuse have also emerged from local research studies; yet domestic workers tend not to report them for fear of losing their job and the chance to work in Hong Kong.[44,45] This refusal to report abuse was found to be associated with increased depression.[45] Suicide data on Filipino female suicides in Hong Kong show that 18.2% and 2.3% were documented with work-related problem and abuse, respectively. However, issues such as conflict and abuse are likely to be underreported by employers.

Poverty and lack of job opportunity at home are common push factors for Filipinos to work abroad as domestic workers.[46] Suicide data reveal that 43.2% of female Filipino suicide victims were documented to have financial issues. Research shows that having serious financial problems is associated with a higher risk of suicide.[47] Local studies also show that debt is a common financial problem encountered by Filipino domestic workers in Hong Kong, which causes them significant mental distress. A recent survey found that 83% of foreign domestic workers interviewed reported being in debt; yet access to formal financial services is very limited for domestic helpers in Hong Kong due to inadequate knowledge or ineligibility. As a result, they resort to borrowing from family, friends, employers, or agencies and loan sharks, taking on average 19 months to clear the debt (Experian and Enrich, 2019).[41]

Bagley *et al.*[44] found that the same group of Filipinos affected by debt were also affected by the stress of separation from family and worrying about their well-being.[47] Yet, fulfilling the purpose of financially supporting the family back home, improving their quality of life and their children's chances of upward social mobility, can be a strong motivation for domestic workers to overcome their struggles.[48] Taken together, the harms and benefits of working to pay off debts and to sustain their family back home may be highly dependent on individual financial and familial situations. However, a resilient family would likely function as a protective factor that improves their chances of coping with distress.[46]

Finally, social connectedness was found to be a major protective factor among Filipinos domestic workers, being associated with a low risk of depression.[44] Such positive social connections are characterized by firm ties with friends and religious organizations in Hong Kong, knowing the local language (Cantonese Chinese), and having satisfactory visits to the Philippines. Sunday gatherings also function as group counselling sessions where Filipino domestic workers can find comfort and release by sharing their problems with one another. Filipino migrant workers also relied greatly on Christian churches for practical help and social support, more so than they did on non-governmental organizations (NGOs) and governmental institutions.[49] This may be because the majority of Filipino domestic helpers attend church every Sunday, and as a result of their frequent gathering, the trust and rapport developed between them and the church community increased their willingness to seek social, emotional, and spiritual support when needed.

In summary, a combination of good health at the beginning of migration, maintenance of a healthy lifestyle, a clear sense of purpose, and being hopeful of improving the quality of life and life chance of their children at home, together with generally favourable conditions that nurture their social connectedness in Hong Kong appear to have strengthened Filipino domestic helpers' resilience against distress caused by work conditions, family separation, and financial difficulties. Therefore, the balance tipping towards the benefits of migration seems to contribute to their reduced suicide risk as migrants in Hong Kong.

Female domestic workers from Indonesia

Indonesian domestic workers share many characteristics with their Filipino counterparts due to their similar job nature and economic migrant status. For example, similar to Filipino domestic workers, Indonesian domestic workers regularly make remittances to their home country, making a large contribution to the economy. They also have the benefit of social support from fellow domestic workers whom they meet regularly on Sundays and with whom they also share a variety of activities organized by the community, as well as by the Indonesian Consulate.[50] Yet, unlike suicide rates among Filipino domestic workers, suicide rates among Indonesian domestic workers are much higher than those of the general population in Indonesia. Therefore, conditions that differ between the two groups of domestic workers warrant further examination.

According to suicide data, as many as 27.5% of Indonesian suicides were documented to be related with work issues, a much higher percentage compared with Filipino suicides. A survey of more than 3000 foreign domestic workers in Hong Kong was conducted by a local NGO,[43] revealing that 72% of Indonesian domestic workers had experienced verbal abuse by their employer, compared to 37% of Filipino domestic workers; 15% and 6% of Indonesian domestic workers also reported physical and sexual abuse by their employer, respectively.

One of the fundamental differences between the two groups of domestic workers lies in the degree to which their recruitment system is monitored and regulated by the labour-sending and receiving governments to protect domestic workers from all kinds of exploitation. Compared to Filipino workers, Indonesian domestic workers in Hong Kong receive much less protection from their government in the recruitment and employment process. Amnesty International[51] published a report that identified treatment of Indonesian domestic workers that amounted to human trafficking, exploitation, and forced labour, condemning both Indonesian and Hong Kong governments for their failures to take adequate legal action to protect the workers. Several factors contribute to the continuation of these practices, but the most crucial one that puts Indonesian workers at severe disadvantage is compulsory use of poorly regulated recruitment agencies. A range of practices are employed by these agencies that make it very difficult for Indonesian domestic workers to terminate their contracts such as charging exorbitant fees for training and other services that would take workers many months to pay off, and then using debt and the two-week rule[iii] to pressure workers into completing the contract, even if they were subjected to threatening and abusive behaviour from the employer.

Shortly after Amnesty International's report was published, the shocking case of Erwiana Sulistyaningsih became internationally known as she escaped from an abusive employer in Hong Kong, who was eventually sentenced to a six-year imprisonment. The high-profile case caused many more domestic workers to speak up about their experiences, exposing the prevalence and seriousness of their plight.[52] Strikingly, suicide data on female Indonesian suicide victims revealed that none were documented with issues of abuse. Noting the limitation of sample size, the finding still brings into question the extent of underreporting abuse among Indonesian suicide victims.

Another factor that makes Indonesian domestic workers more vulnerable than their Filipino counterparts is their lower proficiency in English and Cantonese.[53] This language barrier can make day-to-day communication, acculturation, and help-seeking when in need much more difficult for Indonesian domestic workers.

Finally, restraint from suicide is strictly observed in Islamic cultures, which may explain the low suicide rate in Indonesia. The degree of stigma around suicide is reflected in the Muslim community's reluctance to carry out religious rites such as prayer and burial for any deceased who died by suicide.[54] In some places, following a person's suicide death, a cleansing ceremony has to be conducted by the family and relatives, even people from the same village, to avoid negative consequences on the community (p. 18).[55] The strong stigmatization of suicide has been accredited with a deterrent effect on suicide attempt; yet suicide criminalization may also push the vulnerable into making more fatal attempts.[56] Further studies are needed to determine whether Indonesian domestic workers would feel equally inhibited about killing themselves while living abroad, away from family, relatives, and the usual community.

[iii] According to the terms of employment, domestic helpers are required to leave Hong Kong within two weeks of the end or termination of their employment contracts, unless they find another employer (available from: https://web.archive.org/web/20080409204616/http://www.immd.gov.hk/ehtml/ID%28E%29989.htm).

In summary, due to weaknesses in the recruitment, support, and employment system, Indonesian domestic workers are vulnerable to negative work conditions that directly threaten their finances, health, and safety. The language barrier also weakens any support system that might be available and accessible for those who speak English or Chinese more proficiently. Despite the availability of peer social support and increased societal awareness of their plight, the harms of migration seem to have increased their risk of suicide as migrants in Hong Kong.

Female migrants from mainland China

As mentioned, recipients of the one-way permit consist of a large proportion of female spouses in cross-border marriages to local Chinese men. In 2006, the male-to-female ratio of new arrivals, who had resided in Hong Kong for less than seven years, was 443:1000, compared to 911:1000 of the general population.[57] A similar ratio was observed in 2016.[58] The healthy migrant effect among the female migrants may, to some extent, be related to marriage selection, assuming health is a quality that increases the likelihood of being selected for cross-border marriage.

On the other hand, a cross-border marriage is not without its challenges, which threaten the well-being of female migrants. For example, cross-border marriage has been heavily stigmatized in the Hong Kong society.[59,60] However, research suggests that financial stress has the most significant influence on cross-border marriages. Men involved in cross-border marriages were found to be lower in socio-economic status, as defined by median monthly income, unskilled work, and education.[61,62] Financial stress reported by cross-border couples was found to be significantly higher compared to local couples, resulting in more frequent marital conflict.[63] Suicide data show that 44.9% and 1.5% of female Chinese migrant victims resided in public housing and subdivided flats, respectively, and as high as 32.3% were documented with family issues. Research also shows that compared to local women, migrant women are more vulnerable to spousal violence and be more socially isolated.[61] Taken together, social and economic conditions can significantly affect marital lives and well-being of female migrants.

Until recently, the relative affluence of Hong Kong, compared to mainland China was one of the reasons that made cross-border marriage attractive to mainlanders.[61] Many cross-border marriages led to the mainland-born spouse's improved economic status (e.g. absolute income), as well as to access to better resources such as the more developed health care and education systems in Hong Kong. For spouses with children, these conditions are all the more important. It is still very much part of the Chinese culture to place high expectations on parents to provide the child with the best resources possible. Likewise, high expectations are placed on the child to excel in education, particularly in academic achievement, as it represents to Chinese parents the passage to a better future.[64] Therefore, sustaining the well-being of family members becomes a strong motivation for the women to survive. A local study has shown that having a dependent and having concern for family members prevented at-risk Chinese migrant women from attempting suicide.[65]

In summary, despite a number of adverse conditions faced by mainland-born female migrants, they appear to be ameliorated by protective factors and conditions as well. Being healthier and more resilient to begin with may have helped them cope with financial stress, a lower socio-economic status compared to the general population in Hong Kong, and the locals' discriminatory attitudes. A cultural perspective highlighted the importance of having access to better health care and education resources in Hong Kong, as securing the well-being and a better future of their offspring appears to be a life purpose that not only sustains the children, but also the migrant women themselves. Together, these protective factors and conditions may have improved mainland-born Chinese migrant women's chances of survival against suicide, resulting in a lower suicide rate compared to the female population in China.

Male migrants from mainland China

Mainland Chinese male migrants defied the healthy migrant theory and presented a contrasting picture to their female migrant counterparts. The finding is in line with a study of migrants in a Chinese city near Hong Kong, which found that being male is independently associated with poor mental health.[11] Similarly, a study of internal migrants and locals in a Shanghai district found that physical illnesses, psychological issues, and interpersonal problems were frequently cited in suicide notes as reasons for suicide.[66] Yet migrants were less likely to correlate their suicides with physical illnesses, which implies that psychosocial factors could be more influential to the suicide of Chinese migrants. Unlike female Chinese migrants, who have a degree of financial security in terms of having a working husband and a place of abode in Hong Kong, male migrants face higher pressure in financially sustaining themselves and their dependants. The expectations on men to be financially independent and the main provider are still prevalent in Chinese societies.[67] Economic determinants, such as unemployment and household income, are significantly associated with mainland-born Chinese migrants' quality of life.[68] According to our suicide data, 22.9% of male Chinese migrants who died by suicide were unemployed and over half (52.7%) had a median monthly income below the poverty line of $4000.

Distress may also arise among Chinese male migrants who are confronted with inequality and perceived discrimination in employment. There is evidence that previously earned skills, qualifications, and work experience of mainland-born Chinese migrants were treated as invalid or irrelevant in Hong Kong.[22] According to a government report,[69] 34% of Chinese migrants were employed in elementary occupations and 31% as service and shop sales workers. The proportion employed as managers and administrators was 9%, much lower than the 30% in the general population. This pattern is reflected in our suicide data, which show that the most common full-time occupations of mainland-born Chinese male were either at the elementary level, namely technician and security guard, or classified as self-employment.[iv]

Due to reasons such as differences in economic structures between Hong Kong and mainland China, and the lack of certification of professional qualifications gained in mainland China, a pattern of downward mobility and lowering of social status was observed among mainland-born Chinese migrants who previously held managerial positions or worked as a professional.[22] In addition, those with a high socio-economic status in mainland China and who aimed to have better quality of life post-migration may find that the socio-economic reality falls short of their expectations, thereby lowering their life satisfaction and psychological well-being. Research shows that this expectation–reality discrepancy could lead to worsening of mental health.[11] More studies are needed to understand male migrants' experiences of goal-striving in Hong Kong, what their expectations were for the migration and how they have played out, and the subsequent impact these conditions have had on their well-being.

Local research studies have shown that perceived availability of social support when needed predicted improved quality of life among depressed Chinese migrants[69] and can ameliorate the effect of perceived discrimination on depressive symptoms.[25] Therefore, functional family and social relations would play an important in protecting male migrants' mental health. Suicide data show that 10.7% of mainland-born male suicide victims were divorced or separated[v] and 26.4% experienced family issues. In Hong Kong, long working hours have been shown to have a negative impact on family relations[70] and are likely to reduce male migrants' opportunities to develop and benefit from social and community connections outside the workplace.

[iv] For 172 of 461 male suicide cases who were classified as employed in the suicide data, no occupation information was available.

[v] Divorce rate in China has risen from 0.96 divorces per 1000 people in 2000 to 3.2 divorces in 2018 (an increase from 9.6% to 32%).

All in all, mainland-born male migrants may be healthier and better resourced at the beginning of migration, but their subsequent work and social lives can be challenging. In Hong Kong, male migrants' opportunities in finding appropriate and satisfying work may be more difficult than expected and long working hours can also have a negative impact on their family and social lives. In traditional Chinese cultures, financial pressure can be perceived as even more stressful for men. Although individual differences in protective factors, such as good socio-economic status, family functioning, and a realistic expectation of life after migration, could lead to differential mental health outcomes, by and large the harmful effects of migration on male Chinese migrants appear to have outweighed the beneficial effects, making the migrants more vulnerable to suicide compared to the general population in mainland China. Their help-seeking behaviours have much room for improvement. Seeking help seems to be a sign of weakness.

Mental health status and help-seeking among Asian migrants in Hong Kong

Generally speaking, Asian migrants bring with them a lack of mental health awareness and perceived stigma around such issues as mental illness and suicidal behaviour. Yet the health care system and social environment in which they find themselves are also not conducive to help-seeking for mental health and suicidal problems. In Hong Kong, mental health care services are underutilized[71] and issues of mental health literacy and stigma are common among the general population.[72,73] Against this backdrop, studies have found insufficient support and incentives for domestic workers to seek professional help for medical issues,[74] much less for mental disorders and suicidal behaviour, which remain to be social and religious taboos in the Philippines and Indonesia.[55,75] Yet, Filipino and Indonesian domestic workers may be more vulnerable than local women of similar age to having acute and transient psychiatric disorders.[76] Suicide data show that 6% of Filipino and 13% of Indonesian suicide victims were diagnosed with psychiatric problem(s) at the time of death. The figures may be underreported due to underutilization of mental health care services. Common reasons for Filipino domestic workers not seeking medical help from a doctor or clinic include not perceiving a need and inability to afford or find the right doctor.[77]

By comparison, a higher percentage (33.8%) of mainland-born Chinese suicide cases were diagnosed with psychiatric problem(s) at the time of death, which may be due to mainland-born Chinese having less of a language barrier in accessing social and health care services. However, there is a general reluctance among the Chinese to seek professional help for mental health problems, preferring to seek informal help from family or the internet instead.[78,79] Some of them have also developed the perception that medical staff would treat them differently if their non-local identity was revealed.[39] Thus, perceived discrimination may be a deterrent to Chinese migrants wanting to seek help.

Given the importance of mental health awareness and help-seeking in suicide prevention, better education in mental health knowledge and greater accessibility of help are needed for migrants, employers, and the community as a whole to make the whole system informed and proactive in suicide prevention.

Conclusion

By comparing the suicide rates of Asian migrants in Hong Kong with those of the general population in their respective countries of origin, mixed patterns have emerged, inviting further examination and analysis. To gain a more accurate picture of contributing factors to the differing suicide rates among ethnic minorities and migrants, the healthy migrant effect must be viewed together with the harms and benefits of migration on their post-migration lives. These have been described as risk and protective factors or conditions that can influence suicide patterns and behaviour and interpreted with the knowledge of both the original culture of the migrants as well as the sociocultural context of Hong Kong.

Work and financial conditions emerged as a group of important determinants. Debt was found to be a prevalent issue among Filipino and Indonesian domestic workers, and abuse was a particularly serious problem affecting many Indonesian domestic workers. Low socio-economic status and financial stress affected many Chinese migrant women in cross-border marriages, whereas finding employment and job opportunities that matched one's expectations were most challenging for male Chinese migrants. For both male and female migrants from mainland China, downward mobility and lowering of social status in Hong Kong could contribute to negative life satisfaction, especially if post-migration reality is worse than anticipated.

On the other hand, migrating from a more to less deprived place socio-economically may also reflect migrants' determination and ability to survive these hardships for a better life. Their goal-striving and hopes may constitute protective factors that reduce suicide risk. A strong theme that emerged from this study was female migrants enduring hardship for the well-being of their family and their children's future. The case study of Hong Kong revealed that traditional family values are still being held in Asian countries and form a primary motivating force for many economic migrants. This endorsement of family values, which underlie many migrants' move and endurance of the immense stress it brings, is fundamental to self-determined behaviours that yield more adaptive outcomes for one's psychological well-being and mental health.[80] Having hope[81] and reasons for living[82] are important protective factors that prevent suicide, and these seem to be particularly evident among female migrants who have dependent family members to support. This observation of resilience among Asian migrants in Hong Kong may also provide an explanation for their lower suicide rate compared to the local-born population in Hong Kong. Further research is warranted to examine this phenomenon.

Social support emerged as another group of important determinants, especially for Filipino and Indonesian domestic workers who are separated from their families for long periods of time. From informal gathering to organized activities, there are abundant opportunities for domestic workers to reach out and find practical and social support. For Chinese migrants, the family is a more important source of support and motivation to live.

Some limitations of this study are noted. Suicide is likely to be underreported in Indonesia and the Philippines due to the stigma attached to it. Misclassification is also common.[83,84] By contrast, suicide data in Hong Kong are collected from a well-established system of reporting and documenting suicide and causes of mortality. Due to this discrepancy, accounting for real suicide figures would further increase the gap in suicide rates between the general population in the Philippines and the migrant population in Hong Kong, making the lower risk among Filipino migrants even more significant. Conversely, the significant gap between Indonesian nationals and migrants would be reduced. Therefore, it would be useful to conduct more extensive and in-depth research in countries where the reporting system is less well established, to gain a better understanding of the prevalence and associations between common risk and protective factors, cultural attitudes to suicide and help-seeking, and suicidality among the general population, as well as among the migrants they export.

Relatively little research has been conducted on the experience of male Chinese migrants in Hong Kong, despite research finding that being male is independently associated with poor mental health among Chinese migrants.[11] Studies in Hong Kong that included both genders also tended to recruit a low percentage of male participants, weakening the generalizability of findings. Therefore, more research to examine the experience of male migrants in Hong Kong and the effects on their suicidality is warranted.

As a global phenomenon, suicide is not just a problem of populated regions or powerful groups. Further, as the Hong Kong case study has illustrated, most societies are increasingly multicultural, making it unlikely for suicide knowledge about the majority to also be representative of the minorities living in the same society. This study has extended the current understanding about suicide among Asian migrants and provided an overview of differential ways in which migration factors and conditions are influential to four migrant groups in Hong Kong. Future research should address the gaps identified in this study and generate the insight needed to inform suicide prevention strategies for the large and growing population of Asian ethnic minorities and migrants.

References

1. **United Nations, Department of Economic and Social Affairs, Population Division** (2017). International Migration Report 2017: highlights (ST/ESA/SER.A/404). Available from: https://www.un.org/en/development/desa/population/migration/publications/migrationreport/docs/MigrationReport2017_Highlights.pdf
2. **International Labour Organization** (2017). *World Employment and Social Outlook: Trends for Women 2017.*
3. **Jain PC, Oommen GZ** (2015). *South Asian Migration to Gulf Countries: History, Policies, Development.* Routledge.
4. **Wickramasekara P.** Labour migration in South Asia: a review of issues, policies and practices. International Migration Working Paper. 2011;**108**.
5. **Guillot M, Khlat M, Elo I, Solignac M, Wallace M.** Understanding age variations in the migrant mortality advantage: an international comparative perspective. PLoS One. 2018;**13**(6).
6. **Kennedy S, Kidd MP, McDonald JT, Biddle N.** The healthy immigrant effect: patterns and evidence from four countries. Journal of International Migration and Integration. 2015;**16**(2):317–22.
7. **Abraido-Lanza AF, Dohrenwend BP, Ng-Mak DS, Turner JB.** The Latino mortality paradox: a test of the 'salmon bias' and healthy migrant hypotheses. American Journal of Public Health. 1999;**89**(10):1543–8.
8. **McDonald JT, Kennedy S.** Insights into the 'healthy immigrant effect': health status and health service use of immigrants to Canada. Social Science and Medicine. 2004;**59**(8):1613–27.
9. **Nielsen SS, Krasnik A.** Poorer self-perceived health among migrants and ethnic minorities versus the majority population in Europe: a systematic review. International Journal of Public Health. 2010;**55**(5):357–71.
10. **Ginsburg C, Bocquier P, Béguy D**, et al. Healthy or unhealthy migrants? Identifying internal migration effects on mortality in Africa using health and demographic surveillance systems of the INDEPTH network. Social Science and Medicine. 2016;**164**:59–73.
11. **Li J, Chang SS, Yip PS**, et al. Mental wellbeing amongst younger and older migrant workers in comparison to their urban counterparts in Guangzhou city, China: a cross-sectional study. BMC Public Health. 2014;**14**(1):1280.
12. **Moullan Y, Jusot F.** Why is the 'healthy immigrant effect' different between European countries? European Journal of Public Health. 2014;**24**(suppl 1):80–6.
14. **Ahmedani BK, Peterson EL, Hu Y**, et al. Major physical health conditions and risk of suicide. American Journal of Preventive Medicine. 2017;**53**(3):308–15.

15. **Conwell Y, Duberstein PR, Hirsch JK, Conner KR, Eberly S, Caine ED.** Health status and suicide in the second half of life. International Journal of Geriatric Psychiatry. 2010;**25**(4):371–9.
16. **Fairweather AK, Anstey KJ, Rodgers B, Butterworth P.** Factors distinguishing suicide attempters from suicide ideators in a community sample: social issues and physical health problems. Psychological Medicine. 2006;**36**(9):1235–45.
17. **MacLean J, Kinley DJ, Jacobi F, Bolton JM, Sareen J.** The relationship between physical conditions and suicidal behavior among those with mood disorders. Journal of Affective Disorders. 2011;**130**(1–2):245–50.
18. **Nock MK, Hwang I, Sampson NA, Kessler RC.** Mental disorders, comorbidity and suicidal behavior: results from the National Comorbidity Survey Replication. Molecular Psychiatry. 2010;**15**(8):868–76.
19. **Dow HD.** An overview of stressors faced by immigrants and refugees: a guide for mental health practitioners. Home Health Care Management and Practice. 2011;**23**(3):210–17.
20. **Chou KL, Wong WK, Chow NW.** Interaction between pre- and post-migration factors on depressive symptoms in new migrants to Hong Kong from Mainland China. Community Mental Health Journal. 2011;**47**(5):560–67.
21. **Wong DFK, Song HX.** The resilience of migrant workers in Shanghai China: the roles of migration stress and meaning of migration. International Journal of Social Psychiatry. 2008;**54**(2):131–43.
22. **Lee WKM.** Ethnic and gender relations in Hong Kong: the work experiences of recent Mainland Chinese immigrant women. Asian and Pacific Migration Journal. 2004;**13**(2):233–53.
23. **Kwan YK, Ip WC.** Suicidality and migration among adolescents in Hong Kong. Death Studies. 2007;**31**(1):45–66.
24. **Bhugra D.** Migration and depression. Acta Psychiatrica Scandinavica. 2003;**108**:67–72.
25. **Chou KL.** Perceived discrimination and depression among new migrants to Hong Kong: the moderating role of social support and neighborhood collective efficacy. Journal of Affective Disorders. 2012;**138**(1–2):63–70.
26. **Chung IW, Caine ED, Barron CT, Badaracco MA.** Clinical and psychosocial profiles of Asian immigrants who repeatedly attempt suicide. Crisis. 2015.
27. **Finch BK, Frank R, Vega WA.** Acculturation and acculturation stress: a social–epidemiological approach to Mexican migrant farmworkers' health 1. International Migration Review. 2004;**38**(1):236–62.
28. **Bhugra D, Gupta S, Bhui K,** et al. WPA guidance on mental health and mental health care in migrants. World Psychiatry. 2011;**10**(1):2–10.
29. **Stillman S, McKenzie D, Gibson J** (2007). *Migration and Mental Health: Evidence from a Natural Experiment*. The World Bank.
30. **Mirsky J.** Mental health implications of migration. Social Psychiatry and Psychiatric Epidemiology. 2009;**44**(3):179.
32. **Wong DFK, Yan P, Lo E, Hung M.** Mental health and social competence of mainland Chinese immigrant and local youth in Hong Kong: a comparison. Journal of Ethnic and Cultural Diversity in Social Work. 2003;**12**(1):85–110.

33. **Yu X, Stewart SM, Liu IK, Lam TH.** Resilience and depressive symptoms in mainland Chinese immigrants to Hong Kong. Social Psychiatry and Psychiatric Epidemiology. 2014;**49**(2):241–9.
34. **Hjelmeland H.** Cultural research in suicidology: challenges and opportunities. Suicidology Online. 2010;**1**(1):34–52.
35. **Hong Kong Special Administrative Region** (2019). LCQ1: operation of one-way permits scheme. Press releases. Available from:https://www.info.gov.hk/gia/general/201903/20/P2019032000536.htm
37. **Chen M, Yip P.** Remarriages and transnational marriages in Hong Kong: implications and challenges. Journal of Ethnic and Migration Studies. 2020;**46**(14):3059–77.
38. **Chen J, Xu D, Wu X.** Seeking help for mental health problems in Hong Kong: the role of family. Administration and Policy in Mental Health and Mental Health Services Research. 2019;**46**(2):220–37.
39. **RTHK** (2019). HK becoming ever more hostile to new migrants. RTHK.hk English News. Available from: https://news.rthk.hk/rthk/en/component/k2/1441355-20190203.htm
40. **Hong Kong Special Administrative Region** (2016). Hong Kong 2016 population by-census thematic report: ethnic minorities. Available fromhttps://www.bycensus2016.gov.hk/data/16bc-ethnic-minorities.pdf
41. **Experian and Enrich** (2019). Key contributions of migrant domestic workers to economic growth and family well-being in Asia. The value of care: full report. Available from: https://enrichhk.org/sites/default/files/2019-09/Final_The-Value-of-Care_Full-Report.pdf
42. **World Health Organization** (2018). Suicide rate estimates, age-standardized estimates by country. Global Health Observatory data repository. Available from:https://apps.who.int/gho/data/view.main.MHSUICIDEASDRv?lang=en
43. **Mission for Migrant Workers** (2013). Live-in policy increases female FDW's vulnerability to various types of abuse. Available from:https://issuu.com/mfmw/docs/primer_live-in_english
44. **Bagley C, Madrid S, Bolitho F.** Stress factors and mental health adjustment of Filipino domestic workers in Hong Kong. International Social Work. 1997;**40**(4):373–82.
45. **Cheung JTK, Tsoi VWY, Wong KHK, Chung RY.** Abuse and depression among Filipino foreign domestic helpers. A cross-sectional survey in Hong Kong. Public Health. 2019;**166**:121–7.
46. **Garabiles MR, Ofreneo MAP, Hall BJ.** Towards a model of resilience for transnational families of Filipina domestic workers. PLoS One. 2017;**12**(8):e0183703.
47. **Wang Y, Sareen J, Afifi TO, Bolton SL, Johnson EA, Bolton JM.** Recent stressful life events and suicide attempt. Psychiatric Annals. 2012;**42**(3):101–8.
48. **Cruz RS.** Figures of migration gender, kinship, and the politics of representation. Philippine Studies: Historical and Ethnographic Viewpoints. 2012;**60**(4):513–54.
49. **Nakonz J, Shik AWY.** And all your problems are gone: religious coping strategies among Philippine migrant workers in Hong Kong. Mental Health, Religion and Culture. 2009;**12**(1):25–38.
50. **Chor HK** (2016). Meanings of working abroad: Aastudy on Indonesian domestic workers in Hong Kong. Hong Kong Anthropologist, Vol. **8**. Available from: http://arts.cuhk.edu.hk/~ant/hka/documents/2016/HKA8_CHOR.pdf

51. **Amnesty International** (2013). Exploited for profit, failed by governments: Indonesian migrant domestic workers trafficked to Hong Kong. Available from:https://www.amnesty.org/download/Documents/12000/asa170292013en.pdf
52. **Liljas P** (2014). Hong Kong government could be sued over maid abuses, says top rights lawyer. TIME.com. Available from: https://time.com/1205/hong-kong-government-may-be-sued-over-maid-abuse/
53. **Lau C** (2015). Language and cultural barriers leave Hong Kong's Indonesian maids 'more vulnerable to abuse'. South China Morning Post. Available from: https://www.scmp.com/news/hong-kong/article/1710008/why-indonesian-helpers-are-victims-hong-kongs-most-horrific-abuse
54. **Allam H** (2018). Suicide is on the rise in the US, and Muslims aren't immune. BuzzFeed News. Available from: https://www.buzzfeednews.com/article/hannahallam/suicide-rate-rising-muslims-mental-health-stigma-haydar
55. **Octaria YC** (2008). *The Role of Health System in Suicide Prevention in Bali: Barriers and Possibilities*. MIH Thesis. Amsterdam: Royal Tropical Institute. Available from: https://bibalex.org/baifa/Attachment/Documents/192377.pdf
56. **Wu K, Cai Z, Chang Q, Chang S, Yip PSF, Chen Y.** Criminalization of suicide and suicide rates in the world. **(3/26/2020). Available at SSRN**: https://ssrn.com/abstract=3564402 or http://dx.doi.org/10.2139/ssrn.3564402
57. **Census and Statistics Department, HKSAR** (2007). Hong Kong 2006 population by-census thematic report: persons from the mainland having resided in Hong Kong for less than 7 years. Hong Kong SAR: Census and Statistics Department. Available from: https://www.censtatd.gov.hk/en/
58. **Census and Statistics Department, HKSAR** (2018). Hong Kong 2006 population by-census thematic report: persons from the mainland having resided in Hong Kong for less than 7 years. Hong Kong SAR: Census and Statistics Department. Available from: https://www.censtatd.gov.hk/en/
59. **Law YW, Chan M, Zhang H**, et al. Divorce in Hong Kong SAR, 1999–2011: a review of 1,208 family court cases. Journal of Divorce and Remarriage. 2019;**60**(5):389–403.
60. **Yip P, Chang SS, Law F, Tai L, Tang S, Chan M.** *A Study on the Phenomenon of Divorce in Hong Kong*. Hong Kong SAR: University of Hong Kong, Centre for Suicide Research and Prevention; 2014.
61. **Choi SY, Cheung YW, Cheung AK.** Social isolation and spousal violence: comparing female marriage migrants with local women. Journal of Marriage and Family. 2012;**74**(3):444–61.
62. **Census and Statistics Department, HKSAR.** *Hong Kong Residents with Spouses/ Children in the Mainland of China (Special Topics Report No. 22)*. Hong Kong SAR: Hong Kong SAR Government; 1999.
63. **Choi SY, Cheung AKL.** Dissimilar and disadvantaged: age discrepancy, financial stress, and marital conflict in cross-border marriages. Journal of Family Issues. 2017;**38**(18):2521–44.
64. **Zhou M, Kim S.** Community forces, social capital, and educational achievement: the case of supplementary education in the Chinese and Korean immigrant communities. Harvard Educational Review. 2006 Apr 1;76(1):1–29.
65. **Ling DC, Holroyd EA, Wong WC, Gray SA.** Handling emerging health needs among a migrant population: factors associated with suicide attempts and suicide ideation

among female street sex workers in Hong Kong. Clinical Effectiveness in Nursing. 2004;**8**(3–4):205–14.

66. **Li F.** *A Comparison Study of Suicides between the Locals and Internal Migrants in China*. PhD Thesis. Hong Kong SAR: University of Hong Kong; 2020.
67. **Choi SYP, Cheung FM,** editors. *Women and Girls in Hong Kong: Current Situations and Future Challenges*. Shatin: Hong Kong Institute of Asia-Pacific Studies, Chinese University of Hong Kong; 2012b.
68. **Wong WK, Chou KL, Chow NW.** Correlates of quality of life in new migrants to Hong Kong from mainland China. Social Indicators Research. 2012;**107**(2):373–91.
69. **Census and Statistics Department, HKSAR.** *Special Report No. 25 on New Arrivals from Mainland China*. Hong Kong SAR: Census and Statistics Department; 2000.
70. **Lau YK, Ma LJ, Wan PS, Wong TKY, Lai LY.** Work–family conflicts, family leisure activities, and family functioning in Hong Kong. International Employment Relations Review. 2012;**18**(1):82.
71. **Lam LCW, Wong CSM, Wang MJ,** et al. Prevalence, psychosocial correlates and service utilization of depressive and anxiety disorders in Hong Kong: the Hong Kong Mental Morbidity Survey (HKMMS). Social Psychiatry and Psychiatric Epidemiology. 2015;**50**(9):1379–88.
72. **Chung KF, Wong MC.** Experience of stigma among Chinese mental health patients in Hong Kong. Psychiatric Bulletin. 2004;**28**(12):451–4.
73. **Hong Kong Council of Social Services and Mental Health Association of Hong Kong.** *Public Attitudes towards Mental Health Patients in Hong Kong: A Follow-up Study over Two Years*. Hong Kong: Hong Kong Council of Social Services; 1996.
74. **Holroyd EA, Taylor-Piliae RE, Twinn SF.** Investigating Hong Kong's Filipino domestic workers' healthcare behavior, knowledge, beliefs and attitudes towards cervical cancer and cervical screening. Women and Health. 2003;**38**(1):69–82.
75. **Coronel R** (2019). There's something wrong with the way Filipinos talk about suicide. CNN Philippines. Available from: https://www.scribd.com/document/707045294/There-s-Something-Wrong-With-the-Way-Filipinos-Talk-About-Suicide
76. **Lau PW, Cheng JG, Chow DL, Ungvari GS, Leung CM.** Acute psychiatric disorders in foreign domestic workers in Hong Kong: a pilot study. International Journal of Social Psychiatry. 2009;**55**(6):569–76.
77. **Holroyd EA, Molassiotis A, Taylor-Pilliae RE.** Filipino domestic workers in Hong Kong: health related behaviors, health locus of control and social support. Women and Health. 2001;**33**(1–2):181–205.
78. **Chen J.** Seeking help for psychological distress in urban China. Journal of Community Psychology. 2012;**40**(3):319–41.
79. **Chen J, Li Z, Xu D, Wu X.** Effects of neighborhood discrimination towards mainland immigrants on mental health in Hong Kong. International Journal of Environmental Research and Public Health. 2019;**16**(6):1025.
80. **Deci EL, Ryan RM.** Self-determination theory: a macrotheory of human motivation, development, and health. Canadian Psychology/Psychologie Canadienne. 2008;**49**(3):182.
81. **Grewal PK, Porter JE.** Hope theory: a framework for understanding suicidal action. Death Studies. 2007;**31**(2):131–54.

82. **Linehan MM, Goodstein JL, Nielsen SL, Chiles JA.** Reasons for staying alive when you are thinking of killing yourself: the Reasons for Living Inventory. Journal of Consulting and Clinical Psychology. 1983;**51**(2):276.
83. **Acuna M.** Growing number of young Filipinos committing suicide: mental health experts say many cases might are likely not being reported. Union of Catholic Asian News; 2018. Available from: https://www.ucanews.com/news/growing-number-of-young-filipinos-committing-suicide/81759
84. **World Health Organization**. Preventing suicide: a global imperative. 2014. Available from: https://apps.who.int/iris/bitstream/handle/10665/131056/9789241564779-ger.pdf

Chapter 9

Suicide prevention in sub-Saharan Africa: Cultural considerations and opportunities to advance research and practice

Jason Bantjes, Elsie Breet, Ashraf Kagee, and Dan J. Stein

Introduction

Suicide prevention has received comparatively little attention in sub-Saharan Africa (SSA), despite growing global awareness of the need to expand suicide prevention research and practice in the global south and in low- and middle-income countries (LMICs), where two-thirds of the world's suicides occur.[1,2,3,4] There is widespread acceptance that suicide prevention research and practice should be context-sensitive and culturally appropriate;[5] mental health interventions developed in high-income Western industrialized, democratic countries are not always directly applicable or appropriate for use in the majority of the world.[6] There are rich examples of how culturally appropriate suicide prevention has been approached in diverse settings, including Sri Lanka,[7] Inuit communities in Arctic Canada,[8] and Ghana.[9] It is within this context that this chapter sets out to explore cultural considerations, contextual challenges, and opportunities for suicide prevention in SSA. We begin the chapter with a brief explanation of what defines SSA and critically discuss the utility of employing this geographical region as a unit of analysis in discussions about suicide prevention, as we have done in this chapter. This is followed by an overview of the epidemiology of suicide and suicide prevention practices in SSA. In the main body of the chapter, we identify examples of common cultural considerations and challenges for suicide prevention in the region. We conclude the chapter by proposing strategies which may be helpful in advancing culturally informed and context-sensitive suicide prevention research and practice in SSA. The strategies we propose are aligned with the core values and philosophy of the global mental health movement and the sustainable development goals.[10]

Sub-Saharan Africa

SSA is an indistinctly demarcated geographical region of the African continent, which is generally considered to consist of countries that are either fully or partially located south of the Sahara Desert. SSA consists of 43 countries in mainland Africa, and six island nations.[i] It is a vast, diverse, and culturally heterogeneous region. With a population of almost 1 billion people, SSA is home to 12% of the world's population.[11] The region is culturally and economically distinct from African countries north of the Sahara, although using the Sahara to divide Africa is somewhat arbitrary and the boundaries demarcating SSA have been redrawn on a number of occasions for political and economic reasons.[12,13]

The utility of conceptualizing the countries in this region as a distinct group has been contested. The concept of SSA has also been critiqued by scholars who consider it to be a relic of colonialism and entangled with racist ideas about skin colour, prejudices about 'primitive cultures', and a lack of technological sophistication.[12] It is argued that the ongoing use of the term 'sub-Saharan Africa' perpetuates unhelpful stereotypes which work against economic and human development on the continent. Many people in Africa reject regional labels altogether, and African-led institutions, such as the African Union and the African Development Bank, comprise all countries on the continent up to the Red Sea.[12] Nonetheless, it appears that countries in SSA share common features beyond their geographical proximity, which may make it useful to consider this region as a unit of analysis in discussions about strategies to promote economic growth, human development, and suicide prevention.

A number of countries in SSA are endowed with rich mineral resources, and many are currently experiencing favourable economic growth with rapidly expanding markets, vibrant development, and increasing international trade.[14] Furthermore, the region is characterized by high cell phone penetration, infrastructure that facilitates digital health interventions, and communities with high social capital and strong extended family networks. Many countries in the region have also made innovative advances in developing strategies to deliver health care services by using community health care workers, non-medical professionals, and assistant physicians[15] within a model of task-sharing.[16,17]

[i] The World Bank list 48 countries in this region, whereas the United Nations Development Programme (UNDP) identifies 46 countries. According to the UNDP, SSA includes all countries on the African continent, except Algeria, Djibouti, Egypt, Libya, Morocco, Somalia, Sudan, and Tunisia. The World Bank includes the Arabic-speaking states of Mauritania and Sudan in SSA, whereas the International Monetary Fund (IMF) does not. Somalia and Djibouti (both of which are in the Horn of Africa) are south of the Sahara, but the IMF considers these as being part of the Middle East and Central Asia region.[12]

However, the region also faces a number of critical challenges, which include: high fertility rates, rapid population growth with a disproportionately high number of young people, widespread poverty,[14] a history of colonization and brutal exploitation by imperialist European powers, rapid urbanization,[18] high levels of internal migration,[19] poor access to education and health care, and a marked prevalence of infectious diseases.[20] Many countries in the region have newly established national governments and can be thought of as 'young democracies'. While some countries in SSA are described as 'post-conflict societies', several areas continue to face serious problems with political instability and ongoing violent conflict.[21] Despite these similarities, SSA is diverse in terms of language, religious beliefs, ethnicity, climate, landscape, and cultural practices.

Given political controversy about the use of the term 'SSA', as well as the considerable geographical size of the area and the sociocultural diversity of countries within the region, it is debatable whether it is useful (or indeed even possible) to employ this concept in productive discussions about suicide prevention. On the one hand, it seems completely inappropriate and potentially harmful to make broad generalizations about suicide prevention across such a vast, culturally heterogeneous region, especially if we acknowledge the need for suicide prevention interventions to be context-specific and culturally sensitive. There is a real danger that, in talking about suicide prevention in SSA, we may fall back on making crude generalizations, which obscure important sociocultural differences across countries and hide significant regional differences within countries. Use of the term can also inadvertently reinforce Western tendencies to 'treat Africa as if it were one country'.[22] On the other hand, it may be helpful to identify themes, challenges, and possibilities that are pertinent to suicide prevention and which are common to many (although not all) countries in SSA. Drawing attention to some of these common contextual challenges and cultural considerations could be helpful in identifying potential areas of collaboration and highlighting how networks within the region may be established to work on similar issues and share intellectual capital to promote suicide prevention. It is with this intention that we turn now to consider some of the common elements and cultural considerations for suicide prevention research and practice in SSA.

Epidemiology of suicide in sub-Saharan Africa

Estimates from the World Health Organization (WHO) suggest that globally approximately 793,000 people died from suicide in 2016, which equates to a global age-standardized prevalence of approximately 10.5:100,000.[23] The prevalence of suicide in Africa is estimated to be 7.4:100,000, but it is unclear what the prevalence of suicide is in SSA. Suicide data from the SSA region are not consistently reported within or across countries, and no data are available for some countries.[3,24] A review of the literature on suicide across the African continent published in 2014 concluded that only 15 of the countries in SSA had suicide mortality data.[25]

Table 9.1 provides an overview of the 2019 prevalence estimates for suicide within SSA countries from the Global Burden of Disease (GBD) online database.[26] As shown clearly in Table 9.1, there is marked variation in suicide prevalence rates across countries in the region and some of the suicide rates are below the GBD 2019 global estimate of 9.4:100,000 (95% confidence interval (CI) = 8.5–10.3). It is remarkable that the 2019 prevalence estimates for Zimbabwe, Eswatini, and Lesotho were, respectively, 23.4, 24.5, and 42.2 per 100,000, which are, for example, markedly higher than the GBD 2019 prevalence estimates for the United States of 11.7:100,000 (95% CI = 11.4–11.9) and Europe 12.0:100,000 (95% CI = 11.1–13.2).

Detailed information on estimates of age- and sex-standardized suicide rates for countries in SSA are available from WHO reports[27] and the GBD database.[26] Historically, these data have shown consistently high rates of suicide among men, compared to women, across most SSA countries where data are available.[4] However, caution needs to be exercised when interpreting prevalence estimates for suicide in SSA, as the accuracy and reliability of these data are compromised by factors such as absence of active suicide surveillance systems and lack of official national-level statistics in many countries.[28] For example, in Kenya, there is no systematic collection of national suicide data, possibly because of suicidal behaviour being illegal in the country.[28] Furthermore, suicide data are not consistently collected from one year to the next in some countries, making it impossible to analyse or establish trends, and prevalence estimates are often based on very small samples in cross-sectional studies which only focus on a small region of the country. Indeed, most suicide prevalence data in the region come from statistical modelling rather than from surveillance systems. The variability in suicide rates observed in Table 9.1 may be a function of issues such as: misclassification of death (e.g. insufficient training of police or forensic specialist);[29] religious prohibitions and legal sanctions against suicide;[28] cultural factors (i.e. deliberate underreporting related to fear of stigmatization); and political or economic factors.[30] Anthropological studies that explore the sociocultural beliefs related to suicide suggest that even within populations that share the same cultural beliefs, people may hold different beliefs about suicide,[31] which could impact the availability and consistent reliable reporting of suicide mortality data in SSA. Given all the problems related to collection of accurate suicide data in SSA, it seems possible that the prevalence rates reported in Table 9.1

Table 9.1 Overview of 2019 prevalence estimates for suicide in sub-Saharan countries from the Global Burden of Disease (GBD) online database

	Prevalence estimates per 100,000 of the population		
	Estimate	**95% CI**	
Angola	12.3	9.4	15.6
Benin	10.9	8.2	14.8
Botswana	19	12.3	27.6
Burkina Faso	12.9	10.0	16.4
Burundi	12.4	9.3	16.8
Côte d'Ivoire	13.2	9.6	17.8
Cabo Verde	16	12.4	20.1
Cameroon	13.3	9.4	18.0
Central African Republic	19.4	13.6	27.5
Chad	13	9.1	17.3
Comoros	7.3	4.7	11.4
Congo	12.4	9.3	16.5
Democratic Republic of the Congo	12.1	9.1	16.0
Djibouti	9.4	6.0	14.5
Equatorial Guinea	10.2	6.9	15.6
Eritrea	14.3	9.9	19.8
Eswatini	24.5	14.9	36.4
Ethiopia	10.1	8.2	12.9
Gabon	13.4	9.4	18.1
Gambia	10	6.6	14.0
Ghana	9.7	7.4	12.6
Guinea	11.1	7.5	15.2
Guinea-Bissau	14.9	10.7	20.0
Kenya	10.9	8.7	14.0
Lesotho	42.2	18.8	65.0
Liberia	8.9	5.9	13.0
Madagascar	9.8	7.2	12.9
Malawi	11.7	9.1	14.7
Mali	8.1	5.4	12.4
Mauritania	6.2	4.1	9.4

Table 9.1 Continued

	Prevalence estimates per 100,000 of the population		
	Estimate	**95% CI**	
Mozambique	16	11.7	20.5
Namibia	13.4	9.4	19.6
Niger	9.1	6.2	13.0
Nigeria	7.1	4.6	11.0
Rwanda	9.5	7.0	12.5
Sao Tome and Principe	2.6	1.8	3.3
Senegal	12.2	9.0	16.1
Sierra Leone	9.9	6.7	13.5
Somalia	12.7	7.8	18.7
South Africa	13.5	11.1	16.2
South Sudan	8.5	5.8	12.5
Togo	11.8	8.6	15.3
Uganda	10.8	8.4	14.1
United Republic of Tanzania	10.1	7.7	12.9
Zambia	13.8	10.4	18.0
Zimbabwe	23.4	16.2	30.0

are gross underestimates of the actual prevalence of suicide in the region. Crucially, the lack of reliable and consistent prevalence rates for suicide across SSA is a serious problem that impedes efforts to develop local, regional, and national suicide prevention policies and strategies, as it became acutely apparent during the global coronavirus disease 2019 (COVID-19) pandemic where a lack of accurate real-time data made it impossible to respond swiftly and appropriately to any changes in suicide risk during the pandemic.[24,32,33]

Suicide prevention in sub-Saharan Africa

Comparatively little attention has been paid to coordinating suicide prevention efforts at a national level in SSA. In 2011, Namibia was the first country in Africa to adopt a national suicide prevention strategy, but very few countries in SSA have followed suit.[34] There have also been remarkably few empirical trials of suicide prevention interventions in the region, and the available evidence from other parts of the world indicates that no single suicide prevention strategy stands above the others as clearly being more effective.[35]

Cultural and contextual considerations for suicide prevention

There are several cultural and contextual factors common across many countries in SSA, which have a direct bearing on suicide prevention research and practice. The examples we have identified below of these common contextual considerations, and the opportunities they present for culturally informed suicide research, are by no means definitive or exhaustive. They simply serve to provide some typical examples of contextual challenges faced by countries in SSA and the opportunities these present for collaboration within the region.[ii,iii]

Definitions of suicide and culturally situated meanings

Definitions of suicide have historically been contested, even in Western English-speaking countries, and consensus on suicide nomenclature within the field of suicidology is fairly recent.[36,37,38] Furthermore, what is defined as suicide and the meaning this behaviour holds are historically situated, culturally determined, and context-sensitive.[39] This presents challenges for suicide researchers anywhere in the world but may be particularly complicated in SSA where there is considerable ethnocultural, ethnolinguistic, and religious diversity within and between countries.[40] Insufficient work has been done to explore culturally situated meanings of suicide and the vocabulary that is used to denote this concept in African languages and cultures. Qualitative and ethnographic research by sociologists, anthropologists, and linguists aimed at exploring African understandings of suicidal behaviour will be an important component of mapping the suicide landscape in the region. Such culturally informed work will also be invaluable for subsequent quantitative and epidemiological studies which will be needed to define, operationalize, and measure suicidal behaviour in a meaningful way. This is not simply a matter of translating standardized instruments, such as the widely used *Colombia Suicide Severity Rating Scale*,[41] into African languages (although this may be useful too). What is needed is research which seeks to understand the different ways in which people in SSA talk about this

[ii] Some of the examples we cite below are also applicable to other LMICs outside the region and may thus not be uniquely 'African'.

[iii] The term 'culture' is notoriously difficult to define,[89] and studying it has been likened to trying to describe 'a moving target'.[90] In this chapter, we have used a broad definition of culture to encompass the sociopolitical and economic contexts in which people live, as well as the ideas, customs, and social behaviours which are distinctive within a particular region or place. Use of the term 'culture' in suicide research is also inherently problematic because it is so difficult to define and operationalize.[91]

phenomenon, the language that is used to describe this behaviour, and the situated meanings this behaviour holds for different communities in the region. There are examples of how researchers have started to approach these issues in Ghana[42,43] and Uganda.[44]

Traditional medicine and witchcraft

In SSA, there is a well-established culture of traditional medicine, defined as 'health practices, approaches, knowledge and beliefs incorporating plant, animal and mineral based medicines, spiritual therapies, manual techniques and exercises, applied singularly or in combination to treat, diagnose and prevent illnesses or maintain well-being'.[45] It is estimated that 80% of the population in many parts of SSA consult traditional healers[46] and that divination is an integral component of practices to promote health and well-being in the region.[47] Concepts of illness and disease in SSA are sometimes associated with ideas about witchcraft and ancestral spirits.[48] Furthermore, some people living in rural areas do not have access to biomedical health services and consequently traditional healers are their only port of call when they are unwell.

Some advances have already been made in SSA to include traditional healers in the health care system. For example, traditional healers have been engaged in human immunodeficiency virus (HIV) and tuberculosis (TB) treatment in Africa.[49,50] A small study from South Africa suggests that traditional healers might be open to contributing to public health interventions to reduce suicidal behaviour, and their practices may be complementary to Western biomedical suicide prevention practices.[51] Similarly, work has begun in Ghana to explore how religious leaders may be more involved in the promotion of mental health and suicide prevention.[52] It may be helpful if similar research is conducted in other parts of SSA, especially as part of a process to design culturally acceptable suicide prevention interventions in the region.

Health and the health care context

Countries in SSA typically face several challenges with the provision of health care, including particular problems related to prevention and treatment of infectious diseases, poor maternal and child health, a significant mental health treatment gap, and inadequate access to affordable health care.[20] It is important to carefully consider this health care context and its implications for suicide prevention in the region. SSA has one of the highest burden of disease in the world,[53,54] with a disproportionately high burden of infectious diseases, compared to the rest of the world.[20] The region accounts for more than 70% of the global burden of HIV infections and deaths.[55] In 2014, it was estimated that 90% of the world's 1.5 million TB deaths occurred in SSA and South East

Asia.[56] Although the African continent has witnessed a long-term decline in transmission of malaria, data suggest that, in the period from 2010 to 2015, the prevalence of infection was 24% in the region,[57] with the prevalence of malaria deaths during 2015 estimated at 5.4:100,000.[58] Infectious diseases not only compromise the physical health of individuals, but also place a significant burden on the health care system and on public health care spending in SSA. Furthermore, life expectancy at birth is significantly lower in SSA, compared to all other regions of the world,[iv] in large part as a result of high rates of infant mortality in the region.[20] Furthermore, health care systems in SSA have been characterized as overburdened, resource-constrained, poorly managed, and inadequate.[59]

There are two important implications of the health care context for suicide prevention in SSA:

1. Suicide prevention research should explore the potential links between poor physical health and suicidal behaviour in the region. Data from high-income countries suggest that physical illness and HIV infection are associated with an increased risk of suicide,[60,61] but it is as yet unclear if this pattern is also widely observed in SSA. There are data from some countries in the region to suggest that rates of suicidal behaviours are higher among persons living with HIV/acquired immune deficiency syndrome (AIDS) and those seeking HIV testing, compared to the general population.[62,63] Establishing clear associations between infectious diseases and suicide risk could have important implications for integrating suicide prevention practices and screening within general medical and primary health care settings. Such models of collaborative care (i.e. integration of mental health interventions into general medical settings) are increasingly used within the region,[64,65,66] providing models for how similar approaches could be used for suicide prevention interventions.
2. Arguments about the need to allocate more resources to suicide prevention in SSA need to be contextualized within the reality of competing public health demands and other urgent health care priorities. Given the scarcity of resources, the prevalence of other health conditions, and the lack of an established evidence base for suicide prevention in SSA, it would seem to be unwise to argue too strongly for reallocation of resources until more data are available. Nonetheless, there is an urgent need to collect reliable epidemiological data on the prevalence and burden of suicidal behaviour in SSA, so

[iv] Between 2000 and 2004, life expectancy at birth in SSA was 45.9 years, compared to a global average of 65.4. Asia has the second lowest life expectancy at birth, at 67.3.

that data can be used to establish the priority of suicide prevention relative to other public health concerns.

Migration, forced displacements, and refugees

There is a marked flow of migration in SSA,[67] with migration patterns in the region heavily influenced by forced displacement (as a result of economic factors, violence, political repression, natural disasters, or changes in weather patterns). Forced displacements have resulted in high numbers of refugees in SSA, many of whom are survivors of trauma.[68] Globally, the share of refugees originating from SSA is estimated to be between 3 and 3.5 million (i.e. 30% of the world's total number of refugees), most of whom remain within the region crossing borders within Africa.[69] SSA is also host to a number of refugees from other countries; indeed the region has been hosting more refugees than sending them since 1990.[69]

Globally, data suggest that migrants and refugees are at increased risk of suicide. A recent literature review of suicide risk among immigrants and ethnic minorities ($n=43$ articles) concluded that although some of the evidence is contradictory, it would seem that migrant populations and ethnic minorities are at increased risk of suicide compared to the native population,[70] although most of these data do not come from countries within SSA. It makes sense that this population would be at increased risk of suicide, given the preponderance of suicide risk factors typically found among migrants and refugees, namely a history of trauma, high rates of psychological distress, economic hardship, and marginalization.

Urbanization and the growth of slums

Rapid urbanization (i.e. the growth of urban populations through the combined effects of migration and natural increase, and the transformation of rural areas into urban areas because of industrial and economic development) is a hallmark of SSA.[71,72] Since early 1970s, SSA had the highest urban growth rate in the world, averaging 5% per annum,[73] although some evidence suggests that the rate of urbanization has slowed in recent years.[74] Crucially, this rapid urbanization is taking place with negligible concurrent industrial growth and without adequate provision of shelter, infrastructure, and basic services (including water and sanitation, education, health care, employment, and transport).[73] The inability of many governments to properly manage the process of urbanization in SSA poses a threat to health, psychological well-being, and sustainable development.[67] Urban slums (i.e. urban areas characterized by some combination of tenuous dwelling structures, overcrowding, and lack of access to adequate water and sanitation facilities) have also become characteristic of many urban mega cities in SSA.[72] It is estimated that 800 million people in Africa, Asia, and Latin America live in slums.[75] Over 60% of people in SSA live in slum conditions, the highest proportion of slum residents of any major world region.[76] While SSA has 13% of the urban population of developing regions, it consists of 25% of the slum population of developing countries.[76] Improving the lives of slum dwellers in the region is one of the most pressing development challenges of the twenty-first century.[75]

There is a long-standing and widely held belief that urbanization leads to improvements in health, although some data from SSA suggest that urban adult mortality rates exceeded rural adult mortality rates and that living in some cities in SSA may be particularly hazardous to one's health.[77] Evidence from high-income countries suggests that living in urban areas is also protective against suicide and that suicide rates are higher in rural areas,[78,79] but it is unclear if this pattern also holds true in SSA. If urbanization increases access to employment, education, and health care, it seems likely that it would also decrease the risk of suicide. However, if urbanization results in cultural discontinuity, disruptions in family relationships, marginalization, poor health, economic hardship, and the creation of slums, then it is more likely to increase the risk of suicide.[68] The impact of urbanization on suicide risk in SSA is an area in the need of extensive exploration, as the lack of data in this area makes it impossible to plan appropriate public health interventions or allocate resources.

Slum dwellers in SSA typically exhibit poor health outcomes, compared to other people living in formal urban areas and those in rural areas, at all stages in the life course.[77,78] For example, child mortality rates are, on average, 65% higher in urban slums than in formal settlements, but child mortality rates in slums are still lower than, or equal to, those in rural places.[77] The psychological and physical health of people living in slums is compromised by four key characteristics of these settlements: (1) poor environmental conditions and infrastructure; (2) limited access to services due to lack of income to pay for treatment and preventive services; (3) reliance on poor quality badly situated and mostly informal and unregulated health services; and (4) health services that are poorly suited to meeting the unique realities and health needs of slum dwellers.[81] It seems highly likely that these characteristics will also result in an increased suicide risk for residents of slums in SSA, but this has yet to be empirically established. Although there have been some efforts to compare patterns of injury and causes of death between formal and informal neighbourhoods in urban SSA,[80,82] data about suicide risk among slum dwellers remain scant. Given the large proportion of people living in these settings, it seems appropriate to investigate the risk of suicide in this population and to collect data needed to identify which residents of slums are at highest risk of suicide in SSA. Slums in SSA are, however, not static and homogenous residential entities; they are dynamic environments, with wide variations in the socio-demographic characteristics and health profile of slum dwellers.[75,81] For example, while slum populations are often highly mobile and poor, as many as half of this population are long-term residents (having lived in slum settlements for over 10 years) and many have stable incomes.[81] Suicide research will thus need to take account of this complexity and variety by employing sophisticated research designs that allow for identification of variations in risk among slum dwellers, regional variations across slums, and identification of particular psychological drivers of suicidal behaviour in this population. Epidemiological studies describing suicide risk profiles in this population will be needed, as well as qualitative studies exploring the sociocultural contexts of suicides in slums. There are particularly apt examples of qualitative research from India, which illustrate how verbal autopsy studies might be productively employed to advance our understanding in this area.[83]

Opportunities for collaborative suicide prevention research in the region

There are a number of universal methodological challenges associated with suicide prevention research, including the fact that the base rate of completed suicide is low (even in high-risk groups), making it difficult to execute studies with sufficient statistical power to make definitive claims about risk factors or the efficacy and effectiveness of interventions.[84] One potential solution to this problem is to extrapolate findings from epidemiological and intervention studies focused on non-fatal suicidal behaviour, to make inferences about what may be effective for suicide prevention. But this is problematic, as non-fatal suicidal behaviour and fatal suicidal behaviour are distinct phenomena which only partially overlap.[84] There are at least two alternative solutions: (1) improving mortuary surveillance systems; and (2) mounting large-scale longitudinal studies over multiple sites, with suicide as the primary outcome, in order to collect large enough data sets to draw meaningful conclusions. However, these kinds of studies are logistically difficult and expensive to implement, requiring large investments of human and financial resources over a protracted period of time. Costs of this kind of research are prohibitively expensive in many parts of SSA where there are a large number of low-income countries. There would seem to be an opportunity here for research collaboration across multiple sites in SSA; this could enable a sharing of intellectual capital, economies of scale, and the possibility of larger studies which have the requisite statistical power. Examples of similar networks in the region include *Partnership for mental health development in Sub-Saharan Africa* (PaM-D),[85] the *Africa Focus on Intervention Research for Mental health* (AFFIRM) collaborative research hub,[86] and the *Programme for Improving Mental health carE* (PRIME).[87] A key challenge in achieving a suicide prevention research network in the region will be securing the necessary financial resources and establishing a collaborative network of researchers across the region. This seems to be an important first step in advancing evidence-based suicide prevention practices in SSA.

Given the common contextual and cultural considerations for suicide prevention discussed above, it would make sense for a collaborative suicide prevention research network in SSA to focus on:

1. Establishing a reliable suicide surveillance system (which includes reporting on non-fatal suicidal behaviour) in the region. Reliable epidemiological data about suicide will be the cornerstone of advocating for the allocation of resources to this public health problem, planning targeted interventions, and monitoring the impact of suicide prevention policies and practices in the region.
2. Exploring culturally situated meanings of suicide in the region and the language that is used to describe this aspect of human behaviour in indigenous African languages.
3. Identifying high-risk groups within populations of migrants and refugees, and exploring how the lived experiences of these groups may contribute to suicide.
4. Exploring how traditional healers, religious leaders, and other non-professional health workers might be effectively engaged to promote the goals of suicide prevention.
5. Investigating how processes such as urbanization and contexts such as living in an urban slum may increase the risk of suicide and what the implications of this may be for suicide prevention. Conversely, it would also be important to explore how strengths within the region (such as cell phone penetration and existence of strong extended family networks) might be employed to promote suicide prevention in the region.
6. Establishing the links between infectious diseases and suicide risk in the region and what the implications of this are for integrating suicide prevention practices within general medical and primary health care settings. Similarly, it may be important to explore links between non-communicable diseases and suicide in the region, especially given the growing burden of non-communicable diseases.
7. Developing and testing culturally informed suicide prevention interventions. Given the scarcity of health care professionals in the region, it would

seem to make sense to prioritize the development of interventions that can be delivered by non-professionals within the model of task-sharing. Related to this is the need to include service users in the design and implementation of suicide interventions in the region, to ensure that interventions are culturally acceptable to the intended recipients of these services.

8. Investigating structural and attitudinal barriers to accessing mental health care services in the region, and the impact this may have on suicide.

Before scarce resources in SSA are spent on suicide prevention interventions, we need to understand what works. This is crucially important, given the other urgent health care priorities in the region and the weaknesses in health care systems. Collecting evidence to inform effective, culturally appropriate suicide prevention will require coordinated efforts and collaboration by a network of researchers across SSA.

Conclusion

In this chapter, we have discussed several cultural considerations and challenges for suicide prevention research and practice in SSA. Our intention in considering countries in SSA collectively was not to reify colonial ideas about 'the dark continent' or perpetuate unhelpful stereotypes about this arbitrarily defined geographical region. Instead, we tried to identify themes that are common to many (but not all) countries in the region—themes which need to be considered when planning and implementing context-sensitive and culturally informed suicide prevention research and practices. In drawing attention to some of these common contextual and cultural considerations, we have argued that this is an opportunity to establish a collaborative network in SSA focused on addressing suicide prevention challenges common across multiple countries in the region. Such a network might enable the economies of scale and the sharing of intellectual capital needed to mount large and coordinated multisite studies and interventions to reduce suicide. Beyond simply collaborating on research, this network might also undertake important advocacy work to raise awareness of suicide in the region, spur politicians and policymakers into action, promote mental health, and reduce stigma. The synergy of collective action and coordinated research efforts across national borders has the potential to advance suicide prevention beyond what any country in SSA could achieve on its own.

References

1. **Bertolote JM, Fleischmann A.** Suicide and psychiatric diagnosis: a worldwide perspective. World Psychiatry. 2002;**1**(3):181–5.

2. **Fleischmann A, De Leo D.** The World Health Organization's report on suicide. Crisis. 2014;**35**(5):289–91.
3. **Bertolote JM, Fleischmann A.** A global perspective in the epidemiology of suicide. Suicidologi. 2015;7(2):6–8. Available from:http://www.journals.uio.no/index.php/suicidologi/article/viewFile/2330/2193
4. **World Health Organization**. *Preventing Suicide: A Global Imperative*. Geneva: World Health Organization; 2014.
5. **Colucci E.** The cultural facet of suicidal behaviour: its importance and neglect. Australian e-Journal for the Advancement of Mental Health. 2006;**5**(3):234–46.
6. **Rathod S, Pinninti N, Irfan M**, et al. Mental health service provision in low- and middle-income countries. Health Services Insights. 2017;**10**:117863291769435.
7. **De Silva SA, Colucci E, Mendis J, Kelly CM, Jorm AF, Minas H.** Suicide first aid guidelines for Sri Lanka: a Delphi consensus study. International Journal of Mental Health Systems. 2016;**10**(1):53.
8. **Kral MJ.** Postcolonial suicide among Inuit in Arctic Canada. Culture, Medicine, and Psychiatry. 2012;**36**(2):306–25.
9. **Osafo J.** Unpacking the stigma of suicide in Ghana through the suicide-morality connection: implications for stigma reduction programs. Suicidology Online. 2016;7(1):11–23.
10. **Patel V, Saxena S, Lund C**, et al. The Lancet Commission on global mental health and sustainable development. The Lancet. 2018;**392**(10157):1553–98.
11. **United Nations** (2017). World population prospects. Microsoft Word - 17-DBooklet V9-11-12-2017-3PM (un.org)
12. **Kampala LT** (2019). What is sub-Saharan Africa? The Economist explains. The Economist. 2019. Available from: https://www.economist.com/the-economist-explains/2019/03/07/what-is-sub-saharan-africa
13. **Collins RO, Burns JM.** *A History of Sub-Saharan Africa*, 2nd edition. Cambridge: Cambridge University Press; 2007.
14. **Adams S, Klobodu EKM.** Remittances, regime durability and economic growth in Sub-Saharan Africa (SSA). Economic Analysis and Policy. 2016;50:1–8.
15. **Dussault G, Cobb NM.** A new generation of physicians in sub-Saharan Africa? Comment on 'Non-physician clinicians in sub-Saharan Africa and the evolving role of physicians'. International Journal of Health Policy and Management. 2016;**6**(1):57–9.
16. **Mijovic H, McKnight J, English M.** What does the literature tell us about health workers' experiences of task-shifting projects in sub-Saharan Africa? A systematic, qualitative review. Journal of Clinical Nursing. 2016;**25**(15–16):2083–100.
17. **Rabkin M, de Pinho H, Michaels-Strasser S, Naitore D, Rawat A, Topp SM.** Strengthening the health workforce to support integration of HIV and noncommunicable disease services in sub-Saharan Africa. AIDS. 2018;**32**:S47–54.
18. **Bocquier P.** Analyzing urbanization in sub-Saharan Africa. In: *New Forms of Urbanization*. Oxfordshire, England, UK: Routledge; 2017. pp. 133–50.
19. **Garcia AJ, Pindolia DK, Lopiano KK, Tatem AJ.** Modeling internal migration flows in sub-Saharan Africa using census microdata. Migration Studies. 2015;**3**(1):89–110.
20. **Jamison DT, Feachem RG, Makgoba MW**, et al. *Disease and Mortality in Sub-Saharan Africa*. 2006.

21. **Prah KK.** African wars and ethnic conflicts: rebuilding failed states. In: *Human Development Report*. New York: United Nations Development Programme; 2004.
22. **Wainaina B** (2018). How to write about Africa. Granta. Available from: https://granta.com/how-to-write-about-africa/
23. **World Health Organization.** Global Health Observatory data: suicide rates (per 100,000 population). Geneva: World Health Organization; 2018.
24. **Knipe D, John A, Padmanathan P,** et al. Suicide and self-harm in low- and middle-income countries during the COVID-19 pandemic: a systematic review. PLoS Global Public Health. 2022;**2**(6):e0000282. Available from:https://journals.plos.org/globalpublichealth/article?id=10.1371/journal.pgph.0000282
25. **Mars B, Burrows S, Hjelmeland H, Gunnell D.** Suicidal behaviour across the African continent: a review of the literature. BMC Public Health. 2014;**14**:606.
26. **Institute for Health Metrics and Evaluation.** Global Burden of Disease (GBD). Available from: https://www.healthdata.org/gbd/2019
27. **World Health Organization.** Global Health Observatory data: suicide rates (per 100,000 population). Geneva: World Health Organization; 2018.
28. **Bitta MA, Bakolis I, Kariuki SM,** et al. Suicide in a rural area of coastal Kenya. BMC Psychiatry. 2018;**18**(1):267.
29. **Bitta MA, Bakolis I, Kariuki SM,** et al. Suicide in a rural area of coastal Kenya. BMC Psychiatry. 2018;**18**(1):267.
29. **Burrows S, Laflamme L.** Assessment of accuracy of suicide mortality surveillance data in South Africa. Crisis. 2007;**28**(2):74–81.
30. **Bachmann S.** Epidemiology of suicide and the psychiatric perspective. International Journal of Environmental Research and Public Health. 2018;**15**(7).
31. **Vaughan M.** The discovery of suicide in Eastern and Southern Africa. African Studies. 2012;**71**(2):234–50.
32. **Pirkis J, John A, Shin S,** et al. Suicide trends in the early months of the COVID-19 pandemic: an interrupted time-series analysis of preliminary data from 21 countries. The Lancet Psychiatry. 2021;**8**(7):579–88. Available from: https://linkinghub.elsevier.com/retrieve/pii/S2215036621000912
33. **Pirkis J, Gunnell D, Shin S,** et al. Suicide numbers during the first 9–15 months of the COVID-19 pandemic compared with pre-existing trends: an interrupted time series analysis in 33 countries. EClinicalMedicine. 2022;**51**:101573.
34. **World Health Organization** (2018). National suicide prevention strategies: progress, examples and indicators. Geneva: World Health Organization.
35. **Zalsman G, Hawton K, Wasserman D,** et al. Suicide prevention strategies revisited: 10-year systematic review. The Lancet Psychiatry. 2016;3(7):646–59.
36. **O'Carroll PW, Berman AL, Maris RW, Moscicki EK, Tanney BL, Silverman MM.** Beyond the Tower of Babel: a nomenclature for suicidology. Suicide and Life-Threatening Behavior. 1996;**26**(3):237–52.
37. **De Leo D, Burgis S, Bertolote JM, Kerkhof AJFM, Bille-Brahe U.** Definitions of suicidal behavior. Crisis. 2006;**27**(1):4–15.
38. **Nock MK.** *The Oxford Handbook of Suicide and Self-Injury*. Oxford: Oxford University Press; 2014.

39. **Colucci E, Lester D**, editors. *Suicide and Culture: Understanding the Context*. Cambridge, MA: Hogrefe Publishing; 2012.
40. **Gershman B, Rivera D.** Subnational diversity in Sub-Saharan Africa: insights from a new dataset. Journal of Development Economics. 2018;**133**:231–63.
41. **Posner K, Brent D, Lucas C**, et al. *Columbia-Suicide Severity Rating Scale (C-SSRS)*. New York, NY: Columbia University Medical Center, 10; 2008.
42. **Osafo J, Hjelmeland H, Akotia C, Knizek B.** Social injury: an interpretative phenomenological analysis of the attitudes towards suicide of lay persons in Ghana. International Journal of Qualitative Studies on Health and Well-being. 2011;**6**(4):8708.
43. **Osafo J, Akotia CS, Quarshie ENB, Andoh-Arthur J, Boakye KE.** Community leaders' attitudes towards and perceptions of suicide and suicide prevention in Ghana. Transcultural Psychiatry. 2019;**56**(3):529–51.
44. **Mugisha J, Muyinda H, Hjelmeland H, Kinyanda E, Vancampfort D, Knizek BL.** Cultural responses towards the aftermath of suicide among the Acholi in Northern Uganda. International Journal of Social Psychiatry. 2018;**64**(6):545–53.
45. **World Health Organization**. Factsheet 134: Traditional medicine. Geneva: World Health Organization; 2003.
46. **King R, Homsy J.** Involving traditional healers in AIDS education and counselling in sub-Saharan Africa: a review. AIDS. 1997;**11:217–25.**
47. **Devisch R.** Perspectives on divination in contemporary sub-Saharan Africa. In: **Wim van Binsbergen, Matthew Schoffeleers**, editors. *Theoretical Explorations in Africa*. London, UK: Routledge; 2013. pp. 60–93.
48. **Grietens KP, Ribera JM, Erhart A**, et al. Doctors and vampires in sub-Saharan Africa: ethical challenges in clinical trial research. American Journal of Tropical Medicine and Hygiene. 2014;**91**(2):213–15.
49. **Shey Nsagha D, Ayima CW, Nana-Njamen T, Clement J, Assob N.** The role of traditional, complementary/alternative medicine in primary healthcare, adjunct to universal health coverage in Cameroon: a review of the literature. American Journal of Epidemiology and Infectious Disease. 2020;**8**:37–47. Available from: http://pubs.sciepub.com/ajeid/8/1/6/index.html
50. **Kayombo EJ, Uiso FC, Mbwambo ZH, Mahunnah RL, Moshi MJ, Mgonda YH.** Experience of initiating collaboration of traditional healers in managing HIV and AIDS in Tanzania. Journal of Ethnobiology and Ethnomedicine. 2007;**3**(1):1–9. Available from: https://link.springer.com/articles/10.1186/1746-4269-3-6
51. **Bantjes J, Swartz L, Cembi S.** 'Our lifestyle is a mix-match': traditional healers talk about suicide and suicide prevention in South Africa. Transcultural Psychiatry. 2018;**55**(1):73–93.
52. **Asamoah MK, Osafo J, Agyapong I.** The role of Pentecostal clergy in mental health-care delivery in Ghana. Mental Health, Religion and Culture. 2014;**17**(6):601–14.
53. **World Health Organization**. Global Burden of Disease Study. Geneva: World Health Organization; 2004.
54. **Naghavi M; Global Burden of Disease Self-Harm Collaborators**. Global, regional, and national burden of suicide mortality 1990 to 2016: systematic analysis for the Global Burden of Disease Study 2016. BMJ. 2019;**364**(194):1–11.

55. **Kharsany ABM, Karim QA.** HIV Infection and AIDS in Sub-Saharan Africa: current status, challenges and opportunities. Open AIDS Journal. 2016;**10**:34–48.
56. **World Health Organization**. Global tuberculosis report. Geneva: World Health Organization; 2014.
57. **Snow RW, Sartorius B, Kyalo D**, et al. The prevalence of *Plasmodium falciparum* in sub-Saharan Africa since 1900. Nature. 2017;**550**(7677):515–18.
58. **Gething PW, Casey DC, Weiss DJ**, et al. Mapping *Plasmodium falciparum* mortality in Africa between 1990 and 2015. New England Journal of Medicine. 2016;**375**(25):2435–45.
59. **Deaton AS, Tortora R.** People in sub-Saharan Africa rate their health and health care among the lowest in the world. Health Affairs. 2015;**34**(3):519–27.
60. **Carrieri MP, Marcellin F, Fressard L**, et al. Suicide risk in a representative sample of people receiving HIV care: time to target most-at-risk populations (ANRS VESPA2 French national survey). PLoS One. 2017;**12**(2):e0171645.
61. **Bachmann S.** Epidemiology of suicide and the psychiatric perspective. International Journal of Environmental Research and Public Health. 2018;**15**(7).
62. **Bantjes J, Kagee A, Saal W.** Suicidal ideation and behaviour among persons seeking HIV testing in peri-urban areas of Cape Town, South Africa: a lost opportunity for suicide prevention. AIDS Care. 2017;**29**(7):919–27.
63. **Bantjes J, Kagee A.** Suicide prevention in HIV treatment centres: population attributable risk analysis of treating common mental disorders. AIDS and Behavior. 2021;**25**(6):1864–72. Available from: https://link.springer.com/article/10.1007/s10461-020-03116-5
64. **Fairall L, Petersen I, Zani B**, et al. Collaborative care for the detection and management of depression among adults receiving antiretroviral therapy in South Africa: study protocol for the CobALT randomised controlled trial. Trials. 2018;**19**(1):1–25.
65. **Adewuya AO, Adewumi T, Momodu O**, et al. Development and feasibility assessment of a collaborative stepped care intervention for management of depression in the mental health in primary care (MeHPriC) project, Lagos, Nigeria. Psychological Medicine. 2019;**49**(13):2149–57.
66. **Kermode M, Morgan A, Nyagero J**, et al. Walking together: towards a collaborative model for maternal health care in pastoralist communities of Laikipia and Samburu, Kenya. Maternal and Child Health Journal. 2017;**21**(10):1867–73.
67. **Mberu B, Béguy D, Ezeh AC.** Internal migration, urbanization and slums in sub-Saharan Africa. In: **Hans Groth, John F. May**, editors. *Africa's Population: In Search of a Demographic Dividend.* Cham: Springer International Publishing; 2017. pp. 315–32.
68. **Conejero I, Lopez-Castroman J, Giner L, Baca-Garcia E.** Sociodemographic antecedent validators of suicidal behavior: a review of recent literature. Current Psychiatry Reports. 2016;**18**(10):94.
69. **Fair D.** Refugees in sub-Saharan Africa from cause to solution. Africa Insight. 1996;**26**(1):36–42.
70. **Forte A, Trobia F, Gualtieri F**, et al. Suicide risk among immigrants and ethnic minorities: a literature overview. International Journal of Environmental Research and Public Health. 2018;**15**:1438. Available from: https://www.mdpi.com/1660-4601/15/7/1438/htm

71. **Hove M, Ngwerume ET, Muchemwa C.** The urban crisis in Sub-Saharan Africa: a threat to human security and sustainable development. Stability. 2013;**2**(1):1–14. Available from: http://www.stabilityjournal.org/articles/10.5334/sta.ap/
72. **Albert G, Yiran B, Dziwornu Ablo A, Asem FE, Owusu G.** Urban sprawl in sub-Saharan Africa: a review of the literature in selected countries. Ghana Journal of Geography. 2020;**12**(1):1–28. Available from: https://www.ajol.info/index.php/gjg/article/view/198012
73. **Todaro MP, Smith SC.** *Economic Development*. Essex, England: Pearson Education Limited; 2000.
74. **Potts D.** Challenging the myths of urban dynamics in sub-Saharan Africa: the evidence from Nigeria. World Development. 2012;**40**(7):1382–93.
75. **Fox S.** The political economy of slums: theory and evidence from sub-Saharan Africa. World Development. 2014;**54**:191–203.
76. **UN-Habitat.** *State of the World's Cities 2010/2011: Bridging the Urban Divide*. London: Earthscan Publications Ltd; 2008.
77. **Günther I, Harttgen K.** Deadly cities? Spatial inequalities in mortality in sub-Saharan Africa. Population and Development Review. 2012;**38**(3):469–86.
78. **Helbich M, Blüml V, de Jong T, Plener PL, Kwan MP, Kapusta ND.** Urban–rural inequalities in suicide mortality: a comparison of urbanicity indicators. International Journal of Health Geographics. 2017;**16**(1):39.
79. **Ivey-Stephenson AZ, Crosby AE, Jack SPD, Haileyesus T, Kresnow-Sedacca MJ.** Suicide trends among and within urbanization levels by sex, race/ethnicity, age group, and mechanism of death: United States, 2001–2015. MMWR Surveillance Summaries. 2017;**66**(18):1–16.
80. **Soura AB, Lankoande B, Millogo R, Bangha M.** Comparing causes of death between formal and informal neighborhoods in urban Africa: evidence from Ouagadougou Health and Demographic Surveillance System. Global Health Action. 2014;**7**(1):25523.
81. **Zulu EM, Beguy D, Ezeh AC,** et al. Overview of migration, poverty and health dynamics in Nairobi City's slum settlements. Journal of Urban Health. 2011;**88**(S2):185–99.
82. **Ziraba AK, Kyobutungi C, Zulu EM.** Fatal injuries in the slums of Nairobi and their risk factors: results from a matched case-control study. Journal of Urban Health. 2011;**88**(2):256–65.
83. **Parkar SR, Nagarsekar BB, Weiss MG.** Explaining suicide: identifying common themes and diverse perspectives in an urban Mumbai slum. Social Science and Medicine. 2012;**75**(11):2037–46.
84. **Nordentoft M.** Crucial elements in suicide prevention strategies. Progress in Neuro-Psychopharmacology and Biological Psychiatry. 2011;**35**(4):848–53.
85. **Gureje O, Seedat S, Kola L,** et al. Partnership for mental health development in sub-Saharan Africa (PaM-D): a collaborative initiative for research and capacity building. Epidemiology and Psychiatric Sciences. 2019;**28**(04):389–96.
86. **Lund C, Alem A, Schneider M,** et al. Generating evidence to narrow the treatment gap for mental disorders in sub-Saharan Africa: rationale, overview and methods of AFFIRM. Epidemiology and Psychiatric Sciences. 2015;**24**(3):233–40.

87. **Lund C, Tomlinson M, Patel V.** Integration of mental health into primary care in low- and middle-income countries: the PRIME mental healthcare plans. British Journal of Psychiatry. 2016;**208**(s56):s1–3.
88. **Kroeber AL, Kluckhohn C.** Culture: A critical review of concepts and definitions. Papers Peabody Museum of Archaeology and Ethnology, Harvard University. 1952;**47**(1):viii, 223.
89. **Medin DL, Unsworth SJ, Hirschfeld L.** Culture, categorization, and reasoning. In: **Kitayama S, Cohen D**, editors. *Handbook of Cultural Psychology*. New York, NY: Guilford Press; 2007. pp. 615–44.
90. **Bantjes J, Swartz L.** The cultural turn in critical suicidology: what can we claim and what do we know? Death Studies. 2017;**41**(8):512–20. Available from: https://www.tandfonline.com/doi/full/10.1080/07481187.2017.1333355

Chapter 10

Suicide risk in Latin America: International migrants, prison populations, and sexual minorities

Adrian P. Mundt, Francesco D. Fritz, and Báltica Cabieses

Suicide risk of international migrants in Latin America

International migration as a global determinant of health

As stated by the United Nations in 2018, international migration is a complex phenomenon that is involved on a multiplicity of economic, social, and security aspects affecting our daily lives in an increasingly interconnected world. Globally, there are 272 million international migrants, which represent almost 4% of the world total population. In 2021, there were 21.3 million refugees, 4.6 million asylum seekers, and 51.3 million internally displaced people.[1] Migration is a broad term that encompasses a wide variety of movements and situations. International migration refers to the movement of people to a different country from their country of origin or current residence, with the expectation of staying temporarily or permanently.[2] Reasons for migration are multiple, including work opportunities, poverty, conflict and war, and even natural disasters due to climate change. More than ever before, migration touches all states and people in an era of deepening globalization.[1]

Migration is intertwined with geopolitics, trade, and cultural exchange, and provides opportunities for states, businesses, and communities to benefit enormously.[1] Migration has helped improve people's lives in both their origin and destination countries, and has offered opportunities for millions of people worldwide to forge safe and meaningful lives abroad. Those movements have also supported the economic development of many high-income countries with ageing populations and emerging middle-income economies. They have also brought cultural diversity to many countries and regions, as well as supported, through economic remittances, the life of millions of families left behind.[3] However, we have in recent years seen some worrisome implications of international migration such as an increase in displacement occurring due to conflict, persecution, environmental degradation and change, and a profound lack of human security and opportunity. While most international migration occurs legally, some of the greatest insecurities for migrants, and much of the public concern about immigration, are associated with unsafe transit, irregular migration, and poor integration to, and protection in, host societies.[1,4]

International and interregional migration in Latin America and the Caribbean has increased in the context of crises and disasters, for example, the ongoing political crisis in Venezuela and the earthquake in Haiti in 2010. Most migrants in Latin America are from other Latin American countries. For example, in Chile, the percentage of migrants in the total population has increased from 2.04% in 2012 to over 6.67% in 2018, and Venezuela, Peru, and Haiti are the most common countries of origin.[5] Migration in Latin America has contributed to socio-economic inequality between countries in the region, as it is often related to the movement of people from poorer, less developed countries to more advantaged and stable ones.[6] The relative increase in intraregional migration has brought great attention to international experts, stakeholders, and media in recent years, which has been accompanied by a growing sense of fear and rejection towards the international migrant population in many groups.[7]

Most migrants globally and in Latin America have a *regularized* legal status and can benefit from social protection and job opportunities available to everyone. However, there is an obscure number of migrants who are moving across countries without a secured visa or guaranteed acceptance at the frontier. These people do not aim for this type of movement but need to do it due to social, political, or financial pressures. In this sense, social protection of all migrants, regardless of their migration status, in Latin America has been inconsistent in the past. There is very little understanding of how the migratory process can affect the health of migrants and what actions should be implemented for their protection, particularly at the stages of transit and arrival in the receiving country.[8] This is especially important to those who experience forced migration, as well as those who transit in socio-economic vulnerability and risk of abuse, including women and children.[9]

According to the national authority, about a third of international migrants are possibly undocumented or live in socio-economic vulnerability in Chile.[5] These migrants tend to work in informal jobs and live in poor-quality and overcrowded buildings.[10] They have limited access to health care and many fear to navigate through the health care system when required.[11] According to recent research evidence, between 20% and 60% of these migrants' income is remitted to their countries of origin, supporting the basic needs of their family left behind.[6] They suffer from a lack of institutional support when applying for refugee status[9] in their destination country and experience various types of discrimination when trying to integrate into the host society (e.g. having migrant status, being undocumented, being poor, with an ethnic background).[12] All these factors increase the risk of poor health and subjective well-being among international migrants, compared to the local population, and therefore underline the significance of the migration process as a global social determinant of health.[13]

Suicidal risk of migrants

According to the World Health Organization (WHO),[14] close to 800,000 people die by suicide every year, which is one person every 40 seconds. Suicide is a global phenomenon and occurs throughout the lifespan, with the highest rates in Europe (15.4 per 100,000 population) and South East Asia (13.2 per 100,000 population), followed by Western Pacific (10.2 per 100,000 population), Americas (9.8 per 100,000 population), Africa (7.4 per 100,000 population), and Eastern Mediterranean countries (3.9 per 100,000 population) in 2016. Chile, for example, had an estimated crude rate of suicide of 10.6 per 100,000 population in 2016, slightly lower than in the year 2000 (10.9 per 100,000), but significantly higher in men (17.2 per 100,000) compared to women (4.0 per 100,000). Suicide rates in other Latin American countries range between 7 (Colombia and Costa Rica) and 14 (Cuba) per 100,000 population. The gender gap is consistent across Latin American countries, regardless of the level of suicide rate. At present time, there are no data describing how suicide rates might vary between international migrants and locals in Latin America. The lack of high-quality data sets for analysis and research evidence is an urgent call to develop robust research in this region on how migration status and migration-related variables (such as country of origin, legal status, length of stay, and assimilation and acculturation processes) might have distinctive impacts on suicide rates among immigrants versus local populations.

As suggested by experts, the aetiology of suicide is complex. Besides psychiatric illness, psychological, environmental, and sociocultural factors, as well as genetic traits, also play a role.[15] International migration has been discussed as a potential risk factor for suicide, as concerns about increased suicide rates among immigrants have been raised.[16] International evidence enlightens on some of the plausible mechanisms to explain why suicide could be higher among some international migrants compared to local populations. These mechanisms are also relevant to the Latin American context and can be organized into four main arguments. Firstly, there is the idea that some *conflict and migration-related experiences*, like war, trauma, or political repression, including torture, may increase the risk of mental disorders later in life.[17,18] This is particular true of refugee and asylum-seeking migrants, as well as those who suffered violence and abuse before migration and during transit. Studies on refugees and asylum seekers in Latin America support this idea.[9] Secondly, some studies indicate that *everyday circumstances* in the destination country can also be stressful. Immigrants are often socio-economically disadvantaged, relative to the majority populations, and might face socio-psychological stressors such as discrimination and marginalization.[19] For example, the lack of institutional support for validation of professional qualifications in the country affects the migrants' work opportunities, income, sense of self and identity, potential to contribute to the host society, and self-esteem on a daily basis. Thirdly, the *country of origin* appears to be a determinant of the risk of suicide. Immigrants to higher-income countries are often disadvantaged in socio-economic terms, compared to the local-born populations. Moreover, they may have experienced severe stress before and during migration, and they may be victims of discrimination and marginalization afterwards.[18] This mechanism might become clearer when paying attention to people who migrate from 'lower-status' countries to more advanced ones. In Chile, self-perceived discrimination is generally higher among international migrants than among locals, but it is even higher when they also report an ethnic background or coming from bordering poorer countries.[12] Also, some countries have higher rates of suicide than the host country. The idea of migrants 'bringing along' the suicide risk with them is challenged by current understanding of the assimilation process, which suggests that immigrants' higher suicide risk dilutes over the time spent in the country[15] but continues to be a under debate. Fourthly, the *migration legal status* is also critical to mental health and in influencing suicide risk of migrants. Migrants living in undocumented contexts do not experience the same opportunities and treatment as regular migrants and locals.[20] Studies from Latin America suggest that the effect of being undocumented on mental health might be severe and long-lasting. Poverty, social marginalization and isolation, and a sense of sacrifice and sadness are often present in these situations. In some countries, these migrants are also prosecuted and incarcerated or deported. In Chile, for example, undocumented migrants live with a higher risk of overcrowding, absolute income poverty, and no access to the health care system.[21] As a qualitative study quoted from a Colombian undocumented migrant living in Chile away from their children: 'I survive here for them, this is my life sacrifice'.[13]

Additional elements for analysis of suicide risks are the complex relationships between international migration and *gender*, and international migration and *ethnic background*. Studies on suicide risk among migrants display relevant differences between men and women. For instance, a systematic review by Spallek and colleagues[18] indicated how the risk of suicide among migrants differs between genders. Also, studies suggest that young female immigrants from some more conservative or heteronormative countries might be particularly at higher risk of suicide in terms of socio-economic status, language barriers, intergenerational acculturation conflicts, or marriages that may be involuntary or arranged.[22] In addition, female migrants tend to maintain their breeding and maternity roles over the distance and often virtually via their phones, which might have mental health implications to them and their offspring. These women continue to look after their children concerning domestic and educational matters, helping them with their school exams and checking on their development and medical care whenever required. This is often reported as a worrying and stressful dimension of their lives, as they are responsible for their children left behind despite not being available daily. A recent systematic review examined the effect of parental migration on the health of left behind-children and adolescents in low- and middle-income countries (LMICs), and found that parental migration is detrimental to the health of left-behind children and adolescents, with no evidence of any benefit.[23] Similar findings have been reported in primary studies from Europe and Latin America.[24,25]

In relation to ethnicity, there is a need to better understand factors influencing suicide behaviours in immigrant and ethnocultural minority communities, in order to inform more responsive and effective prevention and intervention services. Ethnocultural identity refers to identification with, and importance placed on, one's cultural heritage and history.[26] This includes adherence to cultural values, beliefs, norms, and practices and meaning attributed to ethnocultural group membership, including pride, belonging, and affirmation, as well as participation in cultural activities and traditions.[27] In contrast to other regions, in Latin America, there is a differentiation between international migrants and ethnic groups. This is because the majority of the population in the region after colonization turned into *mestizos* ('half-blood') that are the historical combination between local aboriginal groups and the Europeans. Hence, nowadays only people who define themselves as members of the indigenous communities that existed before colonization are considered truly ethnic. Given this cultural complexity, it is possible to identify international migrants and locals with and without ethnic background labelling throughout the Latin American region. Studies conducted in the past on this continent indicated that there might be a higher risk of suicide in ethnic minority groups in the region,[28] but there have been no studies focusing on international migrants in Latin America. A recently published systematic review on suicide rates among indigenous peoples worldwide found that suicide rates in these populations vary globally, and that suicide rate disparities between indigenous and non-indigenous populations are substantial in some settings, but not universal. No additional data on international migrants were available for analysis in this study. To sum up, suicide risk, gender, and ethnic-related dimensions in international migrant groups in Latin America need to be better investigated and incorporated into ongoing research and the global mental health agenda.

Preventive strategies

Suicide is a global health problem that needs further understanding and investigation. International migration has been raised as a potential risk factor for suicide in the past decades, with conflicting evidence from local studies. Available systematic reviews suggest that international migration could lead to higher suicide rates in some subgroups of migrant populations such as refugees and asylum seekers, people with socio-economic disadvantages, women, and some ethnic minority groups. Underlying causal mechanisms continue to be developed and discussed, as the global health agenda demands for evidence-based action in this complex matter. We need to improve our understanding of how migration status and migration-related variables (such as country of origin, legal status, length of stay, and assimilation and acculturation processes) might have distinctive impacts on suicide rates among immigrants compared to local populations. The lack of high-quality data sets for analysis and research is a growing concern in Latin America and globally. Nevertheless, some interventions have been developed, with some degree of success, a number of which were developed in Latin America in recent years and will be described below.

According to a recent study of grey literature and governmental websites,[29] over 100 health initiatives to protect the health of migrants in the Latin American region have been conducted. While most of these health initiatives are local efforts focusing on providing food, shelter, and health attentions to migrants, some are part of integrated national health policy plans. In Chile, a national policy to improve the health of migrants was launched in October 2017, with the aim of shortening the gaps in access to health care between immigrants and locals over time. The country allows access to the health care system to all documented, regular migrants living in the country, but those with an irregular visa situation remain disadvantaged. Hence, a special treatment offer to undocumented migrants was promoted, allowing them to register to the public health system in the country with a temporary code until the availability of a visa (Decree 67). This has been a landmark effort of the country to bring the needs of migrants closer to the health care system, especially of those who are often left behind and experience greater socio-economic and emotional vulnerability such as undocumented migrants. Recent evaluations of this measure have proven that Decree 67 has allowed prompter and safer incorporation into the health care system of migrants waiting for a visa in Chile.[30] Additionally, and in collaboration with academia, some boroughs developed a welcome migrant health programme for international migrants living in Chile for less than a year or who have never received healthcare attention before. This low-cost and simple programme, based on a structured interview of migrants and conducted by a trained health professional, has been successful in increasing health literacy and satisfaction with the health care system among international migrants in Chile and has improved the effective rate of referrals to specialists, including referrals to mental health services.[31,32] These strategies are not focused on suicide but are useful to shed light on how structural measures (i.e. health policies) and local interventions (i.e. welcoming health programmes) can play a key role in prevention of this health issue and many others. We believe there is an opportunity for implementing, evaluating, and sharing various successful efforts to support the life of people living in disadvantaged, challenging contexts, including vulnerable international migrants. This is an urgent public health and social justice matter that requires more global attention and consistent effort.

Suicidal behaviour in South American prisons

A world of incarceration

The world prison population was estimated to exceed 10.8 million people in 2020.[33] Prisoners are overrepresented in certain regions and countries. The United States constitute 4.3% of the world population but held about 20% of the world prison population, an estimated 2 million people in 2020. China has the second largest prison population, with 1.69 million people, 15.9% of the world prison population, although this number may be an underestimation as, to this day, full counts of imprisoned individuals in the People's Republic may not be publicly available. Brazil follows, ranking third with 811,000 prisoners, then India and the Russian Federation with, respectively, 478,000 and 471,000 prisoners. Since the turn of the century, the world prison population increased by 24%, from 8 million to 10.8 million, in 2020.[33] This was slightly slower than the growth of the world population; thus, incarceration rates have remained stable. However, worldwide trends mask great regional disparities.

In the United States, a high increase of incarceration rates occurred between late 1970s and late 1990s, from about 100 to 600 per 100,000 people.[34] Since 2000, the rates have remained consistently high, amounting to 683 prisoners per 100,000 people in 2000 and 672 per 100,000 in 2015. In Europe, incarceration rates have remained mostly stable, with the exception of Russia. In 2000,

Russia held one million people imprisoned. That population was reduced to 471,000 in 2020, an ongoing trend since the collapse of the Soviet Union, and incarceration rates were brought down from 724 per 100,000 in 2000 to 326 per 100,000 population in 2022.[33]

These downward trends in Europe and the United States are in contrast to the trend in other regions of the world. In Oceania and Asia, prison populations grew by 82% and 38%, respectively. In South America, the focus of this chapter, prison populations have increased by 200% since 2000, exceeding the general population growth rate, which was 24%. Accordingly, incarceration rates doubled in Colombia, Ecuador, Peru, and Uruguay, and even tripled in Brazil, Paraguay, and Venezuela, thus increasing continent-wide from 132 prisoners per 100,000 population to 219 per 100,000.

However, this increase in South American prison population was not followed by an equivalent growth in prison infrastructure and legal services. Overcrowding in prisons has therefore become increasingly common in the region. In 2017, average prison occupancy was 220% in Peru and 190% in Brazil. In the region as a whole, the occupancy rate was 140%. Remand prisoners who have not yet received a sentence have continued to constitute a high proportion of the prison population. In 2010, in South America, 40% of the prison population was on remand.

Suicide in prisons

Suicide in prisons is a particularly delicate issue because governments hold the responsibility for the safety of individuals while they serve sentences. It may be difficult to imagine how in a supervised environment, such as a prison facility, the conditions as well as the means to die by suicide can be available to prisoners. However, in those countries where mortality in prison populations has been investigated, suicide rates in prisons are higher than among age-standardized general populations. In Europe, suicide is one of the most common causes of death among prisoners, alone accounting for about 28% of all deaths among those in detention in 2020.[35] Accordingly, the odds of dying by suicide in prison are between two and seven times higher than in the general population. In the United States, suicide is the most common cause of death in local jails with 372 deaths in 2014,[36] and the fourth most common cause of death in prisons with 239 deaths in the same year,[37] revealing suicide rates in prisons and jails in the United States about four times higher than in the general population. Worldwide, the suicide mortality in custody was estimated be 2-6 times higher among imprisoned men and 10-32 times higher among imprisoned women compared to the corresponding community population.[38]

Self-harm and suicidal behaviour are also highly prevalent among prison populations. In England and Wales, 5–6% of male prisoners, and 20–24% of female prisoners, were found to self-harm every year. Subsequent suicide was more common among prisoners who self-harmed than among those who did not, and more than half of all deaths in these prisoners occurred within one month of self-harm.[39]

Research on suicidal behaviour and completed suicides in prison populations has brought to light several risk factors that could explain the considerable discrepancy in suicide rates between general and prison populations. Firstly, as it is the case in the general population, psychiatric morbidity has consistently been found to be the factor most often associated with suicide in prison. Specifically, recent suicidal ideation, a history of suicidal behaviour, the presence of a mental disorder, and treatment with psychotropic medications have been found to be associated with suicidal behaviour among prisoners.[40,41,42] In turn, these factors are overrepresented among prison populations. Recent investigations have reported a high prevalence of severe mental illness among prisoners worldwide.[43,44,45,46] In a comprehensive review investigating a set of high- and middle-income countries, 10% of male prisoners were found to be affected by major depression and 4% by psychotic disorders, whereas the prevalence of major depression and psychotic disorders among female prisoners was 14% and 4%, respectively. In low- and middle-income countries, the prevalence of psychotic disorders was about 7% in male and 6% in female prisoners; the prevalence of major depression was 16% in male and 19% in female prisoners.[46] Further, comorbid severe mental illness and substance use disorders were common.[47,48,49]

The most relevant criminological risk factors associated with suicide in prison were being charged with a violent crime,[40] serving a life sentence, and being on remand.[42] This explains the disproportionately high suicide rates in jails in the United States which hold prisoners prior to sentencing or prisoners sentenced to less than a year, when compared to American state and federal prisons which hold sentenced prisoners with sentences of at least one year.

Some risk factors related to the prison environment have also been consistently found to be associated with suicide incidence, the most relevant being placement in single-use or isolation cells. In contrast, high levels of prison overcrowding were found to be negatively associated with suicide rates in prison. A possible explanation for this phenomenon could be that although overcrowding constitutes a highly stressful environment for prisoners, and arguably a violation of human rights, it prevents the isolation necessary to complete suicide. Other research studies assessing the impact of overcrowding in prisons found that it negatively influences both physical and mental health of prisoners, as it can increase the prevalence of infectious diseases and psychiatric disorders.[50] However, it must be noted that several studies have also found a positive association, or none at all, between prison population density and suicide rates.[51,52]

Furthermore, it has been proposed that in countries with low rates of incarceration, prison populations have more severe criminological and psychiatric characteristics, that is a population more vulnerable to suicidal behaviour. This means that the higher incarceration rates are in a country, the more representative of the general population the prison population of that country will be, diluting down, so to speak, the rates at which suicidal behaviour and completed suicides occur. In countries with lower incarceration rates, prison suicide rates will be higher. However, findings of a negative association are still inconclusive[41] and were not consistent across all studies.[53]

Prison suicides in South America

In South America, a continuously growing prison population has put the continent's prison and legal infrastructure under strain. Overcrowding is becoming increasingly common and severe.[54] Prison conditions range from poor to extremely harsh:[55] correctional staff often do not control the internal organization of prison sectors and limit their control to the perimeter of the facilities; although health care should be provided by law to the same standards as provided to the general population, access to timely and adequate services, including mental health, is often unavailable. Many prisons in the regions do not meet international prison standards. Purposeful activities are often lacking, and human rights violations have been repeatedly reported.

Fewer research publications on the mental health and suicidal behaviour of South American prisoners are available, compared to Europe or North America, since the turn of the century and mostly originate from four countries: Brazil, Chile, Colombia, and Ecuador.

In Brazil, along with several studies that consistently found a high prevalence of substance use disorders among prisoners,[56] two relevant studies were conducted that further investigated mental health parameters.[57,58] In São Paulo, investigators found a 12-month prevalence of mental disorders of 39% among imprisoned women and of 22% among imprisoned men. In the city of Salvador (Bahia), the prevalence rates in closed and semi-open prison systems were, respectively, 17.6% and 18.8% for depression, 19.7% and 34.8% for borderline personality disorder, 27.9% and 32.4% for psychosis.

In Chile, there were several studies of interest conducted between 2013 and 2019. In one study, a 12-month prevalence of 27% of any mental disorder was found among prisoners.[59] In another study, 49% of prisoners presented with major depression, and 16% with psychosis, at intake into prison facilities.[60]

Of those prisoners with major depression, 47% presented with a high risk of suicide, which decreased to 14% at follow-up one year later.[61] The prevalence of any suicide risk decreased from 62% at intake to 48% in a group that was followed up after three years of imprisonment.[62] A further study reported 162 completed suicides between 2006 and 2015, of which 65% occurred within the first year of imprisonment.[63] Prison personnel, as well as fellow prisoners, reported that 43% of prisoners who had completed suicide suffered from depressive symptoms prior to their death.

In Colombia, five studies between 2009 and 2015 were conducted, respectively, in single prisons in the departments of Boyacá, Quindío, Tolima, and Antioquia, and one across all departments, investigating mental health and suicidal behaviour in prisoners.[64,65,66,67,68] Investigators found moderate to severe suicide risk among between 20% and 75% of prisoners, and moderate or severe depressive symptoms among between 11% and 56%. When tested, these two variables were positively associated. Between 7% and 12% of prisoners had previously attempted suicide. One study found remand status to be associated with suicide risk, and two studies found that most suicide attempts occurred within the first year of imprisonment.

In Ecuador, a 50% prevalence of depression and 26% prevalence of psychosis were reported in the prison population. Comorbid depression and psychosis were present in 22%.[69]

All studies, except the one conducted in Chile, found higher prevalence rates of mental disorders and suicide risk among prisoners, compared to their respective country's general population.

Only two studies have been conducted on the continent investigating completed suicides and suicide rates in prisoners, in comparison with rates in the general population.[55,70] The first study was conducted in the province of Buenos Aires in 2003 and found prison suicide rates 10 times higher than in the general population. The second study investigated all South American countries, except French Guyana, Suriname, and Venezuela, from 2000 to 2017. In the region as a whole, the mean suicide rate in prison was 40 per 100,000 prisoners, meaning prisoners were four times more likely to die by suicide than the South American general population. Significantly higher suicide rates in prison compared to age-standardized community based populations were also found in each country individually (i.e. Argentina, Bolivia, Brazil, Chile, Colombia, Ecuador, Paraguay, Peru, and Uruguay). Imprisoned women were, on average, 13.5 times more likely to die by suicide than the age-standardized female general population, whereas this ratio in men was 2.4.

In summary, current data on mental health and suicidal behaviour among South American prisoners are scant and findings may not be generalizable outside the countries where data have been collected (i.e. Brazil, Chile, Colombia, and, to some extent, Argentina). Further research needs to be conducted in the remaining countries of the continent to inform on local prison contexts. Nevertheless, data available to us so far on South American prisoners indicate a high prevalence of mental disorders and suicide risk, as well as high incidence rates of completed suicides. Although these rates in South America are lower than in Western Europe and North America, they are significantly higher than the rates in the community-based population. Also, some of the previously reported associations between suicidal behaviour and psychiatric and criminological factors, such as psychiatric disorders and remand status, could be reproduced in the region. With a growing prison population in the region, suicide prevention strategies specifically targeted to prisoners, provision of effective health, including mental health, services, and provision of adequate and humane prison infrastructure are public health necessities.

Suicidal behaviour in sexual and gender minorities in South America

Sexual and gender minorities across the world

There are an estimated 339 million people in the world who are part of sexual or gender minorities (SGMs). In this chapter, the term 'sexual and gender minority' is used to refer to people whose sexual orientation is non-heterosexual and those identifying with, or expressing as, a different gender than the one assigned at birth, as well as intersex individuals. SGMs will therefore include sexual minorities such as lesbian, gay, bisexual, asexual, pansexual, and polysexual people, as well as gender minorities such as transgender, intersex, queer, gender non-conforming, and two-spirit people.

Much has changed over the past three decades in the legal and social status of individuals belonging to SGMs. It is now possible for same-sex couples to marry and adopt children in 26 countries. Further, SGMs are granted broad legal protection against discrimination in 56 countries. However, 67 countries in the world still criminalize same-sex conducts, and in six countries, these acts are punishable by death.[71] On a societal level, in countries where same-sex conducts are illegal, surveys found that only 46% of the population think that equal rights and protections should be given to sexual minorities, and 36% disagree, whereas in non-criminalizing countries, these figures are, respectively, 60% and 19%.[72] Regarding transgender people, only seven countries allow legal gender recognition and gender-affirming surgery without the need for irreversible sterilization or a psychiatric diagnosis.[73]

While civil rights have slowly improved, violence against people belonging to transgender minorities and other SGMs has also increased over the past years.[74] Between 2017 and 2018, 369 killings of transgender individuals were reported worldwide, more than double the number in 2008. Several studies found an increased prevalence of physical (including murder, beating, kidnapping, rape, and sexual assault) and psychological violence (including harassment, threats, coercion, and arbitrary deprivation of liberty) against lesbian, gay, bisexual, and transgender (LGBT) people when compared to the general population.[75,76] Further, a recent review covering 50 countries found a lifetime prevalence of 12–68% of physical violence against transgender people specifically motivated by the perception of sexual orientation and gender identity. The lifetime prevalence of sexual violence ranged between 7% and 49%. Among lesbian, gay, and bisexual (LGB) people, the lifetime prevalence of physical violence was 3–31%, and the prevalence of sexual violence 2–9%.[77] Most research studies on SGMs separately consider LGBT individuals. Other SGMs have mostly been unrepresented in past and current research.

In summary, although many countries provide legal protection to people belonging to SGMs, a hostile and stigmatizing environment may still be present. In addition, in countries without legal protection for SGMs, public institutions even enact and legitimize this stigma. This could mean the absence of protection from aggression as well as restricted access to health and social services.

Mental health and suicidal behaviour in sexual and gender minorities

The discriminatory environment in which SGMs often live can be related to mental health problems and suicide risk. The minority stress theory (MST), a theoretical approach also applied in research to racial and gender discrimination, provides an explanatory link between discrimination of minorities, in this case SGMs, and health disparities such as increased prevalence of mental illness and substance use disorders. According to this explanatory framework, health disparities in relation to SGMs reflect a stigmatizing environment, which leads to an increased risk of discrimination, harassment, victimization, physical and psychological abuse, and possibly limited access to health and social services. Within this framework, psychological research investigating the mental health of SGMs has focused on MST factors such as experience of prejudice, expectations of rejection, and internalized homophobia. The latter describes, in lesbian and gay individuals, the personal acceptance and endorsement of social stigma as part of their value system and self-concept, that is 'the gay person's direction of negative social attitudes toward the self, leading to a devaluation of the self and resultant internal conflicts and poor self-regard'.[78] A corresponding concept has been proposed for transgender individuals called internalized transphobia, which refers to a negative self-concept about gender identity, including self-hate or shame.

Studies directly investigating the mental health of SGMs found a higher risk of mental disorders, such as depression, anxiety, bipolar disorder, and post-traumatic stress disorder, compared to the general population. In surveys from the United States, up to 31% of LGBT, and specifically up to 52% of transgender, individuals screened positive for depression, a rate many times higher than in the general population.[79,80] When directly compared to the general population, LGB people were found to have a significantly higher prevalence of depression[81] and 12-month risk of depression and anxiety disorders. Alcohol and other substance dependence disorders was 50% higher than in the general population.[82]

The prevalence of suicidal behaviour and non-suicidal self-injury was also consistently elevated in SGM populations. The lifetime prevalence of a history of suicide attempt was between 10% and 29% in LGB people, and the risk of attempting suicide was more than twofold higher compared to the general population. One study investigating over 15,000 LGB youth in the United States found a 1-year prevalence of 40% for suicidal ideation (15% among heterosexual youth), 35% for planning suicide (12% among heterosexual youth), and 24.9% for attempted suicide (6% among heterosexual youth).[83]

Among transgender people, the lifetime prevalence of self-harm was estimated to range between 19% and 38%,[84] suicidal ideation between 16% and 69%,[85,86] and suicide attempt between 14% and 52%.[84,87,88,89] To better inform on the specific risk of suicidal behaviour in transgender people, comparisons were made not only between transgender and general or cis-gender populations, but also between transgender and LGB people. Studies separately analysing transgender and LGB participants in the United States reported a lifetime prevalence of attempted suicide of between 41% and 52% in transgender populations, whereas the prevalence in the LGB sample was lower, ranging from 10% to 29%, compared to 5% among the general population.[84,90] Current data indicate that transgender people may be at even greater risk of suicidal behaviour than LGB sexual minorities.

South America

In South America, several countries have recently passed legislation to provide more extensive civil rights to sexual minorities, and to prevent discrimination against sexual minorities in the job market and in provision of health services. Same-sex marriage is now legal in Argentina, Brazil, Ecuador, and Uruguay. Some degree of legal protection against discrimination is provided in all South American countries, except Guyana and Paraguay. However, LGBT people in the region still face hostile environments, with frequent reports of aggressions and discrimination.

As in other regions of the world, SGM status is rarely recorded in police reports, or judicial and health care statistics, making public data on violence against individuals and on health outcomes scarce. For instance, of 1864 suicides reported in Colombia in 2010, only one was registered as belonging to a sexual minority.[91] It is therefore often left to non-governmental organizations (NGOs) and SGM advocacy groups to collect these data.

As previously mentioned, a recent report released by Transgender Europe, together with other worldwide advocacy groups, found that between 2017 and 2018, 369 transgender and gender-diverse people were killed worldwide, which add up to 2982 killings since 2008.[74] More than half of these killings (i.e. 1679) occurred in South America, of which 73% in Brazil only.

Surveys showed that between 77% and 80% of South Americans belonging to SGMs self-reported to have experienced some form of discrimination, with 32% reporting physical aggression.[92,93] Regarding access to health care, an investigation commissioned by the municipality of Bogota (Colombia) found that SGMs were systematically discriminated against in the provision of health services when their sexual orientation or gender identity was revealed to health care providers. This resulted in poor attendance of individuals belonging to SGMs at health care facilities, with only 50% of male-to-female transgender individuals attending a facility within the last six months.[94]

With regard to mental health and suicidal behaviour of SGMs, very little research is available in South America, solely originating from Argentina, Brazil, Chile, and Colombia. To our knowledge, only five studies were conducted on the subject of suicidal behaviour in SGMs in these four countries.

Two studies investigated homosexual men and women; one study investigated homosexual men; and two investigated transgender individuals. These studies found a prevalence of mental disorders of between 10% and 38% among homosexual men and women,[92,95] with the most prevalent mental illnesses being major depressive disorder (15%) and generalized anxiety disorder (13%). Although these rates were higher than in the local general population, one study that directly compared homosexual individuals with heterosexual controls found no significant difference in the prevalence of mental illness between the two groups.[95] Both studies found 8% of the lesbian and gay participants to be at risk of suicide.

The third study investigated gay adolescents and reported a 30% prevalence of suicidal ideation at the time of investigation.[96] The two studies that controlled for factors associated with the prevalence of suicidal behaviour found a strong association with internalized homophobia and past sexual abuse.[95,96]

The two studies investigating transgender individuals found a prevalence of anxiety symptoms and depressive symptoms of 98% and 82%, respectively, and between 33% and 73% of participants had at least one suicide attempt in their lifetime.[97,98] As with studies conducted in homosexual men, one of the two studies found a significant association between prevalence rates of lifetime suicide attempts and internalized stigma in the transgender participants.

Much of the research so far conducted in South America has relevant limitations to the external validity of findings, mostly because of strong sampling bias. Three of the aforementioned studies used snowball sampling techniques,[92,95,96] whereas another study recruited its sample from a clinical population.[98] Although non-probabilistic methods are sometimes unavoidable to investigate SGMs, which often are difficult to access, this limits result generalizations and our understanding of suicidal behaviour in SGMs. In order to better understand the extent of suicidal behaviour in LGBT people in South America, further research is needed by using representative samples, including underrepresented SGMs, addressing associated factors, and involving countries where no studies have been conducted so far.

Nevertheless, data available today indicate a much higher risk of suicidal behaviour in lesbian, gay, and transgender populations in South America. Targeted policies for provision of mental health services to sexual minorities should be developed and implemented.

Acknowledgements

APM received funding from the Agencia Nacional de Investigación y Desarrollo in Chile, FONDECYT Regular 1240624

References

1. **United Nations High Commissioner for Refugees.** *Global Report 2021.* Geneva: United Nations High Commissioner for Refugees; 2021.
2. **International Organization for Migration.** Snapshot: **making migration work for all.** 2023. Available from: https://www.iom.int/sites/g/files/tmzbdl486/files/documents/2023-08/iom-snapshot-digital.pdf
3. **Van del Laat C.** La migración internacional como determinante social. In: **Cabieses B, Bernales** M, **McIntyre AM,** editors. *La Migración Internacional como Determinante Social de la Salud en Chile: Evidencia y Propuestas para Políticas Públicas.* Santiago: Universidad del Desarrollo; 2017. Chapter 2; pp. 29–38.
4. **Spallek J, Zeeb H, Razum O.** What do we have to know from migrants' past exposures to understand their health status? A life course approach. Emerging Themes in Epidemiology. 2011;**8**(1):6.
5. **Departamento de Extranjería y Migración del Ministerio del Interior y Seguridad Pública** (2016). Migración en Chile 2005–2014. Anuario Estadístico Nacional 2016,

Santiago, Chile. Available from: https://serviciomigraciones.cl/wp-content/uploads/2022/12/DEM-2016-Migracion-en-Chile-2005-2014.pdf

6. **Cabieses B, Bernales M, McIntyre AM.** *La Migración Internacional como Determinante Social de la Salud en Chile: Evidencia y Propuestas para Políticas Públicas.* Santiago: Universidad de Desarrollo; 2017.
7. **Williams AM, Baláž V.** Migration, risk, and uncertainty: theoretical perspectives. Population, Space and Place. 2012;**18**(2):167–80.
8. **Larenas D, Cabieses B.** Acceso a salud de la población migrante internacional en situación irregular: la respuesta del sector salud en Chile. Access to health services for international migrant population. Cuadernos Médico Sociales (Chile). 2018;**58**(4):97–108.
9. **Carreño A, Ajraz N, Cabieses B.** *Ser Refugiado en Chile: Trayectorias Institucionales y Experiencias de Salud de Solicitantes Latinoamericanos de Protección Internacional.* Santiago, Chile: Universidad del Desarrollo; 2019.
10. **Cabieses B.** La compleja relación entre posición socioeconómica, estatus migratorio y resultados de salud. Value in Health Regional Issues. 2014;**5**:1–6.
11. **Cabieses B, Tunstall H, Pickett KE, Gideon J.** Understanding differences in access and use of healthcare between international immigrants to Chile and the Chilean-born: a repeated cross-sectional population-based study in Chile. International Journal for Equity in Health. 2012;**11**:68.
12. **Urzua A, Cabrera C, Carvajal CC, Caqueo-Urizar A.** The mediating role of self-esteem on the relationship between perceived discrimination and mental health in South American immigrants in Chile. Psychiatry Research. 2019;**271**:187–94.
13. **Cabieses B, Bernales M, van der Laat C.** Health for all migrants in Latin America and the Caribbean. The Lancet Psychiatry. 2016;**3**(5):402.
14. **World Health Organization** (2019). World health statistics 2019: monitoring health for the SDGs. Available from: https://reliefweb.int/report/world/world-health-statistics-2019-monitoring-health-sdgs
15. **Calliess IT, Machleidt W, Ziegenbein M, Haltenhof H.** Transcultural aspects of suicidal behaviour. Fortschritte der Neurologie Psychiatrie. 2007;**75**(11):653–64.
16. **Voracek M, Loibl LM.** Consistency of immigrant and country-of-birth suicide rates: a meta-analysis. Acta Psychiatrica Scandinavica. 2008;**118**(4):259–71.
17. **Mirsky J, Kohn R, Dolberg P, Levav I.** Suicidal behavior among immigrants. Social Psychiatry and Psychiatric Epidemiology. 2011;**46**(11):1133–41.
18. **Spallek J, Reeske A, Norredam M, Nielsen SS, Lehnhardt J, Razum O.** Suicide among immigrants in Europe: a systematic literature review. European Journal of Public Health. 2015;**25**(1):63–71.
19. **Norredam M, Olsbjerg M, Petersen JH, Laursen B, Krasnik A.** Are there differences in injury mortality among refugees and immigrants compared with native-born? Injury Prevention. 2013;**19**(2):100–5.
20. **Martinez O, Wu E, Sandfort T**, et al. Evaluating the impact of immigration policies on health status among undocumented immigrants: a systematic review. Journal of Immigrant and Minority Health. 2015;**17**(3):947–70.
21. **Cabieses B, Pickett KE, Tunstall H.** What are the living conditions and health status of those who don't report their migration status? A population-based study in Chile. BMC Public Health. 2012;**12**:1013.

22. **Ratkowska KA, De Leo D.** Suicide in immigrants: an overview. Open Journal of Medical Psychology. 2013;**2**(3):124–33.
23. **Fellmeth G, Rose-Clarke K, Zhao C**, et al. Health impacts of parental migration on left-behind children and adolescents: a systematic review and meta-analysis. The Lancet. 2018;**392**(10164):2567–82.
24. **Zapata Martínez A.** Familia transnacional y remesas: padres y madres migrantes. Revista Latinoamericana de Ciencias Sociales, Niñez y Juventud. 2009;7(2):1749–69.
25. **Oso Casas L.** Migración, género y hogares transnacionales. In: **García Roca J, Lacomba Vázquez J**, editors. *La inmigración en la sociedad española: una radiografía multidisciplinar*. 2008, ISBN 978-84-7290-407-1, pp. 561–86.
26. **Kennedy MA, Parhar KK, Samra J, Gorzalka B.** Suicide ideation in different generations of immigrants. Canadian Journal of Psychiatry. 2005;**50**(6):353–6.
27. **Winterrowd E, Canetto SS, Chavez EL.** Friendships and suicidality among Mexican American adolescent girls and boys. Death Studies. 2010;**34**(7):641–60.
28. **Azuero AJ, Arreaza-Kaufman D, Coriat J**, et al. Suicide in the indigenous population of Latin America: a systematic review. Revista Colombiana de Psiquiatría. 2017;**46**(4):237–42.
29. **Larenas D, Cabieses B.** Salud de migrantes internacionales en situación irregular: una revisión sistemática de iniciativas. Revista Peruana de Medicina Experimental y Salud Pública. 2019;**36**(3):487–97.
30. **Cabieses B, Alarcón A, Bernales M, Astorga S, Martínez F** (2018). Informe final estudio licitación sistematización y evaluación del piloto nacional de salud de inmigrantes. Ministerio de Salud (Minsal), Organización Internacional para las Migraciones & Universidad del Desarrollo. Available from: https://repositorio.udd.cl/handle/11447/2487
31. **Cabieses B.** Health of migrants: simple questions can improve care. The Lancet. 2019;**393**(10188):2297–8.
32. **Cabieses B, Bernales M, Chepo M, Escobar MT, Bersano P** (2017). Plan de atención inicial integral de salud de migrantes internacionales. Proyecto Piloto. Santiago: Universidad del Desarrollo. Available from: http://repositorio.udd.cl/handle/11447/1902
33. **Walmsley R** (2021). World prison population list (13th edition). The Institute for Criminal Policy Research (ICPR) at Birkbeck, University of London. Available from: https://www.prisonstudies.org/sites/default/files/resources/downloads/world_prison_population_list_13th_edition.pdf
34. **Bureau of Justice Statistics** (2021). Corrections Statistical Analysis Tool (CSAT). Available from: https://bjs.ojp.gov/data-collection/national-prisoner-statistics-nps-program
35. **Council of Europe** (2021). SPACE I Report 2021. Available from: http://wp.unil.ch/space/space-i/annual-reports/
36. **Noonan ME** (2016). Mortality in local jails, 2000–2014: statistical tables. US Department of Justice. Available from: https://www.bjs.gov/content/pub/pdf/mlj0014st.pdf
37. **Noonan ME** (2016). Mortality in state prisons, 2001–2014: statistical tables. US Department of Justice. Available from: https://www.bjs.gov/content/pub/pdf/msp0114st.pdf

38. **Mundt AP, Cifuentes-Gramajo PA, Baranyi G, Fazel S.** Worldwide incidence of suicide in prisons: a systematic review. The Lancet Psychiatry in press. doi: 10.1016/S2215-0366(24)00134-2
39. **Hawton K, Linsell L, Adeniji T, Sariaslan A, Fazel S.** Self-harm in prisons in England and Wales: an epidemiological study of prevalence, risk factors, clustering, and subsequent suicide. The Lancet. 2014;**383**(9923):1147–54.
40. **Fruehwald S, Matschnig T, Koenig F, Bauer P, Frottier P.** Suicide in custody: case-control study. British Journal of Psychiatry. 2004;**185**:494–8.
41. **Fazel S, Ramesh T, Hawton K.** Suicide in prisons: an international study of prevalence and contributory factors. The Lancet Psychiatry. 2017;**4**(12):946–52.
42. **Zhong S, Senior M, Yu R**, et al. Risk factors for suicide in prisons: a systematic review and meta-analysis. The Lancet Public Health. 2021;**6**(3):e164–74.
43. **Fazel S, Seewald K.** Severe mental illness in 33,588 prisoners worldwide: systematic review and meta-regression analysis. British Journal of Psychiatry. 2012;**200**(5):364–73.
44. **Rivlin A, Hawton K, Marzano L, Fazel S.** Psychiatric disorders in male prisoners who made near-lethal suicide attempts: case-control study. British Journal of Psychiatry. 2010;**197**(4):313–19.
45. **Fazel S, Hayes AJ, Bartellas K, Clerici M, Trestman R.** Mental health of prisoners: prevalence, adverse outcomes, and interventions. The Lancet Psychiatry. 2016;**3**(9):871–81.
46. **Baranyi G, Scholl C, Fazel S, Patel V, Priebe S, Mundt AP.** Severe mental illness and substance use disorders in prisoners in low-income and middle-income countries: a systematic review and meta-analysis of prevalence studies. The Lancet Global Health. 2019;**7**(4):e461–71.
47. **Mundt AP, Baranyi G, Fazel S.** Incomplete discussion of bipolar disorder and comorbid substance use disorder. Authors' reply. The Lancet Global Health. 2019;**7**(7):e847.
48. **Baranyi G, Fazel S, Langerfeldt SD, Mundt AP.** The prevalence of comorbid serious mental illnesses and substance use disorders in prison populations: a systematic review and meta-analysis. The Lancet Public Health. 2022;**7**(6):e557–68.
49. **Mundt AP, Baranyi G.** The unhappy mental health triad: comorbid severe mental illnesses, personality disorders, and substance use disorders in prison populations. Frontiers in Psychiatry. 2020;**11**:804.
50. **García-Guerrero J, Marco A.** [Overcrowding in prisons and its impact on health]. Revista Española de Sanidad Penitenciaria. 2012;**14**(3):106–13.
51. **Duthe G, Hazard A, Kensey A, Shon JL.** Suicide among male prisoners in France: a prospective population-based study. Forensic Science International. 2013;**233**(1–3):273–7.
52. **Fruehwald S, Frottier P, Ritter K, Eher R, Gutierrez K.** Impact of overcrowding and legislational change on the incidence of suicide in custody experiences in Austria, 1967–1996. International Journal of Law and Psychiatry. 2002;**25**(2):119–28.
53. **Fazel S, Grann M, Kling B, Hawton K.** Prison suicide in 12 countries: an ecological study of 861 suicides during 2003–2007. 2011;**46**(3):191–5.
54. **Fritz FD, Fazel S, Benavides Salcedo A**, et al. 1324 prison suicides in 10 countries in South America: incidence, relative risks, and ecological factors. Social Psychiatry and Psychiatric Epidemiology. 2021;**56**(2):315–23.

55. **Almanzar S, Katz CL, Harry B.** Treatment of mentally ill offenders in nine developing Latin American countries. Journal of the American Academy of Psychiatry and the Law. 2015;**43**(3):340–9.
56. **Mundt AP, Baranyi G, Gabrysch C, Fazel S.** Substance use during imprisonment in low- and middle-income countries. Epidemiologic Reviews. 2018;**40**(1):70–81.
57. **Andreoli SB, Dos Santos MM, Quintana MI,** et al. Prevalence of mental disorders among prisoners in the state of Sao Paulo, Brazil. PLoS One. 2014;**9**(2):e88836.
58. **Ponde MP, Freire AC, Mendonca MS.** The prevalence of mental disorders in prisoners in the city of Salvador, Bahia, Brazil. Journal of Forensic Science. 2011;**56**(3):679–82.
59. **Mundt AP, Alvarado R, Fritsch R,** et al. Prevalence rates of mental disorders in Chilean prisons. PLoS One. 2013;**8**(7):e69109.
60. **Mundt AP, Kastner S, Larrain S, Fritsch R, Priebe S.** Prevalence of mental disorders at admission to the penal justice system in emerging countries: a study from Chile. Epidemiology and Psychiatric Sciences. 2015.
61. **Baier A, Fritsch R, Ignatyev Y, Priebe S, Mundt AP.** The course of major depression during imprisonment: a one year cohort study. Journal of Affective Disorders. 2016;**189**:207–13.
62. **Gabrysch C, Fritsch R, Priebe S, Mundt AP.** Mental disorders and mental health symptoms during imprisonment: a three-year follow-up study. PLoS One. 2019;**14**(3):e0213711.
63. **Ceballos-Espinoza F, Chávez-Hernández A-M, Padilla-Gallegos G-M, Leenaars AA.** Suicidio en las cárceles de Chile durante la década 2006–2015. Revista Criminalidad. 2016;**58**:101–18.
64. **Rubio LA, Cardona-Duque DV, Medina-Pérez ÓA, Garzón-Olivera LF, Garzón-Borray HA, Rodríguez-Hernández NS.** Riesgo suicida en población carcelaria del Tolima, Colombia. Revista de la Facultad de Medicina. 2014;**62**:33–9.
65. **Medina Pérez Ó, Cardona Duque DV, Arcila López SC.** Riesgo suicida y depresión en un grupo de internos de una cárcel del Quindío (Colombia). Investigaciones Andina. 2011;**13**:268–80.
66. **Jaramillo Gutiérrez MR, Silva Vallejo C, Rojas Arango BP, Medina-Pérez ÓA.** Ideación suicida y factores asociados en internos de un establecimiento penitenciario de Antioquia (Colombia). Revista Colombiana de Psiquiatría. 2015;**44**:100–5.
67. **Mojica CA, Sáenz DA, Rey-Anacona CA.** Riesgo suicida, desesperanza y depresión en internos de un establecimiento carcelario colombiano. Revista Colombiana de Psiquiatría. 2009;**38**:681–92.
68. **Larrotta Castillo R, Luzardo Briceño M, Vargas Cifuentes S, Rangel Noriega K.** Características del comportamiento suicida en cárceles de Colombia. Revista Criminalidad. 2014;**56**:83–95.
69. **Benavides A, Chuchuca J, Klaic D, Waters W, Martin M, Romero-Sandoval N.** Depression and psychosis related to the absence of visitors and consumption of drugs in male prisoners in Ecuador: a cross sectional study. BMC Psychiatry. 2019;**19**(1):248.
70. **Folino JO, Marchiano S, Sanchez Wilde A.** [Suicide in convicts in Buenos Aires Province]. Vertex. 2003;**14**(54):286–91.
71. **Mendos LR** (2019). State-sponsored homophobia report, 13th edition. Geneva: International Lesbian, Gay, Bisexual, Trans and Intersex Association. Available from: https://ilga.org/state-sponsored-homophobia-report

72. **Carroll A, Robotham G** (2017). Minorities report 2017: attitudes to sexual and gender minorities around the world. Geneva: International Lesbian, Gay, Bisexual, Trans and Intersex Association. Available from: https://ilga.org/downloads/ILGA_RIWI_Minorities_Report_2017_Attitudes_to_sexual_and_gender_minorities.pdf
73. **Chiam Z, Duffy S, González Gil M** (2017). Trans legal mapping report 2017: recognition before the law. Geneva: International Lesbian, Gay, Bisexual, Trans and Intersex Association. Available from: https://ilga.org/downloads/ILGA_Trans_Legal_Mapping_Report_2017_ENG.pdf
74. **Transrespect versus Transphobia Worldwide (TvT).** Trans Day of Remembrance (TDoR) 2018. Press release. Available from: https://transrespect.org/en/tmm-update-trans-day-of-remembrance-2018/
75. **Rothman EF, Exner D, Baughman AL.** The prevalence of sexual assault against people who identify as gay, lesbian, or bisexual in the United States: a systematic review. Trauma, Violence, and Abuse. 2011;**12**(2):55–66.
76. **Stotzer RL.** Violence against transgender people: a review of United States data. Aggression and Violent Behavior. 2009;**14**(3):170–9.
77. **Blondeel K, de Vasconcelos S, García-Moreno C, Stephenson R, Temmerman M, Toskin I.** Violence motivated by perception of sexual orientation and gender identity: a systematic review. Bulletin of the World Health Organization. 2018;**96**(1):29–41L.
78. **Meyer IH.** Prejudice, social stress, and mental health in lesbian, gay, and bisexual populations: conceptual issues and research evidence. Psychological Bulletin. 2003;**129**(5):674–97.
79. **Yarns BC, Abrams JM, Meeks TW, Sewell DD.** The mental health of older LGBT adults. Current Psychiatry Reports. 2016;**18**(6):60.
80. **Espelage DLA, Aragon SR, Birkett M, Koenig BW.** Homophobic teasing, psychological outcomes, and sexual orientation among high school students: what influence do parents and schools have? School Psychology Review. 2008;**37**(2):202–16.
81. **Yi H, Lee H, Park J, Choi B, Kim S-S.** Health disparities between lesbian, gay, and bisexual adults and the general population in South Korea: Rainbow Connection Project I. Epidemiology and Health. 2017;**39**(0):e2017046–0.
82. **King M, Semlyen J, Tai SS,** et al. A systematic review of mental disorder, suicide, and deliberate self harm in lesbian, gay and bisexual people. BMC Psychiatry. 2008;**8**(1):70.
83. **Caputi TL, Smith D, Ayers JW.** Suicide risk behaviors among sexual minority adolescents in the United States, 2015. JAMA. 2017;**318**(23):2349–51.
84. **Mustanski B, Liu RT.** A longitudinal study of predictors of suicide attempts among lesbian, gay, bisexual, and transgender youth. Archives of Sexual Behavior. 2013;**42**(3):437–48.
85. **Chen R, Zhu X, Wright L,** et al. Suicidal ideation and attempted suicide amongst Chinese transgender persons: national population study. J Affective Disorders. 2019;**245**:1126–34.
86. **Mereish EH, O'Cleirigh C, Bradford JB.** Interrelationships between LGBT-based victimization, suicide, and substance use problems in a diverse sample of sexual and gender minorities. Psychology, Health and Medicine. 2014;**19**(1):1–13.
87. **Toomey RB, Syvertsen AK, Shramko M.** Transgender adolescent suicide behavior. Pediatrics. 2018;**142**(4):e20174218.

88. **Maguen S, Shipherd JC.** Suicide risk among transgender individuals. Psychology and Sexuality. 2010;**1**(1):34–43.
89. **Mathy RM.** Transgender identity and suicidality in a nonclinical sample. Journal of Psychology and Human Sexuality. 2003;**14**(4):47–65.
90. **Haas AP, Eliason M, Mays VM,** et al. Suicide and suicide risk in lesbian, gay, bisexual, and transgender populations: review and recommendations. Journal of Homosexuality. 2011;**58**(1):10–51.
91. **Pineda Roa CA.** Factores asociados con riesgo de suicidio de adolescentes y jóvenes autoidentificados como lesbianas, gays y bisexuales: estado actual de la literatura. Revista Colombiana de Psiquiatría. 2013;**42**:333–49.
92. **Barrientos J, Gómez F, Cárdenas M, Gúzman M, Bahamondes J.** Health and wellbeing of sexual minorities. Revista Médica de Chile. 2017;**145**(9):1115–21.
93. **Ripoll JL.** El amor en tiempos de cólera: Derechos LGBT en Colombia. Sur Revista Internacional de Derechos Humanos. 2009;**6**(11):79–97.
94. **Rocha-Buelvas A.** El riesgo suicida y los significados de las minorías sexuales: un nuevo reto para la salud pública. Revista de la Facultad de Medicina. 2015;**63**:537–44.
95. **Ceará AdT, Dalgalarrondo P.** Transtornos mentais, qualidade de vida e identidade em homossexuais na maturidade e velhice. Archives of Clinical Psychiatry (São Paulo). 2010;**37**:118–23.
96. **Carlos Alejandro P-R.** Factores de riesgo de ideación suicida en una muestra de adolescentes y jóvenes colombianos autoidentificados como homosexuales. Revista Colombiana de Psiquiatría. 2019;**48**(1):2–9.
97. **Marshall BD, Socías ME, Kerr T, Zalazar V, Sued O, Arístegui I.** Prevalence and correlates of lifetime suicide attempts among transgender persons in Argentina. Journal of Homosexuality. 2016;**63**(7):955–67.
98. **Lerri MR, Romão APMS, dos Santos MA, Giami A, Ferriani RA, da Silva Lara LA.** Clinical characteristics in a sample of transsexual people. Revista Brasileira de Ginecologia e Obstetrícia. 2017;**39**:545–51.

Chapter 11

Suicidal behaviour and sociocultural factors among immigrants of Turkish origin in Germany

Özlem Eylem-van Bergeijk and Mehmet Eskin

Introduction

Suicide is a complex phenomenon with multiple factors. One of the long-standing patterns in suicide epidemiology is the differences between and within countries worldwide.[1] There is also evidence for further variation, particularly when stratified by region (whether urban or rural area), age, and gender.[2] These differences have led to research on the factors that predispose some people in these countries to an increased risk of suicide.[3]

For instance, suicide rates in the European region (10.5 per 100,000) were higher than the global average (9.0 per 100,000).[4] In Germany, approximately 10,284 people die by suicide every year (12.3 per 100,000 population in 2019),[4] and the completed suicide rates are estimated to be almost three times higher among males compared to females (18.6 vs 6.2 per 100,000). Germany reported the highest absolute suicide rates (10,284 deaths), alongside France (8961 deaths), in 2019 in Europe.[4]

Up until now, suicide in Muslim countries has not received much attention.[5] The main reason is that suicide is strongly prohibited by Islam, which is therefore expected to be protective against suicide.[5] For instance, the completed suicide rates in Turkey are low (2.4 per 100,000) and the gender variation in completed suicide rates (3.6 per 100,000 among males vs 1.2 per 100,000 among females) is in line with the global pattern.[4] However, there are exceptions to this when stratified by region and age. The gender ratio for suicide in Eastern Turkey (a rural and rather traditional region) is reversed compared to the general pattern, with young females reporting almost twice the suicide rate of young males.[6] In particular, young Turkish women aged between 15 and 24 years seem to be at high risk of suicide in Eastern Turkey[7] and Germany.[8] There is a cross-national consistency in rates and characteristics of suicidal behaviours between the Turkish population in Turkey and the Turkish migrant population in Europe,[6] and this is counterintuitive to the protective role of Islam against suicide.[5]

To help prevent future suicide attempts and suicide, it is important to further the current understanding of suicidality in populations that are at elevated risk and have not yet received enough attention. This would also result in improvement in provision of mental health services in the treatment of suicidal behaviours. Thus, this chapter is aimed at furthering the current understanding of social and cultural risk and precipitating factors for suicidal behaviours among Turkish migrants in Germany. These factors are outlined in relation to the research on suicidal behaviours among Turkish populations in Europe and in Turkey. How identified risk and precipitating factors lead to suicidal behaviours are discussed in the context of religion and migration. Additionally, in this chapter, we use the terms *precipitating factors* when referring to perceived causes or important contributors to suicidal behaviour, and the term *characteristics* when referring to aspects that increase the likelihood of a suicidal crisis, which may be 'causal' (e.g. psychiatric or physical illness), whereas others are not necessarily 'causal' (e.g. socio-demographic factors).[9]

Turkish migrants in Germany

Turkish migrants are the largest migrant group in Germany. It is revealed that out of an estimated 14.16 million migrant population in Germany in 2021, 1.313 million (9.2%) have Turkish background.[10]

The history of the Turkish population in Germany dates to 1961 when a convention between Germany and Turkey was signed. This allowed labour migration from Turkey to Germany. At first, most of the migrants came as 'guest labourers' because of a shortage of (low-skilled) workers at that time. The reasons for migration of Turks were mostly economic, and even though their contracts were temporary at first, many of these got prolonged and most of the workers stayed in Germany. Initially, migration from Turkey took place from urban areas, but the majority of migrants came from rural areas in central Anatolia.[11] Migration of Turkish 'guest labourers' continued in large numbers until around the mid seventies. However, migration from Turkey is nowadays still ongoing because of family reunification and children, or even grandchildren, of Turkish 'guest labourers' quite often marry someone from Turkey. In recent years, there has also been a dramatic increase in the number of refugees from Turkey in Germany due to deterioration in the political and economic situation.[12] Thus, the Turkish migrant population in Germany is highly heterogeneous.[12]

Turkish people's migration status often coincides with social adversities. In 2016, they were the immigrant group with the lowest income, with a poverty risk rate of 36%.p. 1.[13] At the same time, education level was often quite low: 45% of Turkish immigrant children grew up with parents who had neither a professional qualification nor a university entrance qualification. Approximately 30% of young immigrants of Turkish descent did not succeed in getting certification from school or finding a job.[14,15] Consequently, the unemployment rate among Turkish migrants was almost three times higher than among Germans.[14] This is the lowest rate among immigrants in Germany.[15,16]

Suicidal behaviours in Turkish migrants in Germany

In Germany, young women of Turkish descent have elevated rates of suicidal ideation, attempted suicide, and suicide.[6,17] The WHO/EURO Multicentre study in Würzburg revealed that the attempted suicide rates were more than five times higher among Turkish females compared to native German women (512 vs 99.9/100,000).[18] The elevated risk of attempted suicide rates was also replicated by a prospective hospital registration study in Berlin.[19] Accordingly, with a rate of 225.4/100,000 in 2009 and 297.0/100,000 in 2010, the youngest female population (aged 18–24 years) had the highest attempted suicide rates compared to the other age groups of women of Turkish descent.[19]

When it comes to suicide, age and gender differences might be even more skewed.[6,20] A study that calculated suicide rates among Turkish immigrant females in Germany indicated that the female-to-male ratio was reversed compared to the global pattern.[8] Girls of Turkish descent aged 10–17 years had an almost twofold elevated risk of suicide (relative risk = 1.79; 95% confidence interval (CI) = 1.41–2.27) compared to same-aged males, as well as to other female and male age groups.[6,8]

Similar patterns of attempted suicide have also been observed in the Netherlands,[21] Switzerland,[22,23] and rural areas in Turkey.[24,25] Turkish migrant women, aged 15–24 years, are 2–3 times more likely to attempt suicide than Dutch native women (545 vs 246/100,000 per year),[21] and 3–4 times more likely than Swiss native women (646 vs 172/100,000 per year).[22,23] In Turkey, examination of hospital registration data in the south-eastern region of Turkey revealed that attempted suicide rates were 4.15 times higher among young females aged 15–24 years compared to same-aged males, as well as to other female and male age groups.[6,7,24,25]

Preceding suicide epidemiology pointed to special risks of suicidal behaviours among Turkish women aged 14–25 years in Europe and Turkey. At present, the most popular explanations of the variation in suicide epidemiology between ethnic minorities and majorities focus on social and cultural factors such as acculturation difficulties in host countries.[3,26] Thus, in the remainder of this chapter, how these factors might lead to an increased risk of suicidal behaviours among Turkish migrants in Germany is discussed.

Social and cultural factors for suicidal behaviours

Religion is one of the most potent factors in the sociocultural context, determining one's accepting and/or rejecting attitudes towards suicide and suicidal people.[26] Migration is another important factor that is heavily investigated to explain the elevated risk of suicidal behaviours among some ethnic groups relative to others.[26–28] Migration is defined as a process of moving from one place to another, either voluntarily or involuntarily, depending on various sociopolitical reasons.[28] On the one hand, it has often been linked to increased psychological well-being, satisfaction, and freedom.[29] On the other hand, it has also been identified as an important contextual factor for mental health problems and suicide among some ethnic groups.[28] In this section, the religious context and migration-related factors are discussed in relation to the increased risk of suicidality among Turkish migrants in Germany.

Religion

Germany's religious landscape has been considered to be dynamic, reflecting the changing political structures. Today, approximately 28.6% of Germans identify as Roman Catholic and 26.6% as Evangelical Christian as a result of Protestant reformations.[30] As a result of the communist regime in East Germany between 1945 and 1990, atheism has been popularized in East Germany and it is estimated that 35.4% of Germans identify as atheists or antagonists.[30] Atheists and antagonists are known to have liberal attitudes towards suicide and are more accepting of those who are thinking of suicide.[31] Historically, the issue of whether Roman Catholics or Protestants have higher suicide rates has been highly debated in suicide literature.[5] The Christian doctrine considers suicide as an act of sin and therefore prohibits it.[31] Islam has been introduced in Germany more recently as a result of migration of guest workers from Muslim countries. The majority of Turkish migrants in Germany are Sunni Muslims.[30] Islam has probably the strongest and the most explicit objection against suicide among the other religions.[31] The Koran prohibits self-killing and those who have committed suicide to be forbidden from entering Paradise.[5,31]

The relationship between Islam and suicide is complicated.[5] Cross-cultural research highlights a more rejecting attitude towards suicide among the Turkish population, compared to their counterparts, in a number of countries in Europe (Slovakia, Austria, and Sweden), reporting more permissive and liberal attitudes towards suicide disclosure of a close friend.[32-34] However, Turkish populations reported feeling more responsible and were more willing to help a suicidal close friend, compared to the majority of populations from Europe.[32-34] These findings could be attributed to differences between individualistic and collectivistic value orientations.[35] It could be argued that Turkish populations who identify themselves more with Islam have more collectivistic value orientations, and therefore are more willing to help a suicidal friend, even though they are more rejecting of disclosure of suicidal intentions.[35]

The impact of the preceding supportive reaction towards a suicidal close friend might be double-edged. A qualitative study by Eylem and colleagues in the Netherlands[36] pointed at the fear of being judged by the informal network (i.e. family and friends) among Turkish migrants because of having suicidal thoughts,[36] and this was highlighted as the main barrier restricting help-seeking among those who are thinking of suicide.[36] Similar findings on the help-seeking patterns for suicidal behaviours among Turkish migrants were reported in another qualitative study in Germany.[37] It could be that the social reactions of the informal network might be perceived as interference and/or rejection by the suicidal individual. It could be that, for instance, people's attempts to keep a suicidal person occupied with fun activities may look like helping but may, in fact, block communication about the real issues causing suicidal thinking.[36] It could also be that those who have suicidal thoughts and are not religious could experience a sense of isolation if they are surrounded by mostly strict believers. This argument is supported by a recent multinational study in various Muslim countries where the freedom of religion is restricted or religion is compulsory, and the protective function of the religion might be limited.[38]

Although religious doctrines are important determinants of suicidal behaviours, their impact cannot be understood without the cultural and individual meanings attributed to religion and suicide. Thus, the next section discusses these meanings. It also highlights how transformations of, and/or continuity in, these meanings could generate distress, leading to suicidal behaviours in the process of migration.

Migration-related factors

Cultural meaning

Douglas recognized the complexity of the cultural meaning of suicide by arguing that 'the meaning of suicide is by no means unidimensional, universally agreed upon, or unchanging among various societies of Europe and certainly not beyond the cultural boundaries of Europe' (p. 178).[39] Accordingly, differences in sociocultural contexts, such as living in a rural or an urban area, and holding cultural beliefs, which would sanction or honour suicide, may have relevance to suicide risk.[3,26,40] Support for the value of the cultural meaning of suicide in explaining the elevated risk of suicidal behaviours comes from a qualitative study by Heredia-Montesinos and colleagues in Germany.[37] Focus group interviews with Turkish migrant women in Berlin highlighted the fear of dishonouring themselves and/or their families by disclosing suicidal thoughts central to their underutilization of psychological services.[37] These findings are also relevant to the findings of other qualitative studies in the Netherlands,[36,41] in which fear of failing responsibilities towards the family and/or the community related to gender role expectations was identified as the main precipitating factor for suicidal behaviours.[36,41] In order to have a better understanding of these culture-specific reactions to mental distress, it is important to understand the gender role conceptualizations among the Turkish diaspora in Germany.

The concepts of *namus* and *seref* (i.e. honour) are relevant to the definition of gender roles in Turkish culture.[11] In a traditional rural family context, these concepts pose powerful mechanisms of social control among members of the family. Family honour is a very important matter among the Turkish diaspora in Germany, many of whom came from traditional rural areas.[11] Accordingly, females are responsible for the honour of the family by maintaining their sexual abstinence until marriage. Failing to do so results in the family's loss of reputation among the Turkish community. This custom brings strong scrutiny to the behaviours of female members of the family. In extreme cases, honour killing is practised by male members of the family when a dishonourable act of a woman jeopardizes the family's reputation in the community.[11,13,14]

Honour-related violence (e.g. domestic violence, physical and emotional abuse), aiming to protect the family *namus*, is often reported as a common precipitating factor for suicidal behaviours among young Turkish migrant women in Germany[14] and the Netherlands,[41] as well as among young Turkish women in rural areas in Turkey.[7,21,24,25] Similar examples have also been observed in other collectivist patriarchal cultures such as young immigrant women of Indian descent in South Africa,[42] young Pakistani women living in rural and/or remote areas of Pakistan,[43] women in rural Iran,[44] young Chinese women in Hong Kong,[45] and South Asian immigrant women in the United Kingdom.[46,47]

Cultural continuity

The above similarities in the cultural meaning of suicide among Turkish migrants in different contexts raise the question: to what extent is there continuity (or change) in the social and cultural factors contributing to suicidal behaviour among Turkish migrants? The cultural continuity theory argues that migrants tend to import the characteristics and precipitating factors for suicidal behaviours from their country of origin into the countries to which they migrate.[3,26]

How the preceding social stressors for suicide (e.g. marital conflict, domestic violence, honour-related violence) consistently precipitate suicidal behaviours among Turkish women in north-west Europe and Turkey could be discussed in reference to Durkheim's fatalistic suicide archetype. Durkheim's theory of suicide is based on the social organization of the community to which the individuals belong.[48] Accordingly, suicide rates are representations of the degree of social integration and regulation in society. Fatalistic suicide is characterized by a lack of control over one's life course, a sense of powerlessness, and the lack of personal autonomy over one's life decisions. When members of a community are forced to abide by harsh sociocultural norms, such as honour, and they do not feel like their own, these rules are experienced as external, demanding, and obtrusive, and are failed to be internalized.[48] A recent systematic literature review by van Bergen and colleagues[6] indicates that autonomy restriction and honour-related issues seem to be more common in the Eastern region of Turkey, which is more traditional and patriarchal, when compared to the rest of the regions in Turkey.[6] The fact that most Turkish immigrants in Germany specifically have migrated from these traditional areas provides further support to the cultural continuity of patriarchy and oppressive practices against women in both Turkish and German contexts, and this finding substantiates Durkheim's fatalistic suicide theory to explain the high rates of suicidality among Turkish women.[6]

Cultural conflict

The elevated risk of suicidal behaviours in a particular ethnic group is also related to the minority and majority experiences, and such experiences are shaped by the diverse climate in a particular society.[49] Thus, in this section, the elevated risk of suicidal behaviours among Turkish migrant females in Germany is discussed from an inter-group relationship perspective.

Migration leads to acculturation—a process when a culture encounters a dominant alternative culture.[50] According to Berry's bi-dimensional acculturation theory, people who are going through the process of acculturation face two fundamental issues: (1) cultural maintenance—the tendency to maintain links with the heritage culture; and (2) participation—the tendency to participate in the culture of other minorities and majorities.[50] Cultural conflict occurs when there is a conflict between the minority and majority groups in terms of the preceding issues, which results in subsequent psychological distress, mental health problems, and suicidal behaviours.[51,-55] The greater the disparity between the demands of the host culture and the minority culture, the greater the risk of psychological distress and subsequent mental health problems.[27]

Support for the relevance of the cultural conflict argument in Turkish migrant females in Germany comes from a cross-sectional study by Aichberger and colleagues.[51] In a representative sample of 205 women of Turkish descent in Berlin, greater perceived ethnic discrimination was related to greater psychological distress only among those who are more oriented to maintaining their heritage culture (i.e. cultural maintenance). This relationship was still significant when well-established demographic characteristics such as unemployment were controlled for.[51] Similar findings come from cross-sectional research from Belgium[54] and the Netherlands.[52] Thus, Turkish migrants with greater cultural maintenance consistently report more psychological distress in their contact with other minority and majority populations, especially when they feel their ethnic identity is incompatible with those of the majority culture.[51,-54]

Overall, the above findings point to the protective role of participation in the host society, which might be linked with more social support and resilience against psychological distress and subsequent suicidal behaviours.[55,56] The protective role of participation in the host country contradicts studies reporting that strong identification with the heritage culture increases resilience against mental health problems.[57] Yet, it is in line with research suggesting that cultural maintenance increases perceived discrimination and subsequent psychological distress.[58] The contradictory findings could be discussed in relation to the sociopolitical contexts of the host countries. The current sociopolitical conditions in Germany and in the rest of Europe are characterized by raising political conservativism, nationalism, racism, and subsequent discriminatory politics, discouraging the continuity of traditional cultural norms and values among migrants. Since Turkish migrants have strong ties with their culture of origin,[27] the perceived pressure to fit in mainstream German society might lead to more perceived discrimination and subsequent psychological distress in inter-group contacts.[59] In light of these findings, it could be argued that the demands for cultural continuity (i.e. maintaining family honour) would be greater among Turkish females in Germany, which would put them in a vulnerable position for greater cultural conflict and subsequent psychological stress and suicidal behaviours.[41,42]

Further, a cross-sectional study in the Netherlands by Eylem and colleagues[52] pointed to a more complex pathway between acculturation and suicidal ideation among Turkish migrants, which might be moderated by the attachment style. Attachment refers to the interaction strategies with others in new situations and is derived from the early emotional experience with primary caretakers.[52] Theoretically, it could be argued that attachment styles in the early years of life predict our attitudes and adaptation strategies in our in-group and out-group interactions later on in life.[60-62] In line with this theoretical insight, the results indicated that those who are less securely attached might be more vulnerable to suicidal ideation, especially if they also have a higher orientation to maintaining their ethnic culture.[52,63]

It is well known that insecure attachment styles are characterized by a sense of unworthiness (unlovability) and the anticipation of rejection by others.[60] It could be that Turkish young women in Germany, who are often exposed to harsh social control within the Turkish migrant community, might be more insecure about making life choices and might be more likely to anticipate rejection in their interpersonal relationships.[6] Additionally, the current sociopolitical context might precipitate this anticipation of rejection by other groups by emphasizing the 'cultural incompatibility' discourse. Arguably, engaging in daily social interactions with members of other minority and majority communities might provide them with positive intergroup contacts, which, in turn, would contradict the anticipation of rejection and reduce the risk of suicidal thinking and attempts.[52,63]

Conclusion and future directions

In light of existing evidence, it could be argued that the patterns and circumstances around suicidal behaviours are intertwined with the processes and consequences of migration among Turkish migrants in Germany. More strikingly, Turkish women aged between 14 and 25 years constitute a specific subgroup, with an elevated risk of suicidal behaviours not only in Germany, but also in Switzerland, the Netherlands, and rural areas in Turkey.[6] The consistency in these sociodemographic characteristics highlights the importance of the role of religion and social and cultural factors, amounting to the elevated risk of suicidal behaviours.

Recent research promises that participation in the social life of the host country might create opportunities for positive intergroup contacts and this, in turn, might reduce psychological distress and the risk of suicidal behaviours. This finding highlights the importance of community-based interventions aiming to improve engagement with this specific group in their help-seeking process. Considering the strong cultural stigma attached to suicide disclosures among Turkish migrants in Germany, prevention efforts should reduce this stigma among those who are at risk of suicide, as well as among their formal (i.e. employers, civil servants, and professionals) and informal networks (i.e. family and friends). Positive social reactions from the informal network in response to suicide disclosures might facilitate a successful social support process.[50]

Even though much has been achieved up until now, there are still important gaps in the literature. For instance, the available research is mainly cross-sectional and does not allow causal interpretations of the preceding associations. Such associations should be tested further by controlled prospective studies. In-depth qualitative studies exist, informing about the cultural meaning attributed to suicide and help-seeking for suicide among Turkish migrants in Germany.[42] However, the sample of the study by Heredia-Montesinos and colleagues,[37] for instance, was recruited from neighbourhood centres and women's organizations and it might be more representative of Turkish migrant women with a long history of settlement in Germany. Recently, there has been an increase in political refugees from Turkey in Germany.[12] This new group of Turkish migrants might have a different cultural meaning of suicide, compared to the Turkish migrant populations with a long history of settlement who have strong ties with their heritage culture.[11,27] Further research is needed to investigate risk and precipitating factors for suicide among Turkish migrants in Germany.

Overall, a strong failure discourse is attached to suicide, especially among young Turkish women. There is also a cultural continuity of patriarchal practices from the country of origin to the host countries through, and/or regardless of, migration. Research findings on the role of religious doctrines are not straightforward. It appears that even though the Islamic doctrines encourage a strong sense of community cohesiveness, this could be double-edged, depending on two major factors: (1) the religiosity of those who are suicidal; and (2) whether those who disclose suicidal intention perceive the social reaction of others as supportive or rejecting. Moreover, research also points to acculturation difficulty as an important migration-related factor precipitating suicidal behaviours. Since harsh moral demands imposed on Turkish migrant women are in conflict with the liberal values and norms of the general German society, it could be that the psychological distress experienced by this subgroup specifically might be greater. Further, Turkish migrants often face social adversities in Germany such as unemployment, low education, and discrimination. In the context of the current sociopolitical climate in Europe in general, the experiences of discrimination within institutions and in social life might be worse and this might have an additive effect on the elevated risk of suicidal behaviours among Turkish migrants in Germany.

The hotline service for suicide crisis, which is specifically tailored for women of Turkish descent in Germany, is a good example of a multimodal intervention not only targeting those who are at risk of suicide, but also their formal and informal networks.[14] The hotline service was supported by a nationwide public awareness campaign raising awareness about the cultural context related to suicidal behaviours among young Turkish women specifically. During the 9 months of the activated telephone hotline, more than 180 calls were received and 44 callers (29.5%) were suicidal or in a crisis at a time.[14] This finding indicates that it is possible to address the cultural needs and expectations of this specific risk group and encourage their participation in their help-seeking process through the mobile health approach (i.e. interventions which are delivered or supported via remote devices such as hotline services, mobile phones, wearable technology, personal digital assistants, or e-mental health interventions).[17,54]

More recently, a systematic review and meta-analysis of individual participant data of existing e-mental health interventions for suicidal thoughts indicated that such interventions are effective in reducing suicidal thoughts, compared to control conditions, post-intervention ($b = -0.247$, 95% CI $= -0.322$ to -0.173; $p < 0.001$).[64] Current evidence suggests that e-mental health interventions based on the principles of cognitive behavioural therapy might be effective, irrespective of participants' age, gender, or history of suicide attempts.[64] Their effectiveness in ethnic minority populations, however, is currently not known.[64] Eylem and colleagues investigated the feasibility and acceptability of a culturally adapted e-mental health intervention in reducing suicidal thoughts among the Turkish migrant community in the Netherlands and the United Kingdom.[65,66] The results indicated that, although the culturally adapted e-mental health intervention was promising in terms of engaging with Turkish migrant communities, there were a number of barriers restricting its usability and acceptability—for instance, not having severe suicidal thoughts and not being able to relate to the culturally adapted content.[66] Thus, in order to optimize such interventions further for ethnic minority populations, cultural adaptations should represent not only the norms and values of the settled communities, but also the norms and values of those who are in the process of settlement.[66] Also, it is important to consider the preferences of the target population in terms of the guidance that they require to follow the e-mental health interventions. For instance, in Eylem and colleagues' study,[66] the majority of the participants reported that they would have preferred more instructions while choosing their exercises.[66] This is in line with the study of Knaevelsrud and colleagues[67] who described how health care professionals in Muslim countries are seen to be authoritative and highly respected figures who give expert advice. Therefore, they tailored their intervention to provide direct instructions and responsibility for therapeutic choices, highlighting how refusal to give explicit advice or lacking assertion could be associated with incompetence and indecisiveness of the therapist, which might lead to the patient becoming irritated or discontinuing their therapy.[67] Additionally, not only the content of the interventions, but also the recruitment strategies need to be tailored and the target population should be involved from the design stage of the research.[68]

To conclude, this chapter highlights gender- and culture-specific issues related to the elevated risk of suicidal behaviours among Turkish migrants in Germany. Prevention efforts should be tailored according to their cultural needs. They should target not only those at risk, but also their informal network to reduce the stigma attached to suicide disclosure. Such multimodal interventions are crucial in facilitating help-seeking. Additionally, mobile health interventions might be possible solutions in engaging with them during the help-seeking process. This has yet to be investigated further in future randomized controlled trials.

References

1. **Haigh M, Kapur N, Cooper J.** Suicidal behaviour among ethnic minorities in England. In: **van Bergen D, Montesinos AH, Schouler-Ocak M,** editors. *Suicidal Behaviour of Immigrants and Ethnic Minorities in Europe.* Gottingen: Hogrefe Publishers; 2015. pp. 45–60.
2. **Cooper J, Murphy E, Webb R,** et al. Ethnic differences in self-harm, rates, characteristics and service provision: three-city cohort study. British Journal of Psychiatry. 2010;**197**:212–18.
3. **Colucci E, San Too L.** Culture, cultural meanings, and suicide among people from migrant and refugee backgrounds. In: **van Bergen D, Montesinos AH, Schouler-Ocak M,** editors. *Suicidal Behavior of Immigrants and Ethnic Minorities in Europe.* Gottingen: Hogrefe Publishers; 2015. pp. 115–33.
4. **World Health Organization.** Global Health Observatory data repository. Suicide rate estimates, age-standardised estimates by country. Available from: https://apps.who.int/iris/rest/bitstreams/1350975/retrieve
5. **Lester D.** Suicide and Islam. Achieves of Suicide Research. 2006;**10**:77–97.
6. **Van Bergen D, Eylem-Van Bergeijk O, Montesinos AH.** Attempted suicide and suicide of young Turkish women in Europe and Turkey: a systematic literature review of characteristics and precipitating factors. PLoS One. 2021;**16**(8):e0253274. https://doi.org/10.1371/journal.pone.0253274
7. **Altindag A, Mustafa O, Remzi O.** Suicide in Batman, South eastern Turkey. Suicide and Life-Threatening Behavior. 2005;**35**:478–82.
8. **Razum O, Zeeb H.** Suicide mortality among Turks in Germany. Der Nervenarzt. 2004;**75**:1092–98.
9. **Heredia Montesinos A.** Precipitating and risk factors for suicidal behaviour among migrants and ethnic minorities in Europe: a review of literature. In: **van Bergen D, Montesinos AH, Schouler-Ocak M,** editors. *Suicidal Behaviour of Immigrants and Ethnic Minorities in Europe.* Gottingen: Hogrefe; 2015. pp. 27–43.
10. **Statistisches Bundesamt.** Bevölkerung und Erwerbstätigkeit. Bevölkerung mit Migrationshintergrund, Ergebnisse des Mikrozensus. [Internet]. Available from: https://www.destatis.de/DE/Themen/Gesellschaft-Umwelt/Bevoelkerung/Migration-Integration/Publikationen/_publikationen-innen-migrationshintergrund.html. [Accessed 3rd July 2022].

11. **Ersanilli E.** *Comparing Integration: Host Culture Adoption and Ethnic Retention among Turkish Immigrants and Their Descendants in France, Germany and the Netherlands.* Unpublished PhD thesis. Amsterdam: VU University Amsterdam; 2010.
12. **Özdemir S, Mutluer SN, Özyürek E.** Exile and plurality in neoliberal times: Turkey's academics for peace. Public Culture. 2019;**31**(2):235–259.
13. **Statistisches Bundesamt.** Bevölkerung und Erwerbstätigkeit. Bevölkerung mit Migrationshintergrund, Ergebnisse des Mikrozensus 2016. Fachserie 1, Reihe 2.2, Wiesbaden 2016.
14. **Schouler-Ocak M.** End your silence, not your life: a suicide prevention campaign for women of Turkish origin in Berlin. In: **van Bergen D, Heredia Montesinos A, Scholer-Ocak M,** editors. Gottingen: Hogrefe Publishing; 2015. pp. 173–85.
15. **Spiegler O, Sonnenberg K, Fassbender I, Kohl K, Leyendecker B.** Ethnic and national identity development and school adjustment: a longitudinal study with Turkish immigrant-origin children. Journal of Cross-Cultural Psychology. April 2018;**49**(7):1009–26.
16. **Statistisches Bundesamt.** Ausstattung privater Haushalte mit Informationsund Kommunikationstechnik: Deutschland. Available from: https://www.destatis.de/DE/ZahlenFakten/GesellschaftStaat/EinkommenKonsumLebensbedingungen/AusstattungGebrauchsguetern/Tabellen/Infotechnik_D.html
17. **Lizardi D, Grunebaum MF, Burke A,** et al. Epidemiologie suizidalen verhaltens von migranten in Deutschland [Epidemiology of suicidal behavior of migrants in Germany]. Suizidprophylaxe. 2006;**33**:171–6.
18. **Löhr C, Schmidtke A, Wohner J, Sell R.** Epidemiologie suizidalen Verhaltens von Migranten in Deutschland. Suizidprophylaxe. 2006;**4**:171–6.
19. **Aichberger MC, Heredia Montesinos A, Bromand Z,** et al. Suicide attempt rates and intervention effects in women of Turkish origin in Berlin. European Psychiatry. 2015;**30**(4):480–5.
20. **Razum O, Zeeb H.** Suicide mortality among Turks in Germany. Der Nervenarzt. 2004;**75**:1092–98.
21. **Burger I, van Hemert AM, Bindraban CA, Schudel WJ.** Parasuicide in The Hague. Incidences in the years 2000–2004 [in Dutch]. Epidemiologisches Bulletin. 2006;**40**:2–8.
22. **Brucker B, Muheim F, Berger P, Riecher-Rossler A.** Charakteristika von Suizidversuchen turkischer Migranten in Kanton Basel-Stadt. Resultate der WHO/EURO-Multizenterstudie [Characteristics of suicide attempts of Turkish migrants in the canton of Basel-Stadt-Results of the WHO/EURO multicentre study.] Nervelheilkunde. 2011;**30**:517–22.
23. **Yilmaz TA, Riecher-Rossler A.** Attempted suicide in immigrants from Turkey: a comparison with Swiss suicide attempters. Psychopathology. 2012;**45**:366–73.
24. **Simsek Z, Demir C, Er G, Munir KM.** Evaluation of attempted suicide in emergency departments in Sanliurfa province, southeastern Turkey. Journal of Public Health. 2013;**21**:325–31.
25. **Turhan E, Inandi T, Aslan M, Zeren C.** Epidemiology of attempted suicide in Hatay, Turkey. Neurosciences (Riyadh). 2011;**16**:347–52.
26. **Lester D.** The cultural meaning of suicide. What does it mean? In: **Lester D, Colucci E,** editors. *Suicide and Culture: Understanding the Context.* Gottingen: Hogrefe Publishers; 2013. pp. 47–57.

27. **Klok J, van Tilburg TG, Suanet B, Fokkema T, Huisman M.** National and transnational belonging among Turkish and Moroccan migrants in the Netherlands: protective against loneliness. European Journal of Ageing. March 2017;**14**(4):341–51.https://doi.org/10.1007/s10433-017-0420-9
28. **Bhugra D, Gupta S.** *Migration and Mental Health*. Cambridge MA: Cambridge University Press; 2011.
29. **Nikolava M, Graham C.** In transit: the well-being of migrants from transition and post-transition countries. Journal of Economic Behavior and Organization. 2015;**112**:164–86.
30. **Sawe BE.** Religious beliefs in Germany. World Atlas. Available from: http://www.worldatlas.com/articles/religious-beliefs-in-germany.html
31. **Gearing RE, Alonzo D.** Religion and suicide: new findings. Journal of Religion and Health. 2018;**57**:2478–99.
32. **Eskin M.** Social reactions of Swedish and Turkish adolescents to a close friends' suicidal disclosure. Social Psychiatry and Psychiatric Epidemiology.1999;**34**:492–7.
33. **Eskin M, Palova E, Krokavcova M.** Suicidal behaviour and attitudes in Slovak and Turkish high school students: a cross-cultural investigation. Archives of Suicide Research. 2014;**18**:58–73.
34. **Eskin M, Schild A, Oncu B, Stieger S, Voracek M.** A cross-cultural investigation of suicidal disclosures and attitudes in Austrian and Turkish university students. Death Studies. 2015;**39**:584–91.
35. **Eskin M.** The effects of individualistic-collectivistic value orientations on non-fatal suicidal behavior and attitudes in Turkish adolescents and young adults. Scandinavian Journal of Psychology. 2013;**54**(6):493–501.
36. **Eylem O, van Bergen DD, Rathod S**, et al. Canına Kıymak 'crushing life energy': a qualitative study on lay and professional understandings of suicide and help-seeking among Turkish migrants in the U.K. and in the Netherlands. International Journal of Culture and Mental Health. 2016;**9**:1–16.
37. **Heredia Montesinos A, Aicherber MC, Temur-Erman S, Bromand Z, Heinz A, Schouler-Ocak M.** Explanatory models of suicidality among women of Turkish descent in Germany: a focus group study. Transcultural Psychiatry. 2019;**22**:1363461518792432.
38. **Eskin M, Poyrazli S, Janghorbani M**, et al. The role of religion in suicidal behavior, attitudes and psychological distress among university students: a multinational study. Transcultural Psychiatry. October 2019;**56**(5):853–77.
39. **Douglas JD.** *The Social Meaning of Suicide*. Princeton, NJ: Princeton University Press; 1967. p. 178.
40. **Hjelmeland H.** Cultural context is crucial in suicide research and prevention. Crisis. 2011;**32**:61–4.
41. **Van Bergen DD, Smit JH, van Balkom AJ, Saharso S.** Suicidal behaviour of young immigrant women in the Netherlands: Can we use Durkheim`s concept of 'fatalistic suicide' to explain their high incidence of attempted suicide? Ethnic and Racial Studies. 2009;**32**:301–22.
42. **Wassenaar DR, Marchiene BW, van der Veen MSS, Pillay AL.** Women in cultural transition: suicidal behavior in South African Indian women. Suicide and Life-Threatening Behavior. 1998;**28**:82–93.

43. **Khan MM, Ahmad A, Khan SR.** Female suicide rates in Ghizer, Pakistan. Suicide and Life-Threatening Behavior. 2009;**39**:227–30.
44. **Aliverdinia A, Pridemore WA.** Women's fatalistic suicide in Iran: a partial test of Durkheim in an Islamic Republic. Violence Against Women. 2009;**15**(3):307–20.
45. **Chen EY, Chan WS, Wong PW**, et al. Suicide in Hong Kong: a case-control psychological autopsy study. Psychological Medicine. 2006;**36**(6):815–25.
46. **Bhugra D, Baldwin DS, Desai M, Jacob KS.** Attempted suicide in west London, II. Inter-group comparisons. Psychological Medicine. 1999;**29**:1131–9.
47. **Bhugra D, Desai M, Baldwin DS.** Attempted suicide in west London, I. Rates across ethnic communities. Psychological Medicine.1999;**29**:1125–30.
48. **Durkheim E.** *Le Suicide* [*Suicide*]. Paris: Felix Alcan; 1897.
49. **Phalet K, Baysu G, Van Acker K.** Ethnicity and migration in Europe. In **Smelser NJ, Baltes PB**, editors. *International Encyclopaedia of the Social and Behavioral Sciences.* 2nd ed. Elsevier; 2015. pp. 142–147. doi: https://doi.org/10.1016/B978-0-08-097 086-8.24040-3.
50. **Berry JW.** Immigration, acculturation, and adaptation. International Journal of Applied Psychology. 1997;**46**(1): 5–68.
51. **Aichberger MC, Bromand Z, Rapp MA**, et al. Perceived ethnic discrimination, acculturation, and psychological distress in women of Turkish origin in Germany. Social Psychiatry and Psychiatric Epidemiology. 2015;**50**(11):1691–700.
52. **Eylem O, Dalgar I, Tok F**, et al. The association between acculturation and suicidal ideation among Turkish migrants in the Netherlands. Psychiatry Research. 2019;**275**:71–7.
53. **Fassaert T, Peen J, van Straten A**, et al. Ethnic differences and similarities in outpatient treatment for depression in the Netherlands. Psychiatric Services. 2010;**61**:690–7.
54. **Güngör D, Bornstein MH.** Gender, development, values, adaptation and discrimination in acculturating adolescents: the case of Turk heritage youth born and living in Belgium. Sex Roles. 2009;**60**:537–48.
55. **Bhui KS, Lenguerrand E, Maynard MJ, Stansfeld SA, Harding S.** Does cultural integration explain a mental health advantage for adolescents? International Journal of Epidemiology. 2012;**41**:791–802.
56. **Schweitzer R, Melville F, Steel Z, Lacherez P.** Trauma, post-migration living difficulties, and social support as predictors of psychological adjustment in resettled Sudanese refugees. Australian and New Zealand Journal of Psychiatry. 2006;**40**:179–87.
57. **Noh S, Kaspar V.** Perceived discrimination and depression: moderating effects of coping, acculturation, and ethnic support. American Journal of Public Health. 2003;**93**:232–8.
58. **Pascoe EA, Smart Richman L.** Perceived discrimination and health: a meta-analytic review. Psychological Bulletin. 2009;**135**:531–54.
59. **Van Bergen DD, Feddes AR, de Ruyter DJ.** Perceived discrimination against Dutch Muslim youths in the school context and its relation with externalising behaviour. Oxford Review of Education. 2021;**47**(4):475–94. https://doi.org/10.1080/03054 985.2020.1862779
60. **Bowlby J.** *Attachment and Loss.* Vol. **2**. Separation. New York, NY: Basic Books; 1973.

61. **Hofstra J, van Oudenhoven JP, Buunk BP.** Attachment styles and majority members' attitudes towards adaptation strategies of immigrants. International Journal of Intercultural Relations. 2005;**29**:601–19.
62. **Van Oudenhoven JP, Hofstra J.** Personal reactions to 'strange situations': attachment styles and acculturation attitudes of immigrants and majority members. International Journal of Intercultural Relations. 2006;**30**:783–98.
63. **Van Acker K, Vanbeselaere N.** Heritage culture maintenance precludes host culture adoption and vice versa. Fleming's perceptions of Turks' acculturation behavior. Group Processes and Intergroup Relations. 2011;**15**:133–45.
64. **Büscher R, Beisemann M, Doebler P**, et al. Digital cognitive-behavioural therapy to reduce suicidal ideation and behaviours: A systematic review and meta-analysis of individual participant data. Evidence-Based Mental Health. 2022;**25**(1):E8–17.
65. **Knaevelsrud C, Brand J, Lange A, Ruwaard J, Wagner B.** Web-based psychotherapy for posttraumatic stress disorder in war-traumatised Arab patients: randomised controlled trial. Journal of Medical Internet Research. 2015;**17**(3):e71. doi: 10.2196/jmir.3582.
66. **Eylem O, van Straten A, Bhui K, Kerkhof AJFM.** Protocol: reducing suicidal thinking among Turkish migrants living in the Netherlands and in the UK: effectiveness of an online intervention. International Review of Psychiatry. 2015;**1**:72–81.
67. **Eylem O, van Straten A, de Wit L**, et al. Reducing suicidal ideation among Turkish migrants in the Netherlands and in the UK: the feasibility of a randomised controlled trial of a guided online intervention. Pilot and Feasibility Studies. 2021;**7**:30. https://doi.org/10.1186/s40814-021-00772-9
68. **Shala M, Morina N, Burchert S**, et al. Cultural adaptation of *Hap-pas-Hapi*, an internet and mobile-based intervention for the treatment of psychological distress among Albanian migrants in Switzerland and Germany. Internet Interventions. 2020;**21**:100339.

Part 3

High risk groups and suicidality

Chapter 12

Suicidal behaviour and sociocultural factors among South Asians in the United Kingdom

Aaron Poppleton, Pooja Saini, Maria Panagioti, and Nusrat Husain

Reasons to consider the British South Asian community

British South Asians (BSAs) form the largest ethnic minority group in the United Kingdom (UK). The BSA population in the UK totalled 3,078,374 (6.9%) in 2021, with individuals identifying with Indian (1,451,862; 3.1%), Pakistani (1,174,983; 2.7%), and Bangladeshi (451,529; 1.1%) ethnic groups.[1] The total community size is likely to be higher, given many second-/third-generation individuals and individuals of mixed-ethnicity heritage may identify as Asian British or 'other Asian background'. There are large cultural, religious, and demographic variations within the BSA community which are important for mental health.[2,3] British Bangladeshi and Pakistani individuals have a lower average age and socio-economic status, and larger family size, and are more likely to lack qualifications and be unemployed, compared to British Indians.[1,4] The Bangladeshi community is said to be the most segregated, with comparatively higher rates of overcrowding (24%) due to a lack of affordable properties and resultant reliance on a limited supply of council or social housing.[4,5]

Epidemiology of suicide and self-harm

Rates of suicide

There is conflicting information regarding the rate and trends of suicide in the BSA community compared to the general population,[6,7,8,9,10,11,12,13] due to poor documentation of ethnicity.[6,14,15] The SANGRA database of South Asian names suggested 1438 suicides (2.6%) in England and Wales from 1993 to 2003 were South Asian.[6] This equated to a suicide rate of 5.5/100,000, lower than the overall population rate (9.31/100,000). The majority of cases were male (79%). Disaggregation suggested a significant variation by surname associated religious affiliation, with a lower rate for Muslims (4.39/100,000) than for Sikhs (7.89/100,000) and Hindus (8.25/100,000).[16] All female BSA groups were reported to have significantly lower rates of suicide when compared to the general population.[13] In comparison, a large UK study considering aggregated data for 1999–2003 reported a marginally raised suicide rate for BSA women when compared to the general population in England and Wales. Older BSA women (aged over 65 years) were identified to be a high-risk group due to experience of migration, acculturation, and bereavement,[6] in keeping with previous figures from the United States showing that older South Asian women have the highest suicide rate of all women.[17]

Rates of self-harm

The strongest predictor of completed suicide is a history of self-harm.[18] Inconsistent findings on the rate of self-harm in the BSA community are likely reflected by varying degrees of disclosure. The UK Ethnic Minority Psychiatric Illness Rates in the Community survey of self-harm and suicide described a 3% BSA lifetime rate of attempted suicide.[19] Such data should be considered alongside reports of higher rates of self-harm[20,21,22] and rates of self-harm comparable to the general population, particularly among female adolescents and young adults.[10,11,23,24] An exploration of self-harm rates among Hindu and Sikh university students found that BSA male students are significantly less likely to self-harm compared to white male students.[25] In contrast, higher rates of self-harm among BSA adolescents have been reported compared to other groups in East London.[26] Gender differences may account for these seemingly inconsistent findings. BSA women have been found to be 17 times more likely to attempt suicide than BSA men in the 16- to 19-year age group,[23] with female BSA attempters more commonly expressing suicidal intent and regret at failure than white females.[11] Self-harm among BSA women decreases with age, with few cases in those aged over 30 years and very few cases in those over 50 years of age. This finding appears to contradict the finding that suicide is more common among older BSA women.[6] Cultural factors have been described as influencing participant study involvement, with female participation prevented by husbands or parents in some cases.[11] Rates of suicide in BSA men may be shaped more by place of birth than by ethnic group.[23,27]

Methods of suicide and self-harm

Methods of self-harm are likely influenced by the degree of acculturation and the availability of means. Overdose with over-the-counter medication was described as the principal method of suicide for BSAs aged 16–64 years in London.[11] BSA individuals often ingested fewer tablets, compared to the general population, due to their uncertainty over the number required for impact. Self-laceration was the second most common form of self-harm (<10%).[11] Less common methods included consumption of non-ingestible substances and use of multiple methods. Other studies reported hanging, consumption of bleach or rat poison, burning, overeating or under-eating, cutting, and hitting.[8,28] Borrill and colleagues[25] reported fewer BSA university students scratching and cutting compared to white students and/or students without a religious affiliation. BSA males were more likely than females to use violent methods.[11] No difference in preparation for a self-harm or suicide attempt has been described, for example writing a suicide note.

Predisposing and protective factors

Suicide and self-harm are major public health problems, with potentially significant physical morbidity, ongoing psychosocial distress, and death by misadventure or progression to suicide. There are unique cultural, religious, and socio-economic factors which increase or reduce the risk of self-harm and suicide in the BSA community. Such areas remain under-researched. Improved understanding of such factors can inform the development of targeted, culturally appropriate suicide prevention strategies for BSA groups.[16,28,29,30]

Stigma and cultural identity

While stigma associated with self-harm and suicide is not unique to the BSA community, its presence impacts family acceptance, the ability of health and social care professionals to work within the community, and the ability to identify gaps in knowledge. BSA individuals admitted to mental health services after a suicide attempt have been found to hold less traditional views on age of marriage, cohabitation, arranged marriages, interracial relationships, and gender roles compared to those managed within general practice.[31] BSA university students have previously demonstrated an avoidance coping style in terms of emotional inhibition, indicating a tendency to inhibit spontaneous action or feelings to avoid disapproval from others, shame, or loss of control.[24] Such findings are in keeping with a suggested lower likelihood of repeating self-harm,[32] and suggest that cultural concordance with traditional and less traditional viewpoints could be a major factor associated with self-harm among BSA women.[31] Such conflict points start during adolescence when a mismatch of traditional cultural roles and individualization and integration within the majority culture become more evident. Resultant isolation and alienation can trigger suicidal ideation as a possible escape from the family environment.[31]

Religion

Durkheim's classical theory of suicide (1897/1951)[33] states that the level of integration within a religious denomination can influence perceptions, and thus the acceptability of suicide.[34] Particular aspects of a religion may have a direct and an indirect influence and a protective role on an individual's suicide risk.[35,36,37] Religious affiliation is far higher among the BSA population than among the general British population. A decreasing rate of suicide incidence among young BSA women may reflect a demographic shift shaped by a higher proportion of Muslims within this age group,[28] for whom suicide is a socially unacceptable act.[38] BSA Muslims are less likely to die by suicide than Hindus or Sikhs,[6] despite higher reported rates of emotional distress. Religious affiliation may prove particularly protective for BSA men.[25]

Marriage and relationships

BSA individuals are more likely to be married than the general population.[23] Marital status has been described as a strong factor in predicting self-harm in BSA individuals.[39] Precipitating life stressors are commonly related to relationship difficulties, family conflict, health and partner life events, and lack of social support, often alongside housing, financial, language, and/or childhood difficulties.[31,40,41] Arranged marriage is not uncommon within the BSA community. Traditional cultural expectations may be placed on the bride, including living with the groom's family, having children, and maintaining family integrity, irrespective of personal cost.[42] Increasingly complex visa arrangements have created a source of stress and inequality within relationships where one partner is a recent migrant from the South Asian subcontinent.[43] Such factors may predispose newly-wed women to isolation, potentially made more complex by the impact of limited privacy on sexual intimacy and the potential for alienation through an inability to have children. While a history of interracial relationships are more common among BSA females who have attempted suicide, this may be a reflection of more extroverted or curious personality traits.[42]

Domestic violence

Domestic abuse and other violence against women and girls are recognized as a precursor to suicide within national[44] and international[45] suicide strategies, although absent from recent gender violence strategies.[46] A recent meta-synthesis found that low self-esteem and interpersonal conflict were key drivers of self-harm among South Asians in the UK.[47] Experiences of domestic violence within ethnic minority groups in the UK are not well researched.[48] Limited translation of data collection questionnaires has led to an under-representation of BSA women, despite their increased vulnerability to abuse secondary to isolation.[49] Associations between suicide risk and cultural practices have been proposed, including concepts of so-called 'honour' and 'shame', and language or community barriers which frustrate help-seeking behaviours.[50] Mental health can be seen as disordered, defective, and threatening to cultural norms and social conformity. Disclosure may risk shame for both the individual and their family, preventing avenues for help-seeking. Female family members may be particularly adversely affected, given their cultural role as the custodians of maintaining family honour.[51]

As many as half of all BSA women living in the UK who attempted suicide or self-harm had also suffered domestic violence.[52] One study of BSA domestic violence reported an average of 11 years of violence, violence on a daily or weekly basis (90%), and contemplation (67%) and attempt of suicide (13%). Ninety-two per cent of study participants reported 'violence by their husband' as the main factor underlying their suicide attempt.[53] In contrast, other data has suggested fewer BSA women who attempt suicide had prior experience of domestic violence, when compared with individuals of mixed, multiple, or other ethnicity. Sensitivities around disclosure, vulnerability of victims, and national variations in predisposing factors within the BSA community including housing, educational and economic situations, may complicate accurate data collection.[54,55]

Mental and physical health factors

BSA individuals with a mental illness have a 5- to 15-fold higher risk of suicide compared to the general population.[56] BSA women who completed suicide were more likely to have a psychiatric history and have previously self-harmed, with around 90% of individuals dying by suicide having suffered with a mental illness. Higher levels of psychotic and depressive symptoms have been reported in BSA individuals who attempted suicide.[27] An association between psychosis and suicide has been reported globally.[57] Recognition of hallucinatory symptoms as part of a mental disorder among BSA individuals may be complicated by multiple explanatory models, including supernatural causes, use of a second language or an interpreter in consultations with clinicians, and difficulties in mapping symptoms to westernized psychiatric frameworks.[58,59] A meta-analysis of pathways to care in England showed that BSAs experienced proportionately higher rates of psychiatric admission, with repeat admissions more likely to be compulsory than for the general population.[60] Strong family ties and 'symptom containment' have been cited as reasons for lower BSA relapse, readmission, and admission via law enforcement than for the general population.[61,62]

Religious and cultural perceptions of alcohol consumption among BSAs mean its use has been associated with disrupted cultural networks and familial relationships.[25] Alcohol abuse by BSA men has been identified as a strong predictor of initial and repeated self-harm among female partners.[10] Conversely, BSAs who abuse alcohol and who do not have a relationship partner may be at increased risk of self-harm and suicide.[9,39]

Service engagement

Access to services

Research has shown that BSAs in the UK underutilize mental health services compared to their white British counterparts.[63] Limited understanding and disillusionment with mental health services, including perceived or actual service unresponsiveness or discrimination against particular needs, care provision outside of the community, difficulty with seeing a psychiatrist of the same religion, and community-specific help-seeking behaviours, have been cited as reasons for lower levels of psychiatric assessment and follow-up after self-harm.[23,39,64]

A number of individual- and community-level factors may influence desire for engagement with UK health services. Historically, mental health stigma within the BSA community has shaped a reluctance to acknowledge mental illness and seek help for psychiatric problems.[64] The reluctance to acknowledge mental illness in BSA communities may be due to the perception that 'madness' is incurable,[65] alongside the notion that prospects of a marriage proposals may reduce.[4,66] Involvement of community members in service provision has raised concerns surrounding disclosure of service user information via the 'community grapevine'.[20] BSA community members have previously described emotional disturbance, distress, and low mood as inappropriate for medical consultation or intervention.[67] The impact of mental health conditions on functional ability and family roles may be negatively perceived as self-centredness (particularly by BSA women), with limited understanding of depression as a disease process.[68] The concept of 'kismet' (fate) can affect perception of problems, with resultant ambivalence and unease towards discussing feelings.[69]

Although the role of general practitioners (GPs) as gatekeepers for access and referral to mental health care is increasingly recognized, primary care research has not specifically considered service availability, access, or targeted risk factor reduction for BSA patients to prevent suicide.[70,71,72] GPs in the UK have reported a range of 'difficulties' in recognizing and managing mental health presentations in BSAs.[68] Many current 'Western' models of depression do not fit particularly well with clinically relatable concepts or culture-specific issues within BSA populations (e.g. '*dil ghirda hai*'—sinking heart (Punjabi)).[65,68,73] Significant variations in prescribing patterns for antidepressants have been reported across practices.[74,75] Routine consultation screening methods risk missing common mental disorders or leading to inappropriate diagnoses of subclinical physical or somatic disorders.[76,77] As such, a lack of availability and inaccessibility of health services for mental health problems may contribute to BSA suicide.[9] A recent meta-synthesis of qualitative studies on self-harm/ suicide experiences among South Asians in the UK reiterated these findings and also proposed that self-harm and suicide prevention strategies for South Asian communities in the UK could be improved via: (1) raising awareness of mental health issues and addressing confidentiality concerns such as shame and secrecy; (2) improving access to mental health services and extending the availability of helplines; and (3) establishing partnerships with community organizations and educational institutions.[47]

Alternative healers

Similar to within South Asian nations, spirituality plays a significant role in many community members' understanding of mental well-being. Belief in 'Jinns'—spiritual beings with the power to possess people, trigger misfortune, and induce mental disturbance—have been reported.[59,78] Traditional and westernized views can coexist to varying degrees, with differing degrees of power attributed to each. While the prevalence and use of traditional healers within BSA populations are unclear, such services are often used alongside, rather than in place of, Western medical provision.[70,79] One study identified a significant proportion of BSA psychiatric inpatients having consulted a traditional healer prior to admission. Of those who had not, many would have done so, given the awareness of a local provider.[80] Traditional healers differ in their methods and often include providing traditional medicine or consultations with a holy person (particularly for Muslims of an older generation). Advertisements for Hakims visiting the UK from Pakistan have been present in a number of local communities' media.[81] Individuals may simultaneously consult several types of healers, employing multiple explanatory models.[59,78] Such care input is often not disclosed to their GP. Traditional healers hold a shared belief system and worldview with the community, often commanding respect and being the preferred option to mental health professionals.[82,83] A diagnosis of mental illness as 'ghost possession' or the outcomes of 'black magic' by traditional healers has been noted to impact perceived relevance of, and to delay access to, psychiatric care.[84] Moreover, use of traditional healers' services can place a significant financial burden on families, with reported costs ranging from £50 to £1000 (€57–1139, $62–1239).[85]

Culturally adapted prevention and care

The need for mental health services to widen access and reflect the population served has been well described.[86] In 2005, the UK Department of Health published a five-year action plan to ensure mental health service provision was appropriate and responsive to the needs of black, Asian, and minority ethnic (BAME) populations.[87] This need to tailor approaches to BAME groups and deliver equitable care was reiterated in the Suicide Prevention Strategy for England.[88] Collaborative prevention research will require work with service users, high-risk spaces, community organizations, workplaces, schools, and policymakers.[89] Psychological autopsy studies, such as those undertaken by the National Confidential Inquiry in Manchester,[90,91,92] require expansion to include information on BSA contact with GPs or emergency departments prior to suicide. Pooling of findings with routinely collected data could support identification of psychosocial features and service usage prior to suicide, directing design and implementation of relevant service provision.

Limited BSA trust in UK mental health services has been identified as a barrier to accessing early support, resulting in crisis presentations.[28] Reports of BSA survivors of suicide describe that individuals often do not feel 'heard' or understood either by their families or by mental health workers.[52] Previous reviews highlight the need for preventative research focused on cultural variations in presentations and ethnic disparities in the management of self-harm and suicide.[20,22,93] As intervention following self-harm is crucial in preventing future episodes of self-harm and suicide,[29,30] existing interventions and mental health services should be tailored to account for the cultural, linguistic, and religious needs of the BSA community.[94,95]

A range of preventative and management strategies have been proposed, which include both universal and targeted approaches. School- and community-based health education programmes may be an avenue to raise awareness on mental health, service provision, and access through printed and electronic resources. Greater collaboration with cultural and religious organizations may aid in the development of tailored, 'non-judgemental' community support approaches to meet the needs of particular at-risk BSA subgroups.[29]

Supporting adaptation of psychological interventions and therapies to become more culturally sensitive, including delivery by alternative methods (e.g. telephone or self-directed), has a realistic potential to improve suicide prevention among BSA communities in the UK. Cultural sensitivity training for key health professionals (e.g. GPs, health visitors) may aid in diagnostic accuracy and appropriate information provision to community members.[89] While higher numbers of BSA counsellors have been proposed, concerns surrounding confidentiality have been raised by some community members. Limited evaluation of such measures has been undertaken, with the exception of educational leaflets on help-seeking attitudes for depression and suicidality.[96] The frequency of family member interpersonal problem/s as a trigger for BSA self-harm and suicide suggests the potential value in an intervention targeted towards such issues. A cognitively based 'problem-solving therapy' would be a potential intervention to address this. A trial protocol has been published, describing adaptation and evaluation of a culturally adapted, manual-assisted problem-solving training (C-MAP) for BSA women who self-harm.[97] The intervention consists of eight sessions of 50 minutes' duration delivered over a 3-month period. Comparison will be made with treatment as usual for self-harm, and outcomes measured in terms of levels of hopelessness and suicidal ideation. Trial of C-MAP in Pakistan among women after self-harm has demonstrated a reduction in suicidal ideation, and thus a potential to reduce future suicide risk.[98]

Conclusion

The BSA community in the UK continues to grow. Despite the natural change and integration of cultural norms over time and generations, a number of differences from the UK general population in terms of mental health, self-harm, and suicide persist. Increasing recognition of the diversity within the community according to class, culture, religion, and geography is providing greater insight into the nature of this phenomenon. Community perceptions of mental health are likely to continue to evolve, as onward generations have less direct contact with South Asian nations, in addition to lower levels of tolerance to racism, socio-economic disparity, and other social problems within the community. For the moment at least, challenges in meeting the mental health needs of the BSA community persist. These include difficulties for UK clinicians to understand culturally unfamiliar presentations, community perceptions of mental health as non-medical, and ongoing use and limited integration of alternative health care providers. Steps to develop greater cultural competence are required.

A number of areas remain open to further research. Recognition of variations and diversity within the population has yet to be translated to targeted strategies for self-harm and suicide prevention, including the place of gender, honour-shame, and religion in suicide. Development and integration of cultural competency training for health care staff offer the potential to increase the understanding of BSA perceptions of mental health. Active recognition of the changing nature of mental health, self-harm, and suicide across generations and among marginalized subgroups of BSAs (e.g. openly homosexual individuals) is required to inform such targeted suicide prevention strategies in the UK.

References

1. **Office for National Statistics**. Population of England and Wales; 2021. Available from: https://www.ethnicity-facts-figures.service.gov.uk/uk-population-by-ethnicity/national-and-regional-populations/population-of-england-and-wales/latest
2. **Robinson L.** Cultural identity and acculturation preferences among South Asian adolescents in Britain: an exploratory study. Children and Society. 2009;**23**(6):442–54.
3. **Dey BL, Balmer JM, Pandit A, Saren M, Binsardi B.** A quadripartite approach to analysing young British South Asian adults' dual cultural identity. Journal of Marketing Management. 2017;**33**(9–10):789–816.
4. **Large P, Ghosh K.** Estimates of the population by ethnic group for areas within England. Population Trends. 2006;**124**:8–17.
5. **Department of Levelling Up, Housing, and Communities**. Overcrowding in South Asian households: a qualitative report; 2022. Available from: https://www.gov.uk/government/publications/overcrowding-in-south-asian-households-a-qualitative-report/overcrowding-in-south-asian-households-a-qualitative-report#reasons-for-remaining-in-overcrowded-accommodation
6. **McKenzie K, Bhui K, Nanchahal K, Blizard B.** Suicide rates in people of South Asian origin in England and Wales: 1993–2003. British Journal of Psychiatry. 2008;**193**(5):406–9.
7. **Neeleman J, Mak V, Wessely S.** Suicide by age, ethnic group, coroners' verdicts and country of birth: a three-year survey in inner London. British Journal of Psychiatry. 1997;**171**(5):463–7.
8. **Patel SP, Gaw AC.** Suicide among immigrants from the Indian subcontinent: a review. Psychiatric Services. 1996;47(5):517–21.
9. **Cooper J, Husain N, Webb R**, et al. Self-harm in the UK. Social Psychiatry and Psychiatric Epidemiology. 2006;**41**(10):782–8.
10. **Bhugra D, Desai M.** Attempted suicide in South Asian women. Advances in Psychiatric treatment. 2002;**8**(6):418–23.
11. **Bhugra D, Desai M, Baldwin DS.** Attempted suicide in west London, I. Rates across ethnic communities. Psychological Medicine. 1999a;**29**:1125–30.
12. **Bhardwaj A.** Growing up young, Asian and female in Britain: a report on self-harm and suicide. Feminist Review. 2001;68(summer):52–67.
13. **Hunt IM, Robinson JO, Bickley H**, et al. Suicides in ethnic minorities within 12 months of contact with mental health services: national clinical survey. British Journal of Psychiatry. 2003;**183**(2):155–60.
14. **Cummins C, Winter H, Cheng KK, Maric R, Silcocks P, Varghese C.** An assessment of the Nam Pehchan computer program for the identification of names of south Asian ethnic origin. Journal of Public Health. 1999;**21**(4):401–6.

15. **Nanchahal K, Mangtani P, Alston M, dos Santos Silva I.** Development and validation of a computerized South Asian Names and Group Recognition Algorithm (SANGRA) for use in British health-related studies. Journal of Public Health. 2001;**23**(4):278–85.
16. **Tuck A, Bhui K, Nanchahal K, McKenzie K.** Suicide rates for different religious groups in the South Asian origin population in England and Wales: a secondary analysis of a national data set. International Journal of Human Rights in Healthcare. 2015;**8**(4):260–6.
17. **Agnew-Davies R, Shah G, Raja F.** Asian women, domestic violence and mental health: a toolkit for health professionals. Publisher EACH [Enabling Change Rebuilding Lives]: Government Office for London; 2009. https://resourcecentre.savethechildren.net/pdf/5774.pdf/
18. **Large M, Corderoy A, McHugh C.** Is suicidal behaviour a stronger predictor of later suicide than suicidal ideation? A systematic review and meta-analysis. Australian and New Zealand Journal of Psychiatry. 2021;**55**(3), 254–67.
19. **Crawford MJ, Nur U, McKenzie K, Tyrer P.** Suicidal ideation and suicide attempts among ethnic minority groups in England: results of a national household survey. Psychological Medicine. 2005;**35**(9):1369–77.
20. **Husain MI, Waheed W, Husain N.** Self-harm in British South Asian women: psychosocial correlates and strategies for prevention. Annals of General Psychiatry. 2006;**5**(1):7.
21. **Baldwin S, Griffiths P.** Do specialist community public health nurses assess risk factors for depression, suicide, and self-harm among South Asian mothers living in London? Public Health Nursing. 2009;**26**(3):277–89.
22. **Al-Sharifi A, Krynicki CR, Upthegrove R.** Self-harm and ethnicity: a systematic review. International Journal of Social Psychiatry. 2015;**61**(6):600–12.
23. **Cooper J, Murphy E, Webb R,** et al. Ethnic differences in self-harm, rates, characteristics and service provision: three-city cohort study. British Journal of Psychiatry. 2010;**197**(3):212–18.
24. **Hunt IM, Richards N, Bhui K,** et al. Suicide rates by ethnic group among patients in contact with mental health services: an observational cohort study in England and Wales. The Lancet Psychiatry. 2021;**8**(12):1083–93.
25. **Borrill J, Fox P, Roger D.** Religion, ethnicity, coping style, and self-reported self-harm in a diverse non-clinical UK population. Mental Health, Religion and Culture. 2011;**14**(3):259–69.
26. **Klineberg E.** *Self-Harm in East London Adolescents* (doctoral dissertation). London: Queen Mary's University; 2010. https://qmro.qmul.ac.uk/xmlui/handle/123456789/521
27. **Bhui KS, McKenzie K.** Rates and risk factors by ethnic group for suicides within a year of contact with mental health services in England and Wales. Psychiatric Services. 2008;**59**(4):414–20.
28. **Chew-Graham C, Bashir C, Chantler K, Burman E, Batsleer J.** South Asian women, psychological distress and self harm: lessons for primary care trusts. Health and Social Care in the Community. 2002;**10**(5):339–47
29. **Hawton K, Bergen H, Cooper J,** et al. Suicide following self-harm: findings from the multicentre study of self-harm in England, 2000–2012. Journal of Affective Disorders. 2015;**175**:147–51.
30. **Radhakrishnan R, Andrade C.** Suicide: an Indian perspective. Indian Journal of Psychiatry. 2012;**54**(4):304.

31. **Bhugra D.** *Culture and Self-Harm: Attempted Suicide in South Asians in London.* London: Psychology Press; 2004.
32. **Cooper J, Steeg S, Webb R,** et al. Risk factors associated with repetition of self-harm in black and minority ethnic (BME) groups: a multi-centre cohort study. Journal of Affective Disorders. 2013;**148**(2–3):435–9.
33. **Durkheim E.** *Suicide: A Study in Sociology.* California: Snowball Public; 2012. pp. 297–325.
34. **Stack S, Kposowa AJ.** Religion and suicide acceptability: a cross-national analysis. Journal for the Scientific Study of Religion. 2011;**50**(2):289–306.
35. **Gearing RE, Lizardi D.** Religion and suicide. Journal of Religion and Health. 2009;**48**(3):332–41.
36. **Kamal Z, Loewenthal KM.** Suicide beliefs and behaviour among young Muslims and Hindus in the UK. Mental Health, Religion and Culture. 2002;**5**(2):111–18.
37. **Colucci E, Martin G.** Religion and spirituality along the suicidal path. Suicide and Life-Threatening Behavior. 2008;**38**(2):229–44.
38. **Khan MM, Islam S, Kundi AK.** Parasuicide in Pakistan: experience at a university hospital. Acta Psychiatrica Scandinavica. 1996;**93**(4):264–7.
39. **Cooper C, Spiers N, Livingston G,** et al. Ethnic inequalities in the use of health services for common mental disorders in England. Social Psychiatry and Psychiatric Epidemiology. 2013;**48**(5):685–92.
40. **Aschan L, Goodwin L, Cross S, Moran P, Hotopf M, Hatch SL.** Suicidal behaviours in South East London: prevalence, risk factors and the role of socio-economic status. Journal of Affective Disorders. 2013;**150**(2):441–9.
41. **Johnston R, Burgess S, Wilson D, Harris R.** School and residential ethnic segregation: an analysis of variations across England's local education authorities. Regional Studies. 2006;**40**(9):973–90.
42. **Vijayakumar L.** Suicide prevention: the urgent need in developing countries. World Psychiatry. 2004;**3**(3):159.
43. **Anitha S.** No recourse, no support: state policy and practice towards South Asian women facing domestic violence in the UK. British Journal of Social Work. 2008;**40**(2):462–79.
44. **Department of Health**. *Preventing Suicide in England: A Cross-government Outcomes Strategy to Save Lives.* London: Department of Health; 2012.
45. **World Health Organization**. *Preventing Suicide: A Global Imperative.* Geneva: World Health Organization; 2014. **World Health Organization**. *Practice Manual for Establishing and Maintaining Surveillance Systems for Suicide Attempts and Self-harm.* Geneva: World Health Organization; 2016.
46. **Home Office**. Strategy to end violence against women and girls: 2016–2020. 2016. Available from: https://www.gov.uk/government/publications/strategy-to-end-violence-against-women-and-girls-2016-to-2020
47. **Ozen-Dursun B, Kaptan S, Giles S, Husain N, Panagioti M.** Understanding self-harm and suicidal behaviour in South Asians in the UK: a systematic review and meta-synthesis. British Journal of Psychiatry Open. 2023;9(3):e82 1–9.
48. **Royal College of Psychiatrists**. Domestic violence Council Report CR102. 2002. https://www.cambridge.org/core/journals/psychiatric-bulletin/article/domestic-viole

nce-council-report-cr102-april-2002-750-44-pp/04920E513A5E9B8D56A9E0C68 8D67B48#article

49. **Barnish M.** Domestic violence: a literature review. HM Inspectorate of Probation; 2004. Available from: https://www.academia.edu/29147259/Domestic_Violence_A_Litera ture_Review
50. **Gill A.** A lethal code of honour. Journal of Community Care. 2004:38–40. Southall Black Sisters. *Safe and Sane: A Model of Intervention on Domestic Violence and Mental Health, Suicide and Self-Harm amongst Black and Minority Ethnic Women*. Middlesex: Southall Black Sisters; 2011.
51. **Sangar M, Howe J.** How discourses of sharam (shame) and mental health influence the help-seeking behaviours of British born girls of South Asian heritage. Educational Psychology in Practice. 2021;**37**(4):343–61.
52. **Chantler K, Burman E, Batsleer J, Bashir C.** *Attempted Suicide and Self-Harm: South Asian Women*. Manchester: Women's Studies Research Centre, Manchester Metropolitan University; 2001. **Newham Asian Women's Project and the Newham Inner-City Multi-Fund.** *Growing Up Young, Asian and Female in Britain: A Report on Self-Harm and Suicide*. 1998.
53. **Belgrave Baheno.** *The Manushi Report 'Beaten But Not Defeated': A Report on Asian Women and Domestic Violence in Leicestershire*. Leicester: Belgrave Baheno; 1996.
54. **McManus S, Walby S, Barbosa EC, Appleby L, Brugha T, Bebbington PE, Cook EA, Knipe D.** Intimate partner violence, suicidality, and self-harm: a probability sample survey of the general population in England. The Lancet Psychiatry. 2022;9(7):574–83.
55. **Hunt IM, Richards N, Bhui K, Ibrahim S, Turnbull P, Halvorsrud K, Saini P, Kitson S, Shaw J, Appleby L, Kapur N.** Suicide rates by ethnic group among patients in contact with mental health services: an observational cohort study in England and Wales. The Lancet Psychiatry. 2021;8(12):1083–93.
56. **Windfuhr K, Kapur N.** Suicide and mental illness: a clinical review of 15 years findings from the UK National Confidential Inquiry into Suicide. British Medical Bulletin. 2011;**100**(1):101–21.
57. **DeVylder JE, Lukens EP, Link BG, Lieberman JA.** Suicidal ideation and suicide attempts among adults with psychotic experiences: data from the collaborative psychiatric epidemiology surveys. JAMA Psychiatry. 2015;**72**(3):219–25.
58. **Pote HL, Orrell MW.** Perceptions of schizophrenia in multi-cultural Britain. Ethnicity and Health. 2002;**7**(1):7–20.
59. **Bhikha A, Farooq S, Chaudhry N, Naeem F, Husain N.** Explanatory models of psychosis amongst British South Asians. Asian Journal of Psychiatry. 2015;**16**:48–54.
60. **Halvorsrud K, Nazroo J, Otis M, Hajdukova EB, Bhui K.** Ethnic inequalities and pathways to care in psychosis in England: a systematic review and meta-analysis. BMC Medicine. 2018;**16**(1):223.
61. **Bhugra D, Leff J, Mallett R, Der G, Corridan B, Rudge S.** Incidence and outcome of schizophrenia in whites, African-Caribbeans and Asians in London. Psychological Medicine. 1997;**27**(4):791–8.
62. **Perera, R, Owen, DG, Johnstone, EC.** Disabilities and circumstances of schizophrenic patients: a follow-up study. Ethnic aspects: a comparison of three matched groups. British Journal of Psychiatry. 1991;**13**(Suppl):40–2, 44–6.

63. **Hussain F, Cochrane R.** Depression in South Asian women living in the UK: a review of the literature with implications for service provision. Transcultural Psychiatry. 2004;**41**(2):253–70.
64. **Bowl R.** The need for change in UK mental health services: South Asian service users' views. Ethnicity and Health. 2007;**12**(1):1–19.
65. **Fazil Q, Cochrane R.** The cultural dimension in a causal model of depression. Bellingham, WA: Fourteenth International Congress of Cross Cultural Psychology; 1998.
66. **Fatemilihin I.** *A Cross-cultural Study of Parents' Attitudes and Beliefs about Mental Handicap*. MSc Dissertation in Clinical Psychology; 1989.
67. **Beliappa J.** *Illness or Distress? Alternative Models of Mental Health*. London: Confederation of Indian Organisations; 1991.
68. **Ineichen B.** Mental illness and suicide in British South Asian adults. Mental Health, Religion and Culture. 2012;**15**(3):235–50.
69. **Anand AS, Cochrane R.** The mental health status of South Asian women in Britain: a review of the UK literature. Psychology and Developing Societies. 2005;**17**(2):195–214.
70. **Hussain F, Cochrane R.** Living with depression: coping strategies used by South Asian women suffering from depression. Mental Health, Religion and Culture. 2003;**5**(3):21–44.
71. **Mason S, Hussain-Gambles M, Leese B, Atkin K, Brown J.** Representation of South Asian people in randomised clinical trials: analysis of trials' data. BMJ. 2003;**326**(7401):1244–5.
72. **Jacob KS, Bhugra D, Lloyd KR, Mann AH.** Common mental disorders, explanatory models and consultation behaviour among Indian women living in the UK. Journal of the Royal Society of Medicine. 1998;**91**(2):66–71.
73. **Husain N, Creed F, Tomenson B.** Adverse social circumstances and depression in people of Pakistani origin in the UK. British Journal of Psychiatry. 1997;**171**(5):434–8.
74. **Hull SA, Cornwell J, Harvey C, Eldridge S, Bare PO.** Prescribing rates for psychotropic medication amongst East London general practices: low rates where Asian populations are greatest. Family Practice. 2001;**18**(2):167–73.
75. **Cornwell J, Hull S.** Do GPs prescribe antidepressants differently for South Asian patients? Family Practice. 1998;**15**:S16–18.
76. **Bhui K, Brown R, Hardie T, Bhugra D, Goldberg D.** Common mental disorders among Punjabi and English subjects in primary care. Prevalence, detection of morbidity and pathways into care. Psychological Medicine. 2001;**81**:815–25.
77. **Bhugra D, Cochrane R.** *Psychiatry in Multicultural Britain*. London: Gaskell; 2001.
78. **Dein S, Alexander M, Napier AD.** Jinn, psychiatry and contested notions of misfortune among East London Bangladeshis. Transcultural Psychiatry. 2008;**45**(1):31–55.
79. **Hussain F, Cochrane R.** Depression in South Asian women: Asian women's beliefs on causes and cures. Mental Health, Religion and Culture. 2002;**6**(1):287–311.
80. **Dein S, Sembhi S.** The use of traditional healing in South Asian psychiatric patients in the UK: interactions between professional and folk psychiatries. Transcultural Psychiatry. 2001;**38**(2):243–57.
81. **Tabassum R, Macaskill A, Ahmad I.** Attitudes towards mental health in an urban Pakistani community in the United Kingdom. International Journal of Social Psychiatry. 2000;**46**(3):170–81.

82. **Malik R.** *Counselling and Ancient Belief Systems. Race and Cultural Education in Counselling*. British Association of Counselling. 1998;**1**(6):12–14.
83. **Sembhi S, Dein S.** The use of traditional healers by Asian psychiatric patients in the UK: a pilot study. Mental Health, Religion, and Culture. 1998;**1**(2):127–33.
84. **Battachaya DP.** *Pagalami: Europsychiatric Knowledge in Bengal*. New York, NY: Syracuse University Press; 1986.
85. **Hussain NO, Dein S.** An exploration of spiritual healing methods amongst the South-Asian Muslim community in the north of England. Journal of Historical Archaeology and Anthropological Sciences. 2018;**3**(2):163–74. doi: 10.15406/jhaas.2018.03.00079
86. **Fernando S.** Multicultural mental health services: projects for minority ethnic communities in England. Transcultural Psychiatry. 2005;**42**(3):420–36.
87. **Department of Health**. Delivering race equality in mental health care: an action plan for reform inside and outside services and the Government's response to the independent inquiry into the death of David Bennett. London: Department of Health; 2005.
88. **Department of Health**. Preventing suicide in England: a cross-government outcomes strategy to save lives. London: Department of Health; 2012.
89. **Husain N, Lunat F, Gire N**, et al. Developing interventions for prevention of self-harm for British South Asian women: a qualitative study. European Psychiatry. 2016;**33**:S749.
90 **Pearson A, Saini P, Da Cruz D**, et al. Primary care contact prior to suicide in individuals with mental illness. British Journal of General Practice. 2009;**59**(568):825–32.
91. **Saini P, Windfuhr K, Pearson A**, et al. Suicide prevention in primary care: general practitioners' views on service availability. BMC Research Notes. 2010;**3**(1):246.
92. **Da Cruz D, Pearson A, Saini P**, et al. Emergency department contact prior to suicide in mental health patients. Emergency Medicine Journal. 2011;**28**(6):467–71.
93. **Bhui K, McKenzie K, Rasul F.** Rates, risk factors and methods of self harm among minority ethnic groups in the UK: a systematic review. BMC Public Health. 2007;**7**(1):336.
94. **Khan F, Waheed W.** Suicide and self-harm in South Asian immigrants. Psychiatry. 2006;**5**(8):283–5.
95. **Husain N, Chaudhry N, Husain M, Waheed W.** Prevention of suicide in ethnic minorities in the UK. Ethnicity and Inequalities in Health and Social Care. 2009;**2**(1):10–17.
96. **Bhugra D, Hicks MH.** Effect of an educational pamphlet on help-seeking attitudes for depression among British South Asian women. Psychiatric Services. 2004;**55**(7):827–9.
97. **Husain N, Chaudhry N, Durairaj SV**, et al. Prevention of self harm in British South Asian women: study protocol of an exploratory RCT of culturally adapted manual assisted Problem Solving Training (C-MAP). Trials. 2011;**12**(1):159.
98. **Husain N, Afsar S, Ara J**, et al. Brief psychological intervention after self-harm: randomised controlled trial from Pakistan. British Journal of Psychiatry. 2014;**204**(6):462–70.

Chapter 13

Suicidality in Black and further non-*white* communities*

Felicia Boma Lazaridou and
Meryam Schouler-Ocak

Introduction

Suicidality is a psychiatric emergency referring to suicidal ideation, which includes talking or thinking about ending one's own life or planning and taking actions to end one's own life.[4] The World Health Organization (WHO)[5] estimates that people from low- and middle-income countries (LMICs) are 3.8 times more likely to take their own life than those from high-income countries (HICs). Disparities in suicide prevalence rates between LMICs and HICs appear to be reproduced among Black and further non-*white* communities migrating from LMICs to HICs.[6] In HICs, people of South Asian descent as well as Black women and Black youth are far more likely to take their own lives than the general population.[6,7,8] Implementing micro-, meso-, and macro-level suicide prevention measures often has to contend with high rates of non-disclosure of suicidal thoughts.[5,9] Research suggests that a pervasive risk factor for suicidality non-disclosure in Black and further non-*white* communities is the worry that suicidality is considered a problem only in the phenomenology of "*white* people's social conditions"; as such, it is often perceived that willingness to disclose suicidality could result in ostracism from one's own community for forgetting one's roots.[10,11,12,13]

Suicidality itself is not a mental illness in its own right according to international medical classifications such as International Classification of Diseases, 11th Revision (ICD-11).[5] However, studies have shown that people

* ...the terms Black and *white*, which are used in this article, are not to be understood as adjectives which refer to biological markers or to skin color, but as categories which point to processes of racialization, to positions in societies and to differences with regard to power. The capitalization of Black and the italicization of *white* is often used in the German context to emphasize this standpoint.[1,2,3] (p. 24)

with mental disorders, including depression, substance use disorders, schizophrenia spectrum disorders, anxiety disorders, personality disorders, and eating disorders, to only name a few, are far more likely to take their own life than people with no mental disorders.[14] In addition to having a greater burden of mental health problems, Black and non-*white* communities in LMICs and HICs often face more barriers to accessing high-quality mental health treatment services than their *white* counterparts.[15,16] In the context of suicidality in Black and further non-*white* communities, while focusing on mental illness is important, the presence of a mental illness is only one piece of the puzzle within the social determinants of health framework (see Figure 13.1).[17,18] There are experiences and processes of racism that touch upon the contexts of governance, macroeconomic, social, and public policies, as well as cultural/ societal values, which negatively impact the physical and mental health of Black and further non-*white* communities in urban and rural environments globally.[19,20,21,22]

For example, food insecurity is a global humanitarian issue, with the highest prevalence in most regions across the world with Black and further non-*white* communities such as sub-Saharan countries (57.9%), Latin American and the Caribbean countries (40.6%), and Asian countries (24.6%).[23] Research has identified that food insecurity is a risk factor for suicidality.[24] A content analysis of the literature on food insecurity has located two meta-narratives explaining the high prevalence of food insecurity in LMICs. The first meta-narrative, which is the most commonly applied in academic articles and aid agency reports, is a 'crisis in food production' narrative, whereas the second meta-narrative is a 'chronic poverty' narrative and is more common in policy documents.[25] In terms of monitoring food insecurity globally, based on thresholds set by the Food and Agriculture Organization of the United Nations, the prevalence of food insecurity is considerably lower in HICs than in LMICs.[26] The United Kingdom is generally a food-secure country. However; the Conservative government's austerity measures since the Great Recession that occurred from 2007 to 2009 resulted in budget cuts across the public sector and higher taxation that have negatively impacted food security levels.[27] Research showed that the prevalence of food insecurity among unemployed people and people with disabilities in the United Kingdom was 27.7% (95% confidence interval (CI) 24.8–30.6%) in 2004 and increased to 45.8% (95% CI 41.6–49.9%) in 2016.[27]

There is evidence that food insecurity affects the mental health of the most deprived groups. Firstly, through a 'social stigma effect' of internalized shame:

> 'The stigma impacts on them in a really significant way, and socially, that's hugely damaging to children. […] they just sniff each other out. They don't speak about it at all, but they all know, and they can read the signs of it, and then they're carrying that

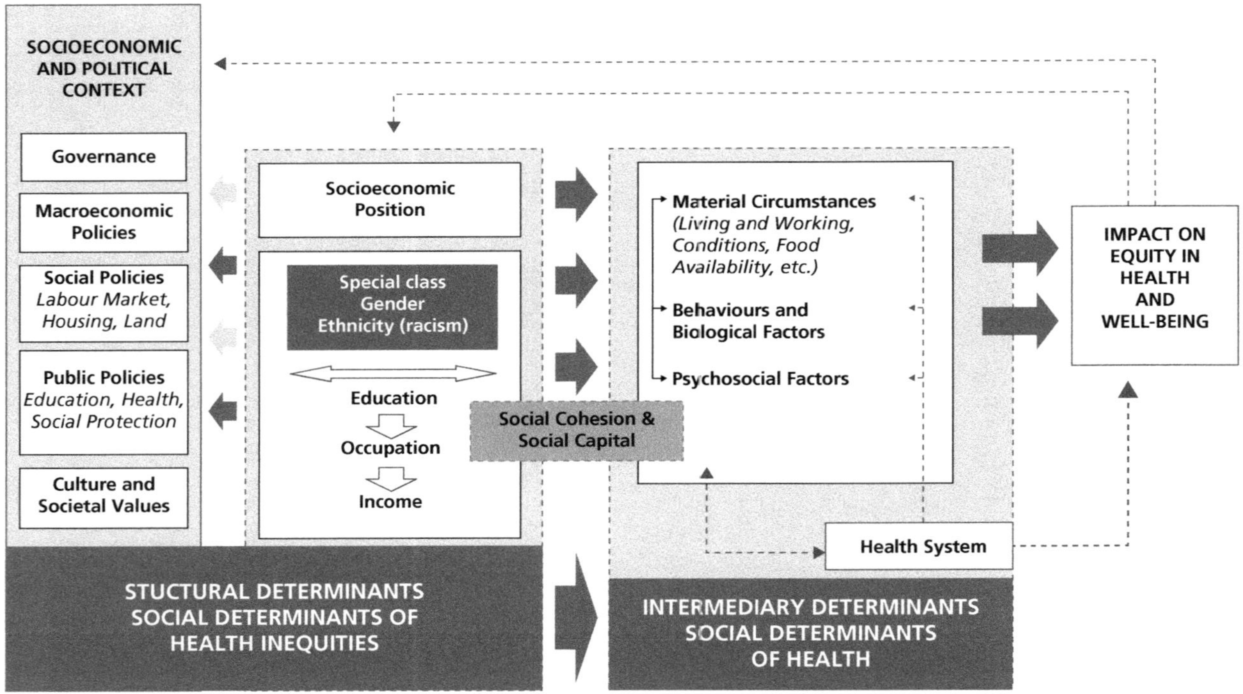

Figure 13.1 The Commission on Social Determinants of Health (CSDH) conceptual framework.
Reproduced from the *A Conceptual Framework for Action on the Social Determinants of Health*, Solar and Irwin, 2010, © World Health Organization (WHO) 2010.

> kind of stigma, and that shame, which is incredibly powerful, and very damaging' (voluntary worker, p. 99).[28]

And secondly, through a 'cycle of deprivation effect' of apathy:

> 'If people absolutely haven't had enough to eat, it's very hard to think straight, it's very hard to make good decisions. If it goes on and on and on, chronically, you tend to just want to go to sleep or sit on the chair or not to do anything, you increasingly lack, literally, the energy to make anything, a change' (independent informant, p. 96).[28]

The coronavirus disease 2019 (COVID-19) pandemic has increased the global prevalence of food insecurity, including in the United Kingdom and European Union countries, and disproportionately so for Black and further non-*white* communities.[23] Countries have been generally reluctant to contextualize the causes of suicidality within a network of precipitating and perpetuating socio-economic and political risk factors. Importantly, however, evidence suggests that suicidality is linked to markers of economic poverty, including unemployment and unaffordable housing.[29,30] Not only is low socio-economic status more strongly associated with suicidality than high socio-economic status,[31] but socio-economic-related depression is also more strongly linked with suicidality than non-socio-economic-related depression.[32] Many other risk factors associated with suicidality, such as low self-esteem and low life satisfaction, are also related to racism.[18]

A social justice approach is required in framing recognition of suicidality among Black and further non-*white* communities because the existence of these groups is resistance as communities having to face struggle.[33] Powerful groups define racialized groups by imposing an 'inferior other' status on them in socially created contrasts to *whiteness*, and racialized groups define themselves in response to the wide range of socially created political neglect resulting from these racist ascriptions.[34,35,36] At the nexus of intersectional and paradoxical social processes, the subjectification of Black and further non-*white* communities emanates from their resistance against racist domination.[37,38,39,40] In terms of preventability, a social justice approach allows the topic to move past understanding suicidality as a problem residing in a sociopolitical vacuum to instead understanding suicidality as a problem residing in the structure of the larger socio-economic and political context.[41]

Racism and suicidality

Social justice approaches are urgently needed if we are to address inequities in complex social meta-problems such as suicidality.[42] Suicidality is conceptualized as a meta-problem in the field of mental health and death studies, especially among 15- to 19-year olds, as it is a leading cause of mortality worldwide.[5] A growing body of anti-racism research associated with, and extending beyond, the rise of the Black Lives Matter movement supports the call for context-specific and targeted decolonial and systemic transformations to support overall health and mental health improvements in Black and further non-*white* communities.[43] What is new about the agentic, relational, and situated power-centric call for anti-racism approaches to suicidality is its focus on structural racism—particularly its contribution to applying analyses of profound, deep-seated racialized structural inequities and exclusion to build upon long-standing knowledge about social disadvantages, such as food insecurity, impoverishment, and endemic violence, and the cumulative impact of these on suicidality.[44] The WHO's structural determinants of health framework imply preventative efforts and strategies through institutional management and responsibility to alleviate all manner of social meta-problems, such as suicidality.

The development and implementation of interventions by Western institutions have, however, been accused of reflecting entrenched interests in keeping hold of power and resources.[45] As such, these institutional interventions tend to be shallow in the sense that they reinforce racialized disadvantages and marginalization, without acknowledging the redistributive gaps and challenges they are exacerbating. The nature of these power imbalances has not been addressed even within psychiatry and clinical psychology's reflexive turn towards an ethos of cultural competency in clinical care interactions. Institutional racism is deeply rooted in the design of global psychiatry and clinical psychology. It stands accused of precipitating and perpetuating structural inequities by default (see Figure 13.2).[46] To combat this issue, we are witnessing a proliferation of calls for structural competency as a force for social justice in psychiatry and clinical psychology.[47] Structural competency advances Fanon's sociogenic perspective on the interrelationship between individuals and society, and provides an alternative lens on suicidality in Black and further non-*white* communities at the interface of social belongingness and anti-Black racism.

The reflexive turn that sought to leave the biological conceptualization of 'race' behind, in favour of embracing social constructions of 'race', acted as a movement against racism and colonialism.[48] Building on theories of intelligence that posited the inferior cognitive capabilities of all Black and non-*white* communities in comparison to *white* people, the internal suicide debate hypothesis was implied. The internal suicide debate hypothesis[49] relays the empirical study of the Freudian psychic tension between Eros and Thanatos—the life drive/instinct and the death drive/instinct.[50] According to Freud, the deliberation between self-destruction and survival that is acutely professed in the suicidal mind is essentially a constant constitution of human selfhood. In that way, beingness and nothingness are deeply embroiled. If, as a deficit model claims,

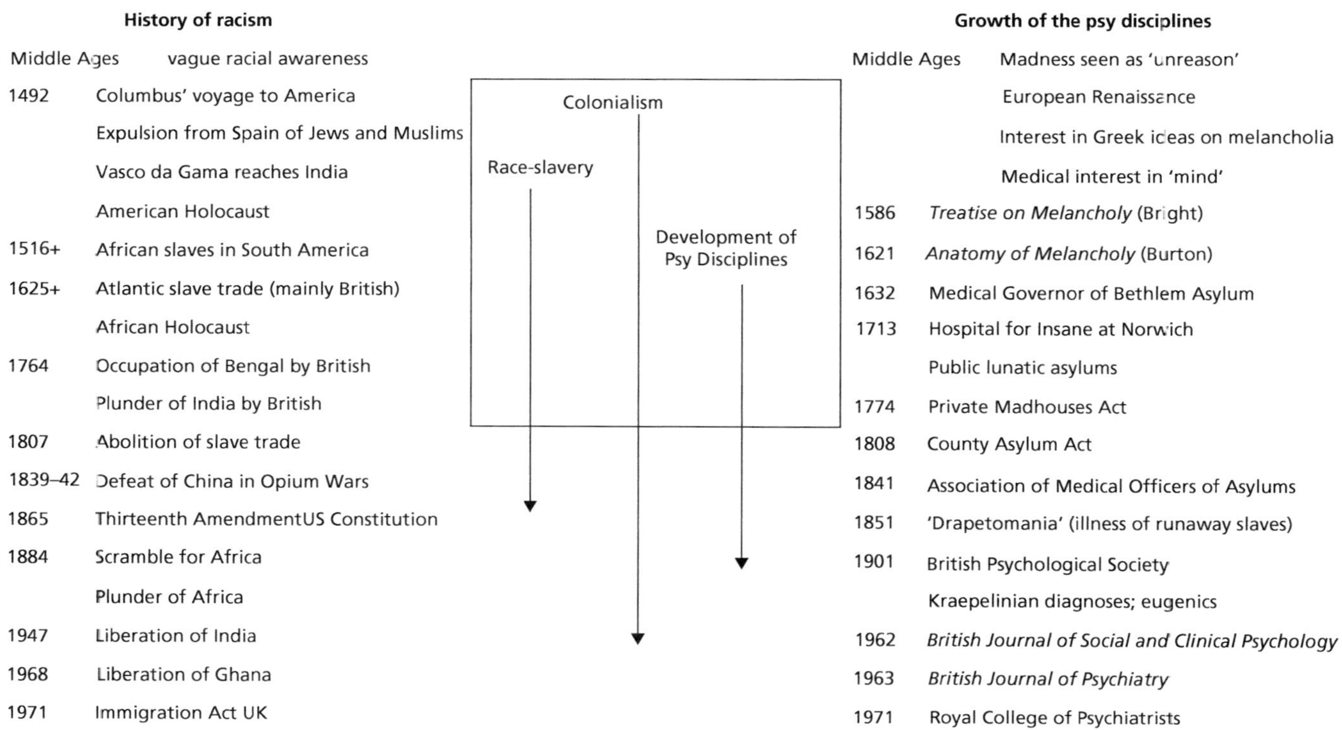

Figure 13.2 Historical context of psychiatry and clinical psychology.

Reproduced from *Institutional Racism in Psychiatry and Clinical Psychology: Race Matters in Mental Health*, 2017, © Palgrave Macmillan/S Fernando.

Black and further non-*white* communities are incapable of the cognitive and rational abilities required to engage in what Freud[50] deems a natural human subjectivity, then, accordingly, Black and further non-*white* communities are sub-human.

According to Fanon, experiencing material and symbolic relegation to 'the zone of non-being', even in the context of highly stigmatizing topics such as suicide, is hellish because people want nothing more than to be humanized. Integrating a conceptualization of inequality and power from the perspective of Bourdieu,[51] 'the zone of being' is the humanizing bridge that can allow the racialized phenomenology of Black and further non-*white* communities' 'weight-of-the-world' experiences of suffering to be structurally recognized. As Fanon outlines, anti-Black racism can be understood as a dual process of racialization. Anti-Black racism naturalizes *whiteness* as humanness, and every racialized category outside of this norm as beneath *whites* or worse. As such, anti-Black racism naturalizes the symbolic violence of identity impositions,[52] the *white* constructivity of which gives rise to a 'one-size-fits-all' Blackness, which is in itself a failure to recognize the fullness and richness of human existence.[53] Anti-racism can give people racialized as Black and as belonging to racistly marked group the benefit of having their suffering recognized as human, without having to live an existence as *white*.[54]

The role of Black and further non-*white* knowledge production in challenging racist suicidality theories

Major work studying suicidality in Black and further non-*white* communities began during the deep fervor of the eugenics movements.[55] In a tripartite understanding of knowledge production processes have significantly improved the state of the literature on this topic, these improvements have also played a role in reducing the stigma of suicidality in Black and further non-*white* communities. Firstly, pervasive attitudes about assumed *white* superiority in terms of intelligence capabilities set the standards of academic demands determining the visibility of research. Despite historical and ongoing racism, researchers from Black and further non-*white* communities—who face stereotyping and being discriminated against in a network of racist struggles in the academic prestige hierarchy—have become heroes. Their ideas, plans, and efforts to elucidate the world around them and give a voice to emotions have changed the literature base in a radical way. This embedded agency has created space for the self-empowerment of researchers through interactions aimed at empowering fellow Black and further non-*white* individuals and their communities.[56] Particularly in community-oriented qualitative methodologies, emotional interactions have enabled Black and further non-*white* communities' perspectives to be heard and understood,[57] thereby stimulating opportunities for intersectional reflexivity and the creation of new intercultural theories.[58]

Secondly, a phenomenology of overwhelming *whiteness* constrains the academic mainstream, limiting structures of opportunity for research and publication to *white* thinkers and *white* knowledge. Despite the fact that researchers from Black and further non-*white* communities have to contend with inhibiting, rather than enhancing, academic milieus, the energy of Black and further non-*white* activism orientations in research is nothing short of inspirational. In spite of the low value placed on Black and further non-*white* knowledge in the academic prestige hierarchy, researchers from Black and further non-*white* communities have negotiated and co-created new understandings about human experiences and the social systems within which they are lived.[59,60] And thirdly, the inevitability of racist interactions in navigating the academic prestige hierarchy is so because the power to productively highlight frictions and tensions is disproportionately centred around people from non-Black and further non-white minority groups. Despite obstacles encountered in terms of access to resources that aid in achieving academic success, researchers from Black and ethnic minority groups have been clear in calling attention to the obstacles that stall or thwart their progress.[61] Research suggests that conversing about suicidality among Black and further non-*white* communities can help prevent suicidality in these communities.[62] Black and further non-*white* activism orientations have received an unprecedented amount of media attention recently. In demanding a greater say in the design of research, developing innovative research methodologies aligned with principles of social justice, and honouring local and indigenous perspectives in mental health and allied fields, a new generation of local expertise are mobilizing anti-racism and decolonial research agendas.[63]

Conceptualizing the cumulativeness and complexity of social stress as a suicide risk factor

In a family systems theory approach, losing someone close through suicide is a significant stress, the repercussions of which can manifest in further loss of life through suicide (adjusted odds ratio 1.65, 95% CI 1.12–2.42; $p = 0.012$).[64] The grieving process of loss survivors of death by suicide appears to be qualitatively distinct from that of loss survivors of other causes of death, requiring qualitatively distinct therapeutic strategies to prevent further suicide.[65] Black and further non-*white* resilience theory is often inquired as a theoretical framework to examine the collectivism of Black and further non-*white* communities as suicide prevention.[66] In a concentric family systems theory approach, most Black and further non-*white* communities that are embedded in their indigenous worldviews are deeply connected to their family, their community, the land, the sacred, and the profane.[67,68] Many Black and further non-white communities posit a collectivistic self that inhabits a ritual space marked by cognitive and affective spiritual resonance.[69] Canons of faith and worship govern the socially mediated and culturally specific philosophical ritual space.[70]

The socialization processes of children and young people in Black and further non-*white* communities, frequently reported as authoritarian, are typically framed within the resilience theory as post-traumatic growth.[71,72,73] Much less time is allocated to analysing the post-traumatic social stress of the actual-self/ideal-self discrepancy perceived in the context of authoritarian demands and expectations. A build-up of post-traumatic social stress is highly regulated by behavioural and normative ideological boundaries pertaining to the social acceptability of emotional expressions.[74] Stunted freedom of emotional expression experiences in said high-power distance cultures only serves to silence feelings of fear and shame that the texture of the community itself plays a role in creating.[75] A post-traumatic accumulation of stress that, particularly within Black and further non-*white* communities in HICs, is augmented by the unpredictability of exposure to racism.[76] Geronimus' weathering theory[77] suggests that excessive demands for psychosocial maturity far beyond the capacities of one's actual age causes an incongruence between external societal expectations and internal perceptions of self.[78] This incongruence is emphasized as a highly subjective perception of age, and in the same way, to Joiner,[79,80] trajectories of belongingness/burdensomeness are highly subjective.

For both the weathering theory[77] and the interpersonal theory of suicide,[79] lived experiences in interactions within the community and larger society are an important contribution to social stress and the development of subsequent mental health symptoms. The weathering theory (1992)[77] is politically relevant in the sense that it was developed in the early 1990s, at a time when conceptualization of 'race' as a biological construct was on the whole publicly shifting towards conceptualizing 'race' as a social phenomenon and, at the same time, Black feminists demands for a shift from normative *whiteness* to intersectionality perspectives began to reach the mainstream. The influence of this social and political milieu on weathering as a theory is clear. In relating Geronimus' work[77] to the intersectionality discourse, the weathering theory resists a single-issue approach to social stress. As the Black feminist Audre Lorde said, 'there is no such thing as a single-issue approach because we do not live single-issue lives' (p. 138).[81] The epigenetic revolution is providing support to this theory, and findings document the embodiment of racism's structural failures biochemically in physiology, typically via repeated episodes of allostasis in response to socially structured stressors experienced in severe duration or amount and the parallel development of allostatic load.[82]

Learning about the history of 'race' and the effects of racism evokes many difficult emotions for Black and further non-*white* communities, and for *white* people too.[83] Experiences of racism are also fraught with psychologically immersive emotions.[84] Powerful personal narratives collected from Black women and those of further non-*white* communities illustrate difficult emotions such as shame/embarrassment and guilt that are completely normal for victims of racism to feel.[85] Experiences of racism are also associated with feelings of shame/embarrassment and guilt, and negative affect in general,[86] and research indicates that[87] shame/embarrassment and guilt activate similar, if not identical, brain regions.[88] Major subcortical components of the fear and shame neurocircuitry are connected in the limbic–hypothalamic–pituitary–adrenal (LHPA) axis.[89] LPHA axis dysregulation is associated with suicidality and food insecurity,[90,91,92] which, at the capitalistic nexus of power, money, and resources, constitute two social issues of great importance disproportionately impacting some of the most vulnerable Black and further non-*white* communities and diasporas across the world.

Studies suggest that racism (traumatization, victimization, discrimination, etc.) and food insecurity (starvation) can dysregulate neurochemical synaptic transmissions in the LHPA axis, leading to hypercortisolaemia.[93,94] The observation of hypersecretion of cortisol in the brain is a consequence of overactivity in the anterior pituitary corticotrophs that are responsible for the production and secretion of adrenocorticotrophic hormones. This results in an increase in synthesis and release of the glucocorticoid hormone hydrocortisone, also known as cortisol, from the brain's adrenal cortex. Studies have shown that racism and food insecurity can cause irreversible HPA axis dysregulation.[95] The evidence base shows that hypercortisolaemia contributes to the future development of, and exacerbates the current existence of, numerous medical and mental health conditions, including suicidality.[96,97]

Centring the thwarted social belongingness of racism's structural denial as a suicide risk factor

Solidarity with the statement 'Black Lives Matter', underpinning the ethos of the movement, as more than a plain rhetoric, hinges on a realization that the fabric of our social and political institutions are not naturally grounded in the assumption that all lives equally matter. For the American Association of Suicidology (AAS), and for many institutions like AAS, this realization resulted in the publication of a position statement on equity and anti-racism under the following overall motto:

> 'We believe that the only way for the field of suicidology to reduce suicide and build lives worth living for BIPOC [Black people, Indigenous people and People of Colour] is to dismantle systems of oppression.'[98]

In addition to the creation of space for expertise on Black and further non-*white* communities,[99,100] in an AAS press release concerning suicide loss in Black communities, Congresswoman Bonnie Watson Coleman stated the following:

> 'It is critical that we open spaces uniquely suited to Black mental health, and that includes Black grief […] our community requires professionals with cultural competence, safe spaces to cover the kinds of challenges we experience, and the comfort of not being the only face of colour in the room. Every step we can take to create more of these spaces, whether its initiatives like this one or resources at the federal level, gets us closer to meeting an urgent need and I am grateful to work together with the American Association of Suicidology on this issue.'[99]

Stigma, and the taboo of talking through psychological pain, results in suicidality being seen as a result of the individual's failure to implement sufficiently helpful mechanisms to cope with their pain.[101]

The racialized inequality and social integration–regulation hypothesis builds on Durkheim's social integration theory of suicidality,[102] which formed the basis of one of the earliest views that society's social conditions may induce suicidality.[103] The main assumption of the social integration theory is furthered in the twofold schema of Van Orden et al.'s interpersonal theory of suicide[104] as thwarted belongingness and perceived burdensomeness. He proposed that thwarted belongingness and perceived burdensomeness induce suicidality somewhat independently, all the while mediated by the individual's capacity for suicide.[79] This notion of capacity for suicide is presumably a reference to the ebbs and flows between the desire for life and the desire for death captured by the internal suicide debate theory mentioned previously.[49,105,106] A critical perspective on suicidality critiques the pathologization of suicidality as well as the dislocations of suicidality from surrounding social interactions to being rooted strictly in the individual.[107] Thus, emphasizing that the individual's capacity for suicide is acquired, this is socially mediated through the 'weight-of-world-suffering' in connection to a lack of social belonginess to one's community, and ultimately to the world.[108]

Social belongingness is the feeling of being meaningfully integrated into one's communities, geopolitical spaces, and institutions.[109,110,111] According to Williams' need–threat model,[112] gratification of social belongingness is cconnected to self-esteem,[113,114,115] control,[116] and meaningful existence.[117] Therefore, social belongingness is related to psychological well-being in general.[118] Well-being is typically conceptualized as the degree of life satisfaction one is experiencing—in other words, the level to which people can say they are living their version of 'the good life'.[119] Furthermore, well-being is the presence of positive affect as compared to the absence of negative affect.[120,121] The overall closeness between social belongingness and social integration firmly places understandings of physical health and mental health in the complexity of historical and current social interactions that impacts how people evaluate their individual progress and development.[122] Globally, suicidality is typically understood in its association with profound, psychologically painful loss and traumatic life events.[123]

The reified fixity of anti-Black racism's structural denial that renders the possibility that Black and further non-*white* communities negotiate social belongingness to many multilayered socio-geographical terrains and objects of attachment impossible is a form of failure.[53] Crenshaw's[124] social and political observation of this structural failure is the most coherent, direct theoretical challenge to the symbolic violence of identity imposition to date.[125] Whether high suicide rates or low suicide rates are being explored, or whether suicide risk factors or protective factors are being explored, it is important to refrain from valorizing differences in cultural value orientations for difference's sake. Problematically, while many cultural theories of suicide exist (e.g. see Chu[126] and Abrutyn),[127] oftentimes cultural theories concerning Black and further non-*white* communities inadvertently attribute experiences of mental distress to 'race'.[53] In centring the cultural value orientations of Black and further non-*white* communities as the problem or the solution, cultural theories of suicidality perpetuate dominant medical and psychological approaches to suicidality that problematize individuals rather than society—in this context, the oppressed individuals rather than the dominating individuals. To clarify, in a social justice approach to suicidality, it could be useful to merge understandings of racism's structural failures with the major tenets of suicide theories within which suicide is understood as a social issue.[41]

Fostering Black and further non-*white* community activism orientations as suicidality resilience

Black and further non-*white* community activism orientations have received an unprecedented amount of media attention recently. At a time when the whole world was in lockdown and contemplating how best to support its communities through the COVID-19 pandemic, the world was stunned by the murder of George Floyd by a police officer in the United States. As the video depicting his death went viral, his death ignited an eruption of physical and digital Black

Lives Matter protests and conversations about anti-Black racism around the world. Despite dozens of murders at the hands of *white* police officers just for being Black, Black and further non-*white* communities and their problems with anti-Black racism have largely been ignored—or worse. Research conducted on the topic of mental health and racism suggests that the mental health of Black and further non-*white* communities is negatively impacted after the news of the death of yet another Black individual at the hands of *white* cops surfaces.[128] A plethora of systematic reviews and meta-analyses offers a panoramic overview of the negative impacts of racism on the mental health of adults, children and youths in Black and further non-*white* communities globally.[129,130] Research suggests that suicidality has increased among Black adolescents in recent years.[131] As a form of social resilience, Black activism orientations are implicated as moderating factors from post-traumatic stress to post-traumatic growth following contexts of anti-Black racism.[132,133]

Bourdieu's social resilience theory[134] is also a socio-ecological understanding of mental health, and suggests that capital (social, economic, cultural, and symbolic) directly supports social integration into social networks, enabling higher-quality psychological functioning. Resilience is typically engineering and physics terminology that, when applied to people, expresses the capacity of said persons to maintain their original condition even after extreme pressure has been exerted on them. The concept of social resilience, as applied in the context of racism and mental health, is a double-edged sword. On one side, social resilience forms the positive value orientations that allow people to cope and manage demands that are creating stress;[135] and on the other side, severe and persistent oppression and saturated disadvantage distort positive coping styles into forms of socially prescribed perfectionism.[136] This is why Huppert and So[119] explained that well-being exists on a spectrum, with flourishing occurring at the positive end and mental disorder occurring at the negative end (see Figure 13.3).

The conceptual closeness of flourishing and social resilience to the well-being literature (e.g. see Jahoda,[137] Antonovsky,[138] Ryan and Deci,[139] and Seligman)[140] leads us to assume that the psychological concepts of flourishing can be understood as value orientations, whereas the ability to access lifestyle factors that support activation and utilization of these value orientations during the most trying times creates a drive towards flourishing and away from mental disorder. In Black Lives Matter, and in various sociopolitical activism orientations, creative historical praxis emerges at the intersection between the value of human life and the value of human death.[141] Awareness that choosing life over death in the face of a sharp reality of racist oppression is the highest form of self-actualization in Black and ethnic minority group activism orientations.

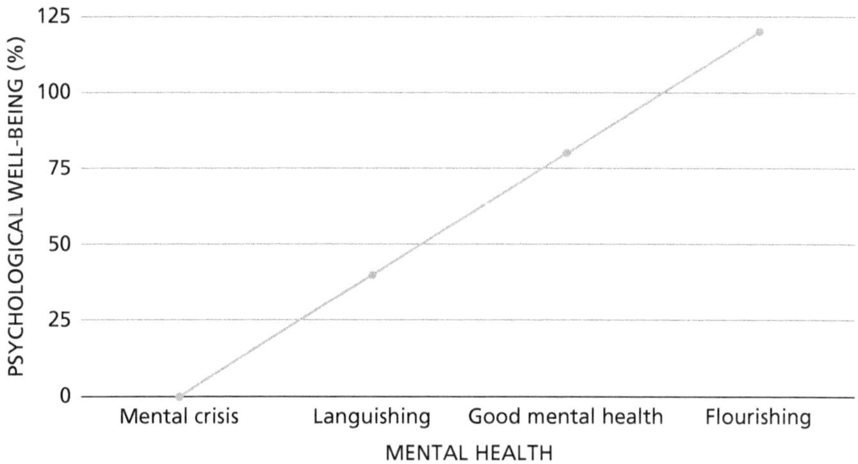

Figure 13.3 The psychological well-being spectrum. As well-being improves, so does mental health, and vice versa.
Adapted from Huppert and So, 2009.

Suicide prevention strategies

According to Morrison and Downey,[142] preventive and protective measures against suicidality, including reasons for living, differ across racialized groups. Black Americans report stronger reasons for living in comparison to European Americans. Marion and Range[143] underlined that social support, religiosity, and negative attitudes towards suicide buffer the relationship between stress and suicidal behaviour among Black Americans. Reasons for living predicted fewer future suicide attempts only among women.[144] Women were influenced more by concerns about death and injury, whereas men scored higher on concerns or fears about social disapproval.[145] Wang et al.[146] found that there is a scarcity of studies that have explicitly examined the intersection of gender and racialization and suicide protective factors such as reasons for living. Wang and colleagues[146] found that gender predicted suicidal thoughts and behaviour, and both depressive symptoms and dissatisfaction with life were stronger predictors of suicidal thoughts and behaviours among men than among women. They also found that among men, only life satisfaction was a significant inverse predictor of suicidal thoughts and behaviour, whereas among women, only reasons for living were a significant inverse predictor of suicidal thoughts and behaviour.

Rockett et al.[147] found that, as shown in official statistics, the racialized suicide gap persists in the lower and upper limit scenarios. The authors found also that suicide data appeared relatively more inadequate for Black women than for Black men. According to Rockett et al.,[147] results strongly indicated greater susceptibility of medico-legal authorities to misclassify suicides among Black people than among *white* people. They recommended to demystify the racialized suicide paradox, and research is needed on medical histories and other biographical information that are accessible by authorities in equivocal cases. Furthermore, to meet the standards of evidence-based medicine and public health, high-quality suicide data are an imperative for: risk group delineation; risk factor identification; policy formulation; programme planning, implementation, and evaluation; and ultimately effective prevention.[147]

Molock et al.[148] discussed suicide prevention programmes for Black American youth in churches, which may have broad appeal because: (1) the Black Church has a strong history of helping community members, regardless of church membership; (2) research suggests Black Americans have the highest level of public and private religiousness; and (3) the church can help to shape cultural norms about mental health and help-seeking. The proposed gatekeeper in this intervention trains lay helpers and clergies to recognize the suicide risk factors, to refer individuals to appropriate community mental health resources, and to deliver a community education curriculum.[148]

References

1. **Ha KN, al-Samarai NL, Mysorekar S.** Einleitung. In: **Ha KN, al-Samarai NL, Mysorekar** S, editors. re/Visionen. *Postkoloniale Perspektiven von People of Color auf Rassismus, Kulturpolitik und Widerstand in Deutschland.* Münster: Unrast Verlag; 2021. pp. 9–22.
2. **Hasters A.** *Was weiße Menschen nicht über Rassismus hören wollen aber wissen sollten.* München: hanserblau; 2019.
3. **Nobis T, Lazaridou F.** Racist stacking in professional soccer in Germany. International Review for the Sociology of Sport. 2023;**58**(1):23–42. https://doi.org/10.1177/101269 02221081125
4. **Oppong Asante K, Kugbey N, Osafo J, Quarshie ., Sarfo JO.** The prevalence and correlates of suicidal behaviours (ideation, plan and attempt) among adolescents in senior high schools in Ghana. SSM Popul Health. 2017 May 6;**3**:427–34. doi: 10.1016/j.ssmph.2017.05.005
5. **World Health Organization.** Suicide. 2019. Available from: https://www.who.int/en/news-room/fact-sheets/detail/suicide
6. **Forte A, Trobia F, Gualtieri F**, et al. Suicide risk among immigrants and ethnic minorities: a literature overview. International Journal of Environmental Research and Public Health. 2018;**15(7):1438.** https://doi.org/10.3390/ijerph15071438
7. **Bridge JA, Horowitz LM, Fontanella CA, Sheftall AH, Greenhouse, J, Kelleher KJ, Campo, JV.** Age-related racial disparity in suicide rates among US youths from 2001 through 2015. JAMA Pediatrics. 2018;**172**(7):697–9. doi:10.1001/jamapediatrics.2018.0399
8. **Couto C, Barreto S, Rolim Neto ML.** Suicide in Black children. International Journal of Social Psychiatry. 2018;**64**(5):506–8. doi:10.1177/0020764018770477

9. **Mérelle S, Foppen E, Gilissen R, Mokkenstorm J, Cluitmans R, van Ballegooijen W.** Characteristics associated with non-disclosure of suicidal ideation in adults. International Journal of Environmental Research and Public Health. 2018. https://doi.org/10.3390/ijerph15050943
10. **Crosby AE, Molock SD.** Introduction: suicidal behaviors in the African American community. Journal of Black Psychology. 2006;**32**(3):253–61. https://doi.org/10.1177/0095798406290552
11. **Early KE, Akers RL.** 'It's a white thing': an exploration of beliefs about suicide in the African-American community. Deviant Behavior. 1993;**14**(4):277–96. https://doi.org/10.1080/01639625.1993.9967947
12. **Kapadia D. Stigma,** mental illness & ethnicity: time to centre racism and structural stigma. Sociology of Health & Illness. 2023 May;**45**(4):855–71. doi/10.1111/1467-9566.13615
13. **Misra S, Jackson VW, Chong J, Choe K, Tay C, Wong J, Yang LH.** Systematic review of cultural aspects of stigma and mental illness among racial and ethnic minority groups in the United States: implications for interventions. American Journal of Community Psychology. 2021 Dec;**68**(3-4):486–512. doi:10.1002/ajcp.12516
14. **Brådvik L.** Suicide risk and mental disorders. International Journal of Environmental Research and Public Health. 2018;**15**(9):2028. https://doi.org/10.3390/ijerph15092028
15. **Cook BL, Hou SS-Y, Lee-Tauler SY, Progovac AM, Samson F, Sanchez MJ.** A review of mental health and mental health care disparities research: 2011–2014. Medical Care Research and Review. 2019;**76**(6):683–710.
16. **Wakida EK, Talib ZM, Akena D,** et al. Barriers and facilitators to the integration of mental health services into primary health care: a systematic review. Systematic Reviews. 2018;7(1):211.
17. **Solar O, Irwin A.** *A Conceptual Framework for Action of the Social Determinants of Health*. Geneva: World Health Organization; 2010.
18. **Paradies Y, Ben J, Denson N,** et al. Racism as a determinant of health: a systematic review and meta-analysis. PLoS One. 2015;**10**(9):e0138511. https://doi.org/10.1371/journal.pone.0138511
19. **Guterres A.** Secretary-General's Nelson Mandela lecture: 'Tackling the inequality pandemic: a new social contract for a new era' [as delivered]. 2020. Available from: https://www.un.org/sg/en/content/sg/statement/2020-07-18/secretary-generals-nelson-mandela-lecture-"tackling-the-inequality-pandemic-new-social-contract-for-new-era"-delivered
20. **Meier BM, Daniely T.** Tlaleng Mofokeng: special rapporteur on the right to health. Health and Human Rights Journal. 2020. https://www.hhrjournal.org/2020/08/tlaleng-mofokeng-special-rapporteur-on-the-right-to-health/
21. **Kampala Initiative Steering Group, Kampala Initiative Task Groups** (2019). Kamapala Initiative Report 2019–2020: cooperation and solidarity for health equity within and beyond aid. Available from: www.medicusmundi.org/kampalainitiative
22. **Medicus Mundi International** (2020). Kampala Declaration on cooperation and solidarity for health equity within and beyond aid. Available from: https://www.medicusmundi.org/kampaladeclaration/
23. **Food and Agriculture Organization of the United Nations,** World Trade Organization and World Bank Organization. Rising global food insecurity: assessing policy

responses, a report prepared at the request of the Group of 20 (G20). April 2023. https://www.fao.org/3/cc5392en/cc5392en.pdf

24. **Koyanagi A, Stubbs B, Oh H**, et al. Food insecurity (hunger) and suicide attempts among 179,771 adolescents attending school from 9 high-income, 31 middle-income, and 4 low-income countries: a cross-sectional study. Journal of Affective Disorders. 2019;**248**:91–8. https://doi.org/10.1016/j.jad.2019.01.033
25. **Legwegoh AF, Fraser EDG.**Food crisis or chronic poverty: metanarratives of food insecurity in sub-saharan Africa. Journal of Hunger & Environmental Nutrition. 2015;**10**:3, 313–42. doi:10.1080/19320248.2014.962777
26. Food and Agriculture Organization of the United Nations. The state of food security and nutrition in the world. 2021. Available from: https://www.fao.org/3/cb4474en/cb4474en.pdf
27. **Loopstra R, Reeves A, Tarasuk V.** The rise of hunger among low-income households: an analysis of the risks of food insecurity between 2004 and 2016 in a population-based study of UK adults. Journal of Epidemiol Community Health. 2019 Jul;**73**(7):668–73. doi:10.1136/jech-2018-211194
28. **Sosenko F, Littlewood M, Bramley G, Fitzpatrick S, Blenkinsopp J, Wood J.** State of Hunger: a study of poverty and food insecurity in the UK. The Trussel Trust; 2019. https://www.stateofhunger.org/wp-content/uploads/2019/11/State-of-Hunger-Report-November2019-Digital.pdf?_ga=2.3105522.310854385.1710760989-1282123478.1710760989
29. **Shand F, Duffy L, Torok M.** Can government responses to unemployment reduce the impact of unemployment on suicide? Crisis. 2022 Jan;**43**(1):59–66. doi:10.1027/0227-5910/a000750
30. **Park GR, Grignon M, Young M, Dunn JR.** The association between housing cost burden and avoidable mortality in wealthy countries: cross-national analysis of social and housing policies, 2000–2017. Journal of Epidemiology and Community Health. 2023 Feb;**77**(2):65–73. doi:10.1136/jech-2022-219545
31. **Näher AF, Rummel-Kluge C, Hegerl U.** Associations of suicide rates with socioeconomic status and social isolation: findings from longitudinal register and census data. Frontiers in Psychiatry. 2020 Jan 14;**10**:898. doi:10.3389/fpsyt.2019.00898
32. **Thekiso TB, Heron EA, Masood B, Murphy M, McLoughlin DM, Kennedy N.** Mauling of the 'Celtic Tiger': clinical characteristics and outcome of first-episode depression secondary to the economic recession in Ireland. Journal of Affective Disorders. 2013 Nov;**151**(2):455–60. doi: 10.1016/j.jad.2013.06.024
33. **Schotten CH.** To exist is to resist: palestine and the question of queer theory. Journal of Palestine Studies. 1 May 2018;**47**(3):13–28. doi: https://doi.org/10.1525/jps.2018.47.3.13
34. **Mohanty CT.** 'Under Western Eyes' revisited: feminist solidarity through anticapitalist struggles. Signs. 2003;**28**(2):499–535. JSTOR, https://doi.org/10.1086/342914
35. **Fanon F.** *Black skin, white masks*. London: Pluto Press; 1986.
36. **Fassin D.** Racialization. In: **Mascia-Lees FE**, editor. *A companion to the anthropology of the body and embodiment*. Wiley-Blackwell; 2011. pp. 419–34. https://doi.org/10.1002/9781444340488.ch24
37. **Foucault M.** The subject and power. In: **James D. Faubion**, editor. *Essential Works of Foucault*, Volume 3 – Power. New York; 1997. pp. 326–49.
38. **Butler J.** 'Conscience Doth Make Subjects of Us All.' Yale French Studies. 1995;**88**:6–26. JSTOR, https://doi.org/10.2307/2930099

39. **Gilroy P.** 'There ain't no black in the Union Jack': the cultural politics of race and nation. Black Literature and Culture. University of Chicago Press; 1991.
40. **Fraser N.** *Justice interruptus: critical reflections on the 'postsocialist' condition* (1st edition). Routledge; 1997. https://doi.org/10.4324/9781315822174
41. **Button ME, Marsh I,** editors. *Suicide and social justice: new perspectives on the politics of suicide and suicide prevention* (1st edition). Routledge; 2019. https://doi.org/10.4324/9780429460494
42. **Hochhauser S, Rao S, England-Kennedy E,** et al. Why social justice matters: a context for suicide prevention efforts. International Journal for Equity in Health. 2020;**19**:76.
43. **Banks C.** Disciplining black activism: post-racial rhetoric, public memory and decorum in news media framing of the Black Lives Matter movement. Continuum. 2018;**32**(6):709–20.
44. **Hassen N, Lofters A, Michael S, Mall A, Pinto AD, Rackal J.** Implementin/g anti-racism interventions in healthcare settings: a scoping review. International Journal of Environmental Research and Public Health. 2021;**18**(6):2993.
45. **Rafi F, Westwood R, Boje DM.** 'I feel like a foreign agent': NGOs and corporate social responsibility interventions into Third World child labor. Human Relations. 2010;**63**(9):1417–38.
46. **Fernando S.** *Institutional racism in psychiatry and clinical psychology*. London: Palgrave Macmillan; 2017.
47. **Marshall-Lee ED, Hinger C, Popovic R, Miller Roberts TC, Prempeh L.** Social justice advocacy in mental health services: consumer, community, training, and policy perspectives. Psychological Services. 2020;**17**(S1):12–21.
48. **Schouler-Ocak M, Bhugra D, Kastrup MC,** et al. Racism and mental health and the role of mental health professionals. European Psychiatry. 2021;**64**(1):e42, 1–15.
49. **Kovacs M, Beck AT.** The wish to die and the wish to live in attempted suicides. Journal of Clinical Psychology. 1977;33(2):361–5. https://doi.org/10.1002/1097-4679(197704)33:2<361::aid-jclp2270330207>3.0.co;2-h
50. **Freud S.** Beyond the pleasure principle. In: **Strachey J.** (Editor & Trans.). *The standard edition of the complete psychological works of Sigmund Freud: Vol. XVIII. (1920–1922).* Hogarth Press; 1955. pp. 3–64.
51. **Bourdieu P.** *The Weight of the World : Social Suffering in Contemporary Society*. Stanford University Press; 1999.
52. **Aouragh M.** 'White privilege' and shortcuts to anti-racism. Race and Class. 2019;**61**(2):3–26.53. **Heinz A, Müller DJ, Krach S, Cabanis M, Kluge UP.** The uncanny return of the race concept. Frontiers in Human Neuroscience. 2014;**8**:836. https://doi.org/10.3389/fnhum.2014.00836
54. **Kendi IX.** *How to be an antiracist*. New York, One World; 2019.
55. **Prudhomme C.** The problem of suicide in the American negro. Psychoanalytic Review. 1938;**25**:187–204; 372–91.
56. **Thomas AL, Brausch AM.** Family and peer support moderates the relationship between distress tolerance and suicide risk in black college students. Journal of American College Health. 2020;**70**(4):1138–45. https://doi.org/10.1080/07448481.2020.1786096
57. **Jason L, Glenwick D.** *Handbook of Methodological Approaches to Community-Based Research: Qualitative, Quantitative, and Mixed Methods*. New York: University Press; 2016.

58. **Opara I, Assan MA, Pierre K,** et al. Suicide among black children: an integrated model of the interpersonal–psychological theory of suicide and intersectionality theory for researchers and clinicians. Journal of Black Studies. 2020;**51**(6):611–31. https://doi.org/10.1177/0021934720935641
59. **Joe S, Scott ML, Banks A.** What works for adolescent Black males at risk of suicide: a review. Research on Social Work Practice. 2018;**28**(3):340–5. https://doi.org/10.1177/1049731517702745
60. **Joe S.** Explaining changes in the patterns of Black suicide in the United States from 1981 to 2002: an age, cohort, and period analysis. Journal of Black Psychology. 2006;**32**(3):262–84.
61. **Banaji MR, Fiske ST, Massey DS.** Systemic racism: individuals and interactions, institutions and society. Cognitive Research. 2021;**6**:82.
62. **Spates K.** 'We have closed our eyes and sealed our lips': black women's accounts of discussing suicide within the black community. Sociological Focus. 2019;**52**(1):34–49. https://doi.org/10.1080/00380237.2018.1484229
63. **Journal of Black Psychology**. (2020). Special issue call for papers: black children and suicide. Journal of Black Psychology, **46**(1):90–1. https://doi.org/10.1177/0095798420901364
64. **Pitman AL, Osborn DP, Rantell K, King MB.** Bereavement by suicide as a risk factor for suicide attempt: a cross-sectional national UK-wide study of 3432 young bereaved adults. BMJ Open. 2016;**6**(1):e009948. https://doi.org/10.1136/bmjopen-2015-009948
65. **Jordan JR.** Lessons learned: forty years of clinical work with suicide loss survivors. Frontiers in Psychology. 2020;**11**:766. https://doi.org/10.3389/fpsyg.2020.00766
66. **Spates K, Slatton BC.** I've got my family and my faith: black women and the suicide paradox. Socius: Sociological Research for a Dynamic World. 2017;**3**:237802311774390. https://doi.org/10.1177/2378023117743908
67. **Sundararajan L, Misra G, Marsella AJ.** Indigenous approaches to assessment, diagnosis, and treatment of mental disorders. In: **Paniagua FA, Yamada A-M,** editors. *Handbook of multicultural mental health: Assessment and treatment of diverse populations* (2nd edition). Elsevier Academic Press; 2013. pp. 69–87. https://doi.org/10.1016/B978-0-12-394420-7.00004-7
68. **Sundararajan L, Yeh KH.** Strong ties and weak ties rationality: theory and scale development. Integrative Psychological and Behavioral Science. 2022 Jun;56(2):405–19. doi:10.1007/s12124-021-09645-5. Epub 2021 Sep 3. PMID: 34478020; PMCID: PMC8413355.
69. **Buchanan MT, Hyde B.** Learning beyond the surface: engaging the cognitive, affective and spiritual dimensions within the curriculum. International Journal of Children's Spirituality. 2008;**13**(4):309–20.
70. **Villani D, Sorgente A, Iannello P, Antonietti A.** The role of spirituality and religiosity in subjective well-being of individuals with different religious status. Frontiers in Psychology. 2019;**10**:1525.
71. **Owusu-Kwarteng L.** Telling a different story: the effect of parenting on the academic and professional achievement of 24 British–Ghanaian high flyers. Power and Education. 2015;7(3):289–305. https://doi.org/10.1177/1757743815600292

72. **Cho PLY, Ong ASE, Cheung HS.** Where authoritarianism is not always bad: parenting styles and romantic relationship quality among emerging adults in Singapore. Current Psychology. 2020;**41**(7):4657–66. https://doi.org/10.1007/s12144-020-00978-9
73. **Akosah-Twumasi P, Alele F, Emeto TI, Lindsay D, Tsey K, Malau-Aduli BS.** 'Preparing them for the road': African migrant parents' perceptions of their role in their children's career decision-making. Education Sciences. 2020;**10**(5). https://doi.org/10.3390/educsci10050138
74. **Heim E, Karatzias T, Maercker A.** Cultural concepts of distress and complex PTSD: future directions for research and treatment. Clinical Psychology Review. 2022;**93**:102143. https://doi.org/10.1016/j.cpr.2022.102143
75. **Matheson K, Foster MD, Bombay A, McQuaid RJ, Anisman H.** Traumatic experiences, perceived discrimination, and psychological distress among members of various socially marginalized groups. Frontiers in Psychology. 2019;**10**:416.
76. **Polanco-Roman L, Chantel TE, Emily NS, Erik MB, Aline ML, Mythili I, Chardée AG.** Racism-related experiences and traumatic stress symptoms in ethnoracially minoritized youth: a systematic review and meta-analysis. Journal of Clinical Child & Adolescent Psychology. 2024. doi:10.1080/15374416.2023.2292042
77. **Geronimus AT.** The weathering hypothesis and the health of African-American women and infants: evidence and speculations. Ethnicity & Disease. 1992;**2**(3):207–21.
78. **Foster H, Hagan J, Brooks-Gunn J.** Growing up fast: stress exposure and subjective "Weathering" in emerging adulthood. Journal of Health and Social Behavior. 2008;**49**(2):162–77. http://www.jstor.org/stable/27638745
79. **Joiner T, Pettit JW, Walker RL, Voelz ZR, Cruz J, Rudd MD**, et al. Perceived burdensomeness and suicidality: two studies on the suicide notes of those attempting and those completing suicide. Journal of Social & Clinical Psychology. 2002;**21**:531–45.
80. **Joiner TE.** *Why people die by suicide*. Cambridge, MA: Harvard University Press; 2005.
81. **Lorde A.** *Sister outsider: essays and speeches.* Trumansburg, NY: Crossing Press; 1984.
82. **McEwen BS, Stellar E.** Stress and the individual. Mechanisms leading to disease. Archives of Internal Medicine. 1993;**153**(18):2093–2101.
83. **Decuir-Gunby JT, Williams MR.** The impact of race and racism on students' emotions: a critical race analysis. In: **Paul A. Schutz, Reinhard Pekrun**, editors. *Emotion in Education*. London: Elsevier; 2007. pp. 205–19. https://doi.org/10.1016/B978-012372545-5/50013-7
84. **Hittner EF, Adam EK.** Emotional pathways to the biological embodiment of racial discrimination experiences. Psychosomatic Medicine. 2020;**82**(4):420–31.
85. **Kalathil J.** *Recovery and resilience: African, African Caribbean and South Asian women's stories of recovering from mental distress.* Mental Health Foundation and Survivor Research; 2011.
86. **Brondolo E, Brady N, Thompson S, Tobin JN, Cassells A, Sweeney M, McFarlane D, Contrada RJ.** Perceived racism and negative affect: analyses of trait and state measures of affect in a community sample. Journal of Social and Clinical Psychology. 2008;**27**(2):150–73. https://doi.org/10.1521/jscp.2008.27.2.150
87. **Gruenewald TL, Kemeny ME, Aziz N, Fahey JL.** Acute threat to the social self: shame, social self-esteem, and cortisol activity. Psychosomatic Medicine. 2004;**66**(6):915–24. doi:10.1097/01.psy.0000143639.61693.ef

88. **Michl P, Meindl T, Meister** F, et al. Neurobiological underpinnings of shame and guilt: a pilot fMRI study. Social Cognitive and Affective Neuroscience. 2014;**9**(2):150–7.
89. **Wagner U, N'Diaye K, Ethofer T, Vuilleumier P.** Guilt-specific processing in the prefrontal cortex. Cerebral Cortex. 2011;**21**(11):2461–70. https://doi.org/10.1093/cercor/bhr016
90. **Berardelli I, Serafini G, Cortese N, Fiaschè F, O'Connor RC, Pompili M.** The Involvement of Hypothalamus-Pituitary-Adrenal (HPA) axis in suicide risk. Brain Sciences. 2020 Sep 21;**10**(9):653. doi:10.3390/brainsci10090653
91. **Chiu DT, Parker JE, Wiley CR, Epel ES, Laraia BA, Leung CW, Tomiyama AJ.** Food insecurity, poor diet, and metabolic measures: the roles of stress and cortisol. Appetite. 2024;107294. Advance online publication. https://doi.org/10.1016/j.appet.2024.107294
92. **McClain AC, Xiao RS, Gao X, Tucker KL, Falcon LM, Mattei J.** Food insecurity and odds of high allostatic load in puerto rican adults: the role of participation in the supplemental nutrition assistance program during 5 years of follow-up. Psychosomatic Medicine. 2018 Oct;**80**(8):733–41. doi:10.1097/PSY.0000000000000628
93. **Giurgescu C, Misra DP, Slaughter-Acey JC, Gillespie SL, Nowak AL, Dove-Medows E, Engeland CG, Zenk SN, Lydic TA, Sealy-Jefferson S, Ford J, Drury S, Stemmer P. Neighborhoods**, racism, stress, and preterm birth among African American women: a review. Western Journal of Nursing Research. 2022;**44**(1):101–10. doi:10.1177/01939459211041165
94. **Jensen SKG, Berens AE, Nelson CA**, 3rd. Effects of poverty on interacting biological systems underlying child development. The Lancet. Child & Adolescent Health. 2017;**1**(3):225–39. https://doi.org/10.1016/S2352-4642(17)30024-X
95. **Odoms-Young A, Bruce MA.** Examining the impact of structural racism on food insecurity: implications for addressing racial/ethnic disparities. Family and Community Health. 2018;**41**(Suppl 2 FOOD INSECURITY AND OBESITY):S3–6.
96. **Qin DD, Rizak J, Feng XL, Yang SC, Lü LB, Pan L, Yin Y, Hu XT.** Prolonged secretion of cortisol as a possible mechanism underlying stress and depressive behaviour. Scientific Reports. 2016;**6**:30187. https://doi.org/10.1038/srep30187
97. **Peters AT, Van Meter A, Pruitt PJ**, et al. Acute cortisol reactivity attenuates engagement of fronto-parietal and striatal regions during emotion processing in negative mood disorders. Psychoneuroendocrinology. 2016;**73**:67–78. https://doi.org/10.1016/j.psyneuen.2016.07.215
98. **American Association of Suicidology** (2020a). American Association of Suicidology partners with Congresswoman Bonnie Watson Coleman to address suicide in black communities. Available from: https://suicidology.org/2021/01/27/missing-matters-release/
99. **American Association of Suicidology** (2020b). Statement on equity and anti-racism. Available from: https://suicidology.org/about-aas/equity-anti-racism/
100. **Boyd RC.** 2.4 Report from the Congressional Black Caucus Taskforce for Black Youth Suicide and Mental Health. Journal of the American Academy of Child and Adolescent Psychiatry. 2020;**59**(10):S269. https://doi.org/10.1016/j.jaac.2020.07.557
101. **Keller S, McNeill V, Honea J, Paulson Miller L.** A look at culture and stigma of suicide: textual analysis of community theatre performances. International Journal of Environmental Research and Public Health. 2019;**16**(3):352.

102. **Lopreato J, Saltzman Chafetz J.** Social integration, regulation of needs, and suicide: an emendation of Durkheim's theory. Revue Européenne des Sciences Sociales. 1979;**17**(47):115–33.
103. **Burr JA, Hartman JT, Matteson DW.** Black suicide in US metropolitan areas: an examination of the racial inequality and social integration–regulation hypotheses. Social Forces. 1999;77(3):1049–80.
104. **Van Orden KA, Witte TK, Cukrowicz KC, Braithwaite SR, Selby EA, Joiner TE,** Jr. The interpersonal theory of suicide. Psychological Review. 2010;**117**(2):575–600. https://doi.org/10.1037/a0018697
105. **Shneidman ES.** Suicide, sleep, and death: some possible interrelations among cessation, interruption, and continuous phenomena. Journal of Consulting Psychology. 1964;**28**(2):95–106. https://doi.org/10.1037/h0048206
106. **Stengel E.** *Suicide and attempted suicide*. Penguin Books; 1964.
107. **Hjelmeland H, Loa Knizek B.** The emperor's new clothes? A critical look at the interpersonal theory of suicide. Death Studies. 2020;**44**(3):168–78. https://doi.org/10.1080/07481187.2018.1527796
108. **Bourdieu P.** *Distinction: A Social Critique of the Judgement of Taste*. London: Routledge; 1984.
109. **Yuval-Davis N.** *The Politics of Belonging: Intersectional Contestations*. London, Sage Books; 2012.
110. **Baumeister RF, Leary MR.** The need to belong: desire for interpersonal attachments as a fundamental human motivation. Psychological Bulletin. 1995;117(3):497–529. https://doi.org/10.1037/0033-2909.117.3.497
111. **Baumeister RF.** Need-to-belong theory. In: **Van Lange PAM, Kruglanski AW, Higgins ET**, editors. *Handbook of theories of social psychology*. Sage Publications Ltd; 2012. pp. 121–40. https://doi.org/10.4135/9781446249222.n32
112. **Williams KD.** Ostracism: a temporal need-threat model. In **Zanna MP**, editor. *Advances in experimental social psychology*. Elsevier Academic Press; 2009. **Vol. 41**, pp. 275–314. https://doi.org/10.1016/S0065-2601(08)00406-1
113. **Wortman CB, Brehm JW.** Responses to uncontrollable outcomes: an integration of reactance theory and the learned helplessness model. In **Berkowitz L**, editor. *Advances in experimental social psychology*. New York: Academic Press; 1975. Vol. 8, pp. 277–336. http://dx.doi.org/10.1016/s0065-2601(08)60253-1
114. **Leary MR.** Making sense of self-esteem. Current Directions in Psychological Science. 1999;**8**(1):32–5. https://doi.org/10.1111/1467-8721.00008
115. **Baumeister RF, Leary MR.** The need to belong: desire for interpersonal attachments as a fundamental human motivation. In **Higgins ET, Kruglanski AW**, editors. *Motivational science: Social and personality perspectives*. Psychology Press; 2000. pp. 24–49.
116. **Bandura A.** *Self-efficacy: The exercise of control*. W H Freeman/Times Books/Henry Holt & Co; 1997.
117. **Solomon S, Greenberg J, Pyszczynski T.** A terror management theory of social behavior: the psychological functions of self-esteem and cultural worldviews. In *Advances in experimental social psychology*. Academic Press; 1991. **Vol. 24**, pp. 93–159. doi:10.1016/S0065-2601(08)60328-7.

118. **Kawachi I, Berkman L.** Social ties and mental health. Journal of Urban Health: Bulletin of the New York Academy of Medicine. 2001;**78**:458–67. 10.1093/jurban/78.3.458.
119. **Huppert FA.** Psychological well-being: evidence regarding its causes and consequences. Applied Psychology: Health and Well-Being. 2009;**1**(2):137–64. https://doi.org/10.1111/j.1758-0854.2009.01008.x
120. **Diener E.** Subjective well-being. Psychological Bulletin. 1984;**95**(3):542–75. https://doi.org/10.1037/0033-2909.95.3.542
121. **Andrews FM, Withey SB.** *Social indicators of well-being*. New York: Plenum Press; 1976. https://doi.org/10.1007/978-1-4684-2253-5
122. **Diener E, Lucas RE, Oishi S.** Subjective well-being: the science of happiness and life satisfaction. In **Snyder CR, Lopez SJ**, editors. *Handbook of positive psychology*. Oxford University Press; 2002. pp. 463–73.
123. **Morales S, Barros J.** Mental pain surrounding suicidal behaviour: a review of what has been described and clinical recommendations for help. Frontiers in Psychiatry. 2022;**12**:750651.
124. **Crenshaw K.** Mapping the margins: intersectionality, identity politics, and violence against women of color. Stanford Law Review. 1991;**43**(6):1241–99. https://doi.org/10.2307/1229039
125. **Yuval-Davis N.** Intersectionality and feminist politics. European Journal of Women's Studies. 2006;**13**(3):193–209. https://doi.org/10.1177/1350506806065752
126. **Chu JP, Goldblum P, Floyd R, Bongar B.** The cultural theory and model of suicide. Applied and Preventive Psychology. 2010;**14**:25–40. https://doi.org/10.1016/j.appsy.2011.11.001
127. **Abrutyn S, Mueller AS.** Toward a cultural-structural theory of suicide: examining excessive regulation and its discontents. Sociological Theory. 2018;**36**(1):48–66. https://doi.org/10.1177/0735275118759150
128. **Bor J, Venkataramani AS, Williams DR, Tsai AC.** Police killings and their spillover effects on the mental health of black Americans: a population-based, quasi-experimental study. The Lancet. 2018;**392**(10144):302–10. https://doi.org/10.1016/S0140-6736(18)31130-9
129. **Priest N, Paradies Y, Trenerry B, Truong M, Karlsen S, Kelly Y.** A systematic review of studies examining the relationship between reported racism and health and wellbeing for children and young people. Social Science and Medicine. 2013;**95**:115–27.
130. **Paradies Y.** A systematic review of empirical research on self-reported racism and health. International Journal of Epidemiology. 2006;**35**(4):888–901. https://doi.org/10.1093/ije/dyl056
131. **Shain BN.** Increases in rates of suicide and suicide attempts among Black adolescents. Pediatrics. 2019;**144**(5):e20191912. https://doi.org/10.1542/peds.2019-1912
132. **Hope EC, Cryer-Coupet QR, Stokes MN.** Race-related stress, racial identity, and activism among young Black men: A person-centered approach. Developmental Psychology. 2020;**56**(8):1484–95. https://doi.org/10.1037/dev0000836
133. **Hope EC, Gugwor R, Riddick KN, Pender KN.** Engaged against the machine: institutional and cultural racial discrimination and racial identity as predictors

of activism orientation among black youth. American Journal of Community Psychology. 2019;63(1-2):61–72. https://doi.org/10.1002/ajcp.12303

134. **Bourdieu P.** The forms of capital. In: **Richardson JG**, editor. *Handbook of Theory and Research for the Sociology of Education*. New York, NY: Greenwood Press; 1986. pp. 241–58.
135. **Lazarus RS, Folkman S.** *Stress, appraisal, and coping*. New York: Springer; 1984.
136. **Etowa JB, Beagan BL, Eghan F, Bernard WT.** 'You feel you have to be made of steel': the strong Black woman, health, and well-being in Nova Scotia. Health Care for Women International. 2017;**38**(4):379–93. https://doi.org/10.1080/07399332.2017.1290099
137. **Jahoda M.** *Current concepts of positive mental health*. New York: Basic Books; 1958.
138. **Antonovsky A.** *Unraveling the mystery of health. How people manage stress and stay well*. San Francisco: Jossey-Bass; 1987.
139. **Deci EL, Ryan RM.** A motivational approach to self: Integration in personality. In: **Dienstbier RA**, editor. *Nebraska Symposium on Motivation, 1990: Perspectives on motivation*. University of Nebraska Press; 1991. pp. 237–88.
140. **Seligman MEP.** *Authentic happiness*. New York, NY: Free Press; 2002.
141. **Mbembe A.** *Necropolitics*. United Kingdom: Duke University Press; 2019. https://doi.org/10.1215/9781478007227
142. **Morrison LL, Downey DL.** Racial differences in self-disclosure of suicidal ideation and reasons for living: implications for training. Cultural Diversity and Ethnic Minority Psychology. 2000;**6**:374–86.
143. **Marion MS, Range LM.** African American college women's suicide buffers. Suicide and Life-Threatening Behavior. 2003;**33**:33–43.
144. **Lizardi D, Currier D, Galfalvy H, Sher L, Burk A, Mann J.** Perceived reasons for living at index hospitalization and future suicide attempt. Journal of Nervous and Mental Disease. 2007;**195**:451–5.
145. **Ellis J, Lamis D.** Adaptive characteristics and suicidal behavior: a gender comparison of young adults. Death Studies. 2007;**31**:845–54.
146. **Wang M-C, Lightsey OR Jr, Tran KK, Bonaparte TS.** Examining suicide protective factors among black college students. Death Studies. 2013;**37**(3):228–47.
147. **Rockett IRH, Samora JB, Coben JH.** The black–white suicide paradox: possible effects of misclassification. Social Science and Medicine. 2006;**63**(8):2165–75.
148. **Molock SD, Matlin S, Barksdale C, Puri R, Lyles J.** Developing suicide prevention programs for African American youth in African American churches. Suicide and Life-Threatening Behaviour. 2008;**38**(3):323–33.

Chapter 14

Suicide in Nepal

Thomas Wenzel and Ajay Risal

Introduction

Nepal is one of the least economically developed countries in the world, with 25.4% of its population 'below the poverty line' in 2010, based on international reference standards, and is only slowly improving.[i] With a developing democratic system, the country, that was 'closed off' until about 1951, has been experiencing further challenges over time,[1] including earthquakes, intake of traumatized refugees from Tibet and Bhutan,[2] a civil war with many civilian victims and child soldiers,[3] Maoist splinter group insurgency and violence,[4] and use of torture.[5] Other problems include trafficking, traditional gender discrimination,[6] and a high rate of further gender-specific health care and safety problems associated with discrimination practices such as 'Chaupadhi' isolation during menstruation in women.[7,8,9,10] Sexual[11] and domestic violence are also common problems that affect women in particular.[6,11,12,13,14,15,16] Only 16.8% of the population were living in urban areas in 2010, with a low three hospital beds per 100,000 population (WHO Global Health Observatory, 2019). The country has very high, if not probably one of the highest, suicide rates in the world.[1,17] At least according to some researchers, suicide is the most frequent cause of death among women,[18,19] although one small study in rural Nepal reported chronic disease as a more common cause of death.[20] Official World Health Organization (WHO) databases reported the suicide index at 9.6–11.4 for men and 8 for women (2016),[ii] as well as an age-standardized suicide rate in Nepal of 24.9 per 100 000 population in 2012, ranking the country seventh in the world.[iii] Discrepancies in reported rates will be discussed later in this chapter

[i] Available from: https://www.thepovertyline.net/nepal

[ii] World Health Organization, Global Health Observatory data repository. Available from: https://www.who.int (accessed 8 November 2019).

[iii] World Health Organization, Global Health Observatory data repository. Suicide rates: data by country. Available from: http://apps.who.int/gho/data/node.main.MHSUICIDE?lang=en (accessed 3 January 2017).

and might be related to the predominant involvement of the police institution in data collection, compared to data collection by health care institutions, as demonstrated by Hagaman et al.[21] It should be noted in this context that Asia in general has been reported to have high suicide rates and the region needs better research due to inconsistent data gathering methodology and partly contradictory or inconclusive data, as observed in a recent review by Jordans et al.[22]

Background: geography, populations, and public mental health in Nepal

Nepal, landlocked between China and India, is highly heterogeneous, both geographically with environments ranging from subtropical terrains to high mountain ranges of the Himalayas, and ethnically with more than 45 main ethnic groups[23], such as the Magar and the Newar, as well as further subgroups, following Hinduism, Buddhism, and also a large range of local ethnic religions and traditions, including shamanism.[24,25] Nepali is the common language, facilitating communication among those who speak the many local languages across the different ethnic groups. The situation is further complicated by the caste system that has been formally abolished, but still remains as a further identifier and distinguishing factor in the social situation and identity of the individual.

The following summary of current knowledge on suicide and suicide-related factors in Nepal should be seen under the precondition that some conclusions or data might not reflect this diversity. Conclusions should not be generalized to all such groups, present in the country and to the different geographical environments.[26]

The health care system has very limited capacity, especially with regard to free-of-charge mental health care,[27,28,29,30] partly due to the geographical location of large parts of the population who live in mountain villages, often days by foot march from major roads or hospitals. Services are provided, if at all, mainly in primary health care centres by nurses or in villages by traditional healers[30] when urban health centres are not accessible. Also, the country has only a very small number of trained psychiatrists, nearly no psychotherapists, no system of advanced psychotherapy training, and a very small number of psychiatric beds. Consequently, it has been proposed that mental health should be closely integrated in primary health care systems.[30]

Suicide: statistics and legal framework

Most researchers exploring suicide in Nepal agree that official statistics and reporting might be unreliable indicators, at least as in terms of total suicide numbers,[1,19,31,32] probably at least partly due to stigma attached to mental health problems in general and to suicidal behaviour in particular.[19] Suicide in Nepal is no longer illegal, as is the case also in neighbouring Bhutan. However, this might lead to problems for the family as survivors in cases of completed suicide, especially if the family are suspected of providing any assistance,[iv] a fact which also could contribute to distorting official examination results and statistics.

Sharma et al.[33] conducted a selective, but systematic, study in the capital of Kathmandu from mid July 2000 to mid July 2004, based on physical autopsy reports of all violent and traumatic death autopsies. Of a total of 4383 autopsies that were conducted by the Department of Forensic Medicine in Kathmandu, there were 1072 (25% of the sample) cases of suicide, 380 (9%) cases of homicide, and 1399 (32%) accident-related deaths. The authors also reported 598 (14%) deaths as a result of natural diseases, and 923 (21%) cases of undetermined causes of death. The number of males was almost twice that of females (sex ratio 2.2:1). Persons aged 15–44 years comprised about two-thirds of the total reported fatalities (65.4%). Suicides were mostly reported being the result of hanging, homicides mostly as being caused by firearms and explosives, and accidents mostly as results of road traffic injuries. The authors recommended increased forensic examination of unclear cases to obtain more reliable data on the cause of death and especially on suicide.

Still, in spite of the above reservations in regard to reliability of data, according to most, Nepal ranks high in the global comparison, with a rate of probably 25 suicides per 100,000 inhabitants.[v] Further, there is a gender imbalance, with suicide being the leading cause of death in women, at least according to some statistics.[1,18,vi] The high rate of suicides among women was confirmed by the official 'National Health Sector Support Programme' report, an initiative co-funded by the United Nations Population Fund (UNFPA),[19] based on Maternal Morbidity and Mortality (MMM)/Maternal Health and Morbidity (MHM) studies (1998, 2008/9), that showed rising numbers of deaths attributable to suicide from 10% to 16%. This report also described an age-specific aspect, with higher risk in women aged 15–34 years, and again above the age of 45 years. Recently, some authors have also drawn attention to the increasing problem of intentional self-harm[34] (independent of suicide attempts with

[iv] Satyal U (2019). Establishment of abetment to suicide no easy task. Available from: https://thehimalayantimes.com/kathmandu/establishment-of-abetment-to-suicide-no-easy-task/

[v] See https://ijmhs.biomedcentral.com/articles/10.1186/s13033-016-0073-7

[vi] World Health Organization. Global Health Observatory database. Available from: https://www.who.int

the intention to die), that is often included in published data on suicide. The methodology used in such cases does not always permit a clear distinction between deliberate self-harm without suicidal intent and actual suicide attempts as defined in the literature,[35] again contributing to the lack of concise data on actual suicide attempts and suicide. Jordan et al. published one of the few international comparative community studies on the subject. The authors noted that the 12-month prevalence of suicidal ideation and suicide plans and attempts, as established from 'community samples ($n = 6689$)' and 'primary care attendees ($n = 6470$)' from districts in Ethiopia, Uganda, South Africa, India, and Nepal by using the Composite International Diagnostic Interview suicidality module were highest in South Africa, and also confirmed high rates in Nepal. The authors also identified consistent risk factors (female, younger age, presence of mental disorders, and lower educational and socioeconomic status) across countries.

Overall, the situation still must be seen as critical and has led to the notion of a 'suicide crisis in Nepal'. This has encouraged a small number of epidemiological and qualitative research studies,[11,21,36] as well as some psychological autopsy studies.[17,36] In a recent systematic review and meta-analysis, Thapaliya et al.[32] concluded that studies on suicide in Nepal so far have been mainly hospital-based and either cross-sectional or retrospective, but also indicated that young persons, women, migrants, and disaster-affected populations, as well as those suffering from mental disorders, especially depression, are at highest risk. Triggers for self-harm and suicidal behaviour include, according to this review, interpersonal and socio-economic issues and marital conflicts.

Two recent major reviews have yielded more information, at least on the prevalence of suicidal ideation.[37,38] Katuwal et al.[37] used, among other instruments, the Beck Scale for Suicide Ideation on 160 psychiatric outpatients in Kathmandu, with 16.9% identified as high risk and 83.1% as low risk. The authors further assessed for protective cognitions, revealing that 91.9% of participants stated strong reasons, including religion or family obligations, as deterrent against suicide. These results underline the importance of careful analysis of actual suicide risk, in addition to suicidal ideation, and of cognitive strategies protecting against suicide.

Dhimal et al.[38] conducted a 'nationwide descriptive cross-sectional community-based prevalence study' of 9200 adults and 5888 adolescents from seven provinces of Nepal by using the Mini International Neuropsychiatric Interview (MINI). They reported suicidality among 7.2% of adults and 4.1% of adolescent participants. The prevalence of suicidal thoughts was 6.5% among adult participants, with a prevalence of lifetime suicidal attempts of 1.1%.[38]

Hospital-based studies

For a long time, studies on suicide in Nepal have predominantly focused on (self-) poisoning cases admitted to hospitals, in particular organophosphorus (OP) poisoning.[39,40,41,42,43,44,45,46,47,48] Most studies make the distinction between intentional (self-) poisoning (suicide attempts) and accidental poisoning. Unfortunately, the methodology used to differentiate between the two forms of poisoning is, in most cases, not clear, and in the majority of studies, no systematic mental health assessment or research protocol to elicit triggering factors or possible background history is included or reported, although some authors include speculations or preliminary data on these aspects in their conclusions. Still, due to a lack of studies focusing on these aspects, we will summarize in the following section those studies on poisoning/self-poisoning published so far.

OP pesticides inhibit the cholinesterase enzyme, leading to overstimulation of cholinergic receptors, which requires immediate treatment by atropine and other measures. Outcome and lethality depend on availability and speed of treatment offered, and mortality/lethality in Nepal are much higher than, for example, in the United States.[49] OP pesticides are cheap and easily available, and are therefore very commonly found, especially among farming communities. They have been described as a key health risk in Asia.[50] Aluminium phosphide is also used as a suicide agent and has a nearly 100% fatality rate.[51] The WHO has started a special programme, including published tools, such as a handbook on prevention of self-poisoning with pesticides,[vii] as the problem is significant not only in Nepal, but also across the world.

Karki et al. conducted two studies analysing records from (general) clinical populations.[43,48] A major retrospective study by Agrawaal and Karki[43] included 2621 patients admitted for poisoning in a tertiary care hospital in Eastern Nepal, the majority of whom ($n = 1661$) had OP poisoning, with a mean stay of 6.7 days. The authors reported that 6.6% of patients died in the first 24 hours, and further noted that most cases 'were under the influence of alcohol'. The authors recommended restrictions on free sale of pesticides. In a retrospective study by Basnet et al.,[52] data collected from hospital records of a total of 134 cases of poisoning from January 2018 to December 2020 were analysed. Of these patients, 71 had consumed OP compounds; the majority of cases were female (59.2%, with a higher percentage of those who used pesticides), and most cases were recorded as suicidal (95.8% in OP groups, 90.5% in non-OP groups), with reasons

[vii] World Health Organization (2019). Preventing suicide, Geneva 2019, Available from: https://www.who.int/publications/i/item/9789241516389

being mostly 'family disputes'. The authors recommended pesticide control and better psychosocial support, especially in family conflicts.[52]

In a retrospective study conducted by Agrawaal and Karki on a large sample of 2621 patients admitted to B.P. Koirala Institute of Health Sciences in Dharan, Nepal from January 2005 to December 2010 for poisoning, 1661 cases were found to be caused by pesticides, usually as a result of ingestion. Further, 6.6% of patients died within 24 hours of admission and 3.54% 48 hours after admission, whereas 0.5% of patients received care in the intensive care unit (ICU). Alcohol was identified as a causative factor in 'most cases'.[43] Referral was usually from primary health care centres, and first-line treatment with atropine was found to be insufficient. Based on psychiatric interviews, but not on systematic evaluation of the cases, the authors concluded that 'impulsive acts' and 'increased indebtedness in the society' were the main reasons. No psychiatric data were reported in the study. The authors recommended better legislation on the sale of toxic agents, as well as better implementation of ICU protocols and an increase in the number of ICU beds.

Self-poisoning has also received special attention in case reports.[53,54] In a 1-year study of poisoning cases in Patan hospital,[46] the authors reported medical drugs as agents used in suicide attempts, in addition to OP compounds (42%), with a peak in summer months and an overall mortality rate of 5%. Aspiration pneumonia and respiratory failure were found to be the most common complications. The authors of this study also reported 75% of the poisoning cases were intentional. Another retrospective hospital record-based study was conducted by Bhattarai et al.[55] including 47 patients admitted to Kathmandu Medical College Teaching Hospital for poisoning between August 2003 and July 2005. Results showed a near-equal distribution, with a peak at age of 33 years (70.2%), and 87.2% of the cases were related to suicide attempts, usually with Metacid, and again most commonly occurred 'after family conflicts'.

Marahatta et al., in a study published in 2009, evaluated 54 poisoning cases in Kathmandu University Teaching Hospital in Dhulikhel over one year.[56] The authors reported a female-to-male ratio of 1.34:1, with 79% of the cases due to self-poisoning. In addition, 40.38% of the cases were farmers and 66.66% had the OP agent stored in their home. The fatality rate was reported to be 5.5%.

Chakrabarti et al., in a review of all poisoning cases admitted to the Nepal Medical College Teaching Hospital Department of Psychiatry via the emergency department from January 2000 to December 2003, found that of the 118 cases (39 male, 58 female), most were related to suicide attempts, usually with use of OP compounds.[57] Most of the cases also suffered from psychiatric disorders (mainly depression and schizophrenia), which might be due to sample selection and the setting of a psychiatric department, and therefore, the findings should not be generalized to the general population.

Shakya et al.[58] analysed data on a similar group of patients admitted to one of the few psychiatric emergency wards in Nepal. The authors found that about 20% of patients had attempted suicide by using different means, with nut poisoning as the most common method.

Pradhan and Adhikary[59] reported on 43 cases of suicide attempts admitted to Kathmandu Medical College Hospital. The severity of suicidal intention was assessed by using the Suicide Intent Scale (SIS). The majority of cases were female ($n = 30$, 69.8%), and the most common mode of suicide was poisoning ($n = 36$, 83.7%). A mean SIS score of 13.88 was obtained, with 58.3% ($n = 21$) as moderate suicide intent, 33.3% ($n = 12$) as mild suicide intent, and 8.3% ($n = 3$) as severe suicide intent ($p < 0.004$). Pesticide (OP) ingestion was the most common method of suicide ($n = 16$, 44.4%), followed by pharmacological drugs ($n = 12$, 33.3%) ($p < 0.267$). Depressive disorders ($n = 27$, 62.9%) were the most common psychiatric diagnosis, which was associated with mainly moderate suicide intent ($n = 19$, 70.4%).

Agrawaal and Karki[43] analysed 1661 inpatient cases of pesticide poisoning that were documented as being mostly suicidal, with the majority of cases having a history of alcohol use at the time of suicide attempt. The authors also reported a high rate of lethal outcomes: 6.6% of patients died within 24 hours of admission, and 3.54% after 48 hours of admission, in spite of the availability of an ICU in the hospital. Patients received psychiatric evaluation and care before discharge, but for which no further details were given by the authors.

Ghimire et al.[60] analysed records of 200 cases of deliberate self-harm (mostly with organophosphates/-chlorides) in a tertiary referral centre in Eastern Nepal from April 2012 to July 2012, most of whom (77%) were below the age of 35 years, with a female-to-male ratio of 1.35:1. The majority of patients were married (73.5%), and 38% were housewives and 25.5% were students. A total of 72.5% of cases had consumed organophosphates/-chlorides. The most common documented reason for deliberate self-harm was interpersonal conflict (72%). Psychiatric disorders according to International Classification of Diseases, Tenth Revision (ICD-10) criteria, were found in 37% of cases, with adjustment disorder in 13.5% and mood disorder in 11% of cases.

Students were a further at-risk group explored by Adhikari et al. in 2017. The authors reported a relatively high rate of depression (29.2%) in a non-clinical sample of students from KIST Medical College, of whom 4.7% 'had seriously considered committing suicide while in medical school'.[61]

Gyenwali et al. reported on 439 acute pesticide poisoning cases (of which 89.5% were suicidal) over a 9-month period in 2015 in four major hospitals in Chitwan District.[42] Vulnerable groups included young adults (111.66 per 100,000 population), women (77.53 per 100,000 population), and individuals from Dalit ethnic groups (98.22 per 100,000 population). Substances used included organophosphates (37.3%) and pyrethroids (36.7%), and the fatality rate was 3.8%.

Qualitative and mixed-method studies and the role of gender as a risk factor

Only a few (semi-)qualitative or mixed-method studies on suicide in Nepal have been published in the international literature so far to explore background and motivations. Hagaman et al., in a recent mixed-method psychological autopsy study,[17] analysed 39 completed suicide cases in one urban and one rural region of Nepal that were randomly sampled from police cases. The authors focused on the quantitative aspects of their (relatively small) sample, and observed that 38.5% of cases met the criteria for depression and 'only 23.1% of the informants believed that the deceased had thoughts of self-harm or suicide before death'. They also observed that 'recent geographic migration, alcohol abuse, and family history of suicide' were warning signs observed in the group included in their study. In a separately published and (we assume) more detailed analysis of the same data, the authors reported further risk factors,[36] including lack of education (72% of cases), poverty (54%), violence (61.1%), migrant labour (33% of men), family disputes 'resulting in isolation or shame' (56.4%), family history of suicidal behaviour (62%), and gender differences. They observed female suicides to 'be attributed to hopeless situations, such as spousal abuse, with high degrees of social stigma'. They further observed male suicides to be most commonly associated with drinking and 'internalized stigma' such as inability to provide for their family. The study also explored justifications for suicide and found attributions to "fate" and personality characteristics such as "stubbornness" and "egoism"' (Note: possible religious aspects will be covered later in this chapter). It was also noted that only '1 out of 3 men and 1 out of 6 women had any communication to family members about suicidal ideation prior to completion'. The authors subsequently went on to conduct a study on everyday life of young mothers, promoting a new data-gathering approach,[62] which, in our opinion, could yield important information on background factors related to suicide, if applied in this area in future studies.

Communication problems and isolation, especially in women, are risk factors related to distress and potential suicidal ideation or behaviour described in a study of Bhutanese refugees living in Nepal. This stresses the importance of family support and care in prevention of suicide in this particular group.[2]

The importance of suicidal ideation and behaviour, especially in women, and possible risk factors in this context, as already noted in the introduction to this chapter, appears to be well established, but not sufficiently explored in the majority of hospital-based studies on self-poisoning. In contrast, studies in samples that are not based on hospital records, such as those by Hagaman et al. and Puri et al.,[14,17] yield more information on the association between gender and suicidal ideation and behaviour. Puri et al., in a qualitative study on gender aspects in 2011, observed suicidal ideation as a reaction among women exposed to sexual violence,[11] which indicates a possible reason for the high rates of suicide among women in Nepal mentioned earlier. Paudhel et al. reported on early learning and deeply ingrained gender bias reflected also in everyday communication and public discourse.[6]

Traditional culture, caste, and help-seeking are further gender-related factors that have also been explored by several authors.

Thapa and Carlough conducted a questionnaire-based psychological mixed-method autopsy study on relatives of 23 confirmed cases of suicide (average age of 33 years, with near-equal gender distribution). They reported Brahmin (the highest caste) to be the most common background with respect to caste (69%), and hanging to be the most common method of suicide (97%) in their sample,[26] with the most common precipitating cause being family disputes (41.5%). Symptoms of depression were observed in 50% of cases. Help-seeking was reported to be rare, according to relatives, and most commonly involved local (shamanistic) healers ('Dhami Jankri'). Consultation in government centres was only sought in 14% of cases. While the results of this study are interesting, they cannot be easily generalized to the whole country.

While qualitative and mixed-method studies published so far indicate the relevance of some possible factors, especially gender, in suicidal behaviour in Nepal, research has been very limited and, as noted earlier, might not give a reliable picture of the situation across all groups and regions. For example, in regard to the method used, self-poisoning has been the primary focus of attention in research on suicide in Nepal so far, which could inform the development of possible targeted interventions. Still, some authors believe that hanging is an equally, if not more, important method of suicide, which might be explained by use of different methodologies or inclusion of different study populations. Results therefore might be seen to yield a controversial picture, underlining the importance of either hanging or self-poisoning, although some authors have also reported on other highly lethal and easily available means of suicide. Many publications, such as the autopsy study by Sharma et al. cited earlier[33] and the study by Atreya et al.,[64] have claimed, in the absence of more general and reliable community-based statistics, that hanging, usually with use of an easily available rope or shawl,[63,64,65] might be the most common method of suicide in Nepal. Atreya and Kanchan examined the records of 10 cases of hanging (mean age 28.8 years) admitted to a tertiary care hospital over a 2-year period, and noted a low lethality rate as all patients survived their suicide attempts.[66] Other methods such as self-stabbing have also been reported, but, to our knowledge, in only one case report and appear to be rare.[67,68]

Intentional burns have been explored by Lama et al.[69] who analysed records of patients treated for burns in the Burns Unit at Bir Hospital in Kathmandu, Nepal during the period 2002–13. The authors reported that intentional burns affected mostly young married women and events were related to interpersonal conflict in about 60% of cases. The rate of suicide attempts with suicidal intention is not clear from the data.

Further, similar to other countries such as Mexico[70] or rural China, suicide by intoxication with use of toxic household substances, such as fertilizers in rural communities, as described earlier, are as demonstrated a characteristic form at least of attempted suicide (47) in women. Such suicide attempts are most frequently triggered by domestic disputes and probably often reflect a situation of dysfunctional communication. It could be argued that it is a cultural (gender-specific) DSM 5 idiom of distress, that is associated with a high risk of fatal outcomes due to the high lethality of substances used and delayed treatment. This could contribute to gender differences between attempted and completed suicide. Availability of highly lethal means has been observed in many studies as a main risk factor. This can therefore be targeted by preventive strategies such as establishing a legal ban on lethal fertilizers,[71] which has been proven to be a successful intervention in a number of countries, such as Bangladesh,[72,73,74] and has been proposed by the authors of several of the studies summarized above. However, the gender-specific aspects also indicate a need to improve the support and protection of women in addition to legal interventions.

Other aspects: mental health, culture, and religion

In the literature over the last decades, a wide range of risk factor, in addition to gender, have been reported to be associated with higher suicide risk and could potentially be explored in the context of Nepal. We want to focus on a few selected issues that might be especially relevant to the understanding of prevalence, possible backgrounds, and different forms of suicide such as 'impulsive' behaviour and the role of religion or of medical disorders, such as severe depression, that, in turn, might reflect different primary factors.

Limited resources and stigma associated with mental health problems and treatment, in combination with frequent depression and post-traumatic stress disorder (PTSD) spectrum disorders and high exposure to poverty and potentially traumatic life events,[4,75,76,77] such as trafficking, political and other types of violence, and earthquakes, as outlined above, are all factors associated with increased suicide risk.[78] They can be considered as potentially relevant, given the high suicide rates in the country. The fact that suicide has been suspected to be most common cause of death in women could be suspected, as noted before, to be, at least partly, due to high social stressor load, sexual and domestic violence, and discrimination in the countrythat is well documented.[11,36] However, given limited available data, no final conclusions can be drawn at present.

Religion and suicide: considerations for Nepal

In general, psychiatric disorders frequently associated with an increased suicide risk, including depression, alcohol abuse, schizophrenia, post-traumatic stress, and sequelae to brain trauma (mostly part of the WHO Mental Health Gap Action Programme),[79] are common problems in Nepal[80,81,82] and insufficiently covered by health care systems in Nepal.[83] A solution towards addressing suicide prevention therefore could also lie in developing measures to improve mental health[30] and reducing the stigma attached to mental health in general.

While suicidal ideation and suicide risk are higher in patients with certain mental disorders, Some forms, especially if permitted by religion (like 'Sati')[84,85,86] should be considered in this context as culturally, and not psychiatrically, related, as proposed, for example, by Bhugra and others,[84,85] and will be discussed later in this chapter.

Social integration

In one of the leading recent models on social factors and suicide risk, Stack and Cao proposed the lack of 'social integration' as a risk factor, especially in 'traditional' cultures.[87] To our knowledge, no studies to date have applied this specific model to Nepal. However, the complexities of the Nepalese society, gender based, and political and ethnic diversities and splits, as outlined in the introduction, could be seen as potentially relevant, according to Stack and Cao's model. A specific factor explored is family separation and women's isolation from their husband working abroad. Shakya conducted a descriptive hospital-based study by using convenience sampling that included 100 female psychiatric patients separated from their husband working abroad. The authors found prior suicide attempts in 10% of the cases.[88] In a recent study, persistent complex bereavement disorder was also observed in a sample of Nepali widows as a significant risk factor for suicidal ideation/suicidality.[89]

Further, Nepali lesbian, gay, bisexual, and transgender (LGBT) persons have been reported to have a higher risk of suicide, according to a study by Kohlbrenner et al., based on a non-clinical survey of 400 TGBT persons.[90] The authors found that 6.8% of the participants had experienced suicidal ideation, 12.0% had made a suicide plan, and 9.0% had attempted suicide.

Students have been reported by some authors to be an at-risk population with respect to suicide in Nepal (see also earlier discussion). A study by Adhikari et al. found that 4.7% of medical students at a university reported suicidal ideation.[61] Findings from the multi-country Global School-based Students Health Survey also confirmed high suicide risk (or suicidal ideation) among students in Nepal.[91]

Self-aspirational models have been shown in a first study by Rai et al.[92] to influence suicidal ideation among Nepalese youths and might be challenged by social fragmentation.

Shrestha et al. reported on the suicide challenge faced by prisons in Nepal in the context of health care provision in this setting.[93] Suicide prevention is a specific obligation as part of health care provision in prisons, as outlined in the United Nations 'Nelson Mandela Rules'.[viii]

Inter-caste relationships or marriages can also lead to social isolation and family conflicts, resulting in suicide. This was demonstrated in a case example of a suicide pact reported by Atreya et al.[94]

A post-Maoist conflict study by Bhardwaj et al.[3] on former child soldiers described interpersonal violence, especially in women, as a risk factor for suicidal ideation, and teacher support as a protective factor in this group. The authors drew attention to the general problems of child soldiers in Nepal who suffer from lack of social (re)integration.[95] The high rate of mental health problems indicates the need for special services that are not limited to suicide prevention at least in this group.[95,96] Kohrt et al.[76] also highlighted the long-term impact of the Maoist insurgency period on mental health when crimes were committed by both governmental forces and insurgents. Such violence has been demonstrated to increase the risk of suicidal ideation and feelings of hopelessness,[97] especially when exposed civilians in villages became trapped in a vicious circle of retaliations between opposing parties. Kohrt et al.[4] conducted a prospective study following a cohort of 298 non-clinical participants, and found an increase in the rate of depression among participants from 30.9% to 40.6%, as well as an increase in anxiety rate from 26.2% to 47.7%. The authors also found

[viii] Available from https://www.unodc.org/documents/justice-and-prison-reform/Nelson_Mandela_Rules-E-ebook.pdf

post-conflict PTSD in 14.1% of participants. This is one of the few prospective studies worldwide investigating the population impact of political violence. It is an important study confirming the importance of taking into account the mental health impact of severe stressors experienced by the Nepalese population, when assessing their health care needs and developing community-based approaches,[98] although the same authors found only limited improvement with use of education reintegration packages (ERPs) for child soldiers.[98] It should be noted that, as part of a therapeutic/transitional justice model, a peace and reconciliation process has begun in the country, including the establishment of a truth and reconciliation committee[99] where the former insurgent group is now part of the government, although the process itself is not without its challenges.[100]

The impact of earthquakes that can, according to some studies, contribute to an increased suicide risk,[101,102,103] should also be considered, as demonstrated by the recent history of Nepal.[104] Kane et al. conducted a population-based survey by using a stratified, multistage cluster sampling design that included 513 participants. The authors found not only increased rates of PTSD and depression in the study sample, but also suicidal ideation among 10.9% of participants.[104]

Religion

As religion plays an important role in daily life of Nepalese people, we will discuss this in more detail. As mentioned earlier, the official government report concluded that data in Nepal are still inconclusive in this regard (p. 4).[19] Religious views are frequently seen as a major factor influencing suicidal behaviour,[105,106,107] in either a positive or negative way, similar to the culture of socially acceptable, or even desired, practice of suicide in Japan[108] or the suicide of widows in neighbouring India (*sati* or *suttee*)[84,85] (the latter not a (recent) common practice in Nepal and mostly obsolete today in India).

In general, global discussion of religion-related factors has led to different models that reflect the complexity of the issue. Colloci et al.[109] have proposed, in a comprehensive issue on the subject, that there are three models present in the discussion on suicide and religion: the 'integration theory' (following Durkheim); Stack's 'religious commitment theory';[110,111] and the 'network theory'.[112] For example, Stack and Lester demonstrated, in a recent study comparing between Protestants and Catholics in Europe by using national data on 1687 respondents, that commitment, as measured by church attendance, is a key protective factor,[110] a discussion that will be taken up in other chapters of this book.

In Nepal, the situation is further complicated by the already described complex building of identity that also affects religious beliefs and identity. The syncretistic melting of (mainly Tibetan) Buddhist and Hindu beliefs and practices, in many regions also with local or shamanistic traditions,[113,114] creates a situation that makes comparison to other countries in this regard more difficult. In this context, Hinduist influence is strong and should be mentioned as a potential influencing factor in the perception of suicidal behaviour, even when its over-interpretation should be avoided. Religion can be expected to at least influence the perception of suicidal behaviour in the community, even if not directly influencing suicidal behaviour itself.

Hinduism

The *Mahabharata*, the traditional epic of Indian Hindu culture, known by heart by nearly everyone in the region, is critical of suicide, noting that suicide prohibits access to blessed regions in heaven.[ix] The risk of consequential reincarnation[115] as an adverse form of life, because of 'selfish violation' of Dharma, the task given in life, is a factor that speaks strongly against suicide and creates stigma attached to individuals dying by suicide in both Hinduism and some forms of Buddhism,[115] although Colucci and Martin,[107] and Vijayakumar and John[116] in their reviews described the Hinduist position in general as 'ambivalent'. Vijayakumar and John[116] contrasted this with the claim that Hinduists 'have a suicide rate of about 21 per 100,000 population compared to the global average of 11.4' and that 'Hindu countries have higher rates of suicide compared to Islamic and Christian countries, but these rates are lower when compared to Atheist and Buddhist countries'. Some authors have proposed that even persons believing in karma might 'give up' any hope of better reincarnation, and therefore are willing to risk dying by suicide in spite of the karmatic consequences.[19]

Authors working on suicide in India have proposed the category of 'altruistic' suicide,[84,86] which includes (at least according to traditional understanding) the already mentioned Sati and, in the only historical context, 'Jauhar, a kind of mass suicide by women of a community when their menfolk suffered defeat in battle'.[86] While these existing cultural 'glorifying' models do actually contribute to the higher rate of suicide in women (as in the 'Werther' model),[117] they remain nevertheless dubious, as both forms are, as noted, obsolete and not really present in the recent public discourse. The government report, based on the Maternal Health Study (MMM) mentioned earlier,[19] discussed such imitation effects, although relying on very limited data.

[ix] *Mahabharata* Book 1, line 17749 in translation by Kisari Mohan Ganguli.

Some forms of suicide are considered acceptable and described not as suicide, but as a selfless act of self-sacrifice (atma huti). Athma Huti can take three forms:

- Self-immolation by entering fire (*agnipravesa*)
- Death by entering a cave and suspending breathing in a state of askesis (*samadhi*)
- Fasting to death (*prayopavesa*).[x]

Also acceptable is dying in battle to save one's honour, as in many cultures, which also would not be described as suicide.

These specific exceptions to the general attitude of condemning suicide as a selfish act are only acceptable in clearly defined situations and settings, related to their meaning in religion, such as Sati, or suttee, of widows,[84,118] which, as noted, is not a significant issue in Nepal.

Buddhism

Buddhism is a religion comprising different forms or sects that can interact with local religions and cultures, especially in Nepal and China. Conclusions on the positive or negative impact of religion on mental health should therefore be considered with caution and not generalized. Keown[119] discussed this issue in a landmark publication in 1981[xi] that led to subsequent discussions in the literature.[110,111] Eskin et al. reported lower suicide risk among further Buddhists than, for example, among followers of Islam in a methodologically limited study of 5572 students from 12 countries based on self-report questionnaires.[112] Many cultural factors might also moderate the interaction between Buddhist denomination and suicidal ideation, and the level of actual religious conviction and lived religious practice should be distinguished from 'on-paper' affiliation. Authors have proposed that some concepts like dukkha (unsatisfactoriness or suffering) and Sati (mindfulness) might be protective against, or even used therapeutically[123] in mental health problems. Jung[124] conducted a survey assessing for variables including depression and suicidal ideation in relation to factors they described as 'organizational religious activity (ORA)', as compared to 'non-ORA (NORA)', and 'intrinsic religiosity' (IR) in a sample of 1180 residents in Gangwon province, South Korea. The authors found that 'ORA was a moderator only among the Buddhist group, and IR only moderated the relationships among the Christians', a difference which would have not been

---

x Jarayam V. About suicides in Hinduism. Available from: https://www.hinduwebsite.com/hinduism/h_suicide.asp

xi Keown D. Buddhism and suicide: the case of Channa. Journal of Buddhist Ethics. 1996;3:19–21. Archived from the original (PDF) on 15 June 2010. Retrieved 29 November 2010.

recognized without the above-mentioned distinction between denomination and actual religiosity and practice, as noted already by Stack.[87] The additional distinction between suicidal ideation (that might actually reflect exhaustion, and not necessarily preparation for actual suicide)[97] and actual suicidal behaviour or completed suicide should also be considered when applying the results to other settings and cultures.[107]

To our knowledge, there have been no reports to date of suicide cults or sects, such as the 'Friends of the Truth' sect in Japan,[125] in Nepal.

Christianity

The proportion of Christians in Nepal is so small that we would not discuss the issue of specific religious factors and suicide in the context of Christianity.

Current interventions and prevention measures

As discussed earlier, overall low availability of resources, stigma attached to mental health problems, and the geographical complexity of Nepal make any interventions or preventive measures difficult to implement. The government has recently established a mental health plan, which has a more general focus and, although it mentions the above issues, it might not be able to offer a sufficiently comprehensive solution that could be expected to make a substantial difference, and some authors have therefore recommended a national health plan specifically targeting suicide.[11] TPO Nepal is an international non-governmental organization (NGO) especially active in this field of research and intervention in Nepal.[3,104,126]

Gender-based violence (GBV) is only insufficiently sanctioned, is firmly embedded in the public discourse,[10] is not really stigmatized, and is, as already noted, seen as one of the main reasons,[19] besides poverty, leading to family conflicts and suicide among women, at least according to the repeatedly cited governmental/United Nations report which also described that men in the study 'openly reported how they treated their wives prior to committing suicide' (p. 4)[19] and consequently help-seeking is discouraged. This is further compounded by the fact that local care centres are 'not aware of the rights of women'.[19] GBV should be seen as part of the general discriminating practices, such as Chaupadhi mentioned earlier, that, in turn, carry a high mortality rate due to snake bites or infections.[7,8,127,128,129] While it is not clear from current data whether general aspects of discrimination and reduced access to health care or specifically violence are the only key factors that can explain higher suicide rates in women, these aspects should obviously be targeted, bearing in mind that change must start first in the perception of women's role or status by the family, through education, and in the public discourse, as proposed recently by Paudhel et al.,[6] as well as in general protection of their human rights.

Media presentation

As noted, the traditional discourse on suicide, as for example in the *Mahabharata*, is ambivalent and includes also a more romanticized presentation of some forms of suicide. This has been identified as a possible target for preventive interventions such as media reporting style contracts or guidelines.[130,131,132] To our knowledge, no such initiatives have yet been effectively implemented or studied in Nepal, unlike in neighbouring India where they have been put into effect recently.[133] A recent research report has indeed underlined the importance of Media reporting guidelines with respect to Nepal.[134]

Hotlines

To our knowledge, several online helplines and telephone hotlines are currently available in Nepal, including National Suicide Prevention Helpline by TPO Nepal, one by the University Teaching Hospital, the Nepal Emergency Hotline, and Patan Hospital Suicide Hotline. It should be considered that access to electricity and each to cell networks is still limited in some regions of Nepal.

Post-suicide intervention programmes

To our knowledge, no data have been published to date on effective post-suicide intervention programmes in Nepal.[135]

Prohibition of poisonous substances

In spite of some controversy in the literature described earlier, ingestion of easily available, but highly dangerous, substances commonly present in farming households appears to be probably the most common method of suicide or suicide attempt in Nepal, at least if we consider data from the large number of retrospective hospital-based studies as an indicator. Women in distress, because of communication problems, conflicts, or violence within the family, are those who are probably the most affected suicide attempts, as discussed earlier. The authors of several of the studies discussed earlier on poisoning in Nepal have recommended for better regulation by distribution of, and access to, these dangerous substances, in addition to improved medical treatment of self-poisoning and its sequelae. As interventions have been demonstrated to be effective, even in countries with a similarly weak economy, this approach should prove realistic and effective also in Nepal, along with changes to legislation and development of alternatives to support rural communities.

Finally, the stigma attached to mental health problems and the very limited availability of low barrier and easily accessible mental health resources especially in the communities, as well as low number of hospital beds and advanced mental health resources such as not only of psychiatric services but also of counselling and psychotherapy constitute key challenges.

Conclusion and perspectives

In short, to tackle a complex process that will require the collaboration of communities, the government, and the health care system, as well as possibly international agencies working in Nepal, such as TPO Nepal,[136] certain actions can be considered that can potentially improve the situation. As discussed above,[137] the complex cultural, geographical, and economic situation of Nepal should be considered,[137] and some authors have advocated for approaches based on consideration of relevant religious beliefs.[107,115] A network analysis by Hagaman et al.[21] found that the police was the main institution responsible for collecting data on suicide, with a minor contribution from health care institutions. The authors proposed that health care institutions should be allowed to play a stronger role in suicide data collection[21] to reduce stigma and improve the database for suicide monitoring.

General measures to be considered based on the above review of limited evidence-based knowledge on suicide in Nepal, and as proposed in recent publications,[1] would require setting up of a national strategic plan[1] that focuses on a number of issues, including dissemination of public information via media channels and training of primary health care providers[136] (in practice, these are often trained nurses in villages in remote rural regions and general practitioners). Further, it would require overall improvement and strengthening of mental health services in Nepal, especially in psychotherapy (e.g. dialectical behaviour therapy specifically adapted to Nepali culture, as described by Ramaiya et al.,[125] and proven to be effective for women in Nepal with suicidal ideation).[137] Community-based counselling services, such as VISHRAM, have also been demonstrated to be effective (with a first positive-outcome study already published).[138] Such efforts might have to be supported by outreach services, including outreach services focusing on suicide prevention and anti-stigma campaigns on depression, suicide, and general mental health (especially in local villages). The READ-MH (responding to experienced and anticipated mental health-related discrimination) programmes could be beneficial in training health care providers, as proposed by Henderson et al., with first data emerging from Nepal and other low-income countries.[139] Agreement with the media channels, or establishing guidelines, on how to report on GBV and suicide,[140] together with changes in legislation discussed earlier to support families and regulate the distribution and sale of toxic fertilizers (or to support use of non-toxic fertilizers), could further contribute to addressing the substantial challenge of suicide in Nepal. Special support might also be necessary for specific groups such as women suffering from abuse, persons in the LGBT community, widows, former child soldiers,[141] victims of trafficking, those from ethnic minorities in rapidly changing environments, and even students.

Due to the lack of infrastructure, innovative solutions that can be implemented also in rural regions that have limited access to electricity and the Internet should be developed. It further would be important to address the lack of trained health care personnel. At the same time, these solutions can be adopted by countries facing similar challenges. Graphical presentations in public spaces, such as on walls, are frequently used to promote awareness of health issues but can only be of limited help in tackling such a complex issue. As discussed earlier, women should receive increased support and protection, both legally and from families and communities. Such supportive measures, in turn, could be expected also to reduce suicidal behaviour, especially as suicide by fertilizer ingestion can be seen as an 'idiom of distress'. The fight against GBV and discriminatory practices should be part of all further measures, as discussed repeatedly in this chapter and recent publications, and perinatal support and women's health care in general should be improved.[11,18,32,36,87,141] Any legal or other sanctions related to suicide should, in our opinion, reflect international standards on suicide prevention and be replaced by other, more supportive measures for families and survivors, as well as by prevention efforts.

Local healers and trusted religious authorities could be recruited, along the establishment of community and women's projects, to support the process. Community health work would require adequate training and monitoring of training outcomes, as demonstrated by certain inadequate competencies among health workers who took part in WHO mental health Gap (mhGAP) training reported by Kohrt et al.[144]

All measures warrant further research, including more reliable statistics and qualitative and psychological, including psychological autopsy, studies. Studies on poisoning, hanging, or other emergency problems should also include in-depth and validated data on social circumstances, as well as mental health data.

References

1. **Marahatta K, Samuel R, Sharma P, Dixit L, Shrestha BR.** Suicide burden and prevention in Nepal: the need for a national strategy. WHO South East Asia Journal of Public Health. 2017;**6**(1):45–9.

2. **Chase L, Sapkota RP.** 'In our community, a friend is a psychologist': an ethnographic study of informal care in two Bhutanese refugee communities. Transcultural Psychiatry. 2017;**54**(3):400–22.
3. **Bhardwaj A, Bourey C, Rai S, Adhikari RP, Worthman CM, Kohrt BA.** Interpersonal violence and suicidality among former child soldiers and war-exposed civilian children in Nepal. Cambridge Prisms: Global Mental Health. 2018;**5**:e9.
4. **Kohrt BA, Hruschka DJ, Worthman CM,** et al. Political violence and mental health in Nepal: prospective study. British Journal of Psychiatry. 2012;**201**(4):268–75.
5. **Tol WA, Komproe IH, Thapa SB, Jordans MJ, Sharma B, De Jong JT.** Disability associated with psychiatric symptoms among torture survivors in rural Nepal. Journal of Nervous and Mental Disease. 2007;**195**(6):463–9.
6. **Paudhel R, Mili A, Kletecka-Pulker M, Wenzel, T.** The construction of power in Nepal: menstrual restriction and rape. Archives of Women Health and Care. 2019;**2**(4):1–7.
7. **Cardoso LF, Clark CJ, Rivers K, Ferguson G, Shrestha B, Gupta J.** Menstrual restriction prevalence and association with intimate partner violence among Nepali women. BMJ Sexual and Reproductive Health. 2018;45(1):38–43.
8. **Atreya A, Nepal S.** Menstrual exile: a cultural punishment for Nepalese women. Medico-Legal Journal. 2019;**87**(1):12–13.
9. **Thapa S, Bhattarai S, Aro AR.** 'Menstrual blood is bad and should be cleaned': a qualitative case study on traditional menstrual practices and contextual factors in the rural communities of far-western Nepal. SAGE Open Medicine. 2019;7:2050312119850400.
10. **Radha P, Adhikari M,** Kletecka-Pulker M, Thomas W. The construction of power in Nepal: menstrual restriction and rape. Archives of Women Health and Care. 2019;**2**(4):1–7.
11. **Puri M, Tamang J, Shah I.** Suffering in silence: consequences of sexual violence within marriage among young women in Nepal. BMC Public Health. 2011;**11**:29.
12. **Acharya K, Paudel YR, Silwal P.** Sexual violence as a predictor of unintended pregnancy among married young women: evidence from the 2016 Nepal demographic and health survey. BMC Pregnancy Childbirth. 2019;**19**(1):196.
13. **Dhakal L, Berg-Beckhoff G, Aro AR.** Intimate partner violence (physical and sexual) and sexually transmitted infection: results from Nepal Demographic Health Survey 2011. International Journal of Women's Health. 2014;**6**:75–82.
14. **Puri M, Frost M, Tamang J, Lamichhane P, Shah I.** The prevalence and determinants of sexual violence against young married women by husbands in rural Nepal. BMC Research Notes. 2012;**5**:291.
15. **Oram S, Stockl H, Busza J, Howard LM, Zimmerman C.** Prevalence and risk of violence and the physical, mental, and sexual health problems associated with human trafficking: systematic review. PLoS Medicine. 2012;**9**(5):e1001224.
16. **Puri M, Shah I, Tamang J.** Exploring the nature and reasons for sexual violence within marriage among young women in Nepal. Journal of Interpersonal Violence. 2010;**25**(10):1873–92.
17. **Hagaman AK, Khadka S, Lohani S, Kohrt B.** Suicide in Nepal: a modified psychological autopsy investigation from randomly selected police cases between 2013 and 2015. Social Psychiatry and Psychiatric Epidemiology. 2017;**52**(12):1483–94.

18. **Karki C.** Suicide: leading cause of death among women in Nepal. Kathmandu University Medical Journal (KUMJ). 2011;**9**(35):157–8.
19. **Pradhan A P, P, Thomas, D., Barnett, S.** A review of the evidence: suicide among women in Nepal. Kathmandu: Family Health Division; 2009.
20. **Pyakurel R, Sharma N, Paudel D**, et al. Cause of death in women of reproductive age in rural Nepal obtained through community-based surveillance: is reducing maternal mortality the right priority for women's health programs? Health Care for Women International. 2015;**36**(6):655–62.
21. **Hagaman AK, Maharjan U, Kohrt BA.** Suicide surveillance and health systems in Nepal: a qualitative and social network analysis. International Journal of Mental Health Systems. 2016;**10**:46.
22. **Jordans MJ, Kaufman A, Brenman NF**, et al. Suicide in South Asia: a scoping review. BMC Psychiatry. 2014;**14**:358.
23. **Thapa S.** The ethnic factor in the timing of family formation in Nepal. Asia-Pacific Population Journal. 1989;**4**(1):3–34.
24. **Albert JP, Crubezy E.** [Shamanic healing in the age of modern medicine]. Médecine Tropicale. 2005;**65**(1):93–9.
25. **Van Ommeren M, Komproe I, Cardena E**, et al. Mental illness among Bhutanese shamans in Nepal. Journal of Nervous and Mental Disease. 2004;**192**(4):313–17.
26. **Thapa B, Carlough MC.** Suicide incidence in the Lalitpur district of Central Nepal. Tropical Doctor. 2000;**30**(4):200–3.
27. **Acharya S, Ghimire S, Jeffers EM, Shrestha N.** Health care utilization and health care expenditure of Nepali older adults. Frontiers in Public Health. 2019;**7**:24.
28. **Acharya Y, Dahal R, Bista NR, Bista S.** Challenges of new Healthcare Reform Act 2017 and possible rise of defensive medicine in Nepal. Journal of Nepal Health Research Council. 2018;**16**(3):357–8.
29. **Adhikari SR, Sapkota D, Thapa A, Pandey AR.** Evaluation of Nepal's Free Health Care Scheme from health system perspective: a qualitative analysis. Journal of Nepal Health Research Council. 2019;**16**(41):372–7.
30. **Acharya B, Tenpa J, Thapa P, Gauchan B, Citrin D, Ekstrand M.** Recommendations from primary care providers for integrating mental health in a primary care system in rural Nepal. BMC Health Services Research. 2016;**16**:492.
31. **Pandit A.** Suicide in Nepal: facts and figures. Tropical Doctor. 2004;**34**(2):125.
32. **Thapaliya S, Sharma P, Upadhyaya K.** Suicide and self harm in Nepal: a scoping review. Asian Journal of Psychiatry. 2018;**32**:20–6.
33. **Sharma G, Shrestha PK, Wasti H, Kadel T, Ghimire P, Dhungana S.** A review of violent and traumatic deaths in Kathmandu, Nepal. International Journal of Injury Control and Safety Promotion. 2006;**13**(3):197–9.
34. **Risal A, Sharma PP.** Psychiatric manifestations of patients admitted for intentional self harm. Journal of the Institute of Medicine. 2011;**33**(1):43–8.
35. **O'Connor E GB, Burda BU**, et al. (2013). Screening for suicide risk in primary care: a systematic evidence review for the U.S. Preventive Services Task Force. Table 1: definitions of suicide-related terms. Rockville, MD: Agency for Healthcare Research and Quality (US). Available from: https://www.ncbi.nlm.nih.gov/books/NBK137739/table/ch1.t1/

36. **Hagaman AK, Khadka S, Wutich A, Lohani S, Kohrt BA.** Suicide in Nepal: qualitative findings from a modified case-series psychological autopsy investigation of suicide deaths. Culture, Medicine, and Psychiatry. 2018;**42**(3):704–34.
37. **Katuwal N, Shrestha DB, Adhikari SP,** et al. Study on prevalence of suicidal ideation and risk factors of suicide among patients visiting psychiatric OPD at Shree Birendra Hospital, Kathmandu Nepal. PLoS One. 2021;**16**(7):e0254728.
38. **Dhimal M, Dahal S, Adhikari K,** et al. A nationwide prevalence of common mental disorders and suicidality in Nepal: evidence from National Mental Health Survey, 2019–2020. Journal of Nepal Health Research Council. 2022;**19**(4):740–7.
39. **Ghimire R, Utyasheva L, Pokhrel M,** et al. Intentional pesticide poisoning and pesticide suicides in Nepal. Clinical Toxicology (Philadelphia, PA). 2022;**60**(1):46–52.
40. **Utyasheva L, Sharma D, Ghimire R, Karunarathne A, Robertson G, Eddleston M.** Suicide by pesticide ingestion in Nepal and the impact of pesticide regulation. BMC Public Health. 2021;**21**(1):1136.
41. **Rajbanshi LK, Arjyal B, Mandal R.** Clinical profile and outcome of patients with acute poisoning admitted in intensive care unit of tertiary care center in Eastern Nepal. Indian Journal of Critical Care Medicine. 2018;**22**(10):691–6.
42. **Gyenwali D, Vaidya A, Tiwari S, Khatiwada P, Lamsal DR, Giri S.** Pesticide poisoning in Chitwan, Nepal: a descriptive epidemiological study. BMC Public Health. 2017;**17**(1):619.
43. **Agrawaal KK, Karki P.** Clinico-epidemiological study on pesticide poisoning in a tertiary care hospital in Eastern Nepal. Journal of Nepal Medical Association. 2014;**52**(196):972–6.
44. **Shrestha B, Singh PM, Bharati U, Dhungel S.** Poisonings at Nepal Medical College Teaching Hospital. Nepal Medical College Journal. 2011;**13**(3):199–204.
45. **Gurung CK, Dahal R, Khanal P, Nepal S, Jaiswal AK.** Pattern of poisoning cases in a hospital in a Terai district of central Nepal. Nepal Medical College Journal. 2011;**13**(3):160–3.
46. **Paudyal BP.** Poisoning: pattern and profile of admitted cases in a hospital in central Nepal. Journal of Nepal Medical Association. 2005;**44**(159):92–6.
47. **Joshi SK.** Pesticides poisoning in Nepal. Kathmandu University Medical Journal. 2003;**1**(3):157.
48. **Karki P, Hansdak SG, Bhandari S, Shukla A, Koirala S.** A clinico-epidemiological study of organophosphorus poisoning at a rural-based teaching hospital in eastern Nepal. Tropical Doctor. 2001;**31**(1):32–4.
49. **Licata C, Liu L, Mole D, Thorp J, Chand R, Chaulagain S.** Social and cultural factors leading to suicide attempt via organophosphate poisoning in Nepal. Case Reports in Psychiatry. 2019;**2019**:7681309.
50. **Bajracharya SR, Prasad PN, Ghimire R.** Management of organophosphorus poisoning. Journal of Nepal Health Research Council. 2016;**14**(34):131–8.
51. **Sharma A, Sharma A, Acharya A,** et al. Extracorporeal membrane oxygenation in aluminum phosphide poisoning in Nepal: a case report. Journal of Medical Case Reports. 2018;**12**(1):311.
52. **Basnet A, Shrestha D, Chaulagain S,** et al. Psychological and clinical-epidemiological profile of poisoning in Nepal: an institutional experience. F1000Res. 2021;**10**:556.

53. **Parajuli S, Jayakumar J, Dham SK.** Intermediate syndrome in organophosphorous poisoning: a case report. Kathmandu University Medical Journal. 2005;**3**(4):421–2.
54. **Pangeni R, Kc RK.** Successfully managed case of celphos poisoning: a case report and review. Journal of Nepal Health Research Council. 2014;**12**(28):200–2.
55. **Bhattarai N, Rauniyar A, Chaudhary D, Jaiswal S, Banthia P, Rana BB.** Patterns of organophosphorous poisoning attending a teaching hospital. JNMA; Journal of the Nepal Medical Association. 2006;**45**(162):228–32.
56. **Marahatta SB, Singh J, Shrestha R, Koju R.** Poisoning cases attending emergency department in Dhulikhel Hospital-Kathmandu University Teaching Hospital. Kathmandu University Medical Journal. 2009;**7**(26):152–6.
57. **Chakrabarti K, Devkota KC.** Retrospective study of suicide cases admitted in Nepal Medical College Teaching Hospital. Nepal Medical College Journal. 2004;**6**(2):116–18.
58. **Shakya M, Singh R, Arya KD, Rure D.** Sociodemography, pattern, and response inhibition in suicide survivors: A case-control study. Industrial Psychiatry Journal. 2023;**32**(Suppl 1):S93–S99.
59. **Pradhan SN, Adhikary SR.** A study of severity of intention of suicide in various psychiatric diagnoses. Kathmandu University Medical Journal. 2009;**7**(25):63–6.
60. **Ghimire S, Devkota S, Budhathoki R, Sapkota N, Thakur A.** Psychiatric comorbidities in patients with deliberate self-harm in a tertiary care center. Journal of Nepal Medical Association. 2014;**52**(193):697–701.
61. **Adhikari A, Dutta A, Sapkota S, Chapagain A, Aryal A, Pradhan A.** Prevalence of poor mental health among medical students in Nepal: a cross-sectional study. BMC Medical Education. 2017;**17**(1):232.
62. **Hagaman A, Lopez Mercado D, Poudyal A,** et al. 'Now, I have my baby so I don't go anywhere': a mixed method approach to the 'everyday' and young motherhood integrating qualitative interviews and passive digital data from mobile devices. PLoS One. 2022;**17**(7):e0269443.
63. **Pradhan A, Mandal BK, Tripathi CB.** Hanging: nature of ligature material applied and type of hanging according to point of suspension. Nepal Medical College Journal. 2012;**14**(2):103–6.
64. **Kanchan T, Raghavendra Babu YP, Atreya A, Acharya J.** Ligature mark on the face: forensic implications. Medico-Legal Journal. 2016;**84**(3):138–41.
65. **Kanchan T, Atreya A.** Duret haemorrhage: an unusual finding in compression of neck structures. Journal of Forensic and Legal Medicine. 2018;**55**:74–5.
66. **Atreya A, Kanchan T.** Clinico-epidemiological study of near-hanging cases: an investigation from Nepal. Journal of Forensic and Legal Medicine. 2015;**33**:35–8.
67. **Atreya A, Rijal D, Kanchan T, Shekhawat RS.** Abdominal self-stabbing: a case report. Medico-Legal Journal. 2017;**85**(2):97–9.
68. **Rabi S, Sulochana J, Pawan S.** Self-inflicted cut injury as common method of deliberate self harm: a retrospective study from Nepal. Indian Journal of Psychological Medicine. 2017;**39**(5):579–83.
69. **Lama BB, Duke JM, Sharma NP,** et al. Intentional burns in Nepal: a comparative study. Burns. 2015;**41**(6):1306–14.
70. **Gonzalez-Santiago O, Morales-San Claudio PC, Cantu-Cardenas LG, Favela-Hernandez JMJ.** Unintentional and self-poisoning mortalities in Mexico, 2000–2012. PLoS One. 2017;**12**(7):e0181708.

71. **Karki RK, Risal A.** Study of poisoning cases in a tertiary care hospital. Kathmandu University Medical Journal. 2012;**10**(40):70–3.
72. **Chowdhury FR, Dewan G, Verma VR**, et al. Bans of WHO Class I pesticides in Bangladesh: suicide prevention without hampering agricultural output. International Journal of Epidemiology. 2018;**47**(1):175–84.
73. **Gunnell D, Knipe D, Chang SS**, et al. Prevention of suicide with regulations aimed at restricting access to highly hazardous pesticides: a systematic review of the international evidence. The Lancet Global Health. 2017;**5**(10):e1026–37.
74. **Eddleston M, Adhikari S, Egodage S**, et al. Effects of a provincial ban of two toxic organophosphorus insecticides on pesticide poisoning hospital admissions. Clinical Toxicology (Philadelphia, PA). 2012;**50**(3):202–9.
75. **Eide AH, Dyrstad K.** PTSD as a consequence of past conflict experience, recent exposure to violence and economic marginalization in post-conflict contexts: study from Nepal, Guatemala and Northern Ireland. International Journal of Social Psychiatry. 2019;**65**(6):488–95.
76. **Jha A, Shakya S.** Rational for conducting PTSD research and challenges of recruiting and training volunteers to screen and treat PTSD among the Nepal 2015 earthquake survivors. Journal of Nepal Medical Association. 2015;**53**(199):202–7.
77. **Kohrt BA, Hruschka DJ.** Nepali concepts of psychological trauma: the role of idioms of distress, ethnopsychology and ethnophysiology in alleviating suffering and preventing stigma. Culture, Medicine, and Psychiatry. 2010;**34**(2):322–52.
78. **Pollock DA.** PTSD and risk of suicide. American Journal of Psychiatry. 1992;**149**(1):142–3.
79. **Fleischmann A, Saxena S.** Suicide prevention in the WHO Mental Health Gap Action Programme (mhGAP). Crisis. 2013;**34**(5):295–6.
80. **Kisely S, Siskind D.** Meeting the mental health needs of low- and middle-income countries: the start of a long journey. BJPsych Open. 2019;**5**(6):e100.
81. **Semrau M, Alem A, Ayuso-Mateos JL**, et al. Strengthening mental health systems in low- and middle-income countries: recommendations from the Emerald programme. BJPsych Open. 2019;**5**(5):e73.
82. **Kudva KG, El Hayek S, Gupta AK**, et al. Stigma in mental illness: perspective from eight Asian nations. Asia-Pacific Psychiatry. 2020;**12**(2):e12380.
83. **Regmi SK, Pokharel A, Ojha SP, Pradhan SN, Chapagain G.** Nepal mental health country profile. International Review of Psychiatry. 2004;**16**(1–2):142–9.
84. **Bhugra D.** Sati: a type of nonpsychiatric suicide. Crisis. 2005;**26**(2):73–7.
85. **India.** Commission of Sati (Prevention) Act, 1987 (No. 3 of 1988), 3 January 1988. Annual Review of Population Law. 1988;**15**:143, 527–30.
86. **Vijayakumar L.** Altruistic suicide in India. Archives of Suicide Research. 2004;**8**(1):73–80.
87. **Stack S, Cao L.** Social integration and indigenous suicidality. Archives of Suicide Research. 2019;**24**(1):1–16.
88. **Shakya DR.** Psychiatric morbidities among mentally ill wives of Nepalese men working abroad. Industrial Psychiatry Journal. 2014;**23**(1):52–7.
89. **Kim J, Tol WA, Shrestha A**, et al. Persistent complex bereavement disorder and culture: early and prolonged grief in Nepali widows. Psychiatry. 2017;**80**(1):1–16.

90. **Kohlbrenner V, Deuba K, Karki DK, Marrone G.** Perceived discrimination is an independent risk factor for suicidal ideation among sexual and gender minorities in Nepal. PLoS One. 2016;**11**(7):e0159359.
91. **Pandey AR, Bista B, Dhungana RR, Aryal KK, Chalise B, Dhimal M.** Factors associated with suicidal ideation and suicidal attempts among adolescent students in Nepal: findings from Global School-based Students Health Survey. PLoS One. 2019;**14**(4):e0210383.
92. **Rai S, Adhikari SB, Acharya NR, Kaiser BN, Kohrt BA.** Elucidating adolescent aspirational models for the design of public mental health interventions: a mixed-method study in rural Nepal. Child and Adolescent Psychiatry and Mental Health. 2017;**11**:65.
93. **Shrestha G, Yadav DK, Sapkota N**, et al. Depression among inmates in a regional prison of eastern Nepal: a cross-sectional study. BMC Psychiatry. 2017;**17**(1):348.
94. **Atreya A, Shrestha M, Acharya J.** Inter-caste lovers' suicide pact: case report from Nepal. Medico-Legal Journal. 2018;**86**(2):103–6.
95. **Kohrt BA, Jordans MJ, Tol WA**, et al. Social ecology of child soldiers: child, family, and community determinants of mental health, psychosocial well-being, and reintegration in Nepal. Transcultural Psychiatry. 2010;**47**(5):727–53.
96. **Kohrt BA, Yang M, Rai S, Bhardwaj A, Tol WA, Jordans MJ.** Recruitment of child soldiers in Nepal: mental health status and risk factors for voluntary participation of youth in armed groups. Peace and Conflict. 2016;**22**(3):208–16.
97. **Wenzel T, Rushiti F, Aghani F, Diaconu G, Maxhuni B, Zitterl W.** Suicidal ideation, post-traumatic stress and suicide statistics in Kosovo. An analysis five years after the war. Suicidal ideation in Kosovo. Torture. 2009;**19**(3):238–47.
98. **Kohrt BA, Burkey M, Stuart EA, Koirala S.** Alternative approaches for studying humanitarian interventions: propensity score methods to evaluate reintegration packages impact on depression, PTSD, and function impairment among child soldiers in Nepal. Cambridge Prisms: Global Mental Health. 2015;**2**:e16.
99. **ICTJ.** Navigating Amnesty and Reconciliation in Nepal's Truth and Reconciliation Commission Bill. In: **International Center for Transitional Justice**, editor. Online Briefing. New York, NY: International Center for Transitional Justice; 2011.
100. **Rausch C.** Reconciliation and transitional justice in Nepal: a slow path. Washington, DC: United States Institute of Peace; 2017.
101. **Lapo-Talledo GJ, Talledo-Delgado JA, Portalanza D, Rodrigues ALS, Siteneski A.** Suicide rates in Ecuador: a nationwide study from 2011 until 2020. Journal of Affective Disorders. 2023;**320**:638–46.
102. **Orui M.** Suicide and suicide prevention activities following the great East Japan earthquake 2011: a literature review. International Journal of Environmental Research and Public Health. 2022;**19**(17):10906.
103. **Inoue K, Kameo S, Murayama Y**, et al. Suicides following an earthquake: Japanese proposals arising from post-earthquake analyses. Medicine, Science and the Law. 2022;**62**(2):158–9.
104. **Kane JC, Luitel NP, Jordans MJD, Kohrt BA, Weissbecker I, Tol WA.** Mental health and psychosocial problems in the aftermath of the Nepal earthquakes: findings from a representative cluster sample survey. Epidemiology and Psychiatric Sciences. 2018;**27**(3):301–10.

105. **Lizardi D, Gearing RE.** Religion and suicide: Buddhism, Native American and African religions, Atheism, and Agnosticism. Journal of Religion and Health. 2010;**49**(3):377–84.
106. **Fang CK, Lu HC, Liu SI, Sun YW.** Religious beliefs along the suicidal path in northern Taiwan. Omega (Westport). 2011;**63**(3):255–69.
107. **Colucci E, Martin G.** Religion and spirituality along the suicidal path. Suicide and Life-Threatening Behavior. 2008;**38**(2):229–44.
108. **Picone M.** Suicide and the afterlife: popular religion and the standardisation of 'culture' in Japan. Culture, Medicine, and Psychiatry. 2012;**36**(2):391–408.
109. **Colucci E, Martin G.** Ethnocultural aspects of suicide in young people: a systematic literature review part 1: Rates and methods of youth suicide. Suicide and Life-Threatening Behavior. 2007;**37**(2):197–221.
110. **Stack S, Lester D.** The effect of religion on suicide ideation. Social Psychiatry and Psychiatric Epidemiology. 1991;**26**(4):168–70.
111. **Stack S.** The effect of religious commitment on suicide: a cross-national analysis. Journal of Health and Social Behavior. 1983;**24**(4):362–74.
112. **Pescosolido BA, Georgianna S.** Durkheim, suicide, and religion: toward a network theory of suicide. American Sociological Review. 1989;**54**(1):33–48.
113. **Jolly A.** Indigenous mental health care among Gurkha soldiers based in the United Kingdom. Journal of the Royal Army Medical Corps. 1999;**145**(1):15–17.
114. **Maskarinec GG.** A shamanic etiology of affliction from western Nepal. Social Science and Medicine. 1992;**35**(5):723–34.
115. **Disayavanish C, Disayavanish P.** A Buddhist approach to suicide prevention. Journal of the Medical Association of Thailand. 2007;**90**(8):1680–8.
116. **Vijayakumar L, John S.** Is Hinduism ambivalent about suicide? International Journal of Social Psychiatry. 2018;**64**(5):443–9.
117. **Jonas K.** Modelling and suicide: a test of the Werther effect. British Journal of Social Psychology. 1992;**31**(Pt 4):295–306.
118. **India.** The Rajasthan Sati (Prevention) Act, 1987 (No. 40 of 1987), 26 November 1987. Annual Review of Population Law. 1987;**14**:477–82.
119. **Keown D.** Suicide, assisted suicide and euthanasia: a Buddhist perspective. Journal of Law and Religion. 1998;**13**(2):385–405.
120. **Florida RE.** A response to Damien Keown's suicide, assisted suicide and euthanasia: a Buddhist perspective. Journal of Law and Religion. 1998;**13**(2):413–16.
121. **Harvey P.** A response to Damien Keown's suicide, assisted suicide and euthanasia: a Buddhist perspective. Journal of Law and Religion. 1998;**13**(2):407–12.
122. **Eskin M, Poyrazli S, Janghorbani M,** et al. The role of religion in suicidal behavior, attitudes and psychological distress among university students: a multinational study. Transcultural Psychiatry. 2019;**56**(5):853–77.
123. **Kelly BD.** Self-immolation, suicide and self-harm in Buddhist and Western traditions. Transcultual Psychiatry. 2011;**48**(3):299–317.
124. **Jung S, Lee D, Park S, Hong HJ.** Subtypes of suicidal ideation in Korean adolescents: A multilevel latent profile analysis. Australian & New Zealand Journal of Psychiatry. 2019;**53**(2):158–67.

125. **Takahashi Y.** Mass suicide by members of the Japanese Friend of the Truth Church. Suicide and Life-Threatening Behavior. 1989;**19**(3):289–96.
126. **Ramaiya MK, Fiorillo D, Regmi U, Robins CJ, Kohrt BA.** A cultural adaptation of dialectical behavior therapy in Nepal. Cognitive and Behavioral Practice. 2017;**24**(4):428–44.
127. **Amatya P, Ghimire S, Callahan KE, Baral BK, Poudel KC.** Practice and lived experience of menstrual exiles (Chhaupadi) among adolescent girls in far-western Nepal. PLoS One. 2018;**13**(12):e0208260.
128. **Ranabhat C, Kim CB, Choi EH, Aryal A, Park MB, Doh YA.** Chhaupadi culture and reproductive health of women in Nepal. Asia Pacific Journal of Public Health. 2015;**27**(7):785–95.
129. **Thapa S.** Early discontinuation of intrauterine device in Nepal: a retrospective study. WHO South-East Asia Journal of Public Health. 2012;**1**(3):309–19.
130. **Tsai JF.** The media and suicide: evidence based on population data over 9 years in Taiwan. Suicide and Life-Threatening Behavior. 2010;**40**(1):81–6.
131. **Utterson M, Daoud J, Dutta R.** Online media reporting of suicides: analysis of adherence to existing guidelines. BJPsych Bulletin. 2017;**41**(2):83–6.
132. **Ziegler W, Hegerl U.** [The Werther effect. Significance, mechanisms, consequences]. Der Nervenarzt. 2002;**73**(1):41–9.
133. **Vijayakumar L.** Media matters in suicide: Indian guidelines on suicide reporting. Indian Journal of Psychiatry. 2019;**61**(6):549–51.
134. **Singh R, Mahato S, Khadka S**, et al. Newspaper reporting of suicide in Nepal: quality assessment against World Health Organization media guidelines. Health Science Reports. 2022;**5**(2):e547.
135. **Szumilas M, Kutcher S.** Post-suicide intervention programs: a systematic review. Canadian Journal of Public Health. 2011;**102**(1):18–29.
136. **Luitel NP, Jordans MJ, Adhikari A**, et al. Mental health care in Nepal: current situation and challenges for development of a district mental health care plan. Conflict and Health. 2015;**9**:3.
137. **Benson J, Shakya R.** Suicide prevention in Nepal: a comparison to Australia—a personal view. Mental Health in Family Medicine. 2008;**5**(3):177–82.
138. **Ramaiya MK, McLean C, Regmi U, Fiorillo D, Robins CJ, Kohrt BA.** A dialectical behavior therapy skills intervention for women with suicidal behaviors in rural Nepal: a single-case experimental design series. Journal of Clinical Psychology. 2018;**74**(7):1071–91.
139. **Shidhaye R, Murhar V, Gangale S**, et al. The effect of VISHRAM, a grass-roots community-based mental health programme, on the treatment gap for depression in rural communities in India: a population-based study. The Lancet Psychiatry. 2017;**4**(2):128–35.
140. **Henderson C, Ouali U, Bakolis I**, et al. Training for mental health professionals in responding to experienced and anticipated mental health related discrimination (READ-MH): protocol for an international multisite feasibility study. Pilot and Feasibility Studies. 2022;8(1):257.
141. **Acosta FJ, Rodriguez CJ, Cejas MR, Ramallo-Farina Y, Fernandez-Garcimartin H.** Suicide coverage in the digital press media: adherence to World Health Organization

guidelines and effectiveness of different interventions aimed at media professionals. Health Communication. 2019;35:1–10.

142. **Jordans MJ**, **Tol WA**, **Susanty** D, et al. Implementation of a mental health care package for children in areas of armed conflict: a case study from Burundi, Indonesia, Nepal, Sri Lanka, and Sudan. PLoS Medicine. 2013;**10**(1):e1001371.

143. **Lee H**, **Lee EY**, **Greene B**, **Shin YJ.** Psychological distress among adolescents in Laos, Mongolia, Nepal, and Sri Lanka. Asian Nursing Research (Korean Society of Nursing Science). 2019;**13**(2):147–53.

144. **Kohrt BA**, **Mutamba BB**, **Luitel NP**, et al. How competent are non-specialists trained to integrate mental health services in primary care? Global health perspectives from Uganda, Liberia, and Nepal. International Review of Psychiatry. 2018;**30**(6):182–98.

Chapter 15

Suicide in Indonesia

Marthoenis Marthoenis, Nani Safuni, Dahlia, and Liza Fathiariani

Introduction

No specific word stands specifically for 'suicide' in Bahasa Indonesia. The term suicide is often mentioned as '*bunuh diri*', which can be translated as 'kill self'. In local languages, such as Acehnese and Sundanese, the exact term for suicide also does not exist. In Acehnese, the term '*poh droe*' is used, which means 'hit or kill self'. Other local languages adopt the national language to refer to suicidality. From a language perspective, it can be said that neither suicide nor suicidal behaviour is part of Indonesian culture. Thus, explaining the problem of suicide in Indonesia is challenging. This chapter describes several issues regarding suicide from the Indonesian viewpoint, including the epidemiology of suicide in Indonesia, suicidal behaviour among adolescents and people with a mental disorder, methods of suicide, mass media reporting of suicide news in Indonesia, Islamic culture and suicide in Indonesia, suicide prevention and interventions in Indonesia, and suicide cases in Gunung Kidul. Several actions to be considered by scientists, health professionals, and policymakers in Indonesia and society at large are also proposed.

Epidemiology of suicide in Indonesia

Suicide is a global phenomenon that exists in all parts of the world and can occur at any point during the lifespan. Every 40 seconds, nearly 800,000 people die by suicide every year. As many as 79% of suicides occurred in low- and middle-income countries in 2016. Suicide accounts for 1.4% of all deaths that occur worldwide, making it the 18th leading cause of death in 2016.[1] Suicide occurs in any country, culture, religion, gender, and social class. The rate of suicide varies across countries and regions. Some countries are considered in the top five in terms of suicide cases, including Lithuania in Eastern Europe (31.9 suicides per 100,000), Russia (31 suicides per 100,000), Guyana in South America

(29.2 suicides per 100,000), South Korea in Asia (26.9 suicides per 100,000), and Belarus in Eastern Europe (26.2 suicides per 100,000).

In contrast, in Western Europe, Belgium ranks 11th in terms of suicide rate (20.7 suicides per 100,000). Interestingly, Bhutan, a country known for its high index of collective happiness and population welfare, has a relatively high suicide rate (11.4 suicides per 100,000). Another interesting point is that worldwide, many countries experiencing significant domestic problems have relatively low suicide rates, for example, Afghanistan (4.7 suicides per 100,000), Iraq (3 suicides per 100,000), and Syria (1.9 cases per 100,000). Reasons explaining these low suicide rates are poorly understood, whether the low suicide rates in these countries are related to mental health problems or deadly diseases, or are due to under-reporting of suicide cases or conflicts that occur in these geographical settings, is unclear. Furthermore, the lowest suicide rates, as well as rarest occurrence of suicide, were recorded in the Caribbean islands of the Bahamas, Jamaica, Grenada, Barbados, and Antigua and Barbuda. In 2018, Barbados was reported to have a suicide rate of 0.8 cases per 100,000, and Antigua and Barbuda 0.5 cases per 100,000.[2]

The global ranking of Indonesia in terms of suicide rate is 158th (3.4 suicides per 100,000), with suicide rates higher among males than among females (4.8 vs 2.0 suicides per 100,000, respectively).[2] This projection means that in 2018, with a population of approximately 265 million inhabitants in Indonesia, the number of deaths by suicide was estimated to reach 9000 cases per year.[3] In contrast, based on the Sample Registration System in 2016, the Indonesian Ministry of Health estimated a suicide rate of 0.71 per 100,000 population or 1800 deaths per year. This inconsistent estimation of the completed suicide rate is simply because of the country's poor registration system for the cause of death.

Furthermore, the Indonesian government survey also found that males are three times more likely to die by suicide than females. Death by suicide frequently occurs among the productive age group: 46% among those aged 25–49 years, or 75% among those aged 15–64 years.[3] In 2015, Indonesian police reported that the highest number of completed suicides occurred in the Province of Jawa Tengah, with 331 cases, followed by Jawa Timur (119 cases), Bali (96 cases), Jogjakarta (59 cases), and Jawa Barat (51 cases), citing depression, bullying, violence, and cultural background as the risk factor for suicide.[4] Still, the actual number of completed suicides is estimated to be higher than that recorded. The lack of a registration system for deaths caused by suicide in Indonesia is responsible for the lower suicide rates reported.

In some cases, suicides are recorded as accidents because of concerns of stigma and community resistance associated with suicide. Autopsy for the cause of death is not part of the Indonesian system. Cases of suicide attempts or other types of incomplete suicides are rarely recorded. The rate of suicide-related behaviour is also rarely studied in Indonesia. Therefore, the country's lack of suicide-related statistical information remains a significant challenge for mental health professionals, policymakers, and the general population.

There has been limited research on suicide-related behaviour in Indonesia. However, studies related to suicide have shown an alarming issue of mental health problems in the country. The Indonesian Basic Health Research conducted in 2018 by the Ministry of Health of the Republic of Indonesia showed that 6.1% of Indonesia's population aged 15 years and above experienced depression, but of whom only 9% underwent treatment or medical care.[5] More research on suicide prevention and management based on cultural reliability is encouraged because Indonesian culture is very diverse and understanding specific local cultural beliefs should help to reduce the suicide rate in Indonesia.

Suicidal behaviour among adolescents

A limited number of studies on suicidal behaviour, suicidal thoughts, and suicide attempts have been conducted in Indonesia. Most of the studies included high-school or university students, which are the most assessable groups for researchers. A comparison study between Indonesian students and those from the Philippines found that approximately 4.8% of Indonesian students ever considered suicide during the past 12 months, which was significantly lower compared to 17.8% of students from the Philippines. Of those Indonesian students who considered suicide, more than half (53.5%) ever made a suicide plan. The authors also found that female students were more likely than their male counterparts to have suicidal behaviour and students with suicidal thoughts were more predisposed to making a suicide plan.[6] Indonesian university students were also reported to have the lowest suicidal ideation rate (6.9%) compared to those from neighbouring countries in South East Asia. However, the rate of suicide attempts among university students in Indonesia was higher (3%) than that in other countries such as Myanmar (1%) and Cambodia (1.6%).[7] Another study on self-injurious behaviour among Indonesian college students found that 38% had at least one intentional suicide during their lifetime. The authors also found that women had more frequency of lifetime self injurious behavior (72%) compared to the man (48%). The first act of self-injury occurred at a mean age of 14 years (standard deviation (SD) = 3.7), whereas the mean age of first suicidal attempts was 15.6 years (SD = 3.4).[8] The lifetime self-injury prevalence of 38% among Indonesian college students found in this study is in agreement with the self-harm rate of 38% previously reported among male college students in the United States.[9]

Data from the Global School-based Student Health Survey (GSHS) in Indonesia suggest that 4.7% of students had suicidal ideation and 2.5% had suicide attempt at least once during the last 12 months. Interestingly, the study found that male students were 59% less likely to consider suicide, and use of tobacco increased suicidal ideation among female students by 5.5 times. Further analysis found that being bullied and physically attacked were significant predictors of suicidal ideation, whereas having a parent who understood the adolescents' problems decreased the likelihood of suicidal ideation.[10]

In conclusion, the rates of suicidal behaviour among Indonesian students and adolescents differ across studies. The rate of suicidal ideation during the last 12 months ranged from 4.7% to 6.9%, whereas the lifetime rate of intentional suicide was 38%. Various socio-demographic and environmental factors have been linked with students' suicidal behaviour. Suicide prevention efforts targeting these groups should consider the determinants of suicidal behaviour among students and adolescents in Indonesia.

Suicide among people with mental disorders

The common occurrence of suicidal behaviour among people with a mental disorder has been widely reported. The phenomenon is even more common in countries or settings where policymaking and implementation of suicide prevention strategies are poor. In Indonesia, as many as 6.1% of people with schizophrenia have ever had suicide ideas at least once in their lifetime. Suicide ideas were significantly associated with a family history of schizophrenia, early age of disease onset, poor concentration, loss of enjoyment, feeling of guilt, nihilistic delusion, and alcohol abuse.[11] Besides schizophrenia, many people with depressive symptoms also experience suicidal or self-harming behaviour.[12] In 2017, approximately 9 million people were diagnosed with depression and had suicidal ideation. The age range for suicide ideas was from 13 years to adulthood, and it is estimated that the number of people with suicide ideas will increase yearly because it also affects younger people. This condition will worsen because of the stigma attached whereby society views suffering from mental illness as an embarrassment, and therefore, many people who experience mental illness hide their condition instead of seeking professional help.[13] Data on suicide among people with other types of mental disorder, such as anxiety and personality disorders, are lacking. Future research should aim to focus on the suicide rate, associated factors, and possible preventive approaches in people with various psychiatric disorders.

Methods of suicide

Various methods of dying by suicide are applied, and different methods are used that have different outcomes for the victim. In general, suicide methods can be classified into two main categories: violent and non-violent. Violent methods include hanging, strangulation and suffocation, drowning, gunshots, cutting or piercing, road-related, and jumping from a height. They are considered violent because of the significantly high risk of complete suicide. Gunshots, for instance, have very low likelihood of survival for the victim.

On the other hand, non-violent methods, including poisoning, are associated with potentially better survival rates. Although the risk factors for both violent and non-violent methods were found to be relatively similar,[14] the risk of death from poisoning varies, depending on the type and dose of the poison used, and on medical treatment given following the suicide attempt.

The choice of different methods of suicide is influenced by culture and tradition. Most suicide attempters from Western countries choose hanging and use of firearms, whereas those from Asian countries choose pesticide poisoning to end their life.[15] Jumping from a height is the most common suicide method used in Singapore and Hong Kong, because most people live in high-rise buildings which are easily accessible and this method is most certainly deadly.[16] On the other hand, use of firearms and hanging are common in the United States and Europe;[17] they accounted for 35% and 36.8%, respectively, of the cause of death among acute alcohol users and are among the three leading methods of suicide in the United States.[18] In Switzerland, data from 2000 to 2004 showed that 33.5% of males died by using firearms, whereas only 0.6% used pesticides.[17] Acknowledging the target population's culture in any suicide prevention programme is therefore significant.

In Indonesia, self-hanging is the most commonly reported method of suicide. In mass media and among the general population, the word self-hanging, or '*gantung diri*' in Bahasa Indonesia, is synonymous with suicide. Our recent content analysis of news reporting by Indonesian mass media on the pattern of suicide suggested that more than 63% of suicide cases used the hanging method. Other methods included jumping from a height, drowning, and poisoning. An earlier report from 1974 suggested that hanging was the most frequently used method of suicide in Jakarta (55.1%), followed by poisoning (7.6%). Furthermore, the study also found that the hanging method was more common among females than among males (72.7% vs 48.9, respectively), whereas poisoning was more common among males than among females (8.7% vs 4.5%, respectively). Poisoning was the most commonly used method among those aged under 25 years (10.3%), followed by shooting (5.1%).[19] Studies on suicide methods in Indonesia have since been scarce and actual data on methods of suicide are lacking.

Suicide news reporting in Indonesian mass media

Most Indonesian mass media do not comply with media guidelines on reporting suicide cases. Online newspaper reporting tends to exaggerate suicide news and does not comply with media guidelines from the World Health Organization (WHO).[20] This problem has also been reported in other Asian countries such as Bangladesh,[21] India,[22] and Thailand.[23] Whether in the news title or news content, Indonesian mass media were found to explicitly report the name, age, and gender of the victims, the methods of suicide, and the possible cause of suicidal behaviour, and to even post a picture of the suicide victim's dead body hanging. Very few of the media channels took the opportunity to educate their readers or audience on suicide prevention or where to seek help when reporting on suicide cases.[20] Such irresponsible reporting on suicide cases could trigger the Werther effect, which is the phenomenon of increased suicide rates following depiction of individual suicides in the media.[24] Indonesian authorities should provide sufficient information to press workers, and develop and implement effective policies and regulation of proper media reporting of suicide cases. Compliance with the WHO media guidelines on suicide reporting should help to improve the appropriateness of suicide-related news content and reduce a possible Werther effect in the Indonesian society.

Islamic culture and suicide in Indonesia

Indonesia has the largest Muslim majority in the world. The 2023 census confirmed that Indonesia has more than 278 million people, of whom more than 86,7% are Muslim. The constitution of Indonesia grants freedom of religion to its citizens, even though, officially, the Indonesian government only recognizes six religions, namely Islam, Protestantism, Roman Catholicism, Buddhism, Hinduism, and Confucianism. Every Indonesian citizen is guaranteed and protected by the government to worship their respective religions.

In carrying out their lives, Muslims are guided by the teachings and laws of Islam (sharia). In Islam, suicide is a sin. According to Islamic teachings, God, Allah the Almighty, has absolute power over human life and affairs. God is the valid owner of man, the creator, and the giver of human life and death. The reality and existence of humans are not only limited to the body, but also the reality and truth of humans are the soul and spirit, which cannot be destroyed by death.[25] Those who violate this means sinning and they will receive eternal punishment for their actions. Islamic teachings also provide rewards for people who do good deeds and stay away from despicable actions. Therefore, suicide in Islam is an act that is highly condemned, whereas preserving life is a commendable act.[26] This belief is also essential to preventing many Indonesian Muslims from developing suicidal behaviour.

The case of the tsunami in 2004 provides an excellent example of how one of the deadliest natural disasters in recorded history did not have a significant impact on the suicide rate. It has been estimated that the tsunami killed more than 160,000 people in the Aceh province of Indonesia. The Acehnese have been known for their firm Islamic religious beliefs. Before the tsunami, they had experienced various calamities, including wars related with European (mainly Portuguese and Dutch) colonization, the enduring local military conflict between the government of Indonesia and the Aceh Freedom Movement, and more recently the devastating tsunami on Boxing day in 2004.[27] These continuous calamities somehow helped to build resilience among the Acehnese. Following the tsunami, there were predictions that the suicide rate could escalate because many had lost their loved ones and belongings. However, suicide cases have never been reported in the province. This situation is similar to that in Sri Lanka, which was also affected by the tsunami in 2004 and where the rate of suicide following the tsunami did not differ from before the tsunami.[28] The Acehnese believe that life and death are God's will, and killing oneself, which is a suicide act, is a great sin and does not solve any problem. This belief perhaps could explain the low suicide rates in this population. Furthermore, it has been widely reported that suicide rates in Muslim-majority populations are lower than in other religious groups.[26,29]

Suicide prevention and interventions in Indonesia

Efforts focused on suicide prevention and interventions in Indonesia began only in the recent decade. Unfortunately, such initiatives targeted larger cities where establishments such as higher educational institutions and NGOs, in particular, have been aware of the burden and impact of suicide on the population. For instance, the Center for Public Mental Health of Universitas Gadjah Mada has issued suicide first-aid guidelines on ways to help suicidal people in Indonesia, which include communicating the problems, being a good listener, knowing what suicidal individuals should and should not do, and setting up protective plans for them. The guidelines also highlight communication issues where women from certain religious and cultural backgrounds usually do not seek professional advice, so their families should be involved in helping with suicidal concerns. Being respectful listeners include, for example, limiting questioning that can cause anxiety, providing high level of encouragement, and showing empathy towards the suicidal person, as well as being aware of high-risk groups such as senior citizens living with chronic diseases, persons suffering from neglect, family assault, and sexual abuse, those with frequent suicide attempts, and individuals with mental disorders. Finally, an important way for others to help suicidal people is to develop a safety strategy. In this context, the helper should set up an agreement with the suicidal person, including advising against dying by suicide and against consuming drugs and alcohol, and to follow the safety strategy. The guidelines recommend that family members and significant elders should be involved in assisting suicidal persons.[30]

The WHO[31] recommended several interventions for persons with risk factors for suicide, including communities providing support and making appropriate and organized referrals to help those at risk of suicide. These interventions have been shown to be effective in reducing the rate of suicide mortality, along with training and education delivered to health care providers, especially emergency care workers. The most important aspect for implementation is ensuring strong psychological support from health care workers in order to provide comprehensive assistance to people with suicidal thoughts and behaviour. Suicide prevention training for health care workers can be undertaken frequently in a year that focuses on objective skills, including improvement in mental health literacy, collaboration among mental health experts, and interviewing competencies.[31] Furthermore, densely populated countries, such as China, India, and Indonesia, have very limited suicidal prevention education and training, although there is a clear need for suicide prevention.[16]

In Indonesia, health care workers could be in the front line to deliver the suicide prevention programme by working in community health centres as they have direct interaction with suicidal people. The religious approach can be used as an effective preventive method for people at risk of self-injury or even suicide. The legislation to restrict alcohol consumption should be strengthened, not only because consumption of alcohol is prohibited in Islam, but also because this would reduce the risk of suicidal behaviour. Other protective measures should be encouraged, including improving cognitive style and personality, strengthening family support, adopting a positive cultural perspective, and improving social and environmental factors for suicide prevention. Addressing cognitive style and personality includes building a high confidence level, improving communication skills, learning how to seek and access assistance if problems arise, and willingness to learn. Family and social factors include having a significant relationship with family and surrounding people, friends, and peers, and receiving family care and support, as well as community support such as from work and sports companions. Environmental factors include good nutritional intake and sufficient sleep, physical activities, sunlight exposure, and no alcohol consumption or smoking.[15] Overall, it can be concluded that suicide plans and suicide attempts can be prevented by using a collaborative approach involving families, village networks, mental health workers, and other health services in Indonesia.

The suicide cases of Gunung Kidul

The District of Gunung Kidul has attracted significant attention due to its significantly high completed suicide rates in Indonesia. The district, which is part of Jogjakarta Province, was reported to have approximately nine suicide cases per 100,000 population,[32] whereas another report estimated a suicide rate of 4.48 cases per 100,000 population.[33] The reported rate was significantly higher than the national suicide rate of 3.4 cases per 100,000 population. Another study found that from 2012 to 2019, there were 242 cumulative completed suicides, suggesting an annual rate of about 30 cases in a population of approximately 736,000 inhabitants in Gunung Kidul.[34]

The high suicide rates in Gunung Kidul have been linked with several factors, including individual, social, and financial factors, physical sickness, and local myths and beliefs. With respect to individual factors, the people of Gunung Kidul tend to be introverted and see it challenging to find the solution to their problems. They tend to keep their problem to themselves and not to share with others.[35] Furthermore, a high rate of depression has also been suggested as another contributor to the high suicide rates in Gunung Kidul.[36] Various social conditions contribute to higher suicide rates among the elderly; for example, many elderly persons live far away from their children who have moved to big cities for better job opportunities or for other reasons, thus leaving the elderly in the remote areas of Gunung Kidul. Some also suffer from chronic physical illness and choose suicide to end their suffering. Most elderly people work as farmers in remote areas, which might hinder them from accessing health information and mental health services. Working as a farmer also provides only lower-than-average incomes. Farmers at times experience crop failure, a situation that generally affects family incomes and increases their stress level, which can lead to suicide.[35] The local myth belief of '*pulung gantung*' has also been investigated and reported to be a possible contributing factor to the high suicide rates in Gunung Kidul.[35,37]

Pulung gantung is a myth believed mostly by the elderly population in Gunung Kidul as an act of suicide. The term *pulung gantung* originates from Javanese, the local language of the Gunung Kidul population. *Pulung* means revelation, guidance, or grace, whereas *gantung* means hanging or suicide by hanging oneself. Locals interpret the term *pulung gantung* as a revelation to commit suicide by hanging oneself.[37,38] *Pulung gantung* is marked by the appearance of a meteor-tailed fireball in the middle of the night. The fireball is a sign of death. When a house is hit by the fireball, the occupants of that house will hang themselves.[39]

Furthermore, the myth of *pulung gantung* is also believed to be 'contagious', spreading to other people. The positioning of the deceased individual's face in cases of suicide by hanging could potentially signify a precursor to future suicide occurrences. To stop this, people usually dig into the ground below the hanging victim. By digging into the ground, people believe that the spread of the 'outbreak' can be stopped.[37] The fact that hanging oneself is the most common, and practically the only, method of suicide in Gunung Kidul[39] is also consistent with a recent report that suggested that hanging oneself is the most common suicide method in Indonesia.[20] The Indonesian mass media use the word suicide synonymously with self-hanging, or *gantung diri*, again reflecting hanging as a common method of suicide used in the country.

Conclusion

Up till 2023, there have been no large, representative, autopsy-based epidemiological studies or reports on suicide rates and suicidal behaviour conducted in Indonesia. Most epidemiological reports are based on estimating or projecting the number of suicidal cases in Indonesia. Indonesia's suicide rate is comparatively lower than that of other countries with high levels of human development. As a Muslim-majority country, Islamic beliefs contribute to this relatively lower suicide rate in Indonesia, together with good social support within the community and close kinship within the family. Nevertheless, local beliefs, such as the myth of *pulung gantung*, consider suicide as part of the local culture. Talking about suicide is also considered taboo by some people, whereas the act of suicide itself is considered a disgrace by the family. Last, but not least, suicide prevention and mental health promotion, in general, have been poor and need further improvement.

References

1. **World Health Organization**. *Suicide in the World: Global Health Estimates*. Geneva: World Health Organization; 2019.
2. **World Health Organization**. *Global Health Observatory Data Repository: Suicide Rate Estimates, Crude Estimates by Bountry*. Geneva: World Health Organization; 2018.
3. **Indonesian Ministry of Health.** *Pedoman Pencegahan dan Penanganan Bunuh Diri.* Jakarta: Ministry of Health; 2021.

4. **Nurjannah R, Kusumadewi A** (2017). Di Balik Angka Bunuh Diri. Available from: https://kumparan.com
5. **Riset Kesehatan Dasar (RISKESDAS)**, 2019. Laporan Nasional Riskesdas 2018. Badan Penelit. dan Pengemb. Kesehat. Ris. doi:1 Desember 2013. https://layanandata.kemkes.go.id/katalog-data/riskesdas/ketersediaan-data/riskesdas-2018
6. **Lie H, Liou J.** Suicide behavior among hunior high school students in Philippines and Indonesia associated with the social factors. GSTF Journal of Biosciences. 2012;**2**:92–7. doi:10.5176/2251-3140_2.1.28
7. **Peltzer K, Yi S, Pengpid S.** Suicidal behaviors and associated factors among university students in six countries in the Association of Southeast Asian Nations (ASEAN). Asian Journal of Psychiatry. 2017;**26**:32–8. doi:10.1016/j.ajp.2017.01.019
8. **Tresno F, Ito Y, Mearns J.** Self-injurious behavior and suicide attempts among Indonesian college students. Death Studies. 2012;**36**:627–39. doi:10.1080/07481187.2011.604464
9. **Gratz KL.** Measurement of deliberate self-harm: preliminary data on the deliberate self-harm inventory. Journal of Psychopathology and Behavioral Assessment. 2001;**23**:253–63. doi:10.1023/A:1012779403943
10. **Putra IGNE, Karin PAES, Ariastuti NLP.** Suicidal ideation and suicide attempt among Indonesian adolescent students. International Journal of Adolescent Medicine and Health. 2019;**33**(5):1–12. doi:10.1515/ijamh-2019-0035
11. **Amir N, Antoni R, Asmarahadi A**, et al. Rates and risk factors for suicide ideas among schizophrenia patients in Indonesia. Open Access Macedonian Journal of Medical Sciences. 2019;7:2579–82. doi:10.3889/oamjms.2019.393
12. **Maramis MM, Pantouw JG, Lesmana CBJ.** Depression screening in Surabaya Indonesia: urgent need for better mental health care for high-risk communities and suicide prevention for men. International Journal of Social Psychiatry. 2021 Aug;**67**(5):421–31. doi: 10.1177/0020764020957359
13. **Pratiwi D, Perdana AS.** Circuit of culture: advocating suicide prevention and eradication of mental illness associated stigma through 'Into The Light Indonesia' campaign. EXPOSE—Jurnal Ilmu Komunikasi. 2019;**2**(**1**):191. doi:10.33021/exp.v2i2.959
14. **Stenbacka M, Jokinen J.** Violent and non-violent methods of attempted and completed suicide in Swedish young men: the role of early risk factors. BMC Psychiatry. 2015;**15**:1–9. doi:10.1186/s12888-015-0570-2
15. **Nock M.** *Oxford Handbook of Suicide and Self-injury*. Oxford: Oxford University Press; 2014.
16. **Chen YY, Chien-Chang Wu K, Yousuf S, Yip PSF.** Suicide in Asia: opportunities and challenges. Epidemiologic Reviews. 2012;34(1):129–44. doi:10.1093/epirev/mxr025
17. **Ajdacic-Gross V, Weiss MG, Ring M,** et al. Methods of suicide: international suicide patterns derived from the WHO mortality database. Bulletin of the World Health Organization. 2008;**86**:726–32. doi:10.2471/BLT.07.043489
18. **Conner KR, Huguet N, Caetano R,** et al. Acute use of alcohol and methods of suicide in a US national sample. American Journal of Public Health. 2013;**104**:171–8. doi:10.2105/AJPH.2013.301352
19. **Rustamdji H.** Some characteristics of suicide in Jakarta. Bulletin Penelitian Kesehatan. 1974;2(2):39–41.

20. **Nisa N, Arifin M, Nur MF, Adella S, Marthoenis M.** Indonesian online newspaper reporting of suicidal behavior: compliance with World Health Organization media guidelines. International Journal of Social Psychiatry. 2020;66(3):259–62. doi:10.1177/0020764020903334
21. **Arafat SMY, Menon V, Bascarane S, Kar SK, Kabir R.** Variations in newspaper reporting of suicidal behavior in the WHO–South-East Asian region. Journal of Public Health (Bangkok). 2021;**43**(4):e684–e688. doi:10.1093/pubmed/fdaa139
22. **Menon V, Kaliamoorthy C, Sridhar VK**, et al. Do Tamil newspapers educate the public about suicide? Content analysis from a high suicide Union Territory in India. International Journal of Social Psychiatry. 2020;66(8):785–91. doi:10.1177/0020764020933296
23. **Marthoenis M, Akter H, Arafat SMY.** Quality of Thai media reporting of suicidal behavior: compliance against the World Health Organization media guidelines. Neurology, Psychiatry and Brain Research. 2020;**38**:39–42. doi:10.1016/j.npbr.2020.09.003
24. **Sisask M, Varnik A.** Media roles in suicide prevention: a systematic review. International Journal of Environmental Research and Public Health. 2012;**9**:123–38.
25. **Ghotbi S, Bozorgmehr A, Razian S.** Suicide from the perspective of Islam and psychology with an emphasize on the models explaining the relationship between impulsivity and suicidal behaviors. International Journal of Multicultural and Multireligious Understanding. 2019;**6**:117. doi:10.18415/ijmmu.v6i3.776
26. **Shah A, Chandia M.** The relationship between suicide and Islam: a cross-national study. Journal of Injury and Violence Research. 2010;**2**:93–7. doi:10.5249/jivr.v2i2.60
27. **Marthoenis M, Yessi S, Aichberger MC, Schouler-Ocak M.** Mental health in Aceh, Indonesia: a decade after the devastating tsunami 2004. Asian Journal of Psychiatry. 2016;**19**:59–65. doi:10.1016/j.ajp.2016.01.002
28. **Rodrigo A, McQjillin A, Pimm J.** Effect of the 2004 tsunami on suicide rates in Sri Lanka. Psychiatric Bulletin. 2009;**33**:179–80. doi:10.1192/pb.bp.108.020743
29. **Eskin M.** Suicidal behavior in the Mediterranean countries. Clinical Practice and Epidemiology in Mental Health. 2020;**16**:93–100. doi:10.2174/1745017902016010093
30. **Center for Public Mental Health**. *Suicide First Aid Guidelines for Indonesia, UGM.* Jogjakarta: Universitas Gadjah Mada; 2020.
31. **World Health Organization**. *Preventing Suicide: A Global Imperative.* Geneva: World Health Organization; 2014.
32. **Rochmawati I.** Nglalu: melihat fenomena bunuh diri dengan hati. Jogjakarta: Jejak Kata Kita; 2009.
33. **Wirasto RT.** Suicide prevention in Indonesia: providing public advocacy. Japan Medical Association Journal. 2012;**55**(1):98–104.
34. **Nurdiyanto FA, Jaroah S.** The characteristics of suicide in Gunungkidul Indonesia. Disease Prevention and Public Health Journal. 2020;**14**:69. doi:10.12928/dpphj.v14i2.2027
35. **Mulyani AA, Eridiana W.** Faktor-Faktor Yang Melatarbelakangi Fenomena Bunuh Diri Di Gunungkidul. Sosietas. 2019;**8**:510–16. doi:10.17509/sosietas.v8i2.14593
36. **Anggraeny K.** Factors causing the increase of suicide in Gunungkidul Regency. Advances in Social Science, Education and Humanities Research. 2019;**317**:134–8. doi:10.2991/iconprocs-19.2019.27

37. **Budiarto S, Sugiarto R, Putrianti FG.** The psychological dynamic of a pulung gantung suicide survivor in Gunung Kidul. Jurnal Psikologi Ulayat. 2020;8(2):174–94. https://doi.org/10.24854/jpu112
38. **Darmaningtyas.** Pulung gantung: menyingkap tragedi bunuh diri di Gunungkidul. Yogyakarta: Salwa Press; 2002.
39. **Fahrudin A.** Fenomena bunuh diri di Gunung Kidul: Catatan tersisa dari Lapangan. Informasi. 2012;**17**(**1**):13–19.

Chapter 16

Suicide scripts of the Nacirema (aka American)

Silvia Sara Canetto

The anthropologist has become so familiar with the diversity of ways in which different peoples behave in similar situations that he is not apt to be surprised by even the most exotic customs. In fact, if all of the logically possible combinations of behavior have not been found somewhere in the world, he is apt to suspect that they must be present in some yet undescribed tribe .... In this light, the magical beliefs and practices of the Nacirema present such unusual aspects that it seems desirable to describe them as an example of the extremes to which human behavior can go. (p. 503)[1]

Many years ago, in an article entitled 'Body ritual among the Nacirema' (American spelt backwards), Miner[1] gave a satirical account of Nacirema/American body-cleaning and body-healing beliefs and rituals from the point of view of a fictional visiting anthropologist. By reversing assumptions on what is normal, and by applying dominant anthropology's gaze and language to 'America', Miner made visible the cultural nature of Nacirema/American beliefs and practices.

Taking Miner's article as a model, in this chapter I provide an account of what dominant Nacirema/American suicide patterns and beliefs may look like from the point of view of an imaginary outsider. Through a playful reversal of perspectives, I aim to engage readers, particularly Nacirema/American readers, into recognizing how in 'America', as everywhere, suicide is a deeply cultural act. This perspective-reversal exercise is also to remind us that science is grounded in culture. Scientists' research interests, questions, methods, and interpretations are shaped by their culture.[2]

This chapter starts with a terminology section. It then describes cultural-scripts-of-gender-and-suicide theory, the framework of this analysis. Next is an account of dominant Nacirema/American suicide scripts as if narrated by an imaginary visitor. In this section, Nacirema/American women's and men's suicide patterns by age and 'race', and dominant Nacirema/American beliefs about these suicide patterns are examined in light of Nacirema/American scripts of femininity and masculinity. The chapter ends with a discussion of the necessity of a cultural perspective in suicide theory, research, and prevention, especially in relation to dominant 'American' suicide theory, research, and prevention, because of how rarely dominant 'American' suicide theory, research, and prevention are the focus of cultural analysis.

Terminology

In this chapter, the term American/Nacirema refers to the United States (US)—and specifically, to US dominant culture. I am aware that the word 'American' also describes the American continent; and that to use the term 'American' for the US renders invisible all other American-continent countries and people, including, for example, the Naidanac (Canadian spelt backwards). The rationale for using here the word American/Nacirema in reference to the US is to connect with Miner's 1956 article.

The suicidality language of this chapter (i.e. non-fatal suicidal behaviour and fatal suicidal behaviour/suicide) is language that I have been using since the 1990s,[3,4] and that only recently is getting established in the field.[5] It is language that avoids the judgemental stance and the gender biases of dominant terminology like 'attempted', 'failed', 'completed', and 'successful' suicide. A problem with the dominant terminology is that it defines surviving a suicidal act as a failure. Calling a death by suicide a 'completed' suicide glorifies killing oneself. The expressions 'attempted suicide' and 'completed suicide' make it difficult to conceive of non-fatal suicidal acts as more successful coping than fatal suicidal acts because fatal suicidal acts represent a failure to survive. These expressions also make it difficult to think of non-fatal suicidal behaviour as courageous behaviour, especially in communities where surviving a suicidal act is stigmatized. With regard to gender biases, it is noteworthy that in the US, where expressions like 'successful suicide' and 'failed suicide' have been widely used, men typically 'succeed' whereas women 'fail' at suicide (for critical analyses of suicide terminology, see Canetto[5,6,7] and Canetto and Lester).[8,9]

Cultural scripts of suicide theory

The framework of this analysis is cultural-scripts-of-gender-and-suicide theory.[5,10,11,12,13,14] This theory builds on the observation that everywhere suicidal behaviour is culturally patterned and regulated. Individuals tend to engage in behaviours that are expected of people like themselves, in their culture.

There is consistency, *within cultures*, in the frequency, forms, and contexts of suicidal behaviours; and there is variability, *across cultures*, in the frequency, forms, and contexts of suicidal behaviours. These within-culture regularities and cross-culture variations are grounded in the suicide scripts of the different cultures.[5,10,12]

A suicide script includes the typical forms and outcomes of the suicidal behaviour (e.g. non-fatal or fatal) to which different people orient as well as the conditions under which the suicidal behaviour typically occurs in a particular community (e.g. the events associated with the suicidal behaviour). The suicide script also involves the characteristics (e.g. sex, age) of the typical suicidal person, the typical suicide methods, and common emotions and motives expressed by, or ascribed to the suicidal person. Furthermore, a suicide script comprises the typical responses to the suicidal behaviour—from the reactions of family and friends to the actions of professional caretakers and community authorities.[10,11,12,15]

The scripts of suicidal behaviour, like the scripts of other behaviours (e.g. the scripts of sexual behaviour), are both descriptive and prescriptive. People implicitly draw upon their culture's suicide scripts, in their choice of when, where, and how to engage in suicidal behaviour. As a result, everywhere suicidal acts have cultural features, meanings, and impact.[10,11,12,15]

The scripts of suicidal behaviour of a culture are not necessarily consistent with the scripts of related behaviours in the same culture. For example, the American/Nacirema scripts of suicidal behaviours are not consistent with the American/Nacirema scripts of depression, even though the American/Nacirema believe that suicidality and depression are related. The American/Nacirema view suicide as a masculine act and death; and depression, together with 'attempted' and 'failed' suicide, as feminine behaviours.[5,10]

The scripts of suicidal behaviour of a culture are not static. Like the scripts of other behaviours, suicide scripts change as the culture changes.

Multiple suicide scripts often coexist in a culture. Some scripts are dominant and other scripts are less common.[10,11,12,15]

The rest of this chapter is written from the point of view of an imaginary visitor of Nacirema/American society. It narrates how an outsider may view dominant Nacirema/American suicide attitudes, beliefs, and practices.

Women and men in Nacirema society

The Nacirema have very peculiar beliefs about women and men, and very strange and contradictory gender norms and practices.

On the one hand, the Nacirema perform rituals that they claim demonstrate (and that could give the impression to outsiders) that women have high status in their society. For example, men are expected to open doors to women. Men are also expected to pull out chairs for women, out of courtesy, in the formal eating areas that the Nacirema call restaurants.[16]

When it comes down to things that matter, however, in Nacirema society women are profoundly discriminated against.[17] Specifically, Nacirema women have substantially lower status and power in the community and in the family, and significantly fewer material and social resources than Nacirema men. For example, nearly all Nacirema chiefs are men. The dominant Nacirema divinity is male and so are most of its shamans. Women spend substantially more time than men taking care (physically, emotionally, and socially) of their kin. At the same time, women have significantly lower access than men to what the Nacirema need for survival and to what they value—for example, money (i.e. special metal, paper, and plastic that the Nacirema use for trade) and material things (e.g. shelter and land, which, among the Nacirema, are by ownership). Women have also considerably less time for themselves. In Nacirema society, women cannot even count on being safe, in their dwellings and outside, because of rampant physical and sexual violence perpetrated against them by Nacirema men, both family and strangers.

Nacirema men control the creation and transmission of community myths and stories. Nearly all Nacirema community myths and stories have men as protagonists. The cultural informants that the Nacirema view as authoritative (and whose opinion is easily accessible to outsiders like me) are men. Given the dominance of men in authority and communication roles, most of what is reported here is from the point of view of Nacirema men.

Finally, a few comments about Nacirema's attitudes and beliefs about culture. I am aware that all people have difficulties in understanding culture—others' and their own. No one holds an objective view of their own culture. Also, perceptions of other cultures are shaped by one's culture.[i]

[i] Of course, the statement about the difficulties in understanding culture, others' and one's own, applies to me as well. Who knows what cultural biases you will catch in my account. Or how I will react to the ideas expressed in this piece, a few years from now, when, with the benefit of time, my cultural frameworks will be less invisible to me.

Still, the Nacirema appear uniquely oblivious to their culture. Most speak only one language: Hsilgne. When asked why, they often say they cannot learn other languages, that other people's languages are difficult, and that, anyway, most outsiders speak Hsilgne. Given these attitudes and behaviours, the Nacirema tend to know less about other cultures than the other way around. The Nacirema also seem unaware of how peculiar their culture appears to outsiders. Many Nacirema insist that they do not have a culture, that they are just people—though they also seem to think of themselves as culturally superior people. At the same time, the Nacirema believe that non-Nacirema people are immersed in culture, and that all people, except them, are ruled by culture.

Suicidality among Nacirema adolescents and young adults

A gender paradox of suicide has been observed among Nacirema adolescents and young adults. Girls and young women have high rates of suicidal ideation and behaviour but low mortality by suicide, whereas boys and young men have low rates of suicidal thinking and behaviour but high suicide mortality. This pattern is a paradox because higher engagement in a life-threatening behaviour is usually associated with both higher morbidity and higher mortality by that behaviour.[14]

The Nacirema think that the gender paradox of suicide results from inborn differences in women's and men's needs, motivations, emotions, and behaviour. Consistent with this idea, in Nacirema language, women and men are referred to as opposite sex. The Nacirema are so convinced that women and men are psychological opposites that they do not seem to notice that the gender-paradox-of-suicide pattern is not universal, even in their community. For example, the gender-paradox-of-suicide pattern does not describe the suicidality of Nacirema older adult women and men. To the non-Nacirema, it is obvious that the gender paradox of suicide is a culturally determined pattern—and one of the many signs of the influence of Nacirema gender ideologies on Nacirema suicidality.[14]

Suicidality among Nacirema girls and young adult women

The Nacirema[ii] have very strange ideas about women. They think that women are inferior to men. For example, they believe that women are, by nature,

[ii] To be precise, I should say 'Nacirema men', not 'the Nacirema', because the very strange ideas described here are Nacirema men's ideas. There are indications that Nacirema women

emotionally and mentally weaker than men. They also assume that women will fail at whatever they do.

The Nacirema have a long tradition of viewing non-fatal suicidal behaviour as a weak, feminine act—and a kind of failure. '[S]uicidal gestures [*sic*] are an expected, and even socially sanctioned behavior in unhappy women,' wrote Neuringer and Lettieri (p. 22).[18] Consistent with these beliefs, the Nacirema call non-fatal suicidal acts 'unsuccessful' suicides—even though the outcome of non-fatal suicidal behaviour is life. Nacirema women are expected to 'fail' at suicide, and at the same time, they are derided for 'failing' to kill themselves. The Nacirema do not seem to appreciate the courage it takes to survive a suicidal act, given the dislike that suicide 'attempters' experience. It is clear that in Nacirema society women are not taken seriously, even when suicidal.[19,20,21]

Among the Nacirema women's suicide is considered an aberration. The Nacirema view female suicide as more wrong, more foolish, weaker, and less permissible than male suicide, independent of precipitant.[23] Women who kill themselves are believed to be more maladjusted than men who kill themselves, independent of suicide context.[24] In other words, the Nacirema assume that only emotionally-disturbed, bad women kill themselves—though they think that normal, good men may suicide, when they experience serious adversities. In Nacirema society, a normal, good woman is a woman whose life centres on serving men (including doing all household and childcare work) in exchange for men's support for material survival. According to Dublin, a Nacirema authority on suicide, women who have 'greater economic and social independence' are at suicide risk. Dublin also stated that women who take their lives must have experienced a 'marked increase in . . . schooling and employment' (p. 23).[25] Consistent with Dublin's ideas, some Nacirema men believe that most women are 'incapable' of suicide—meaning that women are unable to conceive and enact a 'successful' suicide. In their view, only men can intentionally take their lives. Suicide is something that the Nacirema think only men, in fact, only superior (e.g. high-status) men are capable of—because presumably only men can overcome the survival instinct. The Nacirema are so certain that women are incapable of intentional suicide that when a female suicide occurs, they often dismiss the suicide as an accident—a woman's miscalculation of method lethality and/or of rescue plans, and a symptom of women's ineptness.[26,27]

do not endorse these beliefs. For example, a Nacirema woman wrote that 'suicide attempts are the grand rites of "femininity" ... [because] women are supposed to "lose" in order to "win." Women who succeed [sic] at suicide are, tragically, outwitting or rejecting their "feminine" role, and at the only price possible, their death' (p. 49).[22]

The Nacirema's negative views of women who kill themselves likely are a social deterrent to female suicide. In other words, the female suicide stigma probably contributes to Nacirema women's low suicide mortality, relative to their number of suicidal acts, and independent of suicide method. The female suicide stigma likely also biases Nacirema's determination of causes of women's death in the direction of undercounting female suicides. Evidence in support of this idea first came from observations of the Naidanac, a community with a social organization similar to that of the Nacirema. Among the Naidanac, there were more undetermined deaths among women than among men.[14] An undetermined death is a death whose cause cannot be established. Recently, similar observations have been made among the Nacirema.[28]

The Nacirema[iii] have a long history of thinking that women's suicidal behaviour is triggered by relatively ordinary psychological and relationship problems. In Nacirema culture, women are believed to be especially likely to engage in suicidal behaviour when they experience 'love' problems, that is, when they have difficulties and losses in their intimate relationships with men (for a full account of this long-standing Nacirema gender myth of suicide, see Canetto).[5,10,21,26] For example, Wold stated that women become suicidal when they are 'discarded by a lover or husband' (p. 21)[29] (for similar ideas, see also Schrut and Michel).[30] Consistent with these notions, the Nacirema describe women's suicidal behaviour as hysterical,[29,30,31] manipulative,[32,33] masochistic,[34] and as the symptom of a dependent[35] or borderline personality[32,36]—rather than an expression of legitimate despair, as the Nacirema view men's suicidal behaviour.[iv]

Many Nacirema think that women's suicidal behaviour is not 'serious'. What the Nacirema consider non-serious is a suicidal act with contrasting motives—for example, a wish to die and a wish to survive.[5,10,19,20,21] The Nacirema

---

[iii] It would be more accurate to say here 'Nacirema men', instead of 'the Nacirema', because the very strange ideas described here are ideas conceived and spread primarily by Nacirema men.

[iv] A different narrative of women's suicidal behaviour is offered by two Nacirema women.[35] Like many Nacirema men, Kaplan and Klein believe that women's suicidal behaviour is a response to relationship problems, and a 'plea for mutual engagement' (p. 260). However, Kaplan and Klein do not view the plea as a symptom of manipulative dependence. For them, the plea for connection is a manifestation of women's 'interacting sense of self'. 'Women will act so as to preserve a relationship, not because of dependency on the other or inadequacy in other realms, but because connection provides them with the fullest context for their own active participation in a growth enhancing situation,' they state (p. 259). The problem, according to them, is that suicidal women often seek 'connection with others in a context that is neither mutual nor empathic. Their behavior is often experienced as controlling by those who, for their own reasons, need to resist it' (p. 271).

assume that only women experience mixed motives when suicidal, presumably because women are weak, mentally and physically.

The Nacirema's deep-rooted belief that women become suicidal when their lover or husband leaves them, presumably because women are emotionally incapable to survive without a man, is inconsistent with what is known about women, at least by the non-Nacirema. Women are not naturally dependent on men, whether emotionally or materially. Among the Nacirema, however, women are expected to centre their lives on men. They are socialized, and in many cases, given no choice but to rely on men for their material survival. Nacirema women who do not conform to this femininity script are socially and materially penalized. Conforming to the femininity script, however, has costs for Nacirema women. Among the costs are depression and suicidality. Suicidality is less common in Nacirema women who step out, at least in part, of the dominant femininity script, and who achieve some social and material independence via participation in what the Nacirema call the paid labour force.[35,36,37,38,39,40] To a non-Nacirema, it is obvious why this is the case. Being in the labour force expands women's social networks beyond the family domain, and with that, their possibilities for personal expression, learning and accomplishment, and sources of meaning and purpose.[40] Few Nacirema, particularly Nacirema men, seem to realize (or perhaps few Nacirema men are willing to consider) the value of paid labour force participation for women's well-being, and as protection against suicide. Most Nacirema men seem to assume that paid work is men's work. They appear to think that only men benefit from (and many think that men actually require) participation in the paid labour force for their well-being, and as a way to prevent suicide.[10,41]

Another odd belief of the Nacirema is that poisoning is a quintessentially feminine suicide method (e.g. see McAndrew and Garrison).[42] This belief is understandable, given that Nacirema women use poisoning in suicide more frequently than Nacirema men. Many Nacirema do not seem to be aware of the fact that in other cultures poisoning is a top suicide method among both men and women. The Nacirema have other strange ideas about suicide by poisoning. For example, they consider poisoning a non-violent method. Some Nacirema even believe that women use poisoning in suicide because they are vain—supposedly because women think that poisoning preserves their beauty post-mortem (for a critique of this idea, see Canetto[5,7]). The Nacirema are so convinced that poisoning is women's first-choice suicide method that they do not seem to realize that in their own community, firearms are the method most used by women in suicide. Many Nacirema also appear unaware of the fact that poisoning is a less common suicide method than suffocation among young Nacirema women.[43,v]

Suicidality among Nacirema boys and young adult men

The Nacirema[vi] have very odd ideas about men. They think that men are superior to women. For example, they believe that men are more emotionally strong, courageous, and rational than women. The Nacirema also assume that men will succeed at whatever they do, or that they have to succeed—to prove themselves different from, and superior to, women.

Likely because of their strange ideas about men, and because suicide is more common among Nacirema boys and men than among Nacirema girls and women, the Nacirema believe that suicide is a strong masculine act. This belief has been in place for a long time.[28,44] The Nacirema do not seem to consider the influence, on men's suicidal behaviour, of their culture's masculinity beliefs. In their society, there is social pressure on men to die, once they engage in a suicidal act, because surviving a suicidal act (an unsuccessful suicide, as they call it) is considered unmanly.[6,15,45] Men who survive a suicidal act are considered fools. 'Just make sure you do it right the first time, cause nothing's worse than a suicide chump,' sang Nacirema bard Frank Zappa.[46,47,vii]

The Nacirema's long-standing negative views of men who survive a suicidal act (e.g. see Neuringer and Lettieri)[18] probably contribute to the low number of non-fatal suicidal acts by men, relative to the number of men's deaths by suicide, and independent of suicide method. The social pressure against surviving a suicidal act likely makes men selective about when to engage in suicidal behaviour. It likely prevents men from allowing themselves room for survival once they engage in suicidal behaviour.[6,15,46] At the same time, the Nacirema's stigma about male non-fatal suicidal behaviour probably interferes with the Nacirema's ability to recognize, and to keep accurate records of, men's 'failed suicide attempts'. Among the Nacirema, a majority of presumably non-suicidal, non-fatal drug overdoses involve men. It is likely that a proportion of these non-fatal overdoses (and a proportion of other, presumably non-suicidal life-threatening

---

[v] This pattern, however, may be an artefact of suicide misclassification. Suffocation suicides are easier for the Nacirema to recognize than suicides by poisoning.[44]

[vi] Here as well, it would be more accurate to say 'Nacirema men', instead of 'the Nacirema', because the very strange ideas described in this section are Nacirema men's ideas.

[vii] A longer sample of the lyrics of Zappa's song *Suicide Chump* is: 'You say there ain't no use in livin', it's all a waste of time, and you wanna throw your life away. Well people that's just fine. Go ahead on and get it over with then. Find you a bridge and take a jump. Just make sure you do it right the first time, 'cause nothing's worse than a suicide chump'.[47]

behaviours, like drinking and driving, in which men especially engage) are unrecognized male suicide 'attempts'.[28,48]

The Nacirema have a history of thinking that men's suicidal behaviour is an extreme, but relatively justified and relatively understandable response to extraordinary impersonal adversities. The impersonal adversities that the Nacirema believe bring normal, good men to suicide are social and economic problems (e.g. unemployment, and what the Nacirema call an economic recession) and physical-health problems (for a full account of this long-standing Nacirema gender myth of suicide, see Canetto).[5,10,15,26] For these reasons, the Nacirema think that men's suicides are deaths of legitimate despair.

The Nacirema assume that men's suicidal behaviour is deliberate and planned (i.e. not impulsive and not 'emotional', as they believe women's suicidal behaviour is). Furthermore, they think that most male suicidal behaviour is 'serious', which they define as unambivalently aimed at death.[6,10,15] The Nacirema believe that suicidal men do not have contrasting motives because the Nacirema associate single-mindedness with sharpness and toughness—and men presumably are the mentally sharper and tougher sex. Nacirema reports about men who killed themselves, however, indicate that around the time of their suicide these men were not particularly sharp of mind or emotionally tough. Rather, they appeared cognitively impaired (e.g. rigid in their thinking) and emotionally fragile. Also, many men who took their life did not seem burdened by extraordinary adversities. It is therefore possible that cognitive and emotional rigidity contributed to these men's suicide, specifically, to their viewing suicide as the only solution to relatively ordinary life challenges.[49,50,51,52]

The Nacirema's deep-rooted belief that men become suicidal when they experience extraordinary impersonal adversities, and that private relationship problems do not matter in men's suicide, is inconsistent with what is known about men, at least, by the non-Nacirema. A reason for this belief is that Nacirema men are valued based on their status in impersonal domains (e.g. their status and power in the community; their material possessions) and also based on their body's strength.[53] Men who do not conform to this masculinity script are socially and materially penalized. Living by the masculinity script gives Nacirema men many advantages but also has costs, including in terms of suicide. Suicide mortality has been found to be lower among Nacirema men who do not conform, at least in part, with the dominant masculinity script, for example, men who do at least some family care work. The suicide protection enjoyed by men who do family care work was maintained during periods of high unemployment (unemployment is a situation that the Nacirema believe drives men to suicide).[54] To a non-Nacirema, it is clear why this is the case. Doing family care work expands men's social networks beyond the employment domain. It broadens their possibilities for personal expression, learning and accomplishment, and also their sources of meaning and purpose. Few Nacirema seem to be aware of (or perhaps, few are willing to consider) the value of men doing family care work (i.e. not just 'having' a family), for men's well-being and for reducing men's suicide vulnerability. Most Nacirema men appear to think that family care work is women's work. They seem to believe that family care work matters only for women's well-being, and in the prevention of women's suicide.[10,41]

Another odd belief of the Nacirema is that firearms are the masculine suicide method par excellence (e.g. see McAndrew and Garrison).[42] This view is likely because, among the Nacirema, firearms are by far the method most commonly used by men in suicide.[43] Many Nacirema do not appear to know that in a neighbouring community, the Naidanac, suffocation (not firearms) is the most common suicide method among men, as among women.[55] Suffocation is also the most common suicide method in Naidanac Tiuni hunting communities where firearms are easily accessible—a fact that suggests the importance, in method choice, of a method's cultural relevance, not just its physical accessibility.[56]

Suicidality among Nacirema older adults

The Nacirema hold negative stereotypes about ageing. Many think that ageing is all about loss. The Nacirema also have negative beliefs about older adults and about persons with illnesses and disabilities. Many think that having a major illness or a significant disability is a fate worse than death.[25,57] Consistent with these beliefs, the Nacirema have a long tradition of believing that it is normal, and even rational, for older adults to be suicidal: 'it is not strange that some old people wish to shake off the infirmities and the boredom of an unsatisfactory existence' via suicide, stated a Nacirema authority on suicide (p. 7).[25] The Nacirema think that suicide is more permissible for individuals who are older adults and for those with serious physical illnesses or disabilities.[58,59,60,61,62]

Given these views, it is not surprising that among the Nacirema, suicide is most common in older adults. Suicide rates, however, are not equally high across all Nacirema older adults. Nacirema older adult women have substantially lower suicide mortality than Nacirema older adult men. Older adults' likelihood of suicide also varies depending on what the Nacirema call 'race'.[viii] Older adult suicide mortality is highest among Etihw men, the highest-status-'race males'.[57]

[viii] The Nacirema believe that there are four kinds of human beings: Etihw, Kcalb, Nacirema-Naidni, and Naisa. These kinds, or 'races' as the Nacirema call them, are based on physical

Some Nacirema communities with a large Etihw population have established formal systems to assist people in killing themselves. In these communities, persons who are sick can receive assistance with carrying out a self-poisoning suicide, following a ritual of oral and written petitions and waiting periods (for an example of, and details about this practice, see Oregon Health Authority[64,65] and Death with Dignity[66]). Shamans decide who gets the poison to be used in the suicide. Access to the poison is granted to petitioners with an illness expected to end their life in six months—a period of time that the Nacirema consider short. The Nacirema cannot predict a sick-person's death six months in advance. Also, the shamans who determine the six-months life expectancy do not need to have experience with the illness of petitioners. My impression is that the six-months-of-life clause is a way to bring divination to the assisted suicide ritual. The Nacirema however believe that the six-months-of-life clause is a way to make the assisted-suicide process evidence-based, and therefore rational. The assisted-suicide system is consistent with Etihw people's belief that it is understandable and rational for sick persons to desire suicide. A major reason for Etihw's investment in assisted suicide is their concerns about excessive and futile care—specifically, about being kept alive by artificial means while in pain, and with no chance for recovery. Another reason is their preoccupation with having choices and control.[ix] Given these cultural values, Etihw people consider assisting in the suicide of sick persons an act of compassion. They also view the death by assisted suicide of sick persons as a choice-, control-, and dignity-affirming death.[x]

Given Etihw Nacirema's framing of assisted suicide, it is not surprising that autonomy and dignity are the most reported reasons for assisted-suicide requests, according to the shamans who approve the requests. Fears of being a burden is a reason recorded in about half of cases.[xi] By contrast, pain is reported as relevant only in about a quarter of cases.[67] It is noteworthy that the top reasons for assisted suicide involve social concerns. Physical-pain concerns do not drive assisted suicide—contrary to what assisted-suicide advocates argue.

features (e.g. hair texture) that are salient to the Nacirema. Nacirema people have substantially different status and resources, depending on the 'race' they are assigned. Their lives differ, depending on 'race' classification.[64]

ix 'Patient Choice and Control at the End of Life' is the name of the initiative that started the assisted-suicide system in the Nacirema community of Tnomrev.

x 'Death with dignity' is the expression used to refer to assisted suicide in several of the Nacirema communities where assisted suicide by poisoning is permitted and enabled.

xi Among the Nacirema, concerns about being a burden are not a disqualifying condition for physician-assisted suicide.

An implication of the framing of assisted suicide as a death-with-dignity for persons who are ill is that the lives of people with serious illnesses or disabilities are, by definition, undignified; and that their deaths are without dignity unless they are hastened.[68]

Most people who apply for, and die via the Nacirema's assisted-suicide system are older adults, and in similar proportion of women and men. Nearly all are Etihw.[69]

Non-Etihw Nacirema appear uninterested in assisted suicide. For example, a report of the opinions of family members of deceased individuals for whom assisted suicide was an option found that none of the Kcalb decedents had considered assisted suicide, as compared to 20 percent of the Etihw decedents.[70] A reason for the disinterest may be that Kcalb people do not fear excessive and futile care. In Nacirema society Kcalb people have to fight to stay alive. The situations that Kcalb women and men dread most, and that they strive to prevent, throughout their lives, are insufficient or bad-quality care and premature deaths from inadequate care.[68,71,72,73,74]

Suicidality among Nacirema older adult women

Among the Nacirema, women across 'races' represent a minority (about one-sixth) of older adult (non-assisted) suicides.[63] Older adult women, however, constitute half of assisted suicides.[69]

A reason for the discrepancy between women's mortality by unassisted versus assisted suicide may be that assisted suicide looks more like what the Nacirema consider feminine behaviour—and therefore a relatively acceptable way for a woman to end her life.[68] Assisted suicide is a suicide by application. Permission needs to be obtained to access the poison. The permission process involves ritualized and specifically-timed oral and written petitions. Having shamans as suicide arbiters strips the suicide of its independence and agency, and of its masculine connotation, at least based on Nacirema gender ideologies. Also, the Nacirema consider poisoning a feminine method.[68]

Etihw women's substantial representation among the decedents by assisted suicide, relative to non-Etihw women, is likely influenced by the mix of privilege and oppression that Etihw women experience. As members of the high-status 'race', Etihw women have more positive experiences with Nacirema medicine than non-Etihw women. Etihw women also live longer but in poorer health than Etihw men. Because Erihw men's morbidity and longevity patterns are taken as the norm in Nacirema society, Etihw women's longer but sicker lives may be viewed as excessive and burdensome—including by Etihw women, as a result of exposure to ideologies that elevate men over women.[75,76] Older adult Etihw women also have substantially more limited material resources than older adult Etihw men, due to norms and systems that favor men in paid work and unpaid family care work. Older adult Etihw women are less likely to have been in the paid labour force full-time and continuously than older adult Etihw men—and also relative to older adult Kcalb women. When they have children, Etihw women tend to leave the full-time paid labour force or go into part-time employment, to take care of the extra family care work. Furthermore, older adult Etihw women are more likely to be married than, for example, older adult Ckalb women. As a result of these differences, older adult Etihw women are more likely than older adult Etihw men, and also more likely than Kcalb women, to rely on material assets accumulated through marriage rather than individually (for a review, see Addo and Lichter).[77] A consequence is that older adult Etihw women may view themselves, and may be perceived by others, as not quite entitled to their family and community resources, even though Etihw women contribute a lifetime of unpaid care work to their family and community. Another experience that likely explains Etihw women having low entitlement to family and community resources, including medical care, is that Etihw women, like most women in Nacirema society, are socialized into low self-worth and into self-sacrifice.[68,78] Via assisted suicide, Etihw women relieve their families and society of the responsibility of their longevity and ill health.

Another likely reason for Etihw women's substantial representation among the decedents by assisted suicide, relative to non-Etihw women, is that assisted suicide is framed in ways that most resonate with Etihw women's experiences and concerns.[68] This includes the narrative that assisted suicide affirms the right to die,[79] and also the narrative that assisted suicide is a death of graceful determination.[80] An example of an Etihw-centred assisted-suicide narrative is found in statements by Girsh, a founder of an association advocating for hastened death: 'Having fought for choice for women in voting, reproductive rights, property ownership … [women] certainly know what they're doing when they fight for the right to have assistance in dying' (p. 289).[81] It is also relevant to Etihw women's substantial representation among the decedents by assisted suicide that Etihw women are the most common assisted-suicide spokespersons.

Suicidality among Nacirema older adult men

Among the Nacirema, men represent a substantial majority of older adult (unassisted) suicides and half of older adult assisted-suicides.[69] Etihw men have the highest suicide mortality of all older adults.[63]

As reported earlier, the Nacirema have long held the belief that older adult suicide is a response to what they describe as the losses and adversities of old age. In old age, '[i]mpairments are accumulated, particularly of chronic and painful diseases. Many older people suffer from … feelings of loneliness and futility as relations with family and friends and productive work drop off. Economic insecurity is often a serious problem, as is also inability or unwillingness to tolerate hardship,' said suicide authority Dublin (p. 22).[25] This explanation does not account for the uniquely-high suicide mortality of older adult Etihw men.

A problem with the loss-and-adversity explanation of older adult suicide is that as a group, older adult Etihw men, relative to older adult men of other 'races' and older adult women across 'races', are least likely to experience the ageing-related losses and adversities (e.g. chronic illnesses, functional disabilities, financial difficulties, widowhood, and living alone) that the Nacirema believe to be the cause of older adult suicide.[15]

There is reason to believe that cultural factors drive older adult Etihw men's high suicide rates. To start with, older adult Etihw men's suicide propensity is likely influenced by dominant scripts of ageing, masculinity, and suicide. As noted earlier, the Nacirema, and in particular Etihw Nacirema, think of suicide as a masculine act. They also view suicide as more permissible and understandable if it involves an older adult or someone with serious illnesses or disabilities.[58,59,60,61,62]

Another cultural factor contributing to older adult Etihw men's suicide mortality is the suicide method. Middle-aged and older adult Etihw men have the highest firearm suicide-rates and the highest firearm ownership.[15,82] Suicidal acts by firearms are more likely to be fatal than suicidal acts by poisoning, independent of intent.[83]

Cultural and psychological clues to older adult Etihw men's suicide vulnerability come from reports of the personality of suicide decedents. In these studies, the (mostly) Etihw, (mostly) older adult, and (mostly) male decedents were described as inflexible and closed to new experiences.[49,50,51,52] Culture plays a role in how personality develops, and in the specific forms of personality that women and men tend to be socialized into, based on their culture's ideologies of femininity and masculinity.[84,85]

Older adult men represent about half of assisted suicides in the Nacirema communities where assisted suicide is officially permitted. Nearly all of these assisted-suicide male decedents are Eithw.[69] Etihw men's dominance among the dead by assisted suicide, relative to men of other 'races,' may be accounted, at least in part, by Etihw men's experiences as the high-status 'race' and sex class. Assisted suicide is presented as a way to prevent excessive and futile medical care. Based on their higher status and greater resources, Eithw men are the group most likely to have access to sustained medical care—and therefore the group most likely to be trapped in excessive and futile medical care. At the same time, because of their high status, Eithw men have disadvantages and vulnerabilities when sick and older adult.[15,86] Etihw men might be less prepared than, for example, non-Etihw men, for the challenges that older age and ill health represent, in terms of the dominant script of masculinity. Up until late life, Etihw men have more chances than men of other 'races' to fulfil the Nacirema's script of masculinity as being in control. By contrast, as a result of racism, non-Etihw men have practice with compromises in masculinity control and dominance. It may be that Etihw men are interested in hastening their death, when older-adult and ill, because assisted suicide is framed as a way to be in charge—a masculinity imperative.[15,87] Via assisted suicide older adult Etihw men exert control over a major event, their death. Via assisted suicide they also expedite their own demise and erase themselves from the living—hardly a powerful outcome. Therefore, in the case of assisted suicide, the Nacirema's dominant script of masculinity as being in control contributes to paradoxical male behaviour.

Summary, implications, and conclusions

I have described here some of the curious suicide patterns, attitudes, beliefs, and practices of the Nacirema. Many of these patterns and practices are grounded on the Nacirema's peculiar ideas about women and men—for example, the idea that women and men are psychological opposites.

The Nacirema say that they want to reduce suicidality in their community. This commitment is evident in the substantial resources that they invest in understanding and preventing suicide. The Nacirema even have an initiative called 'Zero Suicide'. Its goal is to eliminate some suicides, specifically the suicide of individuals 'under the care of health and behavioral health systems'.[88]

Yet suicide mortality continues to increase among the Nacirema. By contrast, suicide mortality has been mostly flat or declining in other communities, including in communities that invest fewer resources in suicide studies and prevention.[89,90]

As noted earlier, Nacirema's suicide patterns vary greatly by sex, age, and 'race'. Nacirema men die at higher rates than Nacirema women. Older adults have the highest suicide mortality of all age groups. Among older adults, men classified as Etihw have the highest suicide mortality.[63]

There is, of course, no single explanation for the continuing growth in Nacirema suicide-rates; and there are no simple explanations for the patterns of suicide by sex, age, and 'race' observed among the Nacirema, relative to the suicide patterns by sex and age other communities. Everywhere suicide is a multidetermined act; and everywhere suicide is a culturally grounded act.

Of all explanations, the one that the Nacirema seem to especially overlook is their suicide culture—including their suicide attitudes, beliefs and practices.

The Nacirema, like other people, act based on the scripts of their culture. This applies to suicide as well. Nacirema women and men, like women and men everywhere, tend to adopt the suicidal behaviours (e.g. non-fatal vs fatal) that are congruent with the scripts of gender and suicide of their culture.[14]

What is most striking about the Nacirema's suicide culture, at least for an outsider, is its broad range of culturally permissible and even glorified suicides.[5,7,23,58,59,62,68,69,91,92,93] The Nacirema's inattention to their permissive suicide culture, and the possible role of their suicide culture in their growing rates of suicidality, is surprising because there are many Nacirema reports indicating that suicidal behaviour is more common in Nacirema communities and among types of individuals (e.g. men) with more permissive suicide attitudes and beliefs (e.g. see Phillips and Luth,[92] Joe et al.,[94] and Kleiman).[95]

To compensate for their tendency to overlook cultural influences in their suicide patterns, the Nacirema might find it valuable to privilege questions of culture in their suicidality studies and in their prevention initiatives. A focus on culture in Nacirema suicidality studies and prevention could include, for example, evaluating the role of the belief that 'attempting' suicide is expected (though presumably weak) feminine behaviour, in terms of enabling non-fatal suicidality in women. The Nacirema might also find it useful to consider how framing suicide as a masculine death, and as a relatively strong male response of legitimate despair in response to external adversities, might enable male suicide.

Nacirema communities committed to reducing suicidality might also assess and target for change their beliefs and practices about firearms. Among the Nacirema, most suicides are by firearms. Nacirema men's suicide mortality is inflated by men's high use of firearms in suicide. Ambivalent and impulsive suicidal acts by Nacirema men are fatal because of men's frequent use of firearms in suicide. Among the Nacirema, middle-aged and older adult Etihw men have the highest firearm suicide rates and the highest firearm ownership.[15,82] Also, gun ownership is growing in Nacirema communities.[96] Given the prominence of firearms in Nacirema suicide, restrictions in firearm access could go a long way in reducing suicide mortality among the Nacirema, especially among men, as demonstrated in various Nacirema studies.[97,98]

Finally, Nacirema communities invested in reducing suicidality might evaluate, and reconsider their assisted-suicide culture—including their assisted-suicide attitudes, beliefs, and practices. The Nacirema's belief that the suicide wish of persons who are ill is rational, and even admirable (as illustrated by Nacirema's expressions like 'death with dignity'), has inspired the creation of community-sponsored assisted-suicide systems. The purported goal of these systems is to offer people who have a serious illness the option of what some

Nacirema consider a 'good' suicide (i.e. a suicide by prescribed poison), and to prevent what the Nacirema consider a 'bad' suicide (i.e. a suicide by firearm). At the same time, the 'death-with-dignity' system normalizes at least some suicides.[68,99] It is conceivable that the assisted-suicide system plays a role in the continued increase in Nacirema suicide rates. In communities that enable assisted suicide, both assisted and non-assisted suicides are on the rise, especially among women and older adults.[69,100] I think it is hard to be persuasive about suicide being a bad choice and a bad death and to be effective at suicide prevention while also promoting suicide as a dignified choice and a good death for individuals who are sick.

Final remarks

Almost 70 years have passed since Miner discovered the Nacirema. In many ways, today as back then, 'the culture of this people is … very poorly understood' (1956, p. 507).

The findings of this investigation of Nacirema's suicide attitudes, beliefs, and practices are consistent with Miner's[1] observations of Nacirema's body beliefs and practices, and with his conclusion that the Nacirema are 'magic ridden people' (1956, p. 507). Almost 70 years since Miner's report it is 'hard to understand how … [the Nacirema] have managed to exist so long under the burdens which they have imposed upon themselves' (p. 507).

Acknowledgements

I am grateful to Luke Flynn, Vidya Gaddy, John McIntosh, Ian Rockett, and Erin Winterrowd for their feedback on an earlier version of this chapter.

References

1. **Miner H.** Body ritual among the Nacirema. American Anthropologist. 1956;**48**(3):503–7.
2. **Gould SJ.** *Ever since Darwin: Reflections in Natural History.* New York, NY: Norton; 1977.
3. **Canetto SS.** Gender and suicide in the elderly. Suicide and Life-Threatening Behavior. 1992;**22**:80–97.
4. **Canetto SS.** Women and suicidal behavior: issues and dilemmas. In: **Canetto SS, Lester D**, editors. Women and Suicidal Behavior. New York, NY: Springer; 1995a. pp. 3–7.
5. **Canetto SS.** Language, culture, gender, and intersectionalities in suicide theory, research, and prevention: challenges and changes. Suicide and Life-Threatening Behavior. 2021a;**51**:1045–54.
6. **Canetto SS.** Men who survive a suicidal act: successful coping or failed masculinity? In: **Sabo D, Gordon D**, editors. *Men's Health and Illness: Gender, Power, and the Body.* Newbury Park, CA: Sage; 1995c. pp. 292–304.

7. **Canetto SS.** Women and suicidal behavior: new directions in theory, research, and prevention. In: **Wasserman D**, editor. *Oxford Textbook of Suicidology and Suicide Prevention*, 2nd edition. Oxford: Oxford University Press; 2021b. pp. 333–51.
8. **Canetto SS, Lester D.** Gender and the primary prevention of suicide mortality. Suicide and Life-Threatening Behavior. 1995;**25**:58–69.
9. **Canetto SS, Lester D.** Gender, culture, and suicidal behavior. Transcultural Psychiatry. 1998;**35**:163–91.
10. **Canetto SS.** Gender and suicidal behavior: theories and evidence. In: **Maris RW, Silverman MM, Canetto SS**, editors. *Review of Suicidology*. New York, NY: Guilford; 1997a. pp. 138–67.
11. **Canetto SS.** Meanings of gender and suicidal behavior among adolescents. Suicide and Life-Threatening Behavior. 1997b;**27**:339–51.
12. **Canetto SS.** Women and suicidal behavior: a cultural analysis. American Journal of Orthopsychiatry. 2008;**78**:259–66.
13. **Canetto SS.** Prevention of suicidal behavior in females: opportunities and obstacles. In: **Wasserman, D, Wasserman, C**, editors. *Oxford Textbook of Suicidology and Suicide Prevention*, 2nd edition. Oxford: Oxford University Press; 2009. pp. 241–47.
14. **Canetto SS, Sakinofsky I.** The gender paradox in suicide. Suicide and Life-Threatening Behavior. 1998;**28**:1–23.
15. **Canetto SS.** Suicide: why are older men so vulnerable? Men and Masculinities. 2017;**20**:49–70.
16. **Kleinman S, Copp M, Sandstrom K.** Making sexism visible: birdcages, martians and pregnant men. Teaching Sociology. 2006;**24**:126–42.
17. **SteelFisher GK, Findling MG, Bleich SN,** et al. Gender discrimination in the United States: experiences of women. Health Service Research. 2019;**54**(Suppl 2):1442–53.
18. **Neuringer C, Lettieri DJ.** *Suicidal Women*. New York, NY: Gardner Press; 1982.
19. **Canetto SS.** Suicidal women: Intervention and prevention strategies. In: **Canetto SS, Lester D**, editors. *Women and Suicidal Behavior*. New York, NY: Springer; 1995b. pp. 237–55.
20. **Canetto SS, Lester D.** Love and achievement motives in women's and men's suicide notes. Journal of Psychology. 2002;**136**:573–6.
21. **Canetto SS.** Suicidal ideation and behaviors in girls and women in the United States and Canada: cultural and intersectional perspectives. In: **Lamis DA, Kaslow NJ**, editors. *Advancing the Science of Suicidal Behavior: Understanding and Intervention*. Hauppauge, NY: Nova Science; 2015. pp. 215–36.
22. **Chesler P.** *Women and Madness*. New York, NY: Doubleday; 1972.
23. **Deluty RH.** Factors affecting the acceptability of suicide. Omega: Journal of Death and Dying. 1988–9b;**19**:315–26.
24. **Lewis RJ, Shepeard G.** Inferred characteristics of successful suicides as function of gender and context. Suicide and Life-Threatening Behavior. 1992;**22**:187–98.
25. **Dublin LI.** *Suicide: A Sociological and Statistical Study*. New York, NY: Ronald; 1963.
26. **Canetto SS.** She died for love and he for glory: gender myths of suicidal behavior. Omega: Journal of Death and Dying. 1992–3;**26**:1–17.
27. **Kushner HI.** *American Suicide: A Psychocultural Exploration*. New Brunswick, NJ: Rutgers University Press; 1989.

28. **Rockett IRH, Caine ED, Connery HS**, et al. Unrecognized self-injury mortality (SIM) trends among racial/ethnic minorities and women in the USA. Injury Prevention. 2020;**26**:439–47.
29. **Wold CI.** Subgroupings of suicidal people. Omega: Journal of Death and Dying. 1971;**2**:19–29.
30. **Schrut A, Michels T.** Suicidal, divorced, and discarded women. Journal of the American Academy of Psychoanalysis. 1974;**2**:329–47.
31. **Char WF.** The hysterical spouse. Medical Aspects of Human Sexuality. 1985;**19**:123–33.
32. **Stone MH.** Paradoxes in the management of suicidality in borderline patients. American Journal of Psychotherapy. 1993;**47**:255–72.
33. **Zich JM.** A reciprocal control approach to the treatment of repeated parasuicide. Suicide and Life-Threatening Behavior. 1984;**14**:36–51.
34. **Furst SS, Ostow M.** The psychodynamics of suicide. In: **Hankoff LD, Einsidler B**, editors. *Suicide: Theory and Clinical Aspects*. Littleton, MA: PSG; 1979. pp. 165–78.
35. **Maltsberger JT, Buie DH.** Common errors in the management of suicidal patients. In: **Jacobs DJ, Brown HN**, editors. *Suicide: Understanding and Responding*. Madison, CT: International Universities Press; 1989. pp. 257–82.
36. **LeGris J, Links PS, van Reekum R, Tannock R, Toplak M.** Executive function and suicidal risk in women with borderline personality disorder. Psychiatry Research. 2012;**196**:101–8.
37. **Kaplan AG, Klein RB.** Women and suicide. In: **Jacobs DJ, Brown H**, editors. *Suicide: Understanding and Responding*. Madison, CT: International Universities Press; 1989. pp. 257–82.
38. **Kposowa AJ, Aly Ezzat D, Breault K.** New findings on gender: The effects of employment status on suicide. International Journal of Women's Health. 2019;**11**:569–75. https://doi.org/10.2147/IJWH.S216504
39. **Chen Y-Y, Fong TCT, Yip PSF, Canetto SS.** Female-labor participation as suicide prevention: a population study in Taiwan. Archives of Suicide Research. In press. https://doi:10.1080/13811118.2024.2337182.
40. **United Nations (UN) Women** (2015). Transforming economies, realizing rights: progress of the world's women 2015–2016 summary. Available from: http://progress.unwomen.org/en/2015/pdf/UNW_progressreport.pdf
41. **Canetto SS.** Gender issues in the treatment of suicidal individuals. Death Studies. 1994;**18**:513–27.
42. **McAndrew FT, Garrison AJ.** Beliefs about gender differences in methods and causes of suicide. Archives of Suicide Research. 2007;**11**:271–9.
43. **Joseph VA, Martínez-Alés G, Olfson M**, et al. Temporal trends in suicide methods among adolescents in the US. JAMA Network Open. 2022 Oct;**5**(10):e2236049.
44. **Rockett IRH, Caine ED, Connery HS**, et al. Discerning suicide in drug intoxication deaths: paucity and primary of suicide notes and psychiatric history. PLoS One. 2018;13(1):e0190200.
45. **Linehan MM.** Suicide and attempted suicide: study of perceived sex differences. Perceptual and Motor Skills. 1973;**37**:31–14.

46. **White H, Stillion JM.** Sex differences in attitudes toward suicide: do males stigmatize males? Psychology of Women Quarterly. 1988;**12**:357–66.
47. **Zappa** F (1981). Frank Zappa lyrics: Suicide Chump. Available from: https://www.azlyrics.com/lyrics/frankzappa/suicidechump.html
48. **Canetto SS.** Gender roles, suicide attempts, and substance abuse. Journal of Psychology. 1991;**125**:605–20.
49. **Clark DC.** Narcissistic crises of aging and suicidal despair. Suicide and Life Threatening Behavior. 1993;**23**:21–6.
50. **Duberstein PR, Conwell Y, Caine ED.** Age differences in the personality characteristics of suicide completers: preliminary findings from a psychological autopsy study. Psychiatry. 1994;**57**:213–24.
51. **Horton-Deutsch SL, Clark DC, Farran CJ.** Chronic dyspnea and suicide in elderly men. Hospital and Community Psychiatry. 1992;**43**:1198–203.
52. **Useda JD, Duberstein PR, Conner KR**, et al. Personality differences in attempted suicide versus suicide in adults 50 years of age or older. Journal of Consulting and Clinical Psychology. 2007;**75**:126–33.
53. **Mahalik JR, Good GG, Englar-Carlson M.** Masculinity scripts, presenting concerns, and help-seeking: implications for practice and training. Professional Psychology: Research and Practice. 2003;**34**:123–31.
54. **Chen Y-Y, Cai ZY, Chang Q, Canetto SS, Yip PSF.** Caregiving as suicide prevention: an ecological 20-country study of men's family carework, unemployment, and suicide. Social Psychiatry and Psychiatric Epidemiology. 2021;**56**:2185–98.
55. **Liu L, Capaldi CA, Orpana HM, Kaplan MS, Tonmyr L.** Changes over time in means of suicide in Canada: an analysis of mortality data from 1981 to 2018. Canadian Medical Association Journal. 2021;**193**(10):E331–8.
56. **Kral MJ.** Postcolonial suicide among Inuit in Arctic Canada. Culture, Medicine and Psychiatry. 2012;**36**:306–25.
57. **Ditto PH, Druley JA, Moore KA, Danks JH, Smucker WD.** Fates worse than death: the role of valued life activities in health state evaluation. Health Psychology. 1996;**15**:332–43.
58. **Deluty RH.** Physical illness, psychiatric illness, and the acceptability of suicide. Omega: Journal of Death and Dying. 1988–9a;**19**:79–91.
59. **Lund EM, Nadorff MR, Winer ES, Seader K.** Is suicide an option? The impact of disability on suicide acceptability in the context of depression, suicidality, and demographic factors. Journal of Affective Disorders. 2016;**189**:25–35.
60. **Uncapher H, Areán PA.** Physicians are less willing to treat suicidal ideation in older patients. Journal of the American Geriatrics Society. 2000;**48**:188–92.
61. **Stice BD, Canetto SS.** Older adult suicide: perceived precipitants and protective factors. Clinical Gerontologist. 2008;**31**(4):1–25.
62. **Winterrowd E, Canetto SS, Benoit K.** Permissive beliefs and attitudes about older adult suicide: a suicide enabling script? Aging and Mental Health. 2017;**21**:173–81.
63. **Centers for Disease Control and Prevention** (2023n.d.). Disparities in suicide. Available from: https://www.cdc.gov/suicide/facts/disparities-in-suicide.html

64. **Smedley A, Smedley BD.** Race as biology is fiction, racism as a social problem is real: anthropological and historical perspectives in the social construction of race. American Psychologist. 2005;**60**:16–26.
65. **Oregon Health Authority** (n.d.). Oregon Revised Statute: Oregon's Death with Dignity Act. Available from http://www.oregon.gov/oha/PH/PROVIDERPARTNERRESOURCES/EVALUATIONRESEARCH/DEATHWITHDIGNITYACT/Pages/ors.aspx
66. **Death with Dignity** (n.d.). Available from: https://www.deathwithdignity.org
67. **Hedberg K, New C.** Oregon's Death with Dignity Act: 20 years of experience to inform the debate. Annals of Internal Medicine. 2017;**167**(8):579–83.
68. **Canetto SS.** If physician-assisted suicide is the modern woman's last powerful choice, why are white women its leading advocates and main users? Professional Psychology: Research and Practice. 2019;**50**:39–50.
69. **Canetto SS, McIntosh JL.** A comparison of physician-assisted/death-with-dignity-act death and suicide patterns in older adult women and men. American Journal of Geriatric Psychiatry. 2022;**30**:211–20.
70. **Tolle W, Tilden VP, Drach LL, Fromme EK, Perrin NA, Hedberg K.** Characteristics and proportion of dying Oregonians who personally consider physician-assisted suicide. Journal of Clinical Ethics. 2004;**15**(2):111–22.
71. **Dula A.** African American suspicion of the healthcare system is justified: what do we do about it? Cambridge Quarterly of Healthcare Ethics. 1994;**3**:347–57.
72. **Dula A, Williams S.** When race matters. Clinics in Geriatric Medicine. 2005;**21**:239–53.
73. **King PA, Wolf LE.** Empowering and protecting patients: lessons for physician-assisted suicide from the African-American experience. Minnesota Law Review. 1997;**82**:1015–43.
74. **Wicher CP, Meeker MA.** What influences African American end-of-life preferences? Journal of Health Care for the Poor and Underserved. 2012;**23**:28–58.
75. **Canetto SS, Hollenshead JD.** Gender and physician-assisted suicide: an analysis of the Kevorkian cases, 1990–1997. Omega: Journal of Death and Dying. 1999–2000;**40**:165–208.
76. **Canetto SS, Hollenshead JD.** Older women and mercy killing. Omega: Journal of Death and Dying. 2000–1;**42**:83–99.
77. **Addo FR, Richter DT.** Marriage, marital history, and black-white women wealth differentials among older women. Journal of Marriage and the Family. 2013;**75**:342–62.
78. **Canetto SS, Hollenshead JD.** Men's mercy killing of women: mercy for whom? Choice for whom? Omega: Journal of Death and Dying. 2002;**45**:275–80.
79. **The World Federation of Right to Die Societies** (n.d.). Mission, vision, statutes. Available from: https://wfrtds.org/mission/
80. **Basta LL.** *A Graceful Exit: Life and Death on Your Own Terms*. New York, NY: Plenum; 1996.
81. **Girsh FJ.** Older women and mercy killing. Letter to the editor. Omega: Journal of Death and Dying. 2002;**45**:289–90.
82. **John A, Azrael D, Miller M.** Access to firearms and adolescent suicide. BMJ. 2020;**370**:m2829.

83. **Spicer RS, Miller TR.** Suicide acts in 8 states: incidence and case fatality rates by demographics and method. American Journal of Public Health. 2000;**90**:1885–91.
84. **Church AT.** Personality traits across cultures. Current Opinion in Psychology. 2016;**8**:22–30.
85. **Weisberg YJ, DeYoung CG, Hirsh JB.** Gender differences in personality across the ten aspects of the Big Five. Frontiers in Psychology. 2011;**2**:178.
86. **Krag E.** Rich, white and vulnerable: rethinking oppressive socialization in the euthanasia debate. Journal of Medicine and Philosophy. 2014;**39**:406–29.
87. **Dransart DAC, Lapierre A, Erlangsen A,** et al. A systematic review of older adults' request for or attitude toward euthanasia or assisted-suicide. Aging and Mental Health 2021;**25**:420–30.
88. **Zero Suicide** (n.d.). Zero suicide is a transformational framework for health and behavioral health care systems. Available from: https://zerosuicide.edc.org
89. **Bernstein L** (2022). Suicides increased in 2021, especially among younger people. Available from: https://www.washingtonpost.com/health/2022/09/29/suicide-increase-2021/
90. **The Economist** (2018, November 16th). Suicides are declining around the world. But the United States is bucking the trend. Available from: https://www.economist.com/graphic-detail/2018/11/26/suicides-are-declining-around-the-world
91. **Andriolo KR.** Gender and the cultural construction of good and bad suicides. Suicide and Life-Threatening Behavior. 1998;**28**:37–49.
92. **Phillips A, Luth EA.** Beliefs about suicide acceptability in the United States: how do they affect suicide mortality? Journal of Gerontology B. 2018;**75**(2):414–25.
93. **Quill TE.** *Death and Dignity: Making Choices and Taking Charge.* New York, NY: Norton; 1993.
94. **Joe S, Romer D, Jamieson PE.** Suicide acceptability is related to suicide planning in US adolescents and young adults. Suicide and Life-Threatening Behavior. 2007;**37**:165–78.
95. **Kleiman EM.** Suicide acceptability as a mechanism of suicide clustering in a nationally representative sample of adolescents. Comprehensive Psychiatry. 2015;**59**:17–20.
96. **Miller M, Zhang W, Azrael D.** Firearm purchasing during the COVID-19 pandemic: results from the 2021 National Firearms Survey. Annals of Internal Medicine. 2022;**175**:219–25.
97. **Betz ME, Thomas AC, Simonetti JA.** Firearms suicide and approaches for prevention. JAMA. 2022;**328**(12):1179–80.
98. **Means Matter** (n.d.). Firearm access is a risk factor for suicide. Available from: https://www.hsph.harvard.edu/means-matter/means-matter/risk/
99. **Golden M, Zoanni T.** Killing us softly: the dangers of legalizing assisted suicide. Disability and Health Journal. 2010;**3**:16–30.
100. **Girma S, Paton D.** Is assisted suicide a substitute for unassisted suicide? European Economic Review. 2022;**145**:104113.

Part 4

Suicidality and mental health

Chapter 17

Suicidality and trauma

Marianne C. Kastrup

Introduction

Definition of target group

According to the *Oxford Dictionary*, trauma is a 'deeply distressing or disturbing experience', which includes a wide range of events from natural disaster to crime or war. Such events may all be associated with suicidal ideation as well as completed suicides. In the present chapter, the field of trauma and the population under investigation are narrowed and we intend to focus on the traumatized population of refugees and asylum seekers and the inflicted trauma upon them from fellow men. The present context uses the United Nations (UN) definition of refugee[1] as a person who, owing to well-founded fear of being persecuted for reasons of race, religion, nationality, membership of a particular social group, or political opinion, is outside the country of his nationality and is unable or, owing to such fear, is unwilling to avail himself of the protection of that country. And further, according to the United Nations High Commissioner for Refugees (UNHCR), an asylum seeker is someone who says he or she is a refugee, but whose claim has not yet been definitively evaluated.

Size of the population

Migrants represent vulnerable populations that require special attention vis-à-vis provision of mental health care. This population is on the rise. According to the World Health Organization (WHO),[2] there is an estimate of 281 million international migrants and more than one billion people are on the move globally. Among migrants, forcibly displaced persons constitute a particularly vulnerable group. According to UNHCR, almost 60 million persons by the end of 2015 had refugee status, the highest number since World War II, which is an increase by about one-third over the last 10 years.[3] In 2021, UNHCR reported an increase to 89.3 million of forcibly displaced persons, of whom 53.2 million were internally displaced, 27.1 had refugee status, and 4.6 million were asylum seekers.[4]

The exact statistics may, however, vary as there are different ways to delineate the population.

To what extent refugees and asylum seekers have been exposed to various traumatic events also varies greatly. According to Quiroga and Jaranson,[5] 3–16% of the population in refugee camps and between 85% and 100% of former detainees remaining in their countries of origin have a history of extreme trauma in the form of torture. Further, they report that in Western settings, the prevalence of reported torture ranges from 7% to 8% among patients in primary care clinics, and up to 70% in refugee psychiatric clinics; and among a selected group of refugees and asylum seekers in the United States and Europe, the prevalence rates of torture varies between 6% and 55%.[5]

In a Swedish study of Syrian refugees, 31% reported exposure to torture, but a total of 70% reported other life-threatening situations.[6] With torture being the ultimate trauma, many more refugees may have experienced significant trauma, but of less severe nature. So even when using a conservative estimate, we are facing a huge population that have been exposed to severe traumata.

Mental health consequences of trauma

Traumatized refugees and asylum seekers may suffer psychiatric illness because of their exposure to adverse conditions prior to, as well as during and after migration. The migration may be forced by adverse life circumstances, such as persecution, discrimination, imprisonment, and genocide, which may all be precursors for mental health problems. There is consistent evidence to suggest that asylum seekers and refugees have higher rates of mental health difficulties than are found within the general population. The process of seeking asylum in Western countries places additional demands on this group.[7] In a systematic review of 29 large heterogenic studies, Bogic et al.[8] reported a prevalence of more than 20% for depression, post-traumatic stress disorder (PTSD), and anxiety. The prevailing symptom manifestations included anxiety, hopelessness, apathy, depression, irritability, emotional instability, cognitive memory and attention problems, personality changes, behavioural disturbances, and neuro-vegetative symptoms.

Asylum seekers who are detained in the host country experience a further and more specific set of stressors, reflecting the detention process itself and the detention centre environment, which may adversely affect their mental health status.[7] Some compare the asylum process with a grief process, comprising losses of family and friends, language, culture, social status, fatherland, contact with community, and exposure to physical risk.[9]

Several of these symptoms may lead to a state of despair with ruminations related to the meaning of life and the diminishing expectations for the future.

And as Ortiz pointed out, contemplating suicide may be seen as the ultimate solution.[10]

The literature about suicide among refugees and asylum seekers is limited, which may be due to a lack of reliable data, unavailable official archives, or direct under-reporting of suicidal behaviour.[11] There are thus ample reasons to analyse to what extent there is an association between exposure to human-made trauma, being a refugee or asylum seeker, and subsequent suicidal ideation.

Suicidality

The chapter will include suicidal behaviour in a wider sense that is both suicide attempts and completed suicides.

It is well known that suicide rates differ around the world and over time. According to the WHO, on a global level, there are about 800,000 suicides annually and about 30 times more suicide attempts, out of which almost 80% take place in low- and middle-income countries.[12]

Refugees and asylum seekers face particular problems as migrants.[13] These adverse life circumstances associated with mental health problems may further lead to a risk of suicidal ideation.

The suicide incidence rate of refugees comprising different groups of refugees and asylum seekers is found to be higher than the rate of the general population.[14,15,16,17,18] Many studies have reported a significantly higher risk of suicide and self-harm in refugees and asylum seekers in various Western countries,[19] and an even higher risk of suicidal behaviour among detained asylum seekers. Living conditions and uncertainty add to the risk, and among long-stay refugees stranded on the Greek island Lesbos, the treatment rate for attempted suicide was as high as 1.4 per 100 person-years.[20] The overall prevalence rate of suicidal behaviour is found to vary between 3.4% and 34%, with considerable differences across studies, depending upon how suicidal behaviour is measured.[14] Goosen and co-workers[21] analysed death registries from Dutch asylum seeker reception centres in 2002–6 and found a suicide rate of 25.6 per 100,000 for men and 4.0 for women. Suicide rates and hospital-treated attempts were higher among men, but not among women, when compared to Dutch nationals.

Risk factors

Risk factors may be described as characteristics that have been demonstrated to be present more likely among those attempting or dying by suicide.[22] Many factors contribute to suicidal ideation and suicidal acts, and certain factors are particularly prominent among refugees and asylum seekers. Here two factors deserve mentioning as contributors to a wish to no longer live: one is a feeling of not belonging to any significant social group, and the second is the feeling of being a burden to those around you.[18]

In refugees and asylum seekers, risk factors are often classified in relation to the migration process as pre-, peri-, or post-migration adversities.

Awareness of such risk factors may help to identify those at particular risk, and research has demonstrated that there exist important predictors of repeated suicide attempts as well as of completed suicides.[23] Some risk factors may be preventable and subject to interventions, whereas others are fixed and beyond intervention.

Looking at the *pre-migratory conditions*, Joshi and Warfa[19] found in their review that being male, being single, having experiences of prior self-harm, and having a prior mental illness all increased the risk of suicide among refugees and asylum seekers. Young age may also be a risk factor, and a recent Swedish report showed an increased risk of self-harm, suicide attempts, and death by suicide among young refugees.[24] Most of these factors, however, are not approachable for any preventive intervention.

Traumatic experiences

In the case of refugees and asylum seekers, traumatic experiences in the country of origin and during the flight may play a decisive role. Among torture survivors in the United States, a combination of three variables were associated with current suicidal ideation at intake into the programme. Here being female and having a history of rape or sexual assault (as well as not having submitted an application for asylum) were all significantly associated with suicidal ideation, also when controlled for other variables.[25]

Sexual violence against women during war or armed conflict is a clear example of how uniform gender discrimination is around the globe.[26] Sexual violence includes rape, forced pregnancy, forced prostitution, and being coerced to exchange sexual services in exchange for food or access to health services. Rape is a weapon of war spreading political terror and ethnic cleansing. Rape humiliates and silences women and their families.

The vulnerability of women is larger when they are faced with a life situation as single providers, with the destiny of their husbands unknown and new and unfamiliar responsibilities placed upon them. Further, life in exile may not provide the shelter and personal security they had looked for; for example, isolated or overcrowded asylum centres and unsafe sleeping facilities leave women without adequate protection.[27] Suicidal ideation is high in women who have been victims of assaults, but gender differences are not studied in detail on refugees.[28]

Ortiz[10] describes in her chapter on survivors that many survivors of trauma contemplate suicide in an attempt to alleviate their pain, their flashbacks, or nightmares or simply because they want to disappear. Mental health professionals or family members may associate such feelings with suicidal ideations and try to protect the person in question by admission—maybe against her/his will—to a psychiatric institution, presenting for the person an experience of losing control and re-traumatization. Dying by suicide may be the ultimate solution, and Ortiz points out that suicide may be the last resort when the total situation is so painful that there is no other way to forget what otherwise could not be forgotten. Suicide thus can be interpreted as the victory of the perpetrators who, in this way, have won over the victim.

Sexual orientation

The sexual orientation or gender identity of asylum seekers as a main reason for their fleeing the country of origin is receiving increased attention. It is well known that homosexuality is not allowed in many countries and may lead to persecution and imprisonment. And yet the issue has not received a lot of scientific attention. Hopkinson et al.[29] studied in the United States asylum seekers persecuted due to their LGBT identity and matched by country of origin and sex with clients persecuted for other reasons. They reported that LGBT asylum seekers have a higher incidence of sexual violence and suicidal ideation, as well as experiences of persecution by family members.

Among *peri-migration adversities*, the asylum process is decisive and a subject for increasing research. All in all, there is still a shortage of studies focusing on the relationship between suicidal behaviour and the legal status as a refugee or an asylum seeker. Leaving one's own country and community can be a significant loss. Language problems may contribute to problems finding a job, which, in turn, may foster a sense of hopelessness. The fact that many refugees experience high levels of stress and loss following resettlement may be one reason why some refugee groups have higher rates of suicide.

In a Swedish study, Sundvall and co-workers[30] compared suicide attempts in asylum seekers and in persons with a Swedish background, and found that asylum seekers had different social risk factors and that the time relation between the suicide attempt and the asylum process suggested the importance of the asylum decision, as well as a possible role of earlier mental health problems and pre-migration stress, for suicidal behaviour.

Detention

Several countries place asylum seekers in detention centres—frequently for extended periods of time despite the fact that there is ample documentation of how harmful this is for the mental health of the detained. This exacerbation of already existing mental health problems is a concern for many professionals working with this population.[31] The Australian government has used such centres, and here male and female rates of suicidal behaviours are calculated to be 41 and 26 times the national average, respectively, and male rates are 1.8 times higher than the male prison rates, and the high self-harm rates reported reflect conditions of detention and the detention environment and are in contrast to the Australian suicide prevention programmes.[32] According to Procter and co-workers,[33] suicide is the leading cause of premature death for people in the Australian immigration detention network.

The UN has criticized the detention policy in Australia, but the detention continues and a recent report by the BBC[34] claims that the situation is getting worse and on Manus Island housing many asylum seekers, the number of incidents of self-harm has escalated among men. Procter and co-workers[35] found that, among asylum seekers placed in Australian detention centres, thwarted belongingness, purpose, and identity, as well as a shortage of available services and barriers to legal support, all increased the likelihood that the mental health of asylees deteriorates with an increased risk of self-harm and suicide.

Insecurity (e.g. asylum phase)

Schoretsanitis and co-workers[36] analysed the use of mental health services in Bern by those who had their asylum application rejected. With regard to referral to psychiatric care, the rates of suicidal ideation and attempted suicide were higher in patients with a rejected application than in those with a pending application, whereas aggressive behaviour was more frequent in patients with a pending application; nevertheless, these differences did not reach statistical significance. Most referred themselves to services frequently due to suicidal ideas. In a Danish retrospective study of asylum seekers who had their application rejected, a long waiting time contributed to the development of suicidal ideation.[37] Also Yilmaz and Riecher-Rössler[38] reported an association between threat of rejection of status as refugee and suicidal attempts.

Once they have reached the new country and obtained asylum, refugees are faced with many *post-migration adversities* that may not have been anticipated and that make life stressful and when stressors accumulate, in some cases, not worth living. This may exacerbate the risk of mental illness and ultimately increase the risk of suicidal behaviour.

Distress

The migration process and the consequences hereof may be alleviated but may continue to be risk factors. We see a relationship between acculturative stressors, social support, and suicidal ideation among refugee populations.[18] These risk factors can affect anyone, but refugees and asylum seekers are more likely to experience specific risk factors. The Refugee Health Screener (RHS) was developed to screen for emotional distress among refugees and can be used to assess distress severity.[39] When used in asylum seekers, the RHS has shown that at moderate and severe levels of distress, they were much more likely to exhibit suicidal ideation than asylees with low levels of distress. This does not mean, however, that asylum seekers with low distress levels do not have suicidal thoughts, and further suicide assessment is needed in asylum seekers with moderate to severe distress levels on the RHS.[39] When assessing the individual, feelings and behaviours need to be seen in relation to past experiences and stressors at other levels of an individual's social ecology.[18] And it is important to be aware of the fact that there are major barriers at an individual level to communicating with others about distress and suicidal thoughts.

In order to gain more insight into the background of Bhutanese refugees dying by suicide in the United States, psychological autopsies were carried out.[40] Language difficulties, separation from the family, and worrying about the family left behind were all crucial factors as well as barriers to education, difficulties in maintaining cultural traditions, and social isolation.

Acculturation and integration difficulties

The process to obtain refugee status is traumatic, and most individuals undergo a series of phases during the process that can be very stressful. Fleeing one's country may result in that you lose your social network, if not close family members. You are deprived of your language, culture, and traditions, to mention but a few of the traumatic factors. Arrival in a new country may not be the 'safe haven', but instead an experience of detention deprived of autonomy and with no prospects of a future, combined with social isolation. Economic difficulties, housing and educational problems, and experiencing ethnic discrimination may all contribute. Low socio-economic status is also a risk.[19] Refugees do often have unfulfilled expectations; many arrive with a social status and previous employment, but realize that they have to adjust their expectations and may be forced to work much below their educational background. This may lead to a feeling of hopelessness and ultimately suicidal ideation.

All this may increase the risk of developing a problem of substance abuse, which is frequently observed as an ultimate resort when you have to accept a life situation that is far from what you had expected.

A Swedish comparison of suicide attempts in asylum seekers and persons with a Swedish background showed that asylum seekers had different social risk factors, but more often a social network, and they received different diagnoses than the controls.[41] Migrant adolescents not living together with their biological parents experience a higher level of suicidal thoughts than their counterparts living with intact families.[42]

Family conflicts and inability to find work in the new country also were contributory factors. Joshi and Warfa[19] found in their review that having contact with mental health services and having a diagnosis of PTSD or depression both increased the risk of suicide among refugees and asylum seekers. A study of 65 refugees in Sweden diagnosed with PTSD showed that 40% had made suicidal attempts, 29% had a detailed suicidal plan, and 31% had recurrent suicidal thoughts.[43]

Suicide is a major cause of maternal mortality, and a study of refugees at the Thailand–Myanmar border demonstrated that maternal suicide accounted for 9% of maternal deaths among the refugees, which was much higher than the pooled figure for low- and middle-income regions.[44] The authors emphasized the need to address socio-economic determinants, including poverty and violence against women, in such vulnerable groups in order to reduce suicidal behaviour.

At the societal level, several factors are significant, including problems related to acculturation, citizenship, employment, and language. Certain issues cut across different levels of the ecosystem such as loss and isolation, and loneliness.[18]

Protective factors

These are characteristics or experiences that make someone less likely to consider suicide. Building up protective factors may thus help to prevent suicide. As is the case with risk factors, some protective factors are not subject to intervention (e.g. sex), whereas others can be modified and thereby reduce the risk of suicide.

Examples of protective factors include the ability to maintain a sense of belonging and be part of a community. Studies of Bhutanese refugees in the United States have shown that those with caretaking responsibilities towards their family less frequently had suicidal ideation.[45] A sense of duty is crucial as a caretaker and has protective abilities. Other important factors include keeping up hope for the future and a feeling that what you do matters.

Studies of Canadian aboriginal youth point out that cultural continuity is critical to identity formation, and further that community-level rates of youth suicide should ordinarily vary according to whether there have been meaningful connections to their traditional past[46]

Among young North Korean refugees in South Korea, Park and co-workers[47] found that those who did not have suicidal ideation had a higher level of family cohesion and self-esteem, as well as resilience (defined as self-perceived ability to bounce back from stress), compared to those with suicidal thoughts.

In the integration process, the attitude of the receiving country is yet another decisive factor and having qualifications recognized as a refugee increases the empowerment and self-esteem.

Access to care

Refugees and asylum seekers may face several underlying barriers contributing to inequity in access to care either when experiencing suicidal ideation or following a suicide attempt. Barriers may be legal, not allowing certain populations (e.g. illegal migrants) access to care, irrespective of their need), or they may be structural if services, for example, are not available to certain groups for linguistic or cultural reasons. But also, financial barriers may be a risk among mentally ill regarding suicidal behaviour with few resources depriving them of adequate treatment.

Following a suicide attempt, asylum seekers in Sweden were referred to less specialized follow-up treatment, compared to Swedish controls, in spite of their health history and previous and current clinical pictures indicating a similar or—in the case of female asylum seekers—more serious mental health condition.[41] When carrying out a content analysis of asylum-seeking women who have attempted suicide in Sweden, the results suggest that clinicians working with this population need to develop an understanding of social and cultural factors and of trauma issues, and to study how mental health professionals may become more competent due to an enhanced integration of context and subjectivity in psychiatric practice.[48]

Understanding the type of persecution experiences and how these influence mental health outcomes is an essential step towards designing and delivering effective treatments. This was stressed upon by Hopkinson et al.[29] in relation to LGBT asylum seekers, but the recommendations are valid for all asylum seekers and refugees.

In a Danish study,[49] suicidal ideation was the most common reason for rejected asylum seekers to seek psychiatric emergency care. Suicide attempts comprised 10% of forensic medical examinations among refugees in Turkey and, unlike other forensic events, were less likely in males and more likely than other events to require intensive care.[50]

Special attention should be paid to persons exhibiting PTSD symptoms. Persons with a high suicide risk require containment and may benefit from medical treatment with antidepressants. However, suicide risk may increase during therapy that might enhance attention to negative experiences. So it is important to treat comorbid depression in PTSD victims, even though such groups may not be able to sustain exposure- and trauma-focused therapy.[51]

Prevention

Preventing suicide in communities of refugees or asylum seekers requires an understanding of risk factors, protective factors, and ways to identify and help those who are acutely in need. What is contributing to the increased rate of suicide among some refugee communities, and what can be done to prevent it? Working broadly in a community to decrease risk factors and promote protective factors can prevent the risk of suicide across whole refugee communities.

Interventions may be of a general nature or more targeted. In general, finding ways to promote social relations, connecting refugees with employment opportunities, and inducing hope and a sense of belonging in the new country will all add to empowerment and may reduce suicidal thoughts.

Targeted interventions should be directed towards individuals who are most at risk of suicide or have had previous suicide attempts. Specific steps can be directed to help them through the relatively brief period where their risk peaks and help them reach beyond that. Certain warning signs of risk of suicide are not just limited to refugee populations such as talks that life is no longer worth living or that there is no future, but also signs of mental illness in the form of, for example, unusual or changed behaviour or expressing depressive symptoms. Targeted interventions can include helping the person at risk, investigating what the stress factors are, trying to offer a sense of hope, and helping him/her to connect to other people and helpers, including contact with a suicide hotline.[22]

Other warning signs may be culture-specific. Here, culture brokers or other members of refugee communities may be useful in helping to disentangle cultural expressions of distress and despair. A Bhutanese study demonstrated that holistic mental health treatment and suicide prevention programmes should move beyond medication and individual psychotherapies, and instead include relational processes as well as the social environment of the included.[18]

Cohen[52] provides a number of recommendations—based upon a study of asylum seekers in the United Kingdom. First of all, faced with deceased persons, coroners should record asylum seeker status and ethnicity. In the community, self-harm monitoring should also record asylum seeker status and ethnicity. Further, health care in immigration centres should meet the same standards as prisons in the United Kingdom as a minimum when it comes to suicide prevention, and allegation of torture by immigration detainees should result in a case management review and risk assessment for continued detention. Finally, interpreters should be used whenever needed.

Others[33] recommend that an approach taking into consideration cultural explanatory models as a starting point for a preventive strategy would be beneficial not least for asylum detainees.

Intervention programmes by community workers may be useful, as documented by Vijayakumar et al.[53] in their study of two groups of Tamil refugees where the use of safety planning cards (CASP) did reduce suicidal behaviour in the intervention group. The WHO recommends selective suicide prevention for vulnerable groups, including those affected by conflict or disaster, and refugees and migrants.[12]

Conclusion

Mental health professionals need to be aware of the increased risk of suicide among refugees and asylum seekers suffering from PTSD or depression and further that the phase following rejection of asylum requires increased attention.

In-depth analyses of suicidal behaviour among refugees is often denied in low- and middle-income countries, which is a politically sensitive issue. In her editorial, Vijayakumar[11] emphasizes the urgent need to acknowledge the magnitude of the problem of suicide in refugees and asylum seekers, and the need for mental health professionals, policymakers, and non-governmental organizations to be more sensitized to the needs of refugees. And she points out that priority should be given to develop a culturally and contextually appropriate tool for assessment of suicidal ideation and behaviour in refugees and asylum seekers.

These considerations are as valid as when they were written.

References

1. **UNHCR** (1951). Convention and protocol relating to the status of refugees. Available from: https://www.unhcr.org/3b66c2aa10
2. **World Health Organization** (2022). Refugee and migrant health. Available from: https://www.who.int/news-room/fact-sheets/detail/refugee-and-migrant-health
3. **UNHCR Philippines** (2016). With 1 human in every 113 affected, forced displacement hits record high. Available from: https://www.unhcr.org/ph/10977-1-human-every-113-affected-forced-displacement-hits-record-high-1-human-every-113-affected-forced-displacement-hits-record-high.html
4. **UNHCR Philippines** (2021). Figures at a glance: global displacement. Available from: https://www.unhcr.org/ph/figures-at-a-glance
5. **Quiroga J, Jaranson J.** Politically-motivated torture and its survivors: a desk study review of the literature. Torture. 2005;**15**:1–111.

6. **Tinghög P, Malm A, Arwidson C, Sigvardsdotter E, Lundin A, Saboonchi F.** Prevalence of mental ill health, traumas and postmigration stress among refugees from Syria resettled in Sweden after 2011: a population-based survey. BMJ Open. 2017;7(12): e018899.
7. **Robjant K, Hassan R, Katona C.** Mental health implications of detaining asylum seekers: systematic review. British Journal of Psychiatry. 2009;**194**:306–12.
8. **Bogic M, Njoku A, Priebe S.** Long-term mental health of war-refugees: a systematic literature review. BMC International Health and Human Rights. 2015;**15**:29.
9. **Carta MG, Bernal M, Hardoy MC, Haro-Abad JM.** Migration and mental health in Europe (The state of mental health in Europe working group: Appendix I). Clinical Practice and Epidemiology in Mental Health. 2005;**1**:13.
10. **Ortiz SD.** The survivors' perspective. In: **Gerrity** E, **Tuma** F, **Keane** TM, et al., editors. *The Mental Health Consequences of Torture.* New York, NY: Kluwer Academic; 2001. pp. 13–34.
11. **Vijayakumar L.** Suicide among refugees: a mockery of humanity. Crisis. 2016;**37**(1):1–4.
12. **World Health Organization** (2014). *Preventing Suicide: A Global Imperative.* Geneva: World Health Organization.
13. **Fortune SA, Hawton K.** Culture and mental disorders: suicidal behaviour. In: **Bhugra D, Bhui K**, editors. *Textbook of Cultural Psychiatry*. Cambridge: Cambridge University Press; 2007. pp. 255–71.
14. **Vijayakumar L, Jotheeswaran AT.** Suicides in refugees and asylum seekers. In: **Bhugra D, Craig T, Bhui K**, et al., editors. *Mental Health of Refugees and Asylum Seekers.* Oxford: Oxford University Press, 2010. pp. 195–210.
15. **Kalt A, Hossain M, Kiss L, Zimmerman C.** Asylum seekers, violence and health: a systematic review of research in high-income host countries. American Journal of Public Health. 2013;**103**:e30–42.
16. **Akinyemi OO, Atilola O, Soyannwo T.** Suicidal ideation: are refugees more at risk compared to host population? Findings from a preliminary assessment in a refugee community in Nigeria. Asian Journal of Psychiatry. 2015;**18**:81–5.
17. **Saunders NR, Chiu M, Lebenbaum M,** et al. Suicide and self-harm in recent immigrants in Ontario, Canada: a population-based study. Canadian Journal of Psychiatry. 2019;64(11):7777–788.
18. **Brown FL, Mishra T, Frounfelker RL,** et al. 'Hiding their troubles': a qualitative exploration of suicide in Bhutanese refugees in the USA. Cambridge Prisms: Global Mental Health. 2019;**6**:e1.
19. **Joshi P, Warfa N.** Suicide and self-harm in refugees and asylum seekers. In: **van Bergen D, Amanda Heredia Montesinos, Meryam Schouler-Ocak**, editorss. *Suicidal Behavior in Immigrants and Ethnic Minorities in Europe*. Göttingen: Hogrefe; 2015. pp. 91–100.
20. **Hermans MPJ, Kooistra J, Cannegieter SC, Rosendaal FR, Mook-Kanamori DO, Nemeth B.** Healthcare and disease burden among refugees in long-stay refugee camps at Lesbos, Greece. European Journal of Epidemiology. 2017;**32**(9):851–4.
21. **Goosen S, Kunst AE, Stronks K, van Oostrum IEA, Uitenbroek DG, Kerkhof AJ.** Suicide death and hospital treated suicidal behaviour in asylum seekers in the Netherlands: a national registry-based study. BMC Public Health. 2011;**11**:484.

22. **Refugee Health TA**. Suicide. Available from: https://refugeehealthta.org/physical-mental-health/mental-health/suicide/
23. **Bachmann S.** Epidemiology of suicide and the psychiatric perspective. International Journal of Environmental Research and Public Health. 2018;**15**(7):1425.
24. **Hagström A, Hollander AC, Mittendorfer-Rutz E.** [*Kartläggning av Självskadebeteende, Suicidförsök, Sucid och Annan Dödlighet Bland Ensamkommande Barn och Unga.*] Stockholm: Karolinska Institute; 2018.
25. **Lerner E, Bonanno GA, Keatley E, Joscelyne A, Keller AS.** Predictors of suicidal ideation in treatment-seeking survivors of torture. Psychological Trauma. 2016;**8**(1):17–24.
26. **Arcel L, Kastrup M.** War, women and health. NORA. 2004;**12**:40–7.
27. **Arcel L.** Sexual torture: still a hidden problem. Torture. 2002;**12**:3–4.
28. **Kastrup M, Arcel L.** Gender-specific treatment. In: **Wilson J, Drozdek B**, editors. *Broken Spirits*. New York, NY: Brunner & Routledge; 2004. pp. 566–84.
29. **Hopkinson RA, Keatley E, Glaeser E, Erickson-Schroth L, Fattal O, Nicholson Sullivan M.** Persecution experiences and mental health of LGBT asylum seekers. Journal of Homosexuality. 2017;**64**(12):1650–66.
30. **Sundvall M, Tidemalm DH, Titelman DE, Runeson B, Bäärnhielm S.** Assessment and treatment of asylum seekers after a suicide attempt: a comparative study of people registered at mental health services in a Swedish location. BMC Psychiatry. 2015;**15**:235.
31. **Procter NG.** Emergency mental health nursing for self-harming refugees and asylum seekers. International Journal of Mental Health Nursing. 2005;**14**:196–201.
32. **Dudley M.** Contradictory Australian national policies on self-harm and suicide: the case of asylum seekers in mandatory detention. Australasian Psychiatry. 2003;**11**:102–8.
33. **Procter NG, de Leo D, Newman L.** Suicide and self-harm prevention for people in immigration detention. Medical Journal of Australia. 2013;**199**(11):730–2.
34. **BBC** (2019). Manus Island: refugee 'suicide attempts' in wake of Australia election. Available from: https://www.bbc.com/news/world-australia-48375120
35. **Procter NG, Kenny MA, Eaton H, Grech C.** Lethal hopelessness: understanding and responding to asylum seeker distress and mental deterioration. International Journal of Mental Health Nursing. 2018;**27**(1):448–54.
36. **Schoretsanitis G, Bhugra D, Eisenhardt S**, et al. Upon rejection: psychiatric emergencies of failed asylum seekers. International Journal of Environmental Research and Public Health. 2018;**15**(7):1498.
37. **Stæhr MM, Munk-Andersen E.** Suicide and suicidal behaviour among asylum seekers in Denmark during the period 2001–2003. A retrospective study. Ugeskrift for Læger. 2006;**168**:1650–3.
38. **Yilmaz TA, Riecher-Rössler A.** Attempted suicide in immigrants from Turkey: a comparison with Swiss suicide attempters. Psychopathology. 2012;**45**:366–3.
39. **Leiler A, Hollifield M, Wasteson E, Bjärtå A.** Suicidal ideation and severity of distress among refugees residing in asylum accommodations in Sweden. International Journal of Environmental Research and Public Health. 2019;**16**(15):2751.
40. **Hagaman AK, Sivilli TI, Ao T**, et al. An investigation into suicides among Bhutanese refugees resettled in the United States between 2008 and 2011. Journal of Immigrant and Minority Health. 2016;**18**(4):819–27.

41. **Sundvall M, Tidemalm DH, Titelman DE, Runeson B, Baarnhielm S.** Assessment and treatment of asylum seekers after a suicide attempt: a comparative study of people registered at mental health services in Swedish location. BMC Psychiatry. 2015;**15**:235.
42. **Pottie K, Dahal G, Georgiades K, Premji K, Hassan G.** Do first generation immigrant adolescents face higher rates of bullying, violence and suicidal behaviours than do third generation and native born? Journal of Immigrant and Minority Health. 2015;**17**(5):1557–66.
43. **Ferrada-Noli M, Åsberg M, Ormstad K, Lundin T, Sundbom E.** Suicidal behaviour after severe trauma. Part one: PTSD diagnosis, psychiatric comorbidity, and assessments of suicidal behaviour. Journal of Traumatic Stress. 1998;**11**:103–12.
44. **Fellmeth G, Paw MK, Wiladphaingern J, Charunwatthana P, Nosten FH, McGready R.** Maternal suicide risk among refugees and migrants. International Journal of Gynaecology and Obstetrics. 2016;**134**(2):223–4.
45. **Ao T, Shetty S, Sivilli T**, et al. Suicidal ideation and mental health of Bhutanese refugees in the United States. Journal of Immigrant and Minority Health. 2016;**18**(4):828–35.
46. **Chandler MJ, Lalonde CE.** Cultural continuity as a protective factor against suicide in First Nations youth. Horizons. 2008;**10**(1), 68–72.
47. **Park S, Rim SJ, Jun JY.** Related factors of suicidal ideation among North Korean refugee youth in South Korea. International Journal of Environmental Research and Public Health. 2018;**15**(8):1694.
48. **Sundvall M, Titelman D, Bäärnhielm S.** Challenges of combining perspectives. Crisis. 2018;**39**(5):326–34.
49. **Reko A, Bech P, Wohlert C, Noerregaard C, Csillag C.** Usage of psychiatric emergency services by asylum seekers: clinical implications based on a descriptive study in Denmark. Nordic Journal of Psychiatry. 2015;**69**:587–93.
50. **Yüzbaşıoğlu Y, Çıkrıkçı Işık G.** Retrospective analysis of forensic cases in refugees admitted to emergency department. American Journal of Emergency Medicine. 2019;**37**:1691–3.
51. **Bryant RA.** Psychological interventions for trauma exposure and PTSD. In: **Stein DJ**, Friedman MJ, Blanco C., editors. *Post-traumatic Stress Disorder*. Chichester: Wiley-Blackwell; 2011. pp. 171–202. https://doi.org/10.1002/9781119998471.ch5
52. **Cohen J.** Safe in our hands? A study of self-harm and suicide in asylum seekers. Journal of Forensic and Legal Medicine. 2008;**15**:235–44.
53. **Vijayakumar L, Mohanraj R, Kumar S, Jeyaseelan V, Sriram S, Shanmugam M.** CASP: an intervention by community volunteers to reduce suicidal behaviour among refugees. International Journal of Social Psychiatry. 2017;**63**(7):589–97.

Chapter 18

Suicide and psychiatric disorders

Isabella Berardelli, Elena Rogante,
Dorian A. Lamis, and Maurizio Pompili

Introduction

Suicide risk is the result of a multifactorial process where different elements interact with each other and should be evaluated considering the individual's distress. In fact, a significant body of literature has emphasized that the extreme sufferance experienced by the individual represents a central element associated with suicide risk.[1] This perturbated state, known as psychache or mental pain, constitutes a strategic construct for the phenomenology of suicide since when it reaches levels of intolerability, it may result in the belief that suicide is the only viable option to escape this condition.[2] In this framework, other factors, such as depressive symptoms, obtain relevance for their association with psychache which is considered a core aspect of suicide. Therefore, factors underlying suicide risk are complex, with multiple relevant domains generated over several years via developmental processes of the individual. According to the World Health Organization (WHO), mental health is a 'state of well-being in which an individual realizes his or her abilities, can cope with the normal stresses of life, can work productively, and can contribute to his or her community'. In this definition, the WHO emphasizes that mental health is 'more than just the absence of psychiatric disorders or disabilities; however, the presence of a psychiatric disorder affects mental health in various ways. In this perspective, it is important to point out that, even if suicide risk is not directly associated with the presence of psychiatric symptoms, up to 90% of people who die by suicide are diagnosed with a psychiatric disorder[3] and suicide risk has been estimated to be 5–8% for several psychiatric disorders.[4] Among the various psychiatric disorders, depression, substance use disorders, and psychosis are considered the most relevant risk factors. Anxiety, personality disorders (PDs), eating disorders, trauma-related disorders, and organic mental disorders also contribute to an increased vulnerability to suicide. Psychological autopsy studies demonstrated that around 90% of suicide decedents have one or more major psychiatric disorders at the time of their death. Specifically, major mood disorders (59–87%), schizophrenia/schizoaffective disorder (10–12%), and substance use disorders (10–15%) are the most common primary diagnoses.[5] Furthermore, comorbid anxiety and PDs are also frequently present but rare.[6] Although studies on psychological autopsies provided important data, it is important to note that scientific literature has also highlighted several limitations of this approach, specifically, the absence of standardized measures for the evaluation of psychopathological features and life events and the various ranges of agreement between the informants as a result of the heterogeneous methodologies used for the interviews.[1]

Despite scientific evidence, most people with psychiatric disorders do not die by suicide,[4] suggesting that a mental disorder is only one of the possible risk factors for suicide and other—genetic, personality, psychosocial, and demographic—risk factors may also contribute to the genesis of suicide risk. Several suicide risk factors in psychiatric disorders overlap with those found in the general population, whereas other factors are characteristic of each disorder (see Figure 18.1).

Furthermore, up to 66% of suicide decedents contact different levels of health care, providers including psychiatrists, during the four weeks before their suicide death;[5] successful and adequate pharmacotherapy for psychiatric disorders is indispensable not only to alleviate patients' clinical symptoms, but also to decrease their suicide risk. Therefore, research on suicide risk factors in people with mental disorders is critical to preventing suicide by implementing adequate suicide prevention strategies, including pharmacological therapies. Moreover, monitoring and assessing for suicidal ideation and attempts, as well as suicide risk factors, are central tasks in the field of suicide prevention. In this chapter, we summarize current knowledge on the association between psychiatric disorders and suicide risk, focusing on major depressive disorder (MDD), bipolar disorder (BD), schizophrenia, PDs, anxiety disorders, and alcohol and substance abuse disorders.

Suicide and bipolar disorder

The lifetime prevalence of BD is reported to be 1.3–1.6% in the general population, but national lifetime prevalence rates for BD type I (BD-I) and BD type II (BD-II) patients are different.[7] Suicide, cardiovascular diseases, and cancer are the three most frequent causes of death among BD patients.[8] The risk of suicide among patients with BD is estimated to be 20–30 times greater than that of the general population,[8,9] and suicide in BD may account for one-quarter of all suicide deaths.[10]

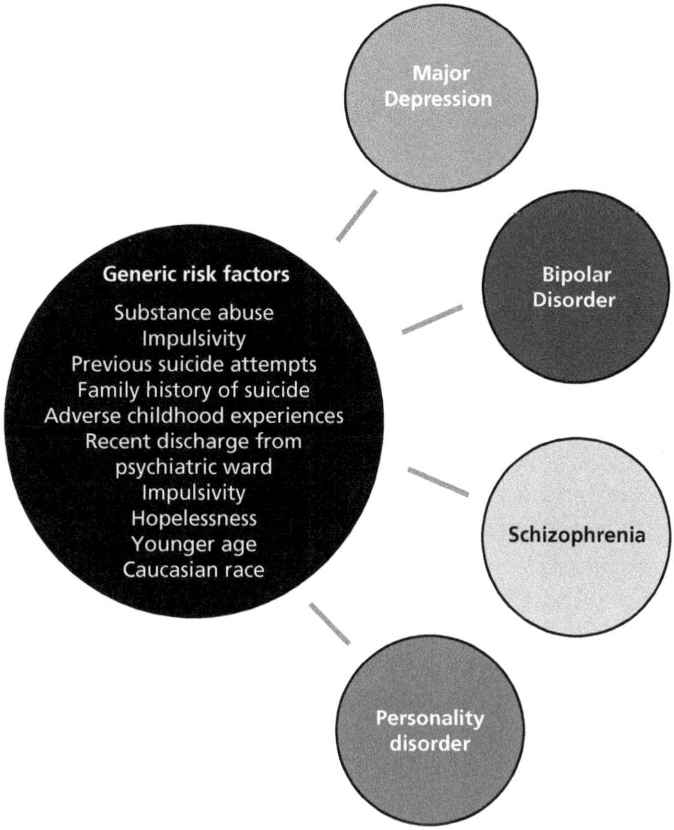

Figure 18.1 Generic risk factors.

Several suicide risk factors in BD overlap with those considered for the general population and for other psychiatric disorders, whereas other factors are characteristic of this disorder (see Figure 18.2). Suicide rates in BD may vary considerably according to gender, previous history of suicide attempts, psychiatric admissions, duration of psychiatric illness, type of medications prescribed, adherence to treatment, recent discharge from a psychiatric hospital, and occupational and interpersonal features.[11] Research has demonstrated that BD patients at highest risk of suicide are generally white, younger, divorced or living alone, and with more frequent hospitalizations. Furthermore, patients with prior suicide attempts, recent discharge from a psychiatric hospital, and occupational problems may also be considered to be at increased risk of suicide. Researchers have demonstrated that suicide risk is higher during the early phase of the disease.[12] A family history of suicide attempts and death increases

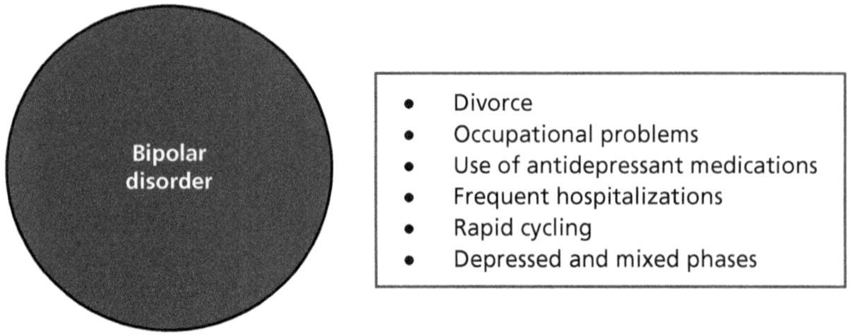

Figure 18.2 Risk factors for bipolar disorder.

suicide risk, especially in first-degree relatives,[13,14] probably in relation to BD heritability (40%) and familial transmission of suicidal behaviour. Regarding other general risk factors for suicide, several researchers have shown that suicide risk is higher among young Caucasian men compared to women.[15,16]

Several clinical features of BD contribute to suicide risk. Studies have demonstrated that suicidal behaviour is mainly related to depressed and mixed phases of BD.[17] Notably, major depressive episodes are associated with the highest risk of suicide, followed by mixed episodes and manic episodes. Furthermore, patients with rapid cycling present with a higher suicide risk than non-rapid cyclers.[9] In light of these observations, the predominant polarity of BD can be used not only to predict the polarity of subsequent episodes, but also to predict suicide risk, with prevailing depression carrying the highest risk of suicide. Mixed states with predominant depression also have a markedly increased association with suicide.[18,19]

In BD, suicidal ideation varies from 14% to 59%. It is related to hopelessness, mixed depression, severe depression, psychotic symptoms, past suicide attempts, alcohol abuse, panic disorder symptoms, and earlier age of onset.[20] In particular, suicidal ideation occurs in 79% of bipolar patients during the depressed phase.[21] Depressive polarity in subsequent episodes is associated with an increased risk of suicidal acts and suicide attempts. Suicidal ideation and behaviour are also common in mixed episodes and dysphoric mania, with 26–55% of patients with dysphoric mania presenting with suicidal ideation.[21] However, BD patients attempt, or die by, suicide mostly during severe, pure, or mixed depressive episodes (78–80%), much less frequently during mixed affective episodes or dysphoric mania (11–20%), and very rarely during states of euphoric mania or euthymia (0–7%).[21] Severe, agitated, or anxious major depression, especially with recurrent insomnia in the presence of a past suicide attempt, is associated with the highest risk of suicide in BD patients.[22] The rapid cycling subtype of BD has also been identified as a risk factor for suicide attempts, with a 54% higher risk of attempted suicide and greater intent and lethality compared to non-rapid cyclers.[23] Other specific features of mood disorders have been associated with suicide, including increased risk at the onset of illness during the first depressive episode, earlier stage in the illness course, longer duration of untreated illness, the number of previous depressive episodes, previous hospitalizations, and concurrent medical comorbidity.[5] There is also an association between the emergence of mood-incongruent psychotic symptoms and increased suicide risk. In addition to clinical characteristics of BD, a comorbid anxiety disorder and a substance abuse disorder are considered important risk factors for suicide death, mainly if related to acute mood episodes.[8]

Among all risk factors for suicide deaths, it is important to highlight the use of antidepressant medications, particularly after abrupt discontinuation of a mood stabilizer[24] or when the patient has stopped taking lithium.[25] It has been estimated that without treatment, about 10 in 1000 BD patients die by suicide every year and 40 in 1000 attempt suicide.[26] Suicide deaths seem to occur more often in the first six months after discharge, particularly in the first three months.[27]

Despite continuing progress in suicide prevention, suicide risk is still mistreated in BD. Assessing suicide risk factors in patients with BD is fundamental to properly managing these patients.[8,28] Furthermore, BD patients use more lethal suicide methods, compared to unipolar patients.[29] In conclusion, several risk factors, including history of past suicide attempt and family history of suicide attempt or death, as well as a predominantly depressive polarity, can be used to assess for, and monitor, suicide risk in patients with BD.

Suicide and major depressive disorder

Major depression and hopelessness are among the most studied risk factors for suicide and are consistently featured in risk factor guidelines developed by major national and international organizations. In addition, many studies have found that the presence of depressive symptoms and hopelessness confers an important risk of suicidal ideation, suicide attempts, and death, even in the absence of a diagnosis of MDD.[30]

The association between a diagnosis of MDD and suicide risk has been well documented; suicidal ideation and suicide attempt were frequently reported during depressive episodes, with a suicide risk rate equivalent to around 15%. Different pathophysiological factors are involved in the relationship between depression and suicidal risk; genetics, exogenous and endogenous stressors

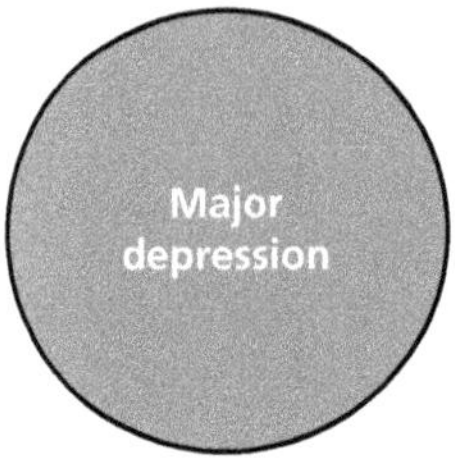

- Exogenous and endogenous stressors
- Alteration in the HPA Axis and in serotoninergic system
- Epigenetic alterations
- Specific neurotrophins
- Insomnia
- Mixed states or agitated depression
- Cyclothymic/irritable/depressive affective temperaments
- Acute psychosocial stressors

Figure 18.3 Risk factors for major depression.

(i.e. interpersonal, professional, and financial stressors, as well as psychiatric disorders), alteration in the hypothalamic–pituitary–adrenal (HPA) stress response system, epigenetics alterations, the monoaminergic neurotransmitter system, particularly serotonergic, and specific neurotrophins are all factors involved in the genesis of suicide risk in MDD[31] (see Figure 18.3). Several clinical features of depression are also involved in suicide risk: early onset of illness, hopelessness, and insomnia, as well as comorbid anxiety, substance use, and PDs.[11,32,33] In addition, depressive mixed states or agitated depression and impulsivity as a personality trait increase suicide risk in depressed patients.[5,34] Current findings also show that cyclothymic/irritable/depressive affective temperaments, characteristic of unipolar disorder and BD, also increase the risk of suicidal behaviour in patients with a depressive episode.[35] Risk factors for suicide in major depression include personal and family history of suicide, family history of suicide among first- and second-degree relatives, past suicide attempt(s), and exposure to childhood physical or sexual abuse.[36,37] Impulsivity seems to be one factor involved in the relationship between childhood abuse and suicidal behaviour, particularly in the case of major depressive episodes.[38]

Furthermore, adverse life events play an important role in a suicidal crisis as predisposing factors (childhood events, including physical and sexual abuse) and precipitating factors (adulthood events).[39,40] Chronic adverse life situations, including unemployment and social isolation, and acute psychosocial stressors (e.g. loss events, financial difficulties) in adult patients with unipolar depression are implicated in suicide risk, mainly if they are present at the same time.[41] In most patients with MDD, if more than one suicide risk factor is present simultaneously, their effect is cumulative; the higher the number of risk factors, the higher the risk of suicide crises.

To better understand specific suicide risk factors in MDD, several studies have investigated the relationship between suicide risk and hospitalization, underlining two different periods of vulnerability: one during the first week after admission to a psychiatric ward and another in the first week following discharge.[42] Furthermore, suicide risk is significantly higher in patients receiving a shorter than the median length of hospital treatment, and an admission history increases the risk relatively more in women patients compared to men.[42]

In contrast to the numerous suicide risk factors, several features are known to have a protective effect in patients with major depression. For example, good family and social support, pregnancy and the post-partum period, having more children, holding strong religious beliefs, restricting lethal suicide methods, and the presence of a hyperthymic temperament seem to have some protective effects against suicide risk in patients with depressive disorders.[43,44,45] However, one of the most extensively studied suicide protective factors in major mood disorders is appropriate acute and long-term pharmacological treatment. Given the strong relationship between depression and suicide risk, detecting suicide risk as early as possible and intervening with proper therapy seem necessary to prevent a suicidal crisis.

Suicide and schizophrenia

Suicide in schizophrenia is a complex and underestimated phenomenon, and a frequent cause of early mortality, affecting nearly 5% of patients with schizophrenia.[46] Furthermore, 25–50% of patients with schizophrenia attempt suicide in their lifetime.[47] Though suicide may occur at any point during the clinical course of schizophrenia, several studies suggested that the first 10 years of illness are the period with higher vulnerability to suicide risk.[48] Evidence has demonstrated numerous individual, clinical, social, and psychological risk factors for suicide in patients affected by schizophrenia (see Figure 18.4).[44,49,50] Patients with suicide risk who are diagnosed with schizophrenia are generally white, young, and unmarried, with good premorbid function, post-psychotic depression, and a history of substance abuse and suicide attempts.[51] Other important suicide risk factors include the presence of hopelessness, social

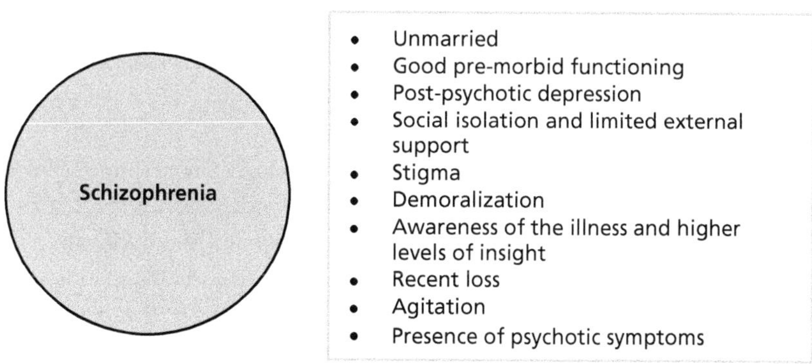

Figure 18.4 Risk factors for schizophrenia.

isolation, limited external support, stigma, demoralization, awareness of the illness, recent loss, agitation, impulsivity, and hospitalization.[52,53] Schizophrenia subtypes, symptom dimensions and severity, global functioning, and alcohol and substance abuse also contribute to an increased suicide risk.[54] Patients with high suicide risk often present with mental deterioration and experience excessive treatment dependence or loss of faith in treatment.[55] Research has also reported suicides due to several psychotic symptoms, including hallucinations, control of thought or thought insertion, loose association, and flight of ideas.[56] Suicide attempts in schizophrenia are often serious; patients typically use highly lethal and violent methods, requiring urgent medical attention and hospitalization.[57]

Dickerson et al.[58] studied 733 patients with a schizophrenia spectrum disorder to examine the role of different variables in suicide risk. This study found that being Caucasian (vs African American) and male was associated with higher hazard rates for suicide. Conversely, a meta-analysis and meta-regression of 96 studies[59] found that being male was a protective factor against suicide in schizophrenia patients.[60] Moreover, several studies demonstrated that younger patients were more likely to attempt suicide.[61,62] Furthermore, in a longitudinal study published in 2017,[63] suicide rates in the unmarried sample were three times higher than in the married sample. Thus, although higher suicide rates have been identified in younger patients, suicide risk tends to remain stable throughout life in individuals with schizophrenia.

Several specific clinical features of schizophrenia are well documented as suicide risk factors. Several authors reported that a longer illness duration was significantly associated with lifetime suicide attempts.[64] Recently, Chang et al.[65] showed that a longer illness duration was a predictor of lifetime suicide attempts in a sample of 263 patients with schizophrenia. Dai et al.[66] replicated this result in a study that compared 908 schizophrenia patients with suicide attempts to those without suicide attempts. The authors identified an indirect path between positive symptoms (hallucinations and delusions) and suicidal ideation through social isolation. Premorbid functioning in psychotic disorders reflects a wide range of social, interpersonal, and occupational skills, which influence clinical and functional outcomes.[67] In a study by Pompili et al.,[54] good premorbid functioning was found to increase the risk of dying by suicide. The authors explained this result as consistent with the 'demoralization syndrome',[68] in which a good level of functioning and insight into the illness may cause hopelessness and suicidal thoughts.[53] Similarly, Bakst et al.[69] assessed premorbid functioning in a sample of 444 individuals with a first psychotic episode and found that a higher likelihood of suicide attempts before the first psychiatric hospitalization was associated with poorer premorbid functioning. Positive and negative symptoms are core manifestations of schizophrenia and may be experienced as enduring and unmanageable. Positive symptoms include delusions, hallucinations, perceptual disturbances, and disorganized speech and behaviour, whereas negative symptoms include anhedonia, lack of emotional experience and expression, and cognitive decline.[70] Evidence regarding the predictive value of positive and negative symptoms in suicide risk is still conflicting.[71,72,73] Andriopoulos et al.[74] found that positive and negative symptoms were increased in individuals with suicidal ideation (vs those without suicidal ideation). Gill et al.[75] examined 42 individuals at high risk of psychosis and found a significant association between suicidal ideation and negative symptoms.

Conversely, Taylor et al.[76] assessed the effect of positive symptoms on suicidal ideation in 78 patients with schizophrenia through the perception of defeat and entrapment. However, the association between specific subtypes of schizophrenia and suicide risk is still controversial. The review conducted by Pompili et al.[77] found no significant differences in suicide risk according to the classical categorization of schizophrenia as catatonic, hebephrenic, or undifferentiated.

Previous suicide attempts are one of the most critical risk factors for suicidal behaviour.[77] Age of schizophrenia onset has a crucial role in understanding the developmental and distinctive features (i.e. genetic and environmental antecedents) of the disease that appear in early adulthood and become chronic and impairing.[78] In particular, suicide risk seems to be associated with an early onset of schizophrenia, as confirmed by Vinokur et al.[79] in a study on 138 patients with schizophrenia. Moreover, in a British follow-up investigation,[80] most suicides were found to occur within the first two years of psychotic disorder onset. Another study by Castelein et al.[73] which followed 424 patients with schizophrenia for 20 years found that suicide rates reduced from 11.0% to 2.4%. Recent discharge from a psychiatric ward is another risk factor for suicide, as noted in a recent study[81] that reported a suicide rate of 178 per 100,000 person-years within the first three months after discharge. In a systematic review by Hawton et al.,[50] agitation or motor restlessness seemed to be associated with suicide risk in patients with schizophrenia. Pompili et al.[82] conducted a retrospective case-control study comparing 20 patients with schizophrenia who died by suicide to 20 living controls. Their results demonstrated that agitation and motor restlessness might significantly predict suicide. Furthermore, guidelines drafted by the European Psychiatric Association[83] highlight the role of agitation in determining suicidal behaviour in patients with schizophrenia.

During the last 15 years, most researchers have defined insight as comprising at least three domains: awareness of the illness; awareness of the need for treatment; and awareness of the consequences of the disorder.[84] Some studies[85,86] demonstrated that hopeless awareness of the severity of psychopathology was one of the most important predictors of suicide death in patients with psychotic disorders. However, it is still unclear whether insight is directly related to suicide or indirectly related to its influence on hopelessness. Several studies have demonstrated that illness awareness is associated with an increased suicide risk in patients with schizophrenia.[87,88,89] In a recent study on 100 psychiatric inpatients, Berardelli et al.[90] showed that patients with higher scores on the insight-high dimension had 1.35 greater odds of having a higher suicide risk, indicating that greater illness insight is involved in suicide risk.

Past and current depressive disorders were strongly associated with suicide in patients diagnosed with schizophrenia.[91,92] More than 50% of patients who died by suicide were depressed at the time of suicide,[50] and it has been suggested that a depressive disorder may trigger suicidal behaviour in vulnerable patients with schizophrenia.[93] Hopelessness is a significant risk factor in people diagnosed with schizophrenia,[94] even without concomitant depression.[68] Insight into the illness is associated with suicide only if it leads to hopelessness.[88] Thus, hopelessness may be an even better marker of suicide death than depression.[95] Several studies have also demonstrated that symptoms of demoralization in patients with schizophrenia are related to suicide risk.[53]

Repeated psychiatric hospitalizations are a common feature of patients with schizophrenia due to the disease's chronic nature and poor medication adherence.[96] Moreover, rehospitalization seems to be strongly associated with suicidal ideation and behaviours, as highlighted by Fleishhacker et al.,[97] who analysed potential baseline risk factors for attempted suicide in 18,154 subjects with schizophrenia. Results showed that a history of more than five hospitalizations was, alongside previous suicide attempts, the strongest variable associated with attempted suicide. Zhang et al.[98] assessed 520 inpatients with schizophrenia and compared suicide attempters to non-attempters. They found that patients who attempted suicide reported significantly more frequent hospitalizations, and logistic regression analysis indicated that suicide attempts were associated with more hospitalizations.

Family functioning (i.e. the ability to adapt to changes), which is determined by cohesion, flexibility, and communication within a family, is often compromised in families of individuals with schizophrenia. Moreover, disrupted relationships with family members may increase suicide risk.[99] Recent loss is often considered a risk factor for suicide in patients with schizophrenia. Gallego et al.[100] investigated 3322 patients diagnosed with schizophrenia and affective disorders, and reported a significant association between recent financial or relational loss and current suicide attempts. In a sample of 180 patients with first-episode psychosis, Fedyszyn et al.[101] demonstrated that one of the strongest risk factors for suicide was a recent negative event such as a traumatic or stressful experience. Social isolation, which consists of disrupted or non-existent interpersonal contacts and relationships, is a well-known suicide risk factor in schizophrenia. Recently, several papers have further addressed this relationship. Bornheimer et al.[102] investigated the relationship between social isolation, psychosis, and suicidal ideation, and confirmed a mediating effect of social isolation in the relationship between psychosis and suicidal ideation.

Adverse childhood experiences (ACEs) that include physical, sexual, and psychological abuse and neglect can impair the sense of security of the individual (i.e. substance-abusing parents, divorce, incarceration of a family member, etc.).[103] ACEs are related to the onset of several psychiatric symptoms and diagnoses.[104] In patients with schizophrenia spectrum disorders, the prevalence of ACEs is almost three times more frequent than in the general population, and ACEs seem to have a key role in suicidal ideation and behaviours.[105] One study[106] found that patients with schizophrenia who had experienced ACEs were more likely to attempt suicide than those who did not report ACEs. Moreover, Prokopez et al.[107] analysed 100 patients with schizophrenia and observed that multiple ACEs were associated with a higher frequency of suicide attempts.

Suicide risk also seems to be associated with poor adherence to treatment. Hering and Erkens[108] analysed 603 patients with schizophrenia and observed a fourfold increased risk of suicide when comparing the group that interrupted their antipsychotic drug treatment to the group that continued treatment. Antipsychotic medications are associated with several movement disorders, acute side effects, late-onset side effects, tardive dyskinesia, and extrapyramidal symptoms (EPS). The latter include acute dystonia and parkinsonism.[109]

Although suicide prevention strategies include drug treatment, administration of pharmacotherapy may be accompanied by increased insight, illness awareness, and demoralization symptoms that could increase suicide risk in patients with schizophrenia. According to the 'insight paradox' in patients with schizophrenia, higher levels of insight are frequently associated with high levels of depression,[110] and therefore with suicide risk. Therefore, appropriate suicide assessment is needed for patients on pharmacological treatment and after a hospital discharge when patients usually present with higher levels of hopelessness and demoralization.[53]

Substance abuse is a common phenomenon among individuals with schizophrenia. Up to 50% of patients with schizophrenia exhibit either alcohol or illicit drug dependence, and more than 70% are nicotine-dependent.[111] In particular, heavy cannabis abuse has been reported to be a stressor, eliciting relapse in patients with schizophrenia and related disorders. Although it is difficult to compare the relative impact of different mental health problems on suicide risk, alcohol and drug use disorders have been strongly related to suicide.[112] Multiple potential links have been discussed, including genetic vulnerability, treatment side effects, and psychosocial factors. Possible explanations for the increased incidence of substance use in schizophrenia include the self-medication hypothesis.[113] Individuals with a substance use disorder (i.e. a diagnosis of either alcohol or drug abuse or dependence) are almost six times more likely to report a lifetime suicide attempt than those without a substance use disorder.[114]

Social support is crucial in maintaining mental health well-being and represents a key factor in managing disabling disorders such as schizophrenia.[115] Several studies have demonstrated the protective role of social support in reducing suicide risk.[116,117] Social support increases feelings of belongingness and prevents negative appraisals after stressful events, and the presence of individuals can physically prevent suicide attempts. Conversely, only a few studies have analysed the role of poor social support in suicide risk in schizophrenia spectrum disorders. Xie et al.[118] reported a significant negative correlation between social support and suicidal ideation in a sample of patients with schizophrenia. In a study on 212 patients with schizophrenia, Pješčić et al.[119] showed a higher prevalence of poor social support and social isolation in patients with suicidal ideation.

Finally, several studies have suggested that a relationship exists between social and cognitive dysfunction and severe health outcomes, premature mortality, and suicide risk in patients with schizophrenia.[120]

Suicide and personality disorders

PDs are enduring, inflexible, and pervasive patterns of behaviour and inner experience that deviate from cultural norms and cause significant distress or impairment in various areas of individuals' functioning.[70] PDs are common in practice and can be found, above and beyond other diagnoses, in up to 45% of all outpatients.[121] PDs are associated with a wide range of psychopathology, including unstable mood, impulsive behaviours, and unstable interpersonal relationships. Research has shown that PDs are often associated with a high risk of suicidal ideation, and suicide attempts and deaths[122] (see Figure 18.5). PDs also increase the risk of self-mutilating behaviours. For example, a study on deliberately self-injuring young inmates showed a high prevalence of PDs and other clinical syndromes in this population compared to inmates without self-mutilating episodes.[123] A review of psychological autopsy studies indicated that up to 57% of individuals who died by suicide were diagnosed with PDs.[122] Data from the World Health Organization/EURO Multicenter Study on Suicidal Behaviour[124] showed that PDs are present in 18% of male, and 15% of female,

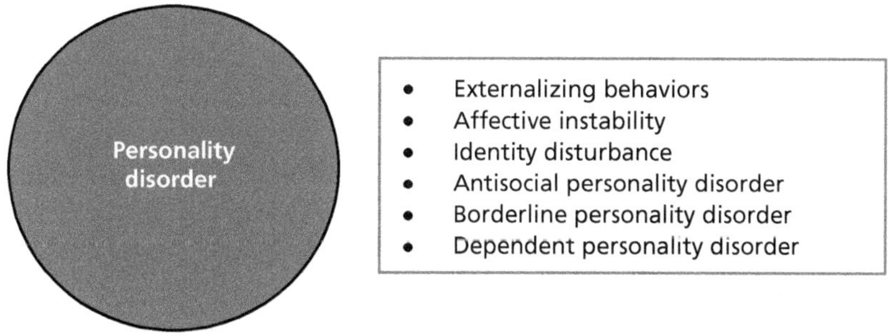

Figure 18.5 Risk factors for personality disorders.

suicide attempters, suggesting that suicide prevention strategies encompass identification and treatment of all mental disorders, including PDs.

Further, studies demonstrated that PDs are related to an increased risk of suicide and self-mutilation in the general population and individuals with other psychiatric diagnosis.[125] A general population study analysing the correlates of 'externalizing' and 'internalizing' psychopathology found that antisocial personality disorder (APD) was related to suicidal behaviour independently of the presence of internalizing symptoms (e.g. depression, anxiety).[126] A report from a 2-year follow-up Collaborative Longitudinal Personality Disorders Study[127] indicated that in individuals with borderline personality disorder (BPD), there might be separate risk factors for suicidal behaviours and suicide attempts. Suicidal behaviours were strongly associated with affective instability, identity disturbance, and impulsivity, and suicidal attempts were linked with affective instability and a history of childhood sexual abuse.

Although most research has focused on BPD and APD, other personality disorders with comorbid depression might be associated with an increased risk of suicidal behaviour.[128] Moreover, most research has focused on single PDs or categorical PD diagnoses without considering the unique influences of different PDs or the severity (sum) of PD criteria on the risk of suicide-related outcomes.

Research has shown that suicide occurs in up to 10% of patients with BPD.[129] However, several discrepancies in suicide rates have been reported in different studies, probably in relation to lower suicide risk in patients who agree to be followed in research studies.[121] Paris et al.[121] observed that suicides in patients with BPD occurred later in the illness and were mostly related to unsuccessful treatment.

Numerous studies examined possible causal pathways between various aspects of the psychosocial functioning of individuals with PDs and suicide risk. Specific recent life events, including love/marriage and crime/legal problems, may increase the imminent risk of suicidal behaviour among individuals with schizotypal, avoidant, borderline, and obsessive–compulsive PDs.[130] Several studies have confirmed the role of childhood sexual abuse as a risk factor for suicide and psychopathology among individuals with BPD.[131,132] In addition, interpersonal problems in individuals diagnosed with BPD, probably related to difficulties in social functioning, represent other suicide risk factors. Poor skills in expressing and understanding non-verbal communication, as well as a relatively high degree of identity confusion in gender roles, represent other suicide risk factors.[133,134] Other mechanisms involved in impulsive suicidal behaviours include deficits in positive future time thinking, which might be related to hopelessness and impulsivity. Further, self-harm in individuals diagnosed with BPD might be related to time perception deficits and orbitofrontal cortex dysfunction.[135] In addition, it has been found that first-degree relatives of BPD individuals who die by suicide present with high levels of aggression and suicidal ideation.[136]

In light of the multifactorial nature of BPD psychopathology,[137,138,139] different theories emphasize various aspects of BPD to explain suicidal risk. Thus, Maltsberger and Lovett[140] emphasized break-up of the self; Gunderson[141] focused on reactivity in the context of insecure attachment and abandonment sensitivity; Linehan[142] and then Stanley and Brodsky[143] highlighted emotional dysregulation and regulatory function of suicide attempts, whereas Kernberg[144] focused mainly on anger, and Singer[145] on emptiness. From an integrative standpoint, Oldham[146] suggested five different types of suicidal BPD patients: affective, impulsive, aggressive, dependent, and empty. These theories match such established clusters of BPD as identity disturbance,[139] interpersonal dysregulation, emotional instability, and impulsivity.[137,138] In conclusion, identifying PD risk factors for suicide attempts is an important research and clinical care consideration.

Suicide and anxiety disorders

Psychic anxiety, agitation, panic attacks, and severe insomnia associated with clinical depression are considered acute high-risk factors that are rapidly modifiable by treatment, and therefore are particularly important to recognize and assess.[147] Suicide risk in patients with anxiety disorders is still unclear, ranging between 6% and 60%. Coryell et al.[148] raised concerns about the high suicide rate among patients with panic disorder—20% when patients were followed for 35 years. On the other hand, Henriksson et al.[149] contended that, based on 1987 autopsy reports in Finland, only 1.2% of suicides had a diagnosis of panic disorder, a figure lower than expected, given the prevalence of panic disorder. Other authors have suggested that the risk of suicide attempt is low in 'pure' panic patients, but relatively high among those with psychiatric comorbidity—depression,[150]

BPD,[151] or substance abuse.[152] Regarding the relation between social anxiety disorder (SAD) and suicide risk, several authors stressed that, given the numerous domains in which individuals with SAD experience impairment, it is not surprising that they are also at greater risk of suicide spectrum disorders.[153] Research suggests that 22% of individuals with SAD have experienced suicidal ideation in the past month and 35% will experience suicidal ideation in their lifetime. A recent meta-analysis[154] showed that several symptoms were associated with suicide risk in patients with panic disorder. Depressive symptoms and agoraphobia were associated with both suicidal ideation and suicide attempt in patients with panic disorder. In addition, anxiety symptoms were directly related to suicidal ideation. Moreover, factors related to the duration of the disorder, such as age of onset and patients' age, were strongly associated with suicide attempts, and the mean length of the disease was associated with suicidal ideation. Finally, patients with panic disorder often have comorbid alcohol or other substance abuse disorders and are more likely to attempt, or die by, suicide.

Several studies on psychiatric patients with anxiety comorbidity demonstrated that the presence of an anxiety disorder increases suicide risk. Panic attacks have been associated with suicide risk in patients with schizophrenia and those with depression.[155] Analysis of a subsample of the STEP-BD study consisting of 120 bipolar patients reported that the presence of a comorbid anxiety disorder doubled the odds of a past suicide attempt. Moreover, the presence of a current anxiety disorder doubled the odds of suicidal ideation and of significantly more severe suicidal ideation.[14] A survey of 7076 subjects found that the presence of any anxiety disorder was significantly associated with both the presence of suicidal ideation and a history of suicide attempts in this epidemiologic sample.[156] Similar results were observed by Wunderlich et al.[157] on 1000 adolescents and young adults aged 16–25 years, and by Boden et al.[158] on 3021 adolescents. Foley et al.[159] found that patients with depression and comorbid anxiety (generalized anxiety disorder) showed the greatest risk of suicidal thoughts and behaviour. Fava et al.[160,161] found that patients with anxious depression were less likely to attain remission with treatment and had more suicidal ideation and more severe symptom patterns. In conclusion, studies on the relationship between anxiety disorders and suicide risk suggest that an assessment of the severity of psychic anxiety, panic attacks, agitation, and insomnia should be a standard element of a suicide risk assessment.

Suicide and dissociative disorders

Dissociative disorders are characterized by sudden or gradual, transient or chronic disturbances, and alterations of memory, identity, perception, or consciousness where the integrative functions of selfhood are dissociated from the mainstream of consciousness of individuals.[162] Several studies have shown that severe dissociative experiences are related to an inclination for self-mutilation and suicidal behaviour.[163] An association between dissociation and suicide risk has been shown in psychiatric and non-psychiatric populations.[164,165,166,167] Several authors have indicated that suicidal individuals experienced dissociation to a higher degree than non-suicidal individuals[168] and hypothesized a common organic basis for both syndromes in right hemisphere dysfunction that manifests itself in general failure of organization, failure to achieve adaptation by using integration of various aspects of functioning and self-representation, lower sensitivity to pain, cognitive constriction, and difficulties in affect regulation.[169] Research indicates that dissociative disorder patients more frequently engage in self-destructive behaviour, use more methods of self-injury, and begin to injure themselves at an earlier age than patients who do not dissociate.[170] Coons and Milstein[171] evaluated 100 consecutive patients with dissociative disorders who were enrolled in a dissociative disorders clinic and found that 36 patients had a history of self-mutilation. Self-mutilation was most common among patients with dissociative identity disorder (48%), as compared to 29% of patients diagnosed with dissociative amnesia and 23% of patients diagnosed with a dissociative disorder 'Not Otherwise Specified'. None of the four patients with a dissociative fugue reported a history of self-injurious behaviour. The above results are consistent with those from Putnam et al.[172] who reported a 34% incidence of self-injurious behaviour in their sample of patients with dissociative identity disorder. More recently, Leonard et al.[173] reported an incidence of 68% of self-injurious behaviour in 55 Australian patients with a dissociative disorder. However, the relationship between dissociative experiences and self-injurious behaviour is complex and more research is needed. Several authors have reported the phenomenon of pain analgesia, a dissociative condition which may facilitate self-harm;[174,175] sometimes self-mutilation can be a method of stopping uncomfortable dissociative experiences,[176] and patients experience amnesia for their episodes of self-mutilation.[168] Most research focuses only on dissociative identity disorder, and only case reports are available for other dissociative disorders. In a clinical investigation of 25 cases of dissociative amnesia, Coons and Milstein[177] reported a 16% incidence of suicide attempts precipitating an amnesic episode. Leonard et al.[173] reported an incidence of 69% of suicide attempts in a sample of 55 patients with dissociative disorders. Tutkun et al.[178] reported rates of 88% of self-mutilation and 82% of suicide attempts among their sample of inpatients. All studies on dissociative identity disorder have reported a high incidence of attempted suicide, ranging from 61% to 91%. For example, Bliss[179] evaluated a sample of 14 patients and found an incidence of 91% of suicide attempts, whereas Putnam et al. [172] found an incidence of 61% of attempted suicide in 100 patients (and also one suicide death).

Suicide and obsessive–compulsive disorder

Several studies have demonstrated that suicide risk in obsessive–compulsive disorder (OCD) is 10 times higher than expected in the general population.[180] More recently, Angelakis and colleagues[181] analysed 48 studies on the association between suicide risk and OCD, demonstrating a significant association between OCD and suicidal ideation and suicide attempts. Furthermore, given that individuals with OCD present with a higher risk of suicidal ideation and suicide attempts than the general population, it is important to determine which patients should be considered at highest suicide risk. Preventive strategies primarily identify and intervene on modifiable risk factors for suicide. Early recognition and diagnosis of OCD and effective pharmacological and psychological treatments of the disorder remain essential for preventing suicide.[182] Studies demonstrated that the association between OCD and suicide risk is independent of the presence of MDD comorbidity; this implies that OCD is associated with a significant risk of suicidal ideation, probably an expression of the disability associated with this disorder.[183] Suicide risk factors in patients with OCD include a history of suicide (previous suicide attempts, previous or current suicidal ideation) and a family history of suicide (increased risk by 78%).[184] More controversy exists about the association between pure OCD (without lifetime comorbid disorders) and suicide attempts.[185]

Suicide and alcohol use disorders, and alcohol intoxication

The relationship between alcohol use disorders (AUDs), alcohol intoxication, and suicide is well documented.[186] Studies reported an almost 10-fold increase in standardized mortality ratios for suicide among patients with AUDs.[187] Furthermore, researchers demonstrated that among suicide decedents who were psychiatrically hospitalized, AUDs in middle-aged males had the highest contribution to the risk of suicide. A meta-analysis of psychological autopsy studies conducted by Yoshimasu et al.[188] demonstrated that substance-related disorders were strongly associated with suicide. The association between AUDs and suicide was stronger in women than in men. Also, acute intoxication is associated with suicidal behaviour. Different mechanisms have been proposed to be involved in this relationship, including increased psychological distress, increased aggressiveness, increased likelihood of translation of ideation into action, (increased impulsivity), and constricted cognition. Cherpitel et al.[189] reviewed studies on acute use of alcohol and suicide, and reported a wide range of results. Between 10–69% of suicide decedents were positive for alcohol and 10–73% of those who attempted suicide were positive for alcohol use. Bagge and colleagues[190] studied 192 recent suicide attempters who presented to a level 1 trauma hospital. They reported that after controlling for acute drug use and negative life events, individuals are at increased risk of suicide attempts soon after drinking. Another recent study by Conner and colleagues[191] using findings from the National Violent Death Reporting System found that among 37,993 decedents who used the three leading methods of suicide (firearm, hanging, and poisoning), alcohol was present in over a third of cases. Although acute intoxication is not the same as alcohol abuse or dependence, the risk of suicide attempts or suicide will intensify during intoxication in individuals with or without a substance use disorder. This also may be particularly important for treatment providers to consider when relapse occurs in a patient to recovery who has a history of mental illness or previous suicidal behaviour. There are various risk factors for suicidal behaviour in those with alcoholism, including gender, family history, and a history of childhood sexual abuse. Higher rates of attempts were associated with females, younger individuals, those with a family history of suicidal behaviour, those on antidepressants, those with higher measures of aggression, and those who began heavy drinking earlier in life.

Further, factors predicting future suicide attempts in individuals with AUD included prior attempts, younger age, separation or divorce, other drug dependence, substance-induced psychiatric disorders, and indicators of severe AUD.[192] Individuals who attempted, or died by, suicide were found to have a more severe form of alcoholism than alcoholics who never attempted suicide. Suicidal behaviour is also associated with a heavier drinking pattern, younger age of onset, and longer duration of alcoholism.[193] Among alcoholics, the greatest risk factor for suicide or a medically severe suicide attempt is the presence of major depression. Recent partner relationship disruption is also a highly significant risk factor for suicide in someone with AUD, and other risk factors include male gender, older age, unemployment, poor social support and increased levels of aggression and impulsivity, comorbid drug abuse, recent heavy drinking and severe alcoholism, serious medical illness, and suicidal communication.[194]

Suicide and drug addiction

For drug addiction, the association with suicidal behaviour is as compelling as that for alcohol. Roy[195] interviewed 527 abstinent opiate-dependent patients in substance abuse treatment sprogrammes and found that 39% had attempted suicide. He reported that significantly more people with opiate dependence who had attempted suicide were female and unemployed. Opiate-dependent suicide attempters were also younger and had significantly more family history of suicide and more childhood trauma than those with opioid dependence who did not attempt suicide. Logistic regression analyses revealed that a family history of suicidal behaviour, alcohol dependence, cocaine dependence, and antidepressant treatment were significant predictors of attempting suicide. Wilcox and colleagues'[186] meta-review of cohort studies on decedents of suicide found that heroin users had a 13.5-fold increase in standardized mortality ratios for suicide compared to a 10-fold increase in those with AUDs.

Roy[195] reported that 43.5% of abstinent cocaine-dependent subjects had attempted suicide. Suicide attempters were more likely to be younger and female and to report childhood trauma. They were also more likely to have a family history of suicidal behaviour, aggression, antidepressant treatment, and comorbidity with alcohol and opiate dependence. In this study, childhood trauma, comorbidity with alcohol dependence, and treatment with antidepressants were significant predictors of attempting suicide.

Landheim et al.[196] studied 260 Norwegian subjects with substance use disorders who sought treatment in inpatient and outpatient settings, and found that 58% of those with polysubstance dependence reported lifetime suicide attempts compared to 38% of those who were only alcohol-dependent. Female polysubstance abusers had the highest frequency of suicide attempts (70%). Wilcox and colleagues,[186] in their meta-analysis, found that polydrug use resulted in a nearly 17-fold increase in suicide rates as compared to the general population.

Suicide risk prevention strategies

Suicide prevention in patients with psychiatric disorders is a complex phenomenon. Inadequate knowledge of suicide risk factors negatively affects the ability of clinicians to recognize patients at risk of suicide. Careful assessment and management of psychotic symptoms, depression, hopelessness, demoralization symptoms, and substance use disorders are necessary to prevent suicide in patients with psychiatric disorders.

Several pharmacological and non-pharmacological strategies are available to reduce suicide risk. Undoubtedly enhancing adherence to medications is critical. For patients with schizophrenia, studies suggested that antipsychotic medications, including clozapine, risperidone, olanzapine, and quetiapine, may reduce mortality and suicide risk.[197,198] In 2002, the US Food and Drug

Administration (FDA) approved clozapine for decreasing suicide risk in patients with schizophrenia. Studies have suggested that use of atypical antipsychotics may be more effective than that of typical antypsychotics.[115,199] Evidence for the ability of clozapine therapy to reduce suicidal behaviours has been highlighted in several studies since the late 1990s. Meltzer and Okayli[200] observed 88 neuroleptic-resistant patients treated with clozapine for 0.5–7.0 years and reported a decrease in suicidal behaviour. Walker and colleagues[201] noted that suicidal behaviour decreased in patients with current clozapine treatment compared to past users. Reinstein et al.,[202] in a retrospective study of 295 patients, confirmed that clozapine treatment reduced suicide risk during continuous drug administration. More recently, Meltzer et al.,[203] in a multicentre, randomized, international 2-year study comparing the risk of suicidal behaviour in patients treated with clozapine to that in patients treated with olanzapine, observed that suicidal behaviour was significantly less frequent in patients treated with clozapine. Several studies conducted by Tiihonen et al. confirmed that antipsychotic medications in general, particularly clozapine, were associated with lower suicide risk.[204,205] Furthermore, the same author observed that long-term treatment with antipsychotic drugs was associated with lower mortality and clozapine seemed to produce substantially lower mortality than any other antipsychotics.[205] However, some antipsychotics, including clozapine, haloperidol, and other antipsychotics, may increase the risk of depression.[206] Tiihonen et al.[207] investigated whether use of benzodiazepines, antidepressants, or multiple concomitant antipsychotics was associated with mortality in patients with schizophrenia. Their results demonstrated that use of two or more antipsychotics was not associated with increased mortality. In contrast, antidepressant use was not associated with a higher risk of mortality and was associated with markedly fewer suicides. However, benzodiazepine use was associated with increased suicide and non-suicide deaths. Haukka et al.[208] observed that olanzapine, and to some degree clozapine, tended to perform well for suicide risk, which is in line with a review on the potential anti-suicidal effects of an atypical antipsychotic.[206] Recently, Taipale et al.[209] investigated the risk of suicide attempts and deaths in schizophrenia patients. The authors confirmed that clozapine is the only antipsychotic associated with a decreased risk of suicide. Several studies have demonstrated that olanzapine, an atypical antipsychotic similar to clozapine, may be effective in reducing both depression and suicide risk in patients with schizophrenia.[210,211] A study of 339 patients with psychotic disorders found that both olanzapine and risperidone were effective for treatment of psychotic symptoms, but that only olanzapine produced a 7-fold lower risk of suicidal behaviours.[212] In addition, olanzapine demonstrated a greater anti-suicidal effect than haloperidol,[213] similar to risperidone.[214]

Furthermore, quetiapine has demonstrated some potential effect for reducing suicidal risk, not only in patients with schizophrenia.[206] Evidence about other atypical antipsychotic drug effects on suicidal risk remains limited, and whether all specific antipsychotics are effective in preventing completed suicides is also unclear. Long-acting injectable antipsychotics (LAIs) have several advantages in terms of efficacy, safety, and tolerability in treating schizophrenia. A better understanding of whether LAI treatment may decrease suicide risk by indirectly acting on a range of risk factors for suicide specific to schizophrenia patients is of significant clinical importance. Pompili et al.[215] suggested that long-acting injections of second-generation antipsychotics can be an effective treatment strategy to improve medication adherence and prevent suicide risk. Furthermore, in addition to antipsychotics, other psychotropic medications, such as antidepressants and mood stabilizers, are often used in patients with schizophrenia.[216] Research suggests that use of antidepressants together with antipsychotic drugs has been associated with a decrease in all-cause mortality, including death by suicide.[208] Tiihonen et al.,[204] in a large cohort study, observed that antidepressant treatment increases the risk of suicide attempts, but not of suicide death. In addition, a cohort study pointed out that antidepressant use in schizophrenia, compared to no use, was associated with a significant reduction in the risk of suicide death.[205] However, two systematic reviews of randomized controlled trials confirmed an increased risk of self-harm or suicidal attempts related to selective serotonin reuptake inhibitors (SSRIs).[199,217] Mood stabilizers have been used to augment the effects of antipsychotic drugs in patients with schizophrenia. Mood stabilizer medications may also effectively reduce depression, aggression, and impulsivity in patients with schizophrenia when administered with antipsychotic therapy. Together with clozapine, lithium is the only drug showing anti-suicidal properties in patients with BD and major affective disorders.[210] A comprehensive meta-analysis of the effect of lithium in reducing suicide risk reported that both suicide attempts and deaths were reduced by nearly 5-fold, or 80%.[218] Recently, several studies have suggested that lithium treatment reduced suicide attempts, suicide deaths, hospitalization for suicide attempts, and other suicide spectrum disorders, compared to treatment with other mood stabilizers.[219,220,221] Although the beneficial effects of lithium on suicide risk in affective disorders are well documented,[222] data on whether this extends to patients with schizophrenia or schizoaffective disorder are lacking.[223] The potential of other mood-stabilizing agents, such as lamotrigine, which has established antidepressant activity, is less well understood than that of lithium, valproate, or carbamazepine.

In a double-blind, randomized controlled multicentre trial on 298 patients with first-episode schizophrenia on treatment with risperidone or haloperidol, suicidal ideation was associated with akathisia, suggesting that EPS may have a promoting effect on suicide risk.[224] However, Reutfors et al.[109] demonstrated a lower suicide risk in patients with a history of EPS. The authors explained their results by noting that better adherence, higher dosages, and a prevalence of polypharmacy characterized these patients.

In patients with BD in general, mood stabilizers and antipsychotics are the mainstay of acute management of mania and depression.[225] Lithium has long been known to reduce rates of suicide attempts and deaths in depressed and bipolar patients. Multiple randomized controlled trials, meta-analyses, and decades of clinical experience have shown that lithium significantly reduces the risk of self-harm and suicide in unipolar depression and bipolar depression.[226] In one study of 50,000 bipolar patients, lithium was found to reduce the rate of suicide deaths and other suicide-related events by 14% relative to treatment with valproate.[221] Long-term lithium use decreases the risk of death by 60–80%.[218] Non-adherence to lithium increases suicidal risk, and discontinuation of lithium treatment increases the risk of death by 13-fold.[227] More rapid treatment of patients at risk for suicide is possible with intravenous and intranasal ketamine for bipolar patients,[228] but ketamine is not widely available.

Although antidepressants significantly reduce the risk of suicide in depressed patients on long-term treatment, no antidepressant medication has demonstrated an anti-suicidal effect.[229] In fact, some studies have suggested that antidepressant treatment might increase suicide risk in a subgroup of bipolar patients, which has not been shown for death by suicide.[22] There also remain concerns that antidepressant medications can worsen the course of the disease by provoking a switch into a hypomanic, manic, or mixed-mood state or by inducing agitation in mixed episodes, possibly contributing to suicidal behaviour.[22] However, the International Society for Bipolar Disorders (ISBD) task force acknowledged that some bipolar patients might benefit from antidepressant medication, with bupropion having the lowest risk of switching, only as long as the antidepressants are prescribed as an adjunct to mood stabilizers.[230]

In addition, current evidence suggests that antipsychotic medications should only be used in addition to mood stabilizers for breakthrough hypomanic or manic episodes, and discontinued as soon as clinically feasible due to long-term metabolic side effects.[231]

Esketamine in major depressive disorder with suicidal ideation and suicidal behaviour

Esketamine is a *N*-methyl-*D*-aspartate (NMDA) receptor antagonist that modulates glutamatergic transmission. Recently, this drug, which is available as an intranasal formulation, has been proposed for treatment-resistant depression and rapid reduction of symptoms of MDD in patients with suicidal ideation with intent.[232] Two major double-blind, randomized controlled studies investigated the effects of esketamine in psychiatric emergencies; these studies involved two groups of patients affected by a moderate or severe major depressive episode and concomitant suicidal ideation with intent.[233,234,235] Fu et al.,[235] in a double-blind, multicentre study (ASPIRE I), enrolled 226 adults having MDD with active suicidal ideation with intent and need for psychiatric hospitalization. Patients were randomized 1:1 to esketamine 84 mg or to placebo nasal spray twice weekly for four weeks. More remarkable improvement in the Montgomery-Asberg Depression Rating Scale (MADRS) total score was observed with esketamine + standard of care versus placebo + standard of care at 24 hours and later time points during the 4-week double-blind treatment. Also, Ionescu et al.,[234] in a double-blind study (ASPIRE II), observed a greater improvement in MADRS total score in patients treated with esketamine and a rapid reduction in Clinical Global Impression-Severity of Suicidality-revised score. Finally, Canuso et al.,[233] combining data from ASPIRE I and ASPIRE II studies, observed that esketamine plus comprehensive standard of care rapidly reduced depressive symptoms in patients with MDD who had acute suicidal ideation or behaviour, especially in those with a history of suicide attempt, providing a new treatment option for this particularly ill and vulnerable population. These studies assessed whether therapy with esketamine could improve the severity of depression, according to MADRS scores and, as a secondary end point, whether such treatment could reduce suicide risk (in terms of scores assessed with a specific evaluation scale, namely the Clinical Global Impression Scale) after 24 hours from administration. It emerged that the group of patients treated with esketamine plus comprehensive standard of care improved in terms of overall depression severity, whereas for the secondary end point, both groups—one group treated with esketamine in addition to oral antidepressant therapy and the other group treated with placebo plus oral antidepressant therapy—improved in terms of severity of suicidal ideation and risk of suicide with no statistically significant difference between the groups. Various hypotheses can be tested about this result. First, the trials on efficacy and safety of esketamine in patients with depression and at risk of suicide include patients normally excluded from clinical studies.

Furthermore, the level of assistance and observation was inevitably enhanced compared to routine care to reduce the suffering of these subjects. Also, the role of hospitalization and medical attention dedicated to those taking esketamine and those taking placebos may have helped reduce the risk of suicide, especially in those taking placebo. In summary, esketamine is not intended as a therapy for management of suicide risk, but as an acute treatment of depressive symptoms, the reduction of which should quickly alleviate the suicidal emergency condition and return the patient to a minor acute condition.

Conclusion

To summarize, suicide is a complex and multifactorial phenomenon involving different interconnected features, including psychiatric disorders. Suicide risk represents a major health care problem, and the relationship between suicide and psychiatric disorders is well documented. Virtually all mental disorders increase the risk of suicidal ideation, suicide attempt, and death by suicide. However, a psychiatric disorder may be an almost necessary, yet insufficient, risk factor for suicide. Suicide most often occurs when stressors and health issues converge to create an experience of hopelessness and despair. Furthermore, suicide risk factors can vary by age group, culture, sex, and other patient characteristics. Depression, BD, schizophrenia, substance use disorder, anxiety disorders, and PDs constitute the most relevant risk factors for suicide. Undertreatment, comorbidity, treatment non-compliance and poor adherence, and a high frequency of non-responders are common problems and challenges in treating suicidal psychiatric patients. On the other hand, treatment adherence is an important factor in medical suicide prevention. Clinicians and practitioners often face difficulties in assessing suicide risk factors and in assimilating the evidence base for suicide prevention interventions, evaluating their effectiveness, and decoding the best practice elements of each approach. Awareness programmes, screening, gatekeeper training, access to means restriction, follow-up care, hotlines, media strategies, and pharmacotherapeutic and psychotherapeutic approaches are indispensable suicide prevention strategies to be adopted in clinical practice.

References

1. **Pompili M.** On mental pain and suicide risk in modern psychiatry. Annals of general psychiatry. 2024;**23**(1):6. doi: 10.1186/s12991-024-00490-5.
2. **Pompili M, Erbuto D, Innamorati M,** et al. The relationship between mental pain, suicide risk, and childhood traumatic experiences: results from a multicenter study. The Journal of clinical psychiatry. 2022;**83**(4):41432. doi: 10.4088/JCP.21m14176.
3. **Pandey GN.** Biological basis of suicide and suicidal behavior. Bipolar Disorders. 2013;**15**(5):524–41. doi: 10.1111/bdi.12089.
4. **Brådvik L.** Suicide risk and mental disorders. International Journal of Environmental Research and Public Health. 2018;**15**(9):2028. doi: 10.3390/ijerph15092028.
5. **Rihmer Z, Rihmer A, Dome P.** Suicidal behaviour in patients with mood disorders. Evidence-Based Psychiatric Care. 2015;**1**:19–26.

6. **Cheng AT, Chen TH, Chen CC, Jenkins R.** Psychosocial and psychiatric risk factors for suicide. Case-control psychological autopsy study. British Journal of Psychiatry. 2000;**177**:360–5. doi: 10.1192/bjp.177.4.360.
7. **Müller-Oerlinghausen B, Berghöfer A, Bauer M.** Bipolar disorder. The Lancet. 2002;**359**(9302):241–7. doi: 10.1016/S0140-6736(02)07450-0.
8. **Pompili M, Gonda X, Serafini G,** et al. Epidemiology of suicide in bipolar disorders: a systematic review of the literature. Bipolar Disorders. 2013;**15**(5):457–90. doi: 10.1111/bdi.12087.
9. **Dome P, Rihmer Z, Gonda X.** Suicide risk in bipolar disorder: a brief review. Medicina (Kaunas). 2019;**55**(8):403. doi: 10.3390/medicina55080403.
10. **Rihmer Z, Kiss K.** Bipolar disorders and suicidal behaviour. Bipolar Disorders. 2002;**4**(Suppl 1):21–5. doi: 10.1034/j.1399-5618.4.s1.3.x.
11. **Pompili M, Rihmer Z, Innamorati M, Lester D, Girardi P, Tatarelli R.** Assessment and treatment of suicide risk in bipolar disorders. Expert Review of Neurotherapeutics. 2009;**9**(1):109–36. doi: 10.1586/14737175.9.1.109.
12. **Osby U, Brandt L, Correia N, Ekbom A, Sparén P.** Excess mortality in bipolar and unipolar disorder in Sweden. Archives of General Psychiatry. 2001;**58**(9):844–50. doi: 10.1001/archpsyc.58.9.844.
13. **Dennehy EB, Marangell LB, Allen MH, Chessick C, Wisniewski SR, Thase ME.** Suicide and suicide attempts in the Systematic Treatment Enhancement Program for Bipolar Disorder (STEP-BD). Journal of Affective Disorders. 2011;**133**(3):423–7. doi: 10.1016/j.jad.2011.04.036.
14. **Simon GE, Hunkeler E, Fireman B, Lee JY, Savarino J.** Risk of suicide attempt and suicide death in patients treated for bipolar disorder. Bipolar Disorders. 2007;**9**(5):526–30. doi: 10.1111/j.1399-5618.2007.00408.x.
15. **Jacobs DG, Baldessarini RJ, Conwell Y,** et al. Assessment and treatment of patients with suicidal behaviors. APA Practice Guidelines. 2010;1:183.
16. **Karch DL, Barker L, Strine TW.** Race/ethnicity, substance abuse, and mental illness among suicide victims in 13 US states: 2004 data from the National Violent Death Reporting System. Injury Prevention. 2006;**12**(Suppl 2):ii22–7. doi: 10.1136/ip.2006.013557.
17. **Isometsä E.** Suicidal behaviour in mood disorders: who, when, and why? Canadian Journal of Psychiatry. 2014;**59**(3):120–30. doi: 10.1177/070674371405900303.
18. **Persons JE, Coryell WH, Solomon DA, Keller MB, Endicott J, Fiedorowicz JG.** Mixed state and suicide: is the effect of mixed state on suicidal behavior more than the sum of its parts? Bipolar Disorders. 2018;**20**(1):35–41. doi: 10.1111/bdi.12538.
19. **Baldessarini RJ, Tondo L.** Suicidal risks in 12 DSM-5 psychiatric disorders. Journal of Affective Disorders. 2020;**271**:66–73. doi: 10.1016/j.jad.2020.03.083.
20. **Abreu LN, Lafer B, Baca-Garcia E, Oquendo MA.** Suicidal ideation and suicide attempts in bipolar disorder type I: an update for the clinician. Brazilian Journal of Psychiatry. 2009;**31**:271–80. doi: 10.1590/s1516-44462009005000003.
21. **Gonda X, Pompili M, Serafini G,** et al. Suicidal behavior in bipolar disorder: epidemiology, characteristics and major risk factors. Journal of Affective Disorders. 2012;**143**:16–26. doi: 10.1016/j.jad.2012.04.041.

22. **Rihmer Z, Gonda X.** Antidepressant-resistant depression and antidepressant-associated suicidal behaviour: the role of underlying bipolarity. Depression Research and Treatment. 2011;**2011**:906462. doi: 10.1155/2011/906462.
23. **Hawton K, Sutton L, Haw C, Sinclair J, Harriss L.** Suicide and attempted suicide in bipolar disorder: a systematic review of risk factors. Journal of Clinical Psychiatry. 2005;**66**:693–704. doi: 10.4088/jcp.v66n0604.
24. **Yerevanian BI, Koek RJ, Mintz J, Akiskal HS.** Bipolar pharmacotherapy and suicidal behavior. Part 2. The impact of antidepressants. Journal of Affective Disorders. 2007;**103**(1–3):13–21. doi: 10.1016/j.jad.2007.05.017.
25. **Yerevanian BI, Koek RJ, Mintz J.** Lithium, anticonvulsants and suicidal behavior in bipolar disorder. Journal of Affective Disorders. 2003;**73**(3):223–8. doi: 10.1016/s0165-0327(02)00302-6.
26. **Gibbons RD, Hur K, Brown CH, Mann JJ.** Relationship between antiepileptic drugs and suicide attempts in patients with bipolar disorder. Archives of General Psychiatry. 2009;**66**(12):1354–60. doi: 10.1001/archgenpsychiatry.2009.159.
27. **Desai RA, Dausey DJ, Rosenheck RA.** Mental health service delivery and suicide risk: the role of individual patient and facility factors. American Journal of Psychiatry. 2005;**162**(2):311–18. doi: 10.1176/appi.ajp.162.2.311.
28. **Dunner DL.** Clinical consequences of under-recognized bipolar spectrum disorder. Bipolar Disorders. 2003;**5**(6):456–63. doi: 10.1046/j.1399-5618.2003.00073.x.
29. **Raja M, Azzoni A.** Suicide attempts: differences between unipolar and bipolar patients and among groups with different lethality risk. Journal of Affective Disorders. 2004;**82**(3):437–42. doi: 10.1016/j.jad.2004.02.001.
30. **Ribeiro JD, Huang X, Fox KR, Franklin JC.** Depression and hopelessness as risk factors for suicide ideation, attempts and death: meta-analysis of longitudinal studies. British Journal of Psychiatry. 2018;**212**(5):279–86. doi: 10.1192/bjp.2018.27.
31. **Orsolini L, Latini R, Pompili M,** et al. Understanding the complex of suicide in depression: from research to clinics. Psychiatry Investigation. 2020;**17**(3):207–21. doi: 10.30773/pi.2019.0171.
32. **Dilsaver SC, Benazzi F, Akiskal HS, Akiskal KK.** Post-traumatic stress disorder among adolescents with bipolar disorder and its relationship to suicidality. Bipolar Disorders. 2007;**9**(6):649–55. doi: 10.1111/j.1399-5618.2007.00396.x.
33. **Sánchez-Gistau V, Colom F, Mané A, Romero S, Sugranyes G, Vieta E.** Atypical depression is associated with suicide attempt in bipolar disorder. Acta Psychiatrica Scandinavica. 2009;**120**(1):30–6. doi: 10.1111/j.1600-0447.2008.01341.x.
34. **Swann AC, Moeller FG, Steinberg JL, Schneider L, Barratt ES, Dougherty DM.** Manic symptoms and impulsivity during bipolar depressive episodes. Bipolar Disorders. 2007;**9**(3):206–12. doi: 10.1111/j.1399-5618.2007.00357.x.
35. **Pompili M, Innamorati M, Rihmer Z,** et al. Cyclothymic-depressive-anxious temperament pattern is related to suicide risk in 346 patients with major mood disorders. Journal of Affective Disorders. 2012;**136**(3):405–11. doi: 10.1016/j.jad.2011.11.011.
36. **Carballo JJ, Harkavy-Friedman J, Burke AK,** et al. Family history of suicidal behavior and early traumatic experiences: additive effect on suicidality and course of bipolar illness? Journal of Affective Disorders. 2008;**109**(1–2):57–63. doi: 10.1016/j.jad.2007.12.225.

37. **Braquehais MD, Oquendo MA, Baca-García E, Sher L.** Is impulsivity a link between childhood abuse and suicide? Comprehensive Psychiatry. 2010;**51**(2):121–9. doi: 10.1016/j.comppsych.2009.05.003.
38. **Brodsky BS, Oquendo M, Ellis SP, Haas GL, Malone KM, Mann JJ.** The relationship of childhood abuse to impulsivity and suicidal behavior in adults with major depression. American Journal of Psychiatry. 2001;**158**(11):1871–7. doi: 10.1176/appi.ajp.158.11.1871.
39. **Serafini G, Muzio C, Piccinini G,** et al. Life adversities and suicidal behavior in young individuals: a systematic review. European Child and Adolescent Psychiatry. 2015;**24**(12):1423–46. doi: 10.1007/s00787-015-0760-y.
40. **Rajalin M, Hirvikoski T, Renberg ES, Åsberg M, Jokinen J.** Exposure to early life adversity and interpersonal functioning in attempted suicide. Frontiers in Psychiatry. 2020;**11**:552514. doi: 10.3389/fpsyt.2020.552514.
41. **Gonda X, Fountoulakis KN, Kaprinis G, Rihmer Z.** Prediction and prevention of suicide in patients with unipolar depression and anxiety. Annals of General Psychiatry. 2007;**6**:23. doi: 10.1186/1744-859X-6-23.
42. **Qin P, Nordentoft M.** Suicide risk in relation to psychiatric hospitalization: evidence based on longitudinal registers. Archives of General Psychiatry. 2005;**62**(4):427–32. doi: 10.1001/archpsyc.62.4.427.
43. **Marzuk PM, Tardiff K, Leon AC,** et al. Lower risk of suicide during pregnancy. American Journal of Psychiatry. 1997;**154**(1):122–3. doi: 10.1176/ajp.154.1.122.
44. **Dervic K, Oquendo MA, Grunebaum MF, Ellis S, Burke AK, Mann JJ.** Religious affiliation and suicide attempt. American Journal of Psychiatry. 2004;**161**(12):2303–8. doi: 10.1176/appi.ajp.161.12.2303.
45. **Driver K, Abed RT.** Does having offspring reduce the risk of suicide in women? International Journal of Psychiatry in Clinical Practice. 2004;**8**(1):25–9. doi: 10.1080/13651500310004506.
46. **McGrath J, Saha S, Chant D, Welham J.** Schizophrenia: a concise overview of incidence, prevalence, and mortality. Epidemiologic Reviews. 2008;**30**:67–76. doi: 10.1093/epirev/mxn001.
47. **Hor K, Taylor M.** Suicide and schizophrenia: a systematic review of rates and risk factors. Journal of Psychopharmacology. 2010;**24**(4 Suppl):81–90. Doi: 10.1177/1359786810385490.
48. **Heilä H, Isometsä ET, Henriksson MM, Heikkinen ME, Marttunen MJ, Lönnqvist JK.** Suicide and schizophrenia: a nationwide psychological autopsy study on age- and sex-specific clinical characteristics of 92 suicide victims with schizophrenia. American Journal of Psychiatry. 1997;**154**(9):1235–42. doi: 10.1176/ajp.154.9.1235.
49. **Pompili M, Girardi P, Ruberto A, Tatarelli R.** Toward a new prevention of suicide in schizophrenia. World Journal of Biological Psychiatry. 2004;**5**(4):201–10. doi: 10.1080/15622970410029934.
50. **Hawton K, Sutton L, Haw C, Sinclair J, Deeks JJ.** Schizophrenia and suicide: systematic review of risk factors. British Journal of Psychiatry. 2005;**187**:9–20. doi: 10.1192/bjp.187.1.9.
51. **Pompili M, Mancinelli I, Ruberto A, Kotzalidis GD, Girardi P, Tatarelli R.** Where schizophrenic patients commit suicide: a review of suicide among inpatients and former inpatients. International Journal of Psychiatry in Medicine. 2005;**35**(2):171–90. doi: 10.2190/9CA1-EL73-1VXD-9F2V.

52. **Roy A.** Depression, attempted suicide, and suicide in patients with chronic schizophrenia. Psychiatric Clinics of North America. 1986;**9**(1):193–206.
53. **Berardelli I, Sarubbi S, Rogante E**, et al. The role of demoralization and hopelessness in suicide risk in schizophrenia: a review of the literature. Medicina (Kaunas). 2019;**55**(5):200. doi: 10.3390/medicina55050200.
54. **Pompili M, Lester D, Innamorati M, Tatarelli R, Girardi P.** Assessment and treatment of suicide risk in schizophrenia. Expert Review of Neurotherapeutics. 2008;**8**(1):51–74. doi: 10.1586/14737175.8.1.51.
55. **Popovic D, Benabarre A, Crespo JM**, et al. Risk factors for suicide in schizophrenia: systematic review and clinical recommendations. Acta Psychiatrica Scandinavica. 2014;**130**(6):418–26. doi: 10.1111/acps.12332.
56. **Zisook S, Byrd D, Kuck J, Jeste DV.** Command hallucinations in outpatients with schizophrenia. Journal of Clinical Psychiatry. 1995;**56**(10):462–5.
57. **Lyu J, Zhang J.** Characteristics of schizophrenia suicides compared with suicides by other diagnosed psychiatric disorders and those without a psychiatric disorder. Schizophrenia Research. 2014;**155**(1–3):59–65. doi: 10.1016/j.schres.2014.02.018.
58. **Dickerson F, Origoni A, Schweinfurth LAB**, et al. Clinical and serological predictors of suicide in schizophrenia and major mood disorders. Journal of Nervous and Mental Disease. 2018;**206**:173–8. doi: 10.1097/NMD.0000000000000772.
59. **Cassidy RM, Yang F, Kapczinski F, Passos IC.** Risk factors for suicidality in patients with schizophrenia: a systematic review, meta-analysis, and meta-regression of 96 studies. Schizophrenia Bulletin. 2018;**44**:787–97. doi: 10.1093/schbul/sbx131.
60. **Canetto SS, Sakinofsky I.** The gender paradox in suicide. Suicide and Life-Threatening Behaviour. 1998;**28**:1–23. doi: 10.1111/j.1943-278X.1998.tb00622.x.
61. **Gohar SM, Dieset I, Steen NE**, et al. Association between leptin levels and severity of suicidal behaviour in schizophrenia spectrum disorders. Acta Psychiatrica Scandinavica. 2019;**139**:464–71. doi: 10.1111/acps.13019.
62. **Woottiluk P, Maneeton B, Jaiyen N, Khemawichanurat W, Kawilapat S, Maneeton N.** Prevalence and associated factors of suicide among hospitalized schizophrenic patients. World Journal of Clinical Cases. 2020;**8**:757–70. doi: 10.12998/wjcc.v8.i4.757.
63. **Ran MS, Wong YI, Yang SY**, et al. Marriage and outcomes of people with schizophrenia in rural China: 14-year follow-up study. Schizophrenia Research. 2017;**182**:49–54. doi: 10.1016/j.schres.2016.10.034.
64. **Baldessarini RJ, Tondo L, Pinna M, Nuñez N, Vázquez GH.** Suicidal risk factors in major affective disorders. British Journal of Psychiatry. 2019;**11**:1–6. doi: 10.1192/bjp.2019.167.
65. **Chang Q, Wu D, Rong H**, et al. Suicide ideation, suicide attempts, their sociodemographic and clinical associates among the elderly Chinese patients with schizophrenia spectrum disorders. Journal of Affective Disorders. 2019;**256**:611–17. doi: 10.1016/j.jad.2019.06.069.
66. **Dai Q, Wang D, Wang J**, et al. Suicide attempts in Chinese Han patients with schizophrenia: cognitive, demographic, and clinical variables. Brazilian Journal of Psychiatry. 2021;**43**:29–34. doi: 10.1590/1516-4446-2020-0900.
67. **Buonocore M, Bosinelli F, Bechi M**, et al. The role of premorbid adjustment in schizophrenia: focus on cognitive remediation outcome. Neuropsychological Rehabilitation. 2019;**29**:1611–24. doi: 10.1080/09602011.2018.1433048.

68. **Drake RE, Cotton PG.** Depression, hopelessness and suicide in chronic schizophrenia. British Journal of Psychiatry. 1986;**148**:554–9. doi: 10.1192/bjp.148.5.554.
69. **Bakst S, Rabinowitz J, Bromet EJ.** Is poor premorbid functioning a risk factor for suicide attempts in first-admission psychosis? Schizophrenia Research. 2010;**116**:210–16. doi: 10.1016/j.schres.2009.11.005.
70. **American Psychiatric Association.** *Diagnostic and Statistical Manual of Mental Disorders*, 5th edition. Arlington, VA: American Psychiatric Association; 2013.
71. **Drake RE, Gates C, Whitaker A, Cotton PG.** Suicide among schizophrenics: a review. Comprehensive Psychiatry. 1985;**26**:90–100. doi: 10.1016/0010-440x(85)90053-7.
72. **Pratt D, Gooding P, Johnson J, Taylor P, Tarrier N.** Suicide schemas in non-affective psychosis: an empirical investigation. Behaviour Research and Therapy. 2010;**48**:1211–20. doi: 10.1016/j.brat.2010.08.005.
73. **Castelein S, Liemburg EJ, de Lange JS,** et al. Suicide in recent onset psychosis revisited: significant reduction of suicide rate over the last two decades: a replication study of a Dutch incidence cohort. PLoS One. 2015;**10**:e0129263. doi: 10.1371/journal.pone.0129263.
74. **Andriopoulos I, Ellul J, Skokou M, Beratis S.** Suicidality in the 'prodromal' phase of schizophrenia. Comprehensive Psychiatry. 2011;**52**:479–85. doi: 10.1016/j.comppsych.2010.10.011.
75. **Gill KE, Quintero JM, Poe SL,** et al. Assessing suicidal ideation in individuals at clinical high risk for psychosis. Schizophrenia Research. 2015;**165**:152–6. doi: 10.1016/j.schres.2015.04.022.
76. **Taylor PJ, Gooding PA, Wood AM, Johnson J, Pratt D, Tarrier N.** Defeat and entrapment in schizophrenia: the relationship with suicidal ideation and positive psychotic symptoms. Psychiatry Research. 2010;**178**:244–8. doi: 10.1016/j.psychres.2009.10.015.
77. **Pompili M, Amador XF, Girardi P,** et al. Suicide risk in schizophrenia: learning from the past to change the future. Annals of General Psychiatry. 2007;**6**:10. doi: 10.1186/1744-859X-6-10.
78. **Hakulinen C, McGrath JJ, Timmerman A,** et al. The association between early-onset schizophrenia with employment, income, education, and cohabitation status: nationwide study with 35 years of follow-up. Social Psychiatry and Psychiatric Epidemiology. 2019;**54**:1343–51. doi: 10.1007/s00127-019-01756-0.
79. **Vinokur D, Levine SZ, Roe D, Krivoy A, Fischel T.** Age of onset group characteristics in forensic patients with schizophrenia. European Psychiatry. 2014;**29**:149–52. doi: 10.1016/j.eurpsy.2012.11.006.
80. **Dutta R, Murray RM, Hotopf M, Allardyce J, Jones PB, Boydell J.** Reassessing the long-term risk of suicide after a first episode of psychosis. Archives of General Psychiatry. 2010;**67**:1230–7. doi: 10.1001/archgenpsychiatry.2010.157.
81. **Olfson M, Wall M, Wang S,** et al. Short-term suicide risk after psychiatric hospital discharge. JAMA Psychiatry. 2016;**73**:1119–26. doi: 10.1001/jamapsychiatry.2016.2035.
82. **Pompili M, Lester D, Grispini A,** et al. Completed suicide in schizophrenia: evidence from a case-control study. Psychiatry Research. 2009;**167**:251–7. doi: 10.1016/j.psychres.2008.03.018.
83. **Wasserman D, Rihmer Z, Rujescu D,** et al. The European Psychiatric Association (EPA) guidance on suicide treatment and prevention. European Psychiatry. 2012;**27**:129–41. doi: 10.1016/j.eurpsy.2011.06.003.

84. **Amador XF, Kronengold H.** Understanding and assessing insight. In: **Amador X, David A**, editors. *Insight and Psychosis*, **2**. New York, NY: Oxford University Press; 2004. pp. 3–30.
85. **Farberow NL, Shneidman ES, Leonard CV.** Suicide among schizophrenic mental hospital patients. In: **Farberow NL, Shneidman ES**, editors. *The Cry for Help*. New York, NY: McGraw-Hill; 1961. pp. 78–109.
86. **Drake RE, Gates C, Cotton PG.** Suicide among schizophrenics: a comparison of attempters and completed suicides. British Journal of Psychiatry. 1986;**149**:784–7. doi: 10.1192/bjp.149.6.784.
87. **Kim CH, Jayathilake K, Meltzer HY.** Hopelessness, neurocognitive function, and insight in schizophrenia: relationship to suicidal behavior. Schizophrenia Research. 2003;**60**:71–80. doi: 10.1016/s0920-9964(02)00310-9.
88. **Bourgeois M, Swendsen J, Young F**, et al. Awareness of disorder and suicide risk in the treatment of schizophrenia: results of the international suicide prevention trial. American Journal of Psychiatry. 2004;**161**:1494–6. doi: 10.1176/appi.ajp.161.8.1494.
89. **Pompili M, Ruberto A, Kotzalidis GD, Girardi P, Tatarelli R.** Suicide and awareness of illness in schizophrenia: an overview. Bulletin of the Menninger Clinic. 2004;**68**:297–318. doi: 10.1521/bumc.68.4.297.56643.
90. **Berardelli I, Innamorati M, Sarubbi S**, et al. Are demoralization and insight involved in suicide risk? An observational study on psychiatric inpatients. Psychopathology. 2021;**54**:127–35. doi: 10.1159/000515056.
91. **Balhara YP, Verma R.** Schizophrenia and suicide. East Asian Archives of Psychiatry. 2012;**22**:126–33.
92. **Large M, Smith G, Sharma S, Nielssen O, Singh SP.** Systematic review and meta-analysis of the clinical factors associated with the suicide of psychiatric in-patients. Acta Psychiatrica Scandinavica. 2011;**124**(1):18–29. doi: 10.1111/j.1600-0447.2010.01672.x.
93. **Carlborg A, Winnerbäck K, Jönsson EG, Jokinen J, Nordström P.** Suicide in schizophrenia. Expert Review of Neurotherapeutics. 2010;**10**:1153–64. doi: 10.1586/ern.10.82.
94. **Nordentoft M, Jeppesen P, Abel M**, et al. OPUS study: suicidal behaviour, suicidal ideation and hopelessness among patients with first-episode psychosis. One-year follow-up of a randomised controlled trial. British Journal of Psychiatry Suppl. 2002;**43**:s98–106. doi: 10.1192/bjp.181.43.s98.
95. **Beck AT, Steer RA, Kovacs M, Garrison B.** Hopelessness and eventual suicide: a 10-year prospective study of patients hospitalized with suicidal ideation. American Journal of Psychiatry. 1985;**142**:559–63. doi: 10.1176/ajp.142.5.559.
96. **Bodén R, Brandt L, Kieler H, Andersen M, Reutfors J.** Early non-adherence to medication and other risk factors for rehospitalization in schizophrenia and schizoaffective disorder. Schizophrenia Research. 2011;**133**:36–41. doi: 10.1016/j.schres.2011.08.024.
97. **Fleischhacker WW, Kane JM, Geier J**, et al. Completed and attempted suicides among 18,154 subjects with schizophrenia included in a large simple trial. Journal of Clinical Psychiatry. 2014;**75**:e184–90. doi: 10.4088/JCP.13m08563.
98. **Zhang XY, Al Jurdi RK, Zoghbi AW**, et al. Prevalence, demographic and clinical correlates of suicide attempts in Chinese medicated chronic inpatients with

schizophrenia. Journal of Psychiatric Research. 2013;**47**:1370–5. doi: 10.1016/j.jpsychires.2013.05.024.

99. **Pompili M, Mancinelli I, Girardi P, Tatarelli R.** Preventing suicide in schizophrenia inside the family environment. Crisis. 2003;**24**:181–2. doi: 10.1027//0227-5910.24.4.181.
100. **Gallego JA, Rachamallu V, Yuen EY, Fink S, Duque LM, Kane JM.** Predictors of suicide attempts in 3,322 patients with affective disorders and schizophrenia spectrum disorders. Psychiatry Research. 2015;**228**:791–6. doi: 10.1016/j.psychres.2015.05.024.
101. **Fedyszyn IE, Robinson J, Harris MG, Paxton SJ, Francey S.** Predictors of suicide-related behaviors during treatment following a first episode of psychosis: the contribution of baseline, past, and recent factors. Schizophrenia Research. 2012;**140**:17–24. doi: 10.1016/j.schres.2012.06.022.
102. **Bornheimer LA, Li J, Im V, Taylor M, Himle JA.** The role of social isolation in the relationships between psychosis and suicidal ideation. Clinical Social Work Journal. 2020;**48**:54–62. doi:10.1007/s10615-019-00735-x.
103. **Norman RE, Byambaa M, De R, Butchart A, Scott J, Vos T.** The long-term health consequences of child physical abuse, emotional abuse, and neglect: a systematic review and meta-analysis. PLoS Medicine. 2012;**9**:e1001349. doi: 10.1371/journal.pmed.1001349.
104. **Stumbo SP, Yarborough BJ, Paulson RI, Green CA.** The impact of adverse child and adult experiences on recovery from serious mental illness. Psychiatric Rehabilitation Journal. 2015;**38**:320–7. doi: 10.1037/prj0000141.
105. **Short AT, Nemeroff CB.** Early life trauma and suicide. In: **Cannon KE, Hudzik TJ**, editors. *Suicide: Phenomenology and Neurobiology*. Cham: Springer; 2014. pp. 187–205.
106. **Hassan AN, Stuart EA, De Luca V.** Childhood maltreatment increases the risk of suicide attempt in schizophrenia. Schizophrenia Research. 2016;**176**:572–7. doi: 10.1016/j.schres.2016.05.012.
107. **Prokopez CR, Vallejos M, Farinola R,** et al. The history of multiple adverse childhood experiences in patients with schizophrenia is associated with more severe symptomatology and suicidal behavior with gender-specific characteristics. Psychiatry Research. 2020;**293**:113411. doi: 10.1016/j.psychres.2020.113411.
108. **Herings RM, Erkens JA.** Increased suicide attempt rate among patients interrupting use of atypical antipsychotics. Pharmacoepidemiology and Drug Safety. 2003;**12**:423–4. doi: 10.1002/pds.837.
109. **Reutfors J, Clapham E, Bahmanyar S,** et al. Suicide risk and antipsychotic side effects in schizophrenia: nested case-control study. Human Psychopharmacology. 2016;**31**:341–5. doi: 10.1002/hup.2536.
110. **Belvederi Murri M, Amore M, Calcagno P,** et al. The 'insight paradox' in schizophrenia: magnitude, moderators and mediators of the association between insight and depression. Schizophrenia Bulletin. 2016;**42**(5):1225–33. doi: 10.1093/schbul/sbw040.
111. **Kavanagh DJ, McGrath J, Saunders JB, Dore G, Clark D.** Substance misuse in patients with schizophrenia: epidemiology and management. Drugs. 2002;**62**:743–55. doi: 10.2165/00003495-200262050-00003.

112. **Carrasco-Farfan CA, Alvarez-Cutipa D, Vilchez-Cornejo J**, et al. Alcohol consumption and suicide risk in medical internship: a Peruvian multicentric study. Drug and Alcohol Review. 2019;**38**:201–8. doi: 10.1111/dar.12897.
113. **Winklbaur B, Ebner N, Sachs G, Thau K, Fischer G.** Substance abuse in patients with schizophrenia. Dialogues in Clinical Neuroscience. 2006;**8**:37–43. doi: 10.31887/DCNS.2006.8.1/bwinklbaur.
114. **Kessler RC, Borges G, Walters EE.** Prevalence of and risk factors for lifetime suicide attempts in the National Comorbidity Survey. Archives of General Psychiatry. 1999;**56**:617–26. doi: 10.1001/archpsyc.56.7.617.
115. **Kasckow J, Felmet K, Zisook S.** Managing suicide risk in patients with schizophrenia. CNS Drugs. 2011;**25**:129–43. doi: 10.2165/11586450-000000000-00000.
116. **Kleiman EM, Liu RT.** Social support as a protective factor in suicide: findings from two nationally representative samples. Journal of Affective Disorders. 2013;**150**:540–5. doi: 10.1016/j.jad.2013.01.033.
117. **Kleiman EM, Riskind JH, Schaefer KE.** Social support and positive events as suicide resiliency factors: examination of synergistic buffering effects. Archives of Suicide Research. 2014;**18**:144–55. doi: 10.1080/13811118.2013.826155.
118. **Xie P, Wu K, Zheng Y**, et al. Prevalence of childhood trauma and correlations between childhood trauma, suicidal ideation, and social support in patients with depression, bipolar disorder, and schizophrenia in southern China. Journal of Affective Disorders. 2018;**228**:41–8. doi: 10.1016/j.jad.2017.11.011.
119. **Pješčić KD, Nenadović MM, Jašović-Gašić M, Trajković G, Kostić M, Ristić-Dimitrijević R.** Influence of psycho-social factors on the emergence of depression and suicidal risk in patients with schizophrenia. Psychiatria Danubina. 2014;**26**:226–30.
120. **Turecki G, Brent DA, Gunnell D**, et al. Suicide and suicide risk. Nature Reviews Disease Primers. 2019;**5**:74. doi: 10.1038/s41572-019-0121-0.
121. **Paris J.** Suicidality in borderline personality disorder. Medicina (Kaunas). 2019;**55**(6):223. doi: 10.3390/medicina55060223.
122. **Pompili M, Ruberto A, Girardi P, Tatarelli R.** Suicidality in DSM IV cluster B personality disorders: an overview. Annali dell'Istituto Superiore di Sanità. 2004;**40**(4):475–83.
123. **Mohino Justes S, Ortega-Monasterio L, Planchat Teruel LM, Cuquerella Fuentes A, Talón Navarro T, Macho Vives LJ.** Discriminating deliberate self-harm (DSH) in young prison inmates through personality disorder. Journal of Forensic Sciencee. 2004;**49**(1):137–40.
124. **Schmidtke A, Bille-Brahe U, De Leo D**, et al. Sociodemographic characteristics of suicide attempters in Europe: combined results of the monitoring part of the WHO/EURO Multicentre Study on Suicidal Behaviour. In: **Schmidtke A, Bille-Brahe U, De Leo D, Kerkhof A**, editors. *Suicidal Behaviour in Europe: Results from the WHO/EURO Multicentre Study on Suicidal Behaviour*. Gottingen: Hogrefe & Huber; 2004. pp. 29–43.
125. **Krysinska K, Heller TS, De Leo D.** Suicide and deliberate self-harm in personality disorders. Current Opinion in Psychiatry. 2006;**19**(1):95–101. doi: 10.1097/01.yco.0000191498.69281.5e.
126. **Verona E, Sachs-Ericsson N, Joiner TE Jr.** Suicide attempts associated with externalizing psychopathology in an epidemiological sample. American Journal of Psychiatry. 2004;**161**(3):444–51. doi: 10.1176/appi.ajp.161.3.444.

127. **Yen S, Shea MT, Sanislow CA,** et al. Borderline personality disorder criteria associated with prospectively observed suicidal behavior. American Journal of Psychiatry. 2004;**161**(7):1296–8. doi: 10.1176/appi.ajp.161.7.1296.
128. **Dervic K, Grunebaum MF, Burke AK, Mann JJ, Oquendo MA.** Cluster C personality disorders in major depressive episodes: the relationship between hostility and suicidal behavior. Archives of Suicide Research. 2007;**11**(1):83–90. doi: 10.1080/13811110600992928.
129. **Paris J, Zweig-Frank H.** A 27-year follow-up of patients with borderline personality disorder. Comprehensive Psychiatry. 2001;**42**(6):482–7. doi: 10.1053/comp.2001.26271.
130. **Yen S, Pagano ME, Shea MT,** et al. Recent life events preceding suicide attempts in a personality disorder sample: findings from the collaborative longitudinal personality disorders study. Journal of Consulting and Clinical Psychology. 2005;**73**(1):99–105. doi: 10.1037/0022-006X.73.1.99.
131. **Söderberg S, Kullgren G, Salander Renberg E.** Childhood sexual abuse predicts poor outcome seven years after parasuicide. Social Psychiatry and Psychiatric Epidemiology. 2004;**39**(11):916–20. doi: 10.1007/s00127-004-0839-0.
132. **Sansone RA, Songer DA, Miller KA.** Childhood abuse, mental healthcare utilization, self-harm behavior, and multiple psychiatric diagnoses among inpatients with and without a borderline diagnosis. Comprehensive Psychiatry. 2005;**46**(2):117–20. doi: 10.1016/j.comppsych.2004.07.033.
133. **McKay D, Gavigan CA, Kulchycky S.** Social skills and sex-role functioning in borderline personality disorder: relationship to self-mutilating behavior. Cognitive Behavior Therapy. 2004;**33**:27–35. doi: 10.1080/16506070310002199.
134. **MacLeod AK, Tata P, Tyrer P,** et al. Personality disorder and future-directed thinking in parasuicide. Journal of Personality Disorders. 2004;**18**(5):459–66. doi: 10.1521/pedi.18.5.459.51329.
135. **Berlin HA, Rolls ET.** Time perception, impulsivity, emotionality, and personality in self-harming borderline personality disorder patients. Journal of Personality Disorders. 2004;**18**(4):358–78. doi: 10.1521/pedi.18.4.358.40349.
136. **Kim CD, Seguin M, Therrien N,** et al. Familial aggregation of suicidal behavior: a family study of male suicide completers from the general population. American Journal of Psychiatry. 2005;**162**(5):1017–19. doi: 10.1176/appi.ajp.162.5.1017.
137. **Sanislow CA, Grilo CM, McGlashan TH.** Factor analysis of the DSM-III-R borderline personality disorder criteria in psychiatric inpatients. American Journal of Psychiatry. 2000;**157**(10):1629–33. doi: 10.1176/appi.ajp.157.10.1629.
138. **Sanislow CA, Grilo CM, Morey LC,** et al. Confirmatory factor analysis of DSM-IV criteria for borderline personality disorder: findings from the collaborative longitudinal personality disorders study. American Journal of Psychiatry. 2002;**159**(2):284–90. doi: 10.1176/appi.ajp.159.2.284.
139. **Hurt SW, Clarkin JF.** Borderline personality disorder: prototypic typology and the development of treatment manuals. Psychiatric Annals. 1990;**20**(1):13–18. doi: 10.3928/0048-5713-19900101-05.
140. **Maltsberger JT, Lovett CG.** Suicide in borderline personality disorder. In: **Silver D, Rosenbluth Madison M,** editors. *Handbook of Borderline Disorders*. Madison, CT: International Universities Press; 1992. pp. 335–87.

141. **Gunderson JG, Ridolfi ME.** Borderline personality disorder: suicidality and self-mutilation. Annals of the New York Academy of Sciences. 2001;**932**:61–73.

142. **Linehan MM.** Dialectische gedragstherapie bij borderline persoonlijkheidsstoornis: theorie en behandeling. Tijdschrift voor Psychiatrie. 2003;**45**:7.

143. **Stanley B, Brodsky BS.** Suicidal and self-injurious behavior in borderline personality disorder: a self-regulation model. In: **Gunderson JG, Hoffman PD**, editors. *Understanding and Treating Borderline Personality Disorder: A Guide for Professionals and Families*. Washington, DC: American Psychiatric Publishing; 2005. pp. 43–63.

144. **Kernberg OF.** Suicidal behavior in borderline patients: diagnosis and psychotherapeutic considerations. American Journal of Psychotherapy. 1993;**47**(2):245–54. doi: 10.1176/appi.psychotherapy.1993.47.2.245.

145. **Singer M.** The experience of emptiness in narcissistic and borderline states. I. Deficiency and ego defect versus dynamic-defensive models. International Review of Psychoanalysis. 1977;**4**:459–69.

146. **Oldham JM.** Borderline personality disorder and suicidality. American Journal of Psychiatry. 2006;**163**(1):20–6. doi: 10.1176/appi.ajp.163.1.20.

147. **Fawcett J, Scheftner WA, Fogg L**, et al. Time-related predictors of suicide in major affective disorder. American Journal of Psychiatry. 1990;**147**(9):1189–94. doi: 10.1176/ajp.147.9.1189.

148. **Coryell W, Noyes R, Clancy J.** Excess mortality in panic disorder: a comparison with primary unipolar depression. Archives of General Psychiatry. 1982;**39**(6):701–3. doi: 10.1001/archpsyc.1982.04290060051010.

149. **Henriksson MM, Isometsä ET, Kuoppasalmi KI, Heikkinen ME, Marttunen MJ, Lönnqvist JK.** Panic disorder in completed suicide. Journal of Clinical Psychiatry. 1996;**57**(7):275–81.

150. **Johnson J, Weissman MM, Klerman GL.** Panic disorder, comorbidity, and suicide attempts. Archives of General Psychiatry. 1990;**47**(9):805–8. doi: 10.1001/archpsyc.1990.01810210013002.

151. **Friedman S, Jones JC, Chernen L, Barlow DH.** Suicidal ideation and suicide attempts among patients with panic disorder: a survey of two outpatient clinics. American Journal of Psychiatry. 1992;**149**(5):680–5. doi: 10.1176/ajp.149.5.680.

152. **Lepine JP, Chignon JM, Teherani M.** Suicide attempts in patients with panic disorder. Archives of General Psychiatry. 1993;**50**(2):144–9. doi: 10.1001/archpsyc.1993.01820140070008.

153. **Arditte KA, Morabito DM, Shaw AM, Timpano KR.** Interpersonal risk for suicide in social anxiety: the roles of shame and depression. Psychiatry Research. 2016;**239**:139–44. doi: 10.1016/j.psychres.2016.03.017.

154. **Tietbohl-Santos B, Chiamenti P, Librenza-Garcia D**, et al. Risk factors for suicidality in patients with panic disorder: a systematic review and meta-analysis. Neuroscience and Biobehavioral Reviews. 2019;**105**:34–8. doi: 10.1016/j.neubiorev.2019.07.022.

155. **Goodwin R, Lyons JS, McNally RJ.** Panic attacks in schizophrenia. Schizophrenia Research. 2002;**58**:213–20. doi: 10.1016/s0920-9964(01)00373-5.

156. **Sareen J, Cox BJ, Afifi TO**, et al. Anxiety disorders and risk for suicidal ideation and suicide attempts: a population-based longitudinal study of adults. Archives of General Psychiatry. 2005;**62**(11):1249–57. doi: 10.1001/archpsyc.62.11.1249.

157. **Wunderlich U, Bronisch T, Wittchen H-U.** Comorbidity patterns in adolescents and young adults with suicide attempts. European Archives of Psychiatry and Clinical Neuroscience. 1998;**248**(2):87–95. doi: 10.1007/s004060050023.

158. **Boden JM, Fergusson DM, Horwood LJ.** Anxiety disorders and suicidal behaviours in adolescence and young adulthood: findings from a longitudinal study. Psychological Medicine. 2007;**37**(3):431–40. doi: 10.1017/S0033291706009147.

159. **Foley DL, Goldston DB, Costello EJ, Angold A.** Proximal psychiatric risk factors for suicidality in youth: the Great Smoky Mountains Study. Archives of General Psychiatry. 2006;**63**(9):1017–24. doi: 10.1001/archpsyc.63.9.1017.

160. **Fava M, Rush AJ, Trivedi MH**, et al. Background and rationale for the sequenced treatment alternatives to relieve depression (STAR*D) study. Psychiatric Clinics of North America. 2003;**26**(2):457–94, x. doi: 10.1016/s0193-953x(02)00107-7.

161. **Fava M, Rush AJ, Wisniewski SR**, et al. A comparison of mirtazapine and nortriptyline following two consecutive failed medication treatments for depressed outpatients: a STAR*D report. American Journal of Psychiatry. 2006;**163**(7):1161–72. doi: 10.1176/appi.ajp.163.7.1161.

162. **American Psychiatric Association.** *Diagnostic and Statistical Manual of Mental Disorders*, 4th edition, text revised. Washington, DC: American Psychiatric Association; 2000.

163. **Demitrack MA, Putnam FW, Brewerton TD, Brandt HA, Gold PW.** Relation of clinical variables to dissociative phenomena in eating disorders. American Journal of Psychiatry. 1990;**147**(9):1184–8. doi: 10.1176/ajp.147.9.1184.

164. **Kaplan MS, Adamek ME, Rhoades JA.** Prevention of elderly suicide: physicians' assessment of firearm availability. American Journal of Preventive Medicine. 1998;**15**(1):60–4. doi: 10.1016/s0749-3797(98)00019-1.

165. **Matsumoto T, Yamaguchi A, Chiba Y, Asami T, Iseki E, Hirayasu Y.** Patterns of self-cutting: a preliminary study on differences in clinical implications between wrist- and arm-cutting using a Japanese juvenile detention center sample. Psychiatry and Clinical Neurosciences. 2004;**58**(4):377–82. doi: 10.1111/j.1440-1819.2004.01271.x.

166. **Maaranen P, Tanskanen A, Honkalampi K, Haatainen K, Hintikka J, Viinamäki H.** Factors associated with pathological dissociation in the general population. Australia and New Zealand Journal of Psychiatry. 2005;**39**(5):387–94. doi: 10.1080/j.1440-1614.2005.01586.x.

167. **Zoroglu SS, Tuzun U, Sar V**, et al. Suicide attempt and self-mutilation among Turkish high school students in relation with abuse, neglect and dissociation. Psychiatry and Clinical Neurosciences. 2003;**57**(1):119–26. doi: 10.1046/j.1440-1819.2003.01088.x.

168. **Orbach I, Kedem P, Herman L, Apter A.** Dissociative tendencies in suicidal, depressed, and normal adolescents. Journal of Social and Clinical Psychology. 1995;**14**(4):393–408.

169. **Weinberg I.** The prisoners of despair: right hemisphere deficiency and suicide. Neuroscience and Biobehavioral Reviews. 2000;**24**(8):799–815. doi: 10.1016/s0149-7634(00)00038-5.

170. **Saxe GN, Chawla N, Van der Kolk B.** Self-destructive behavior in patients with dissociative disorders. Suicide and Life-Threatening Behaviour. 2002;**32**(3):313–20. doi: 10.1521/suli.32.3.313.22174.

171. **Coons PM, Milstein V.** Self-mutilation associated with dissociative disorders. Dissociation. 1990; **3**(2):81–87.
172. **Putnam FW, Guroff JJ, Silberman EK, Barban L, Post RM.** The clinical phenomenology of multiple personality disorder: review of 100 recent cases. Journal of Clinical Psychiatry. 1986;**47**(6):285–93.
173. **Leonard D, Brann S, Tiller J.** Dissociative disorders: pathways to diagnosis, clinician attitudes and their impact. Australia and New Zealand Journal of Psychiatry. 2005;**39**(10):940–6. doi: 10.1080/j.1440-1614.2005.01700.x.
174. **Orbach I.** Dissociation, physical pain, and suicide: a hypothesis. Suicide and Life-Threatening Behaviour. 1994;**24**(1):68–79.
175. **Orbach I, Palgi Y, Stein D**, et al. Tolerance for physical pain in suicidal subjects. Death Studies. 1996;**20**(4):327–41. doi: 10.1080/07481189608252786.
176. **Favazza AR, Favazza B.** *Bodies under Siege: Self-Mutilation in Culture and Psychiatry.* Baltimore, MD: Johns Hopkins University Press; 1987.
177. **Coons PM, Milstein V.** Psychogenic amnesia: a clinical investigation of 25 cases. Dissociation. 1992;**5**(2):73–9.
178. **Tutkun H, Sar V, Yargiç LI, Ozpulat T, Yanik M, Kiziltan E.** Frequency of dissociative disorders among psychiatric inpatients in a Turkish university clinic. American Journal of Psychiatry. 1998;**155**(6):800–5. doi: 10.1176/ajp.155.6.800.
179. **Bliss EL.** Multiple personalities: a report of 14 cases with implications for schizophrenia and hysteria. Archives of General Psychiatry. 1980;**37**(12):1388–97. doi: 10.1001/archpsyc.1980.01780250074009.
180. **Harris EC, Barraclough B.** Suicide as an outcome for mental disorders: a meta-analysis. British Journal of Psychiatry. 1997;**170**:205–28. Doi: 10.1192/bjp.170.3.205.
181. **Angelakis I, Gooding P, Tarrier N, Panagioti M.** Suicidality in obsessive compulsive disorder (OCD): a systematic review and meta-analysis. Clinical Psychology Review. 2015;**39**:1–15. Doi: 10.1016/j.cpr.2015.03.002.
182. **Turecki G, Brent DA.** Suicide and suicidal behaviour. The Lancet. 2016;**387**:1227–39. doi: 10.1016/S0140-6736(15)00234-2.
183. **Fernández de la Cruz L, Rydell M, Runeson B**, et al. Suicide in obsessive–compulsive disorder: a population based study of 36 788 Swedish patients. Molecular Psychiatry. 2017;**22**:1626–632. http://dx.doi.org/10.1038/mp.2016.115
184. **Velloso P, Piccinato C, Ferrão Y**, et al. The suicidality continuum in a large sample of obsessive–compulsive disorder (OCD) patients. European Psychiatry. 2016;**38**:1–7. doi: 10.1016/j.eurpsy.2016.05.003.
185. **Albert U, De Ronchi D, Maina G, Pompili M.** Suicide risk in obsessive–compulsive disorder and exploration of risk factors: a systematic review. Current Neuropharmacology. 2019;**17**(8):681–96. doi: 10.2174/1570159X16666180620155941.
186. **Wilcox HC, Conner KR, Caine ED.** Association of alcohol and drug use disorders and completed suicide: an empirical review of cohort studies. Drug and Alcohol Dependence. 2004;**76** Suppl:S11–19. doi: 10.1016/j.drugalcdep.2004.08.003.
187. **Flensborg-Madsen T, Knop J, Mortensen EL, Becker U, Sher L, Grønbaek M.** Alcohol use disorders increase the risk of completed suicide irrespective of other psychiatric disorders: a longitudinal cohort study. Psychiatry Research. 2009;**167**:123–30. doi: 10.1016/j.psychres.2008.01.008.

188. **Yoshimasu K, Kiyohara C, Miyashita K; Stress Research Group of the Japanese Society for Hygiene.** Suicidal risk factors and completed suicide: meta-analyses based on psychological autopsy studies. Environmental Health and Preventive Medicine. 2008;**13**:243–56. doi: 10.1007/s12199-008-0037-x.

189. **Cherpitel CJ, Borges GL, Wilcox HC.** Acute alcohol use and suicidal behavior: a review of the literature. Alcohol, Clinical and Experimental Research. 2004;**28**(5 Suppl):18S–28S. doi: 10.1097/01.alc.0000127411.61634.14.

190. **Bagge CL, Lee HJ, Schumacher JA, Gratz KL, Krull JL, Holloman G Jr.** Alcohol as an acute risk factor for recent suicide attempts: a case-crossover analysis. Journal of Studies on Alcohol and Drugs. 2013;**74**:552–8. doi: 10.15288/jsad.2013.74.552.

191. **Conner KR, Huguet N, Caetano R,** et al. Acute use of alcohol and methods of suicide in a US national sample. American Journal of Public Health. 2014;**104**:171–8. doi: 10.2105/AJPH.2013.301352.

192. **Yuodelis-Flores C, Ries RK.** Addiction and suicide: a review. Focus. 2019;**17**:193–9. doi: 10.1176/appi.focus.17203.

193. **Roy A, Janal. MN.** Risk factors for suicide among alcohol-dependent patients. Archives of Suicide Research. 2007;**11**:211–17. doi: 10.1080/13811110701250150.

194. **Conner KR, Beautrais AL, Conwell Y.** Risk factors for suicide and medically serious suicide attempts among alcoholics: analyses of Canterbury Suicide Project data. Journal of Studies on Alcohol and Drugs. 2003;**64**:551–4. doi: 10.15288/jsa.2003.64.551.

195. **Roy A.** Risk factors for attempting suicide in heroin addicts. Suicide and Life-Threatening Behaviour. 2010;**40**:416–20. doi: 10.1521/suli.2010.40.4.416.

196. **Landheim AS, Bakken K, Vaglum P.** What characterizes substance abusers who commit suicide attempts? Factors related to Axis I disorders and patterns of substance use disorders. A study of treatment-seeking substance abusers in Norway. European Addiction Research. 2006;**12**:102–8. doi: 10.1159/000090430.

197. **Reutfors J, Bahmanyar S, Jönsson EG,** et al. Medication and suicide risk in schizophrenia: a nested case-control study. Schizophrenia Research. 2013;**150**(2–3):416–20. doi: 10.1016/j.schres.2013.09.001.

198. **Tiihonen J, Mittendorfer-Rutz E, Torniainen M, Alexanderson K, Tanskanen A.** Mortality and cumulative exposure to antipsychotics, antidepressants, and benzodiazepines in patients with schizophrenia: an observational follow-up study. American Journal of Psychiatry. 2016;**173**(6):600–6. doi: 10.1176/appi.ajp.2015.15050618.

199. **Khan A, Khan SR, Leventhal RM, Brown WA.** Symptom reduction and suicide risk among patients treated with placebo in antipsychotic clinical trials: an analysis of the food and drug administration database. American Journal of Psychiatry. 2001;**158**(9):1449–54. doi: 10.1176/appi.ajp.158.9.1449.

200. **Meltzer HY, Okayli G.** Reduction of suicidality during clozapine treatment of neuroleptic-resistant schizophrenia: impact on risk–benefit assessment. American Journal of Psychiatry. 1995;**152**(2):183–90. doi: 10.1176/ajp.152.2.183.

201. **Walker EF, Diforio D.** Schizophrenia: a neural diathesis-stress model. Psychological Review. 1997 Oct;**104**(4):667–85. doi: 10.1037/0033-295x.104.4.667.

202. **Reinstein MJ, Chasonov MA, Colombo KD, Jones LE, Sonnenberg JG.** Reduction of suicidality in patients with schizophrenia receiving clozapine. Clinical Drug Investigation. 2002;**22**:341–6.

203. **Meltzer HY, Alphs L, Green AI**, et al. Clozapine treatment for suicidality in schizophrenia: International Suicide Prevention Trial (InterSePT). Archives of General Psychiatry. 2003;**60**(1):82–91. doi: 10.1001/archpsyc.60.1.82. Erratum in: Archives of General Psychiatry. 2003;60(7):735.

204. **Tiihonen J, Wahlbeck K, Lönnqvist J**, et al. Effectiveness of antipsychotic treatments in a nationwide cohort of patients in community care after first hospitalisation due to schizophrenia and schizoaffective disorder: observational follow-up study. BMJ. 2006;**333**(7561):224. doi: 10.1136/bmj.38881.382755.2F.

205. **Tiihonen J, Lönnqvist J, Wahlbeck K**, et al. 11-year follow-up of mortality in patients with schizophrenia: a population-based cohort study (FIN11 study). The Lancet. 2009;**374**(9690):620–7. doi: 10.1016/S0140-6736(09)60742-X.

206. **Pompili M, Baldessarini RJ, Forte A**, et al. Do atypical antipsychotics have antisuicidal effects? A hypothesis-generating overview. International Journal of Molecular Sciences. 2016;**17**(10):1700. doi: 10.3390/ijms17101700.

207. **Tiihonen J, Suokas JT, Suvisaari JM, Haukka J, Korhonen P.** Polypharmacy with antipsychotics, antidepressants, or benzodiazepines and mortality in schizophrenia. Archives of General Psychiatry. 2012;**69**(5):476–83. doi: 10.1001/archgenpsychiatry.2011.1532.

208. **Haukka J, Tiihonen J, Härkänen T, Lönnqvist J.** Association between medication and risk of suicide, attempted suicide and death in nationwide cohort of suicidal patients with schizophrenia. Pharmacoepidemiology and Drug Safety. 2008;**17**(7):686–96. doi: 10.1002/pds.1579. Erratum in: Pharmacoepidemiology and Drug Safety. 2011;20(10):1113.

209. **Taipale H, Lähteenvuo M, Tanskanen A, Mittendorfer-Rutz E, Tiihonen J.** Comparative effectiveness of antipsychotics for risk of attempted or completed suicide among persons with schizophrenia. Schizophrenia Bulletin. 2021;**47**(1):23–30. doi: 10.1093/schbul/sbaa111.

210. **Baldessarini RJ, Tondo L, Hennen J.** Lithium treatment and suicide risk in major affective disorders: update and new findings. Journal of Clinical Psychiatry. 2003;**64** Suppl 5:44–52.

211. **Ringbäck Weitoft G, Berglund M, Lindström EA, Nilsson M, Salmi P, Rosén M.** Mortality, attempted suicide, re-hospitalisation and prescription refill for clozapine and other antipsychotics in Sweden-a register-based study. Pharmacoepidemiology and Drug Safety. 2014;**23**(3):290–8. doi: 10.1002/pds.3567.

212. **Tran PV, Hamilton SH, Kuntz AJ**, et al. Double-blind comparison of olanzapine versus risperidone in the treatment of schizophrenia and other psychotic disorders. Journal of Clinical Psychopharmacology. 1997;**17**(5):407–18. doi: 10.1097/00004714-199710000-00010.

213. **Tollefson GD, Beasley CM Jr, Tran PV**, et al. Olanzapine versus haloperidol in the treatment of schizophrenia and schizoaffective and schizophreniform disorders: results of an international collaborative trial. American Journal of Psychiatry. 1997;**154**(4):457–65. doi: 10.1176/ajp.154.4.457.

214. **Barak Y, Mirecki I, Knobler HY, Natan Z, Aizenberg D.** Suicidality and second generation antipsychotics in schizophrenia patients: a case-controlled retrospective study during a 5-year period. Psychopharmacology (Berlin). 2004;**175**(2):215–19.

doi: 10.1007/s00213-004-1801-2. Erratum in: Psychopharmacology (Berlin). 2010;210(3):449.

215. **Pompili M.** Adding suicide prevention to the triple advantages of injectable long-acting second-generation antipsychotics. Frontiers in Psychiatry. 2020;**10**:931. doi: 10.3389/fpsyt.2019.00931. Erratum in: Frontiers in Psychiatry. 2020;11:101.
216. **Vares M, Saetre P, Strålin P, Levander S, Lindström E, Jönsson EG.** Concomitant medication of psychoses in a lifetime perspective. Human Psychopharmacology. 2011;**26**(4–5):322–31. doi: 10.1002/hup.1209.
217. **Gunnell D, Saperia J, Ashby D.** Selective serotonin reuptake inhibitors (SSRIs) and suicide in adults: meta-analysis of drug company data from placebo controlled, randomised controlled trials submitted to the MHRA's safety review. BMJ. 2005;**330**(7488):385. doi: 10.1136/bmj.330.7488.385. Erratum in: BMJ. 2006;333(7557):30.
218. **Baldessarini RJ, Tondo L, Davis P, Pompili M, Goodwin FK, Hennen J.** Decreased risk of suicides and attempts during long-term lithium treatment: a meta-analytic review. Bipolar Disorders. 2006;**8**(5 Pt 2):625–39. doi: 10.1111/j.1399-5618.2006.00344.x. Erratum in: Bipolar Disorders. 2007;9(3):314.
219. **Lauterbach E, Felber W, Müller-Oerlinghausen B**, et al. Adjunctive lithium treatment in the prevention of suicidal behaviour in depressive disorders: a randomised, placebo-controlled, 1-year trial. Acta Psychiatrica Scandinavica. 2008;**118**(6):469–79. doi: 10.1111/j.1600-0447.2008.01266.x.
220. **Hayes JF, Pitman A, Marston L**, et al. Self-harm, unintentional injury, and suicide in bipolar disorder during maintenance mood stabilizer treatment: a UK population-based electronic health records study. JAMA Psychiatry. 2016;**73**(6):630–7. doi: 10.1001/jamapsychiatry.2016.0432.
221. **Song J, Sjölander A, Joas E**, et al. Suicidal behavior during lithium and valproate treatment: a within-individual 8-year prospective study of 50,000 patients with bipolar disorder. American Journal of Psychiatry. 2017;**174**(8):795–802. doi: 10.1176/appi.ajp.2017.16050542.
222. **Cipriani A, Pretty H, Hawton K, Geddes JR.** Lithium in the prevention of suicidal behavior and all-cause mortality in patients with mood disorders: a systematic review of randomized trials. American Journal of Psychiatry. 2005;**162**(10):1805–19. doi: 10.1176/appi.ajp.162.10.1805.
223. **Leucht S, Helfer B, Dold M, Kissling W, McGrath JJ.** Lithium for schizophrenia. Cochrane Database of Systematic Reviews. 2015;**2015**(10):CD003834. doi: 10.1002/14651858.CD003834.pub3.
224. **Seemüller F, Schennach R, Mayr A**, et al. Akathisia and suicidal ideation in first-episode schizophrenia. Journal of Clinical Psychopharmacology. 2012;**32**:694–8. doi: 10.1097/JCP.0b013e3182677958.
225. **Shah N, Grover S, Rao GP.** Clinical practice guidelines for management of bipolar disorder. Indian Journal of Psychiatry. 2017;**59**(Suppl 1):S51–66. doi: 10.4103/0019-5545.196974.
226. **Cipriani A, Hawton K, Stockton S, Geddes JR.** Lithium in the prevention of suicide in mood disorders: updated systematic review and meta-analysis. BMJ. 2013;346:f3646. doi: 10.1136/bmj.f3646.

227. **Smith EG, Austin KL, Kim HM**, et al. Suicide risk in Veterans Health Administration patients with mental health diagnoses initiating lithium or valproate: a historical prospective cohort study. BMC Psychiatry. 2014;**14**:357. doi: 10.1186/s12888-014-0357-x.
228. **Dadiomov D, Lee K.** The effects of ketamine on suicidality across various formulations and study settings. The Mental Health Clinician. 2019;**9**(1):48–60. doi: 10.9740/mhc.2019.01.048.
229. **Pompili M, Serafini G, Innamorati M**, et al. Antidepressants and suicide risk: a comprehensive overview. Pharmaceuticals (Basel). 2010;**3**(9):2861–83. doi: 10.3390/ph3092861.
230. **Pacchiarotti I, Bond DJ, Baldessarini RJ**, et al. The International Society for Bipolar Disorders (ISBD) task force report on antidepressant use in bipolar disorders. American Journal of Psychiatry. 2013;**170**(11):1249–62. doi: 10.1176/appi.ajp.2013.13020185.
231. **Vieta E, Sanchez-Moreno J.** Acute and long-term treatment of mania. Dialogues in Clinical Neuroscience. 2008;**10**(2):165–79. doi: 10.31887/DCNS.2008.10.2/evieta.
232. **Pompili M.** Intranasal esketamine and current suicidal ideation with intent in major depression disorder: beat the clock, save a life, start a strategy. Frontiers in Psychiatry. 2020;**11**:325. doi: 10.3389/fpsyt.2020.00325.
233. **Canuso CM, Ionescu DF, Li X**, et al. Esketamine nasal spray for the rapid reduction of depressive symptoms in major depressive disorder with acute suicidal ideation or behavior. Journal of Clinical Psychopharmacology. 2021;**41**(5):516–24. doi: 10.1097/JCP.0000000000001465.
234. **Ionescu DF, Fu DJ, Qiu X**, et al. Esketamine nasal spray for rapid reduction of depressive symptoms in patients with major depressive disorder who have active suicide ideation with intent: results of a phase 3, double-blind, randomized study (ASPIRE II). International Journal of Neuropsychopharmacology. 2021;**24**(1):22–31. doi: 10.1093/ijnp/pyaa068.
235. **Fu DJ, Ionescu DF, Li X**, et al. Esketamine nasal spray for rapid reduction of major depressive disorder symptoms in patients who have active suicidal ideation with intent: double-blind, randomized study (ASPIRE I). Journal of Clinical Psychiatry. 2020;**81**(3):19m13191. doi: 10.4088/JCP.19m13191.

Chapter 19

Bullying, cyberbullying, and suicide

Tania Nadeem, Sahar N. Hamid, Fauzia Mahr, and Nargis Asad

Bullying

Bullying is defined as the intent to harm another with repeated aggressive behaviour in the presence of a power imbalance, and the perpetrator usually has stronger physical ability and power compared to the victim.[1,2,3] It can be categorized in many different ways. Verbal bullying is the use of threats, insults, or sarcasm to humiliate the victim. Physical bullying is using physical force or unwanted sexual touching towards a victim. Exclusion, backbiting, or damaging someone else's reputation falls under social bullying.[4,5] Social bullying tends to be more covert and indirect, and is more frequently seen in females. Verbal and physical bullying tends to be overt and more direct, and is frequently used by males.[3] In most cases, the victim of bullying suffers various forms of bullying concurrently.[6] With the introduction of the World Wide Web and higher availability of smartphones, there has been the advent of a new type of bullying called cyberbullying.

Cyberbullying is defined as the use of technology like smartphones, messaging apps, and websites to intentionally humiliate, embarrass, intimidate, or harass a victim.[7] Cyberbullying works in many ways: it can practise exclusion by not adding an individual to specific online groups or chats that everyone else is talking about or involved in; a cyberbully can also hack into a victim's online accounts and release private information or spread fake or embarrassing rumours about the victim to negatively impact and damage relationships and the reputation of the victim. A cyberbully can also send intimidating and threatening messages to the victim online.[8] There is also appearance-related cyberbullying, in which the focus is on disparaging a victim's appearance and shaming them for the way they look; for example, for girls, it would focus on looking overweight or 'ugly', and for boys, it would focus on looking effeminate or not manly enough. For adolescents, this can have a significant impact on their self-esteem.[9] The victim suffers from a feeling of helplessness, as they cannot control the actions of the cyberbully.[10]

Research carried out in Canadian high schools showed that 77% of adolescents had experienced some form of bullying.[11] In the United States, the 2011 Youth Risk Behavior Surveillance (YRBS) survey showed that 20.1% of high school students had been bullied,[12] whereas 16.2% had experienced cyberbullying.[13] There is wide variation in reported levels of bullying across Europe. The Health Behaviour in School-aged Children (HBSC) survey showed results as low as 3% in Armenia to above 20% in Lithuania.[14] Nordic countries tend to have the lowest rates of reported bullying,[15] and African nations tend to have the highest rates of reported bullying.[16] In Arab nations, there is also variation in the reporting of bullying, ranging from 20.9% in the United Arab Emirates to 44.2% in Jordan.[17] Modecki et al. in their meta-analysis analysed about 80 studies and found a 35% prevalence of traditional bullying and specifically a 15% prevalence of cyberbullying.[18] China, Singapore, and India had the highest self-reports of perpetrators and victims of cyberbullying in Asia.[19] Malaysia had 33% of self-reports, Pakistan 26%, and Japan 11% for cyberbullying. In the African countries Botswana, Guyana, Kenya, Namibia, Swaziland, Uganda, and Zimbabwe, self-reports of cyberbullying ranged from 21% to 60%.[20] Girls were more likely to report being cyber victims and cyberbullies.[21] In Delhi, India, the results stated the opposite, with males being more likely to report being cyber victims and cyberbullies.[22] Data across the world consistently show that bullying as a whole is a problem for adolescents of all countries, cultures, and religions.

Bullying tends to start from a younger age. It usually peaks at around the age of 13–14 years and starts to decrease by the age of 15–16 years.[23] Cyberbullying usually occurs during adolescence, when adolescents get access to their own mobile phones[24] and make their own online profiles on social apps.[25] Cyberbullying allows the perpetrator to have a wider audience and more anonymity. Contents online can be seen across the world, and absolute strangers can join in by liking or adding comments that further humiliate and embarrass the victim. Moreover, these bystanders participate in spreading the material by reposting and sharing embarrassing information.[26] The audience of a cyberbully also has more anonymity to actively support and cooperate with the perpetrator. In traditional bullying, there is less anonymity for the perpetrator and the onlookers. A traditional bully also needs the victim to be close by for them to successfully humiliate a victim, and the victim has an escape from the bully by physically taking themselves out of the same environment. On the other hand, cyberbullying is all invasive and there are very few avenues of escape for the victim, as the rumours, intimidation, or embarrassing information follows the victim everywhere, regardless of whether they are at home, with friends, or in any place that they consider safe or comfortable.[23] In traditional bullying, everyone is physically present and peer pressure plays a big part in how the bystanders react due to their need to fit in.[27] In traditional bullying, it has been seen that the larger the number of bystanders, the further strengthening of the perpetrator's bullying behaviour as the bully feels supported and goaded on.[28] However, if the bystanders decide to support the victim, it can threaten the bully's status and put an end to the bullying.[29] In most cases, research on online bystanders looks at how they decide to help or not to help the victim. A study on Israeli adolescents showed that a bystander was more likely to help if they were older girls and had a good social support network themselves.[30] Flemish bystanders who helped were likely to be younger adolescents and more likely to have been victims of cyberbullying themselves.[31] Adolescents from the Czech Republic were more likely to help if there were very few bystanders to the bullying taking place.[32] The effect of bystanders, active or passive, in cyberbullying needs to be researched in more detail.[33]

Bullying is a significant public health issue for adolescents across the world. Bullying in all its forms takes its toll on the mental health of all: the perpetrator, the bystander, and the victim. There is a large amount of research that shows a strong link between increased suicidal ideation for victims and perpetrators of traditional bullying.[34,35,36] Traditional bullies and their victims across the world show low self-esteem, feelings of loneliness, and issues with their mental and physiological health.[37,38,39] Common factors seen across cultures for victims of traditional bullying include being from a lower socio-economic background, belonging to a minority group, having learning disability,[40] or having dissatisfaction with their body image,[41] as well as a higher likelihood for mental health issues like anxiety and depression.[42] Perpetrators also show a higher likelihood of criminal offending later on in life and a higher probability of risk-taking behaviour.[43]

In the case of cyberbullying, Garaigordobil in his study in northern Spain found adolescent victims and perpetrators showed a range of common traits such as neuroticism, antisocial behaviour, poor academic performance, psychosomatic symptoms, and low scores on traits of agreeableness, social adjustment, and responsibility.[44] Bottino et al. also reported that cyber victims and cyberbullies had feelings of being unsafe at school and emotional problems such as substance abuse, depression, suicidal ideation, and suicide attempts.[45] Higher levels of psychosomatic complaints and depression were also seen in cyberbullies and cybervictims in Turkish schools.[46] Adolescents who have been victims of cyberbullying reported feelings of depression, hopelessness, loneliness, frustration, humiliation, and trauma.[35,47] Cyberbullies show high levels of aggression and low levels of empathy or emotional regulation.[44] Cyberbullies and cybervictims both have parents who have higher levels of stress and are either too permissive or authoritarian in their approach to parenting.[47]

Suicide

All forms of bullying are directly and indirectly associated with high vulnerability for suicidal ideation and suicide attempts.[48] Increased depression and anxiety, due to bullying, are important mediators elucidating the bullying perpetration–victimization–suicide sequence.[49] Cyberbullies and victims are also at higher risk of self-harm and suicidal ideation.[50,51] There is evidence that gender differences prevail in the intersection between cyberbullying and mental health, as studies have reported that depression mediates the relationship between cyberbullying and suicide attempts, but only in females.[52,53] Kowalski et al. found similar gender associations among bullying victimization (traditional and cyber) with depression and suicidal thinking.[54] However, data on gender-associated risk of suicidality are conflicting, as some studies have reported no difference between the genders.[55,56] Kowalski et al.[54] also found age to be an important, though less researched, determinant of the association among cyberbullying victimization, depression, and suicide attempts; the authors found that younger adolescents, such as ninth graders, were more likely to report suicide attempts rather than older adolescents. More than two-thirds of female patients who presented to the paediatric emergency department with suicidal ideation had a history of cyberbullying.[57] Risk factors for bullying and suicidality include individual traits, family turmoil, and social and other environmental difficulties.[58] Poverty, living in disadvantaged neighbourhoods, easy accessibility of firearms, feelings of fear due to perceived threat at school and home, perception of poor relationship with schoolteachers and peers, academic difficulties, social isolation, and difficulty assimilating as an immigrant are other risk factors for self-harm.[56,58] It has been suggested that childhood bullying continues to be associated with increased suicidality in later life as adults.[55] Interestingly, a study on Spanish adolescents showed that if cyberbullies had high self-esteem or high emotional intelligence, then they had a lower risk of suicidal ideation.[51]

Understanding bullying-linked suicide from the perspective of widespread shame in collectivistic cultures of low- to middle-income countries (LMICs) is important. 'Collectivistic' cultures foster and encourage interdependency and relatedness, unlike individualistic autonomous cultures. At a personal level, collectivism is manifested by concern about interpersonal bonds and a greater awareness of, and responsiveness to, the needs of others, reflecting a sense of interconnectedness and interdependence.[59] However, in this complex matrix of interrelatedness, the consequences of disparaging rumours, triggered by bullying, regarding any family member can cause a threat to the whole family's integrity and social stature, leading to an amplification of the trauma suffered by the victim when compared to individualistic cultures. This is especially pertinent when girls' intimate and private information/photographs are shared online. Considering the cultural context, these girls carry immense shame not only for themselves, but also for undermining their family's reputation; hence, the focus changes from blaming the perpetrator to blaming the victim. DeSmet et al. discussed that acute humiliation and embarrassment secondary to bullying can cause suicidal ideation and suicide attempt in victims.[60] Therefore, in collectivistic practices, there is a magnification of shame, which could contribute further to suicidality.

Assessment

Various health care professionals can come into contact with bullies or bully-victims, as both can present with physical injuries, aggression, somatic complaints, psychological symptoms, and suicidality.[61,62] In view of the high incidence of bullying, its association with suicide, and the variability in medical presentation, it is crucial that in every contact that children and adolescents have with medical professionals, they should be assessed for exposure to bullying in the role of a perpetrator, bystander,[63] or victim; otherwise there is a high reluctance to disclose this information.

Standardized screening tools, such as the Olweus Bully/Victimization Questionnaire (OBVQ) and the California Bullying Victimization Scale (CBVS), can be helpful assessment tools for physicians. The OBVQ is an older self-report scale that has 40 questions, with some about bullying or being bullied. It had been translated and validated in many countries, including Pakistan[64] and Turkey,[65] and has been used by teachers, researchers, and medical professionals. Felix et al. developed the CBVS, a self-report scale, which does not use the term bullying but tries to assess its three main fundamentals: repetition, intention, and power imbalance.[66] Interestingly, Kert et al. had shown that scales that did not use or define the term bullying showed a higher yield of positive responses.[67] The CVBS was validated in Turkish middle schools students and showed a positive correlation with bullying and a negative correlation with life satisfaction.[68] These scales did not assess specifically for cyberbullying or the role of bystanders. Alavi et al. had recommended asking further targeted questions about cyberbullying because children often do not consider it as bullying, resulting in it being the least reported.[69] Most cyberbullying scales have limited validity and reliability, as they do not account for the variability in different forms of social media and have minimal psychometric information.[63] Similarly, assessment tools for bystanders are limited and specific questions about running away, cheering the bully, or not responding while witnessing bullying should be explored. Likewise, following online pages where someone is being bullied and liking or sharing those comments can be given as examples of cyberbullying bystanders.[70,71]

Subsequently, after detailed questioning about bullying and victimization, suicide risk assessment should be done. A history of previous depression or anxiety symptomatology, prior self-harm behaviour, aggression, incidents of running away from home, a history of previous criminal acts, and chronic illness or disability should be taken as they increase the risk of bullying and victimization.[56,58,72] Perceived body weight when individuals believe that they are 'fat', sexual orientation differences such as being part of the lesbian, gay, bisexual, and transgender (LGBT) community, a previous history of abuse and substance abuse are additional factors which increase the occurrence of self-harm.[56,58] Parental conflict or violence, separation or divorce, and serious illness or death of a parent are contributing factors for suicidality in bullies and bully-victims, which thus should be explored. Some parents are ashamed of their child being a victim or proud of their offspring being an aggressor. Thus, these attitudes need to be explored further.[73] Inquiries regarding family history of suicide should also be made.[56,58,72] In addition to suicidality, bully-victims should be assessed for low self-esteem, homicidal ideation and attempts, and detailed symptoms of depression, post-traumatic stress disorder, and anxiety disorders.[6]

The aforementioned detailed assessments can be executed by mental health professionals. Therefore, other physicians should refer to psychiatrists/psychologists if they find bullying and extreme distress in a child or adolescent.

Management

Prevention programmes against bullying should take priority and can focus on interventions within the community, family, and school. Community awareness programmes have been shown to help by educating the population and promoting unity.[74] Community programmes can focus on encouraging empathy, building positive relationships, accepting differences, assimilating immigrants, and being more mindful of the effects of an individual's words and actions on others, while also showing intolerance towards bullying.[72,75] Discussions on 'what is bullying?' can be initiated and should highlight different forms of bullying, especially cyberbullying.[19,23] Print and broadcast media can be important tools in developing nations for such awareness programmes. Another factor to consider in LMICs would be unplanned urbanization resulting in exacerbating inequalities, which can increase the likelihood of bullying.[76]

Family interventions should focus on promoting harmony between family members and enabling parents to discuss this topic with their children. A supportive family structure is protective against the suicidal effects of bullying, and this can be a focus of preventive programmes.[77] Collectivistic cultures of developing nations can be helpful in this perspective. A research study on cyberbullying and suicide in Hong Kong adolescents found that children who had higher life satisfaction with family were more resilient compared to children with peer satisfaction or high academic achievements.[77] Focus on family support and religion/spirituality in collectivistic cultures are supposed to be beneficial for individuals facing bullying.[78] A research study on Indian adolescents and cyberbullying showed that children coming from individualistic values had a higher incidence of being a bully or victim, whereas collectivistic values had a negative correlation with the two.[79]

It is important that parents are taught to talk to their children about responsible behaviour on social media: to think about what they say, not to send messages while angry, to show problematic messages to adults, to keep rigid privacy settings, to block individuals who are bullying them, and not to send compromising pictures.[75] Children should be educated about the permanence and repetitiveness of anything that is posted on the Internet. They should be informed that bystanders play a crucial role in perpetuating bullying and cyberbullying by providing an audience, directly encouraging a bully, and spreading rumours. Parents should regularly check their child's phone to monitor this behaviour.[75] Adults should be aware that children fear that their phones will be taken away if they report any problematic behaviours, as parents will blame technology rather than individuals.[72] Thus, to encourage safe disclosures, such punitive actions should not be implemented.[80]

Additionally, schools can play a vital role in anti-bullying initiatives, as most of these behaviours start among students who know one another at academic institutes. All such initiatives should have a suicide prevention aspect.[80] School administration, teachers, peers, families, and individuals all need to be involved.[56] The curriculum should focus on improving awareness about bullying in easily understandable terms[80] and encouraging positive personality traits like kindness, respect, and fairness[75] in pupils. Schools should ensure that children are well assimilated in a safe and inclusive school environment,[75,81] their strengths, and not just their weaknesses, are highlighted, and toxic competition is discouraged. Cassidy et al.[23] discussed how increasing extracurricular activities in schools can alleviate cyberbullying by decreasing time spent on the Internet by children. As many children are merely bystanders while bullying occurs, they should also be enabled to speak up in the face of such deviant behaviour. Victims can be enabled to make presentations on bullying in their classrooms to empower them to speak against the aggressor. One supportive adult in school can protect from the harmful effects of bullying;[75] schools with lower student:teacher ratios and a structure where one teacher can be assigned to a mentor or supervise a group of children can be studied to assess the benefit against bullying. A positive teacher–student relationship was found to buffer from the effects of bullying in Chinese youth.[82] Clear consequences should be implemented, and academic institutes should show zero tolerance towards bullying.[75] Shaikh discussed that only 50% of victims report bullying. Thus, school reporting systems should be looked at.[81] Systems to encourage anonymous reporting of bullying can be considered, along with methods of seeking support from peers, as it has been shown to have a buffering effect on depression.[74,75] Essential counselling services should be easily accessible to children in schools, and referrals to psychiatrists should be made if needed.

Proper legislation and guidance by governments are crucial to aid in the implementation of an anti-bullying programme. In Hong Kong, the Education Bureau has provided guidelines to schools on how to address bullying by creating a clear policy and providing resources.[83] In 2012, the Ministry of Education (MOE) in Taiwan passed the 'Regulations on the Prevention of School Bullying' policy, which provides definitions, guidelines, and procedures for schools to prevent and manage school bullying. In Taiwan, parents are held liable for their children's cyberbullying activities.[84]

Ultimately, focus should be paid on building resilience in a child by increasing levels of positive mental health, which is a buffer between cyberbullying and suicide, by initiating well-being programmes.[85] Children should be aided in communicating effectively—being able to identify their feelings as alexithymia is more prevalent in both bullies and victims.[86] Critical thinking skills like problem-solving should be encouraged to enable children to find a resolution to their predicament and empower them.[74] Relaxation techniques like mindfulness and exercise can aid in dealing with the stress of bullying and also help in putting things into perspective.[19] Family strengthening interventions and parent training to improve violent and delinquent behaviour in children should be implemented to reduce risk factors.[56]

In summary, encouraging protective factors, which include connectedness to a parent or another adult, perceiving friends as caring, living and studying in safer environments, and promoting acceptance of a child's strengths and weaknesses, consequently encouraging positive self-esteem,[56,72] are the main themes for anti-bullying programmes.

The main limitations for anti-bullying interventions in LMICs with high fertility rates (documented total fertility rate of 3.72 from 2010 to 2015 by the United Nations secretariat) and poverty (24.3% living below the national poverty line, according to Asian Development Bank statistics) are a lack of resources.[86] Families live in derelict surroundings and parents usually work all day long, returning home late in the evening and continuously worrying about finances, a situation which is not conducive to a healthy parent–child bond. Unsupervised children can be out on the streets and have easy access to social media via cell phones, providing ample opportunity for physical and cyberbullying or victimization. Furthermore, parents are not as educated or as competent at using social media as their children, making it difficult for them to monitor use; thus, interventions to improve media literacy are needed.[83] Moreover, parents place immense academic pressures on children as a pathway to a better life, but there are limited or absent resources for children with academic difficulties and minimal opportunities for extracurriculars, resulting in poor self-esteem and an increased risk of bullying or victimization for children with differences.[56,72] Physical punishments, including beatings, are very common and again a risk factor. Chang et al. discussed how Chinese schools have placed emphasis on academic achievement at the expense of socialization, resulting in an increased likelihood of bullying. Developing nations have gravely limited budgets for education and minimally monitored governmental school systems, poorly trained teachers, and high student:teacher ratios, which can increase the risk of bullying. Limited behaviour management capacity of teachers can create immense frustration at all ends and results in causing conflict between schools and parents, which is then displaced as anger towards both the victim and the perpetrator, ultimately worsening the situation.

Conclusion

Finally, at the level of a mental health professional, specialized services should be provided, but taboo against psychiatric care in LMICs can be a limiting factor. Individual counselling can help to provide support and build confidence in tackling this problem in the child. Family counselling can aid in improving communication and support within the family. Parenting skills session to encourage setting clear rules, a healthy structure with limited Internet time, and a parent–child open and flexible dialogue can be beneficial.[56] Couples therapy in cases where the parental relationship is creating stress within the household should be explored, as this is commonly seen in households of bullies.[72] A healthy routine with balanced sleep, physical activity, time with family, and limited screen time can be encouraged.[75] Extracurriculars, to help with confidence and social opportunities, can be promoted as social isolation and low self-esteem are risk factors for bullying. Peer-led support groups are also beneficial.[72] If the child is suffering from other psychiatric comorbidities, then medications can be considered.

References

1. **Furlong MJ, Sharkey JD, Felix ED, Tanigawa D, Green JG.** Bullying assessment: a call for increased precision of self-reporting procedures. In: **Jimerson SR, Swearer SM, Espelage DL**, editors. *Handbook of Bullying in Schools: An International Perspective.* New York, NY: Routledge; 2010. pp. 329–45.
2. **Pittet I, Berchtold A, Akré C, Michaud P, Surís J.** Are adolescents with chronic conditions particularly at risk for bullying? Archives of Disease in Childhood. 2010;**95**(1):711–16.
3. **Romero AJ, Wiggs CB, Valencia C, Bauman S.** Latina teen suicide and bullying. Hispanic Journal of Behavioral Sciences. 2013;**35**(2):159–73.
4. **Holt M, Vivolo-Kantor A, Polanin J**, et al. Bullying and suicidal ideation and behaviours: a meta-analysis. American Academy of Pediatrics. 2015;**135**(2):496–509.
5. **Hinduja S, Patchin JW** (2014). *Bullying beyond the Schoolyard: Preventing and Responding to Cyberbullying.* United States of America: Corwin Press.
6. **Roh BR, Yoon Y, Kwon A**, et al. The structure of co-occurring bullying experiences and associations with suicidal behaviors in Korean adolescents. PLoS One. 2015;**10**(11):e01.
7. **Nansel TR, Craig W, Overpeck MD, Saluja G, Ruan WJ; Health Behaviour in School-aged Children Bullying Analyses Working Group**. Cross-national consistency in the relationship between bullying behaviors and psychosocial adjustment. Archives of Pediatrics and Adolescent Medicine. 2004;**158**(8):730–6.
8. **Rémond JJ, Kern L, Romo L.** A cyberbullying study: analysis of cyberbullying, comorbidities and coping mechanisms. L'Encéphale. 2014;**41**(4):287–94.
9. **Berne S, Frisén A, Kling J.** Appearance-related cyberbullying: a qualitative investigation of characteristics, content, reasons, and effects. Body Image. 2014;**11**(4):527–33.
10. **Dooley JJ, Pyżalski J, Cross D.** Cyberbullying versus face-to-face bullying: a theoretical and conceptual review. Zeitschrift für Psychologie/Journal of Psychology. 2009;**217**(4):182–8.
11. **Alavi N, Reshetukha T, Prost E**, et al. Relationship between bullying and suicidal behaviour in youth presenting to the emergency department. Journal of the Canadian Academy of Child and Adolescent Psychiatry. 2017;**26**(2):70–7.
12. **Centres for Disease Control and Prevention** (2012). Youth Risk Behavior Surveillance—United States, 2011. Available from: https://www.cdc.gov/mmwr/pdf/ss/ss6104.pdf
13. **Bhatta M, Shakya S, Jefferis E.** Association of being bullied in school with suicide ideation and planning among rural middle school adolescents. Journal of School Health. 2014;**84**(11):731–8.

14. World Health Organization. **Health-Behaviour in School-Aged Children (HBSC) Study, 2023.** Available from: https://www.who.int/europe/initiatives/health-behaviour-in-school-aged-children-(hbsc)-study
15. **Craig W, Harel-Fisch Y, Fogel-Grinvald H,** et al.; **HBSC Violence & Injuries Prevention Focus Group; HBSC Bullying Writing Group**. A cross-national profile of bullying and victimization among adolescents in 40 countries. International Journal of Public Health. 2009;**54**(Suppl 2):216–24.
16. **Richardson D, Hiu CF.** Developing a global indicator on bullying of school-aged children. Innocenti Working Papers, no. 2018-11. Florence: UNICEF Office of Research; 2018.
17. **Kazarian S, Ammar J.** School bullying in the Arab world: a review. Arab Journal of Psychiatry. 2013;**24**:37–45.
18. **Modecki KL, Minchin J, Harbaugh AG, Guerra NG, Runions KC.** Bullying prevalence across contexts: a meta-analysis measuring cyber and traditional bullying. Journal of Adolescent Health. 2014;**55**(5):602–11.
19. **Bhat C, Chang S-H, Ragan MA.** Cyberbullying in Asia. Education about Asia. 2013;**18**(2):36–9.
20. **Fleming LC, Jacobsen KH.** Bullying among middle-school students in low and middle income countries. Health Promotion International. 2010;**25**(1):73–84.
21. **Rice E, Petering R, Rhoades H,** et al. Cyberbullying perpetration and victimization among middle-school students. American Journal of Public Health. 2015;**105**(3):e66–72.
22. **Sharma D, Kishore J, Sharma N, Duggal M.** Aggression in schools: cyberbullying and gender issues. Asian Journal of Psychiatry. 2017;**29**:142–5.
23. **Cassidy WEM, Jackson M, Brown KN.** Sticks and stones can break my bones, but how can pixels hurt me?: students' experiences with cyber-bullying. School Psychology International.2009, **30**(4):383–402.
24. **Suzuki K, Asaga R, Sourander A, Hoven CW, Mandell D.** Cyberbullying and adolescent mental health. International Journal of Adolescent Mental Health. 2012;**24**(1):27–35.
25. **Kowalski RM, Limber SP.** Electronic bullying among middle school students. Journal of Adolescent Health. 2007;**41**(6 Suppl 1):S22–30.
26. **Vaillancourt T, Faris R, Mishna F.** Cyberbullying in children and youth: implications for health and clinical practice. Canadian Journal of Psychiatry. 2017;**62**(6):368–73.
27. **Nickerson A, Taylor D, Princiotta D.** Attachment and empathy as predictors of roles as defenders or outsiders in bullying interactions. Journal of School Psychology. 2009;**46**:687–703.
28. **Fonagy P, Twemlow SW, Sacco FC, Gies ML, Hess D.** Improving the social and intellectual climate in elementary schools by addressing bully-victim-bystander power struggles. In: **Cohen J**, editor. *Caring Classrooms/Intelligent Schools: The Social Emotional Education of Young Children.* Teachers College Press, Columbia University, New York & London; 2001. pp. 162–82.
29. **Pepler D, Craig W, O'Connell P.** Peer processes in bullying: informing prevention and intervention strategies. In: **Jimerson SR, Swearer SM, Espelage DL**, editor. *Handbook of Bullying in Schools: An International Perspective.* Routledge: New York; 2009. pp. 469–79.

30. **Olenik-Shemesh D, Heiman T.** Cyberbullying victimization in adolescents as related to body esteem, social support, and social self-efficacy. Journal of Genetic Psychology. 2017;**178**(1):28–43.
31. **Van Cleemput K, Vandebosch H, Pabian S.** Personal characteristics and contextual factors that determine 'helping,' 'joining in,' and 'doing nothing' when witnessing cyberbullying. Aggressive Behavior. 2014;**40**(5):383–96
32. **Machackova H, Dedkova L, Mezulanikova K.** Brief report: the bystander effect in cyberbullying incidents. Journal of Adolescence. 2015;**43**:96–9.
33. **Garett R, Lord LR, Young SD.** Associations between social media and cyberbullying: a review of the literature. mHealth. 2016;**2**:46.
34. **Baldry AC, Winkel FW.** Direct and vicarious victimization at school and at home as risk factors for suicidal cognition among Italian adolescents. Journal of Adolescence. 2003;**26**(6):703–16.
35. **Hinduja S, Patchin J.** Bullying, cyberbullying, and suicide. Archives of Suicide Research. 2010;**14**:206–21.
36. **Kim YS, Koh Y-J, Leventhal B.** School bullying and suicidal risk in Korean middle school students. Pediatrics. 2005;**115**:357–63.
37. **Prinstein MJ, Boergers J, Vernberg EM.** Overt and relational aggression in adolescents: social-psychological adjustment of aggressors and victims. Journal of Clinical Child Psychology. 2001;**30**:479–49.
38. **Prinstein MJ, Boergers J, Spirito A, Little TD, Grapentine WL.** Peer functioning, family dysfunction, and psychological symptoms in a risk factor model for adolescent inpatients' suicidal ideation severity. Journal of Clinical Child Psychology. 2000;**29**:392–405.
39. **Mills C, Guerin S, Lynch F, Daly I, Fitzpatrick C.** The relationship between bullying, depression and suicidal thoughts/behaviour in Irish adolescents. Irish Journal of Psychological Medicine. 2004;**21**:112–16.
40. **Alavi N, Roberts N, Sutton C, Axas N, Repetti L.** Bullying victimization (being bullied) among adolescents referred for urgent psychiatric consultation: prevalence and association with suicidality. Canadian Journal of Psychiatry. 2015;**60**(10):427–31.
41. **Rech RR, Halpern R, Tedesco A, Santos DF.** Prevalence and characteristics of victims and perpetrators of bullying. Jornal de Pediatria. 2013;**89**:164–70.
42. **Schwartz D, Lansford J, Dodge K, Pettit G, Bates J.** Peer victimization during middle childhood as a lead indicator of internalizing problems and diagnostic outcomes in late adolescence. Journal of Clinical Child and Adolescent Psychology. 2014;**53**:44.
43. **Liang H, Flisher A, Lombard C.** Bullying, violence, and risk behavior in South African school students. Child Abuse and Neglect. 2007;**31**:161–71.
44. **Garaigordobil M.** Cyberbullying in adolescents and youth in the Basque Country: prevalence of cybervictims, cyberaggressors, and cyberobservers. Journal of Youth Studies. 2015;**18**:569–82.
45. **Bottino S, Bottino C, Regina C, Correia A, Ribeiro W.** Cyberbullying and adolescent mental health: systematic review. Cadernos de Saude Publica. 2015;**31**:463–75.
46. **Hesapçıoğlu ST, Ercan F.** Traditional and cyberbullying co-occurrence and its relationship to psychiatric symptoms. Pediatrics International. 2016;**59**:16–22.

47. **Garaigordobil M, Machimbarrena J.** Stress, competence, and parental educational styles in victims and aggressors of bullying and cyberbullying. Psicothema. 2017;**29**:335–40.
48. **Cash SJ, Bridge JA.** Epidemiology of youth suicide and suicidal behavior. Current Opinion in Pediatrics. 2009;**21**(5):613–19.
49 **Aoyama I, Saxon T, Fearon D.** Internalizing problems among cyberbullying victims and moderator effects of friendship quality. Multicultural Education and Technology Journal. 2011;5:92–105.
50. **John A, Glendenning AC, Marchant A,** et al. Self-harm, suicidal behaviours, and cyberbullying in children and young people: systematic review. Journal of Medical Internet Research. 2018;**20**(4):e129.
51. **Extremera N, Quintana-Orts C, Mérida-López S, Rey L.** Cyberbullying victimization, self-esteem and suicidal ideation in adolescence: does emotional intelligence play a buffering role? Frontiers in Psychology. 2018;**9**:367.
52. **Bauman S.** Cyberbullying: what does the research tell us? Theory into Practice. 2013;**52**:249–56.
53. **Bonanno R, Hymel S.** Cyber bullying and internalizing difficulties: above and beyond the impact of traditional forms of bullying. Journal of Youth and Adolescence. 2013;**42**:685–97.
54. **Kowalski R, Limber S.** Psychological, physical, and academic correlates of cyberbullying and traditional bullying. Journal of Adolescent Health. 2013;**53**:S13–20.
55. **Bhatta MP, Shakya S, Jefferis E.** Association of being bullied in school with suicide ideation and planning among rural middle school adolescents. Journal of School Health. 2014;**84**(11):731–8.
56. **Borowsky IW, Taliaferro LA, McMorris BJ.** Suicidal thinking and behavior among youth involved in verbal and social bullying: risk and protective factors. Journal of Adolescent Health. 2013;**53**(1 Suppl):S4–12.
57. **Roberts N, Axas N, Nesdole R, Repetti L.** Pediatric emergency department visits for mental health crisis: prevalence of cyber-bullying in suicidal youth. Child and Adolescent Social Work Journal. 2016;**33**:469–72.
58. **Jimerson S, Swearer S, Espelage D.** *Handbook of Bullying in Schools: An International Perspective.* Routledge: New York and UK; 2010.
59. **Hui C, Triandis H.** Individualism–collectivism: a study of cross-cultural researchers. Journal of Cross-Cultural Psychology. 1986;**17**:225–48.
60. **DeSmet A, Deforche B, Hublet A, Tanghe A, Stremersch E, De Bourdeaudhuij I.** Traditional and cyberbullying victimization as correlates of psychosocial distress and barriers to a healthy lifestyle among severely obese adolescents: a matched case-control study on prevalence and results from a cross-sectional study. BMC Public Health. 2014;**14**:224.
61. **Owusu A, Hart P, Oliver B, Kang M.** The association between bullying and psychological health among senior high school students in Ghana, West Africa. Journal of School Health. 2011;**81**(5):231–8.
62. **Gini G.** Associations between bullying behaviour, psychosomatic complaints, emotional and behavioural problems. Journal of Paediatric Child Health. 2008;**44**(9):492–7.

63. **Berne S, Frisén A, Schultze-Krumbholz A, Scheithauer H, Naruskov K, Luik P, Katzer C, Erentaite R, Zukauskiene R.** Cyberbullying assessment instruments: A systematic review. Aggression and Violent Behavior. 2013;**18**(2):320–34.
64. **Khawar R, Malick F.** Bullying defined in Pakistani school context: an Urdu translation of Olweus Bully Victim Questionnaire. Journal of Behavioural Sciences. 2018;**28**(2):85–111.
65. **Dölek N.** *An Investigation of Bullying Behaviors among Elementary and High School Students and the Effect of Program Developing Bullying Prevention Attitudes.* (Unpublished doctoral dissertation). Istanbul: Marmara University; 2002.
66. **Furlong MJ, Sharkey JD, Bates MP, Smith DC.** An examination of the reliability, data screening procedures, and extreme response patterns for the Youth Risk Behavior Surveillance Survey. Journal of School Violence. 2004;**3**(2–3):109–30.
67. **Kert A, Codding R, Tryon G, Shiyko M.** Impact of the word 'bully' on the reported rate of bullying behavior. Psychology in the Schools. 2009;**47**:193–204.
68. **Atik G, Guneri OY.** California bullying victimization scale: validity and reliability evidence for the Turkish middle school children. Procedia—Social and Behavioral Sciences. 2012;**46**:1237–41.
69. **Vandebosch H, Cleemput K.** Cyberbullying among youngsters: profiles of bullies and victims. New Media and Society. 2009;**11**:1349–71.
70. **Brown K, Jackson M, Cassidy W.** Cyber-bullying: developing policy to direct responses that are equitable and effective in addressing this special form of bullying. Canadian Journal of Educational Administration and Policy. 2006;**57**.
71. **Bhat CS.** Proactive cyberbullying and sexting prevention in Australia and the USA. Journal of Psychologists and Counsellors in Schools. 2018;**28**(1):120–30.
72. **Field T.** Cyberbullying: a narrative review. Journal of Addiction Therapy and Research. 2018;**2**:10–27.
73. **Besag V.** *Bullies and Victims in Schools.* Milton Keynes: Open University Press; 1989.
74. **Sampasa-Kanyinga H, Roumeliotis P, Xu H.** Associations between cyberbullying and school bullying victimization and suicidal ideation, plans and attempts among Canadian schoolchildren. PLoS One. 2014;**9**(7):e102145.
75. **Mental Health Commission of Canada.** Bullying and suicide. Available from: https://mentalhealthcommission.ca/wp-content/uploads/2017/11/Bullying-and-suicide-prevention.pdf
76. **Wilson M, Dunlavy A, Berchtold A.** Determinants for bullying victimization among 11–16-year-olds in 15 low-and middle-income countries: a multi-level study. Social Sciences. 2013;**2**(4):208–20.
77. **Chang Q, Xing J, Ho RTH, Yip PSF.** Cyberbullying and suicide ideation among Hong Kong adolescents: the mitigating effects of life satisfaction with family, classmates and academic results. Psychiatry Research. 2019;**274**:269–73.
78. **Hu Q, Bernardo AB, Lam SW, Cheang PK.** Individualism–collectivism orientations and coping styles of cyberbullying victims in Chinese culture. Current Psychology. 2018;**37**(1):65–72.
79. **Wright MF, Kamble SV, Soudi SP.** Indian adolescents' cyber aggression involvement and cultural values: the moderation of peer attachment. School Psychology International. 2015;**36**(4):410–27.

80. **Van Geel M, Vedder P, Tanilon J.** Relationship between peer victimization, cyberbullying, and suicide in children and adolescents: a meta-analysis. JAMA Pediatrics. 2014;**168**(5):435–42.
81. **Shaikh AM.** Bullying victimization among school-attending adolescents in Pakistan. Journal of the Pakistan Medical Association. 2013;**63**(9):1202.
82. **Han Z, Zhang G, Zhang H.** School bullying in urban China: prevalence and correlation with school climate. International Journal of Environmental Research and Public Health. 2017;**14**(10):1116.
83. **Bhat C, Chang S-H, Linscott J.** Addressing cyberbullying as a media literacy issue. New Horizons in Education. 2010;**58**(3):34–43.
84. **Chen LM.** School-based anti-bullying strategies in Taiwan and their effects. Studies in Educational Evaluation. 2018;**59**:218–23.
85. **Brailovskaia J, Teismann T, Margraf J.** Cyberbullying, positive mental health and suicide ideation/behavior. Psychiatry Research. 2018;**267**:240–2.
86. **Murshid NS.** Bullying victimization and mental health outcomes of adolescents in Myanmar, Pakistan, and Sri Lanka. Children and Youth Services Review. 2017;**76**:163–9.

Chapter 20

The influence of religion on euthanasia and physician-assisted suicide

Shahnaz Savani, Anil Arora, Marcus Brown, Ying Ma, and Robin Edward Gearing

Introduction

Euthanasia is defined as the act of hastening the death of an individual to prevent suffering, sometimes with assistance from a physician.[1] Physician-assisted suicide (PAS) can be explained as death that occurs with the help of a physician providing the means or knowledge, or both, to a person to end their own life, usually because of terminal or debilitating illness, or unbearable pain.[2] In the literature, euthanasia and PAS are often used interchangeably and have further evolved into the more nuanced terms of active and passive euthanasia. Active euthanasia is understood as an act that would actively cause someone's death, whereas passive euthanasia is understood as withholding medical treatment so that death is allowed to occur.[3] The term 'active euthanasia' is further developed into terms like 'voluntary active euthanasia', 'involuntary active euthanasia', and 'non-voluntary active euthanasia', with more specific definitions. Voluntary active euthanasia is categorized as an act by a physician wherein the physician administers a medication to end a patient's life at the patient's explicit request.[2] Involuntary active euthanasia is conceptualized as an act by a physician administering medication to end a patient's life who is not mentally competent, with the act being carried out without the patient's request.[2] Non-voluntary active euthanasia occurs when an individual administers a medication to end the life of a non-competent person unable to give informed consent (e.g. a child or a patient with Alzheimer's disease).[2] Although rarely acknowledged, passive euthanasia is common and practised freely around the world, despite euthanasia and PAS being illegal in most countries around the world.

Suicide, euthanasia, and PAS are complex phenomena that intersect and possess the common characteristic of being voluntary actions that lead to unnatural death. Further, suicide, euthanasia, and PAS can be understood on a spectrum with much overlap in their meaning, practice, and interpretation.[4] A deeper understanding of euthanasia and PAS is critical in way of contributing to suicide assessment, prevention, and intervention efforts among vulnerable and chronically ill populations.

Religious beliefs and attitudes play a key role in how individuals navigate complex issues in their life. Most world religions have a strong prohibitionary stance against suicide and, by extension, against euthanasia and PAS. Religious ideology, beliefs, and practices exert a significant amount of influence on attitudes towards, perspectives on, and understanding of individuals and groups on the ethics, permissibility, and acceptability of euthanasia and PAS in society.[5] The intersection of religion and euthanasia remains important in research on suicide, and obtaining a more accurate and nuanced understanding of religious perspectives on the issue are critical in advancing the science on suicide prevention and intervention.

This chapter provides an analysis of the current state of knowledge regarding the relationship between religion and euthanasia across the five dominant world religions: Buddhism, Christianity, Hinduism, Islam, and Judaism. Research on religion and euthanasia is scant and primarily focused on examining attitudes, beliefs, and understanding of people on euthanasia and PAS. Further, research on this topic is mostly conducted with medical doctors, nurses, allied health professionals, medical and nursing students, religious leaders of various denominations, and patients and their loved ones. Most research on the topic is specific to the local context and is quantitative, mainly conducted through self-reported responses to questionnaires. Research outcomes examining the influence of religion on euthanasia and PAS are mixed and inconsistent, with no clear understanding or depth on the topic.

Method

Researchers reviewed search results on PAS and euthanasia with religion by using PsycINFO, MEDLINE, and PubMed databases. Keywords included from the Boolean search were broken down into two key areas: religion and euthanasia. Religious terms included: Buddhism, Buddhist, Buddhists; Christian, Christianity, Christians; Hindu, Hinduism; Islam, Islamic, Muslim; and Jewish, Judaism, Jew. Euthanasia terms included: physician-assisted suicide; physician-assisted death; euthanasia; and assisted suicide. Based on Figure 20.1, created by the research team examining the database searches, the total records identified were 4086 articles, with an additional set of 10 articles identified and included for further analysis from references. In total, 2334 duplicates were identified

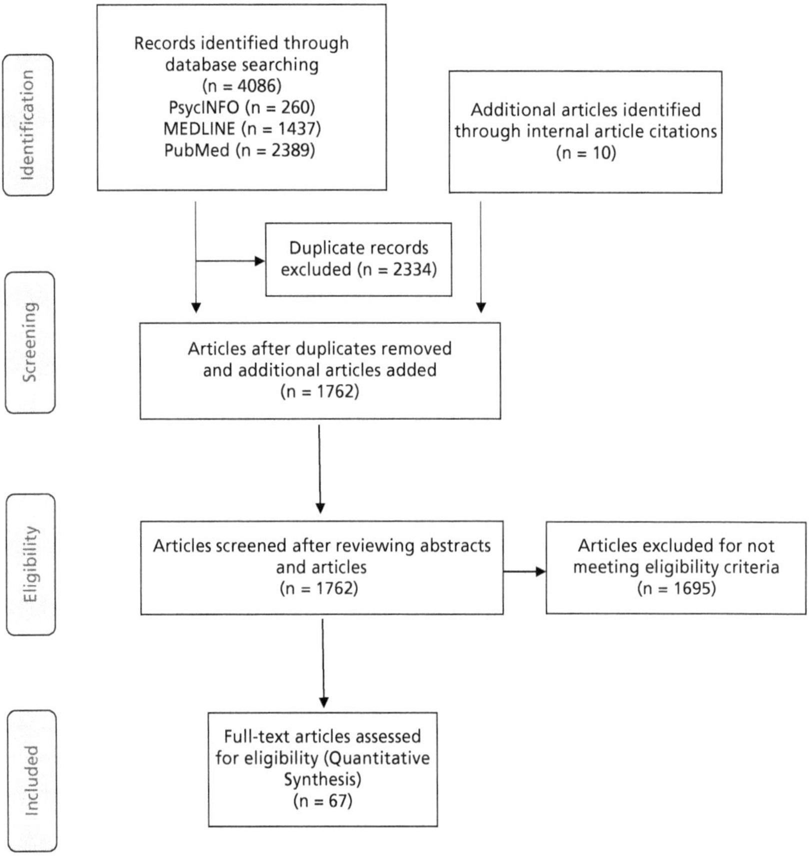

Figure 20.1 Review and selection of articles approximately.

and removed. The resulting 1762 eligible abstracts were reviewed by the research team. After removing 1695 articles, a total of 67 full-text articles were included in the review.

Buddhism

Euthanasia and PAS are an important social, medical, legal, and religious issue in contemporary society.[6] About 7% of the world's population identify as Buddhist and live predominantly in East and South East Asia.[6] Buddhism has branched into several sects, with some differences in both interpretation of Buddha's teachings and practice, making it difficult to describe a universal Buddhist view on euthanasia and PAS. Regardless of the denomination, Buddhism does seem to influence individual beliefs and attitudes towards euthanasia and PAS, in keeping with major values of Buddhism to do no harm to any forms of living beings.[7] This section of the chapter summarizes the extant literature examining the Buddhist perspectives on euthanasia and PAS.

Buddhism and euthanasia and PAS research

Grove and colleagues (2002) analysed secondary texts from 44 articles, including the ancient scriptural texts of the Bible, the Quran, the Veda, and the Pali Canon to learn the understandings and interpretations of the official teachings on euthanasia and PAS of the four major world religions.[6] Buddhists understand euthanasia and PAS from the perspectives of life and suffering, and karma and rebirth. The Four Noble Truths in Buddhism are the foundation of the Buddhist doctrine, which are described in the Pali Canon and various other scriptures.[6] Based on these four Truths, suffering is an innate part of life and an undeniable reality; removing all desires is a way to end suffering, rather than ending life.[6] Thus, euthanasia and PAS are at odds with the Buddhist philosophy.

Only three empirical studies were found that reported data on Buddhism, euthanasia, and PAS (See Table 20.1). A cross-sectional study in China surveying attitudes towards suicide among lawyers ($n = 77$), Buddhists ($n = 56$), and medical staff ($n = 296$) demonstrated that only one-third of Buddhists, 69.6% of medical personnel, and 50.5% of lawyers were accepting of euthanasia.[8] This study did not delineate the religious affiliation of the lawyers or medical staff. A second study was conducted with 43 Chinese older adults at a day care centre in Singapore.[9] The predominant religion of this population was Taoism/Buddhism, and the median age of participants was 71 years. Results revealed that 51.2% of participants were supportive of euthanasia, whereas 34.9% were against it.[9] Further, 53.5% of participants reported that they would consider a doctor as a surrogate decision-maker, followed by a family member (34.9%).[9]

A third study by Tanida (2000) surveying 144 leaders and 23 theologians through case analyses in 388 Japanese religious corporations included Shintos ($n = 53$), Buddhists ($n = 66$), Christians ($n = 33$), and others ($n = 15$).[10] This study found that over 70% of respondents accepted passive euthanasia and indirect euthanasia, whereas fewer than 20% favoured active euthanasia. Additionally, Christians were less supportive of active euthanasia than Buddhists.

Affiliation with Buddhism seems to render less support for active euthanasia. Also, the limited research indicates that doctors appear to play an important role in euthanasia decision-making. Existing empirical studies ($n = 3$) investigating the Buddhist perspectives on euthanasia and PAS are very limited, and the impact of Buddhism on this issue remains unclear. Further, there is a complete lack of evidence from other Asian countries such as Korea and Thailand. Research is

Table 20.1 Buddhism: Euthanasia and Physician Assisted Suicide

Author	Year	Population	Country	N	Age (years)	Female (%)	Euthanasia	PAS
Low et al.	2000	Older Adults	Singapore	43	71*	58.1%	✓	✓
Tanida	2000	Clergy & Theologians	Japan	167	—	—	✓	
Yang et al.	1999	Lawyers & Doctors	China	429	30.3	42.2%	✓	✓
Total: 3 Articles				**Avg.: 213 Range: 43-429**	**Avg.: 50.7**	**Avg.: 50.2%**	**Total: 3**	**Total: 2**

* Mean calculated from data in article

needed to better understand the relationship between Buddhism and euthanasia/PAS, including the role of age, region, gender, and race or ethnicity.

Christianity

Death and dying occur around the world. However, individual opinions on euthanasia and PAS are regarded differently, based on geographical location and religious influence. Balboni et al. (2018) found that religious practices help people form opinions on care at the end of life, leading to moral stances about euthanasia and PAS.[11] This section will review the literature on Christianity and euthanasia and/or PAS to describe how different populations develop their impressions of end-of-life decisions. Research on Christianity and euthanasia/PAS is centred around examining attitudes, views, understandings, preferences, desires, perceptions, and affiliation of the clergy and other religious leaders, doctors, nurses, students, and patients on euthanasia and PAS in different geographical locations. This section summarizes the research grouped according to subpopulations and geographical locations.

Christianity and euthanasia and PAS research

A total of 24 empirical studies were found supporting Christianity, euthanasia, and PAS (See Table 20.2). Maclean and colleagues (2003) described Americans' dependence on their religious beliefs during difficult life challenges, serious illness, or old age.[12] Among Christian populations, the clergy tends to have influence on how religious beliefs are shaped, and understanding the views of clergy members with regard to euthanasia and PAS is important.[11,13] Balboni et al. (2018) collected data from August 2014 to February 2015 at The National

Clergy Project on End-of-Life Care funded by the National Cancer Institute.[11] The study included an eight-page self-administered questionnaire that was mailed to a random sample of 2000 clergies in the United States from all different houses of worship.[11] The questionnaire asked about end-of-life decisions that the clergy would make if an individual became ill, physician aid in dying, or specifically PAS.[11] Ninety-eight per cent of religious leaders who responded to the questionnaire ($n = 1005$) identified with Christianity; 83.1% were male, with a mean age of 54.3 years (standard deviation (SD) 13.2) and 85% identifying as white or Caucasian. The results were conflicting, as 80% of respondents agreed that 'sometimes there are circumstances where a patient should be allowed to die',[11] in comparison with only under two-thirds (66%) stating that physician aid in dying and PAS are immoral no matter the situation. Interestingly, 22% of the clergy felt that physician aid in dying and PAS should be a person's legal right. Multivariate statistical tests with variables of race and denominational affiliation predicted that 58% of Hispanic and 60% of black religious leaders were less likely than white religious leaders (88%) to agree with allowing a person to die. Regression analysis adjusted for gender, age, years in ministry, race, and geographical location, along with other variables, found that affiliation was a strong predictor of moral and legal views for clergy members. Other findings indicated that clergy members who had more medical knowledge were 1.5 times more likely to agree that physician aid in dying and PAS are immoral. This study found that discussion among clergies in the United States about the idea of individuals who are terminally ill being allowed to die is ongoing, with most clergies in the study stating that this is immoral and should not be legal.

Two other studies involving religious leaders were reviewed: one in Oregon (where PAS was legal) with chaplains[14] and the other in Cleveland with clergies.[13] Results from the Oregon study found that the discourse on this topic is akin to conversations with clergy around immorality of PAS.[14] Under two-thirds (65%) of potential participants responded to the mailed survey ($n = 50$). Chaplains were asked about their views regarding PAS and results found that their views were most influenced by morals and theological beliefs. Results were mixed, with some chaplains believing that God makes decisions on taking life, whereas others believe in self-determination, with the quality of an individual's life being a factor for PAS.[14] In their research, Goy et al. (2006) highlighted that most individuals (86%) who requested PAS in Oregon were in hospice care.[14] In the Cleveland study involving Catholic and Protestant clergies ($n = 275$), Nagi and Lazerine (1982) defined the different types of euthanasia as voluntary euthanasia with either active or passive interaction.[13] Active voluntary euthanasia is defined as a doctor using lethal substances to induce death,[13] and passive voluntary euthanasia is when an individual discontinues any type of

Table 20.2 Christianity: Euthanasia and Physician Assisted Suicide

Author	Year	Population	Country	N	Age (years)	Female (%)	Euthanasia	PAS
Balboni et al.	2018	Clergy	USA	1005	54.3	17%		✓
Balslev et al.	2020	Doctors	Denmark	911	48.9	42.5%	✓	✓
Baume et al.	1995	Doctors	Australia	1238	—	—	✓	✓
Bülow et al.	2012	Nurses, Patients, Families	Sweden, Netherlands, UK, Czech Republic, Israel, Portugal	304	38*	—	✓	
Davidson et al.	2022	Nurses	USA	2043	52.4	91.5%	✓*	
Davidson et al.	2022	Nurses	USA	1213	54.2	90.2%	✓*	
Engelhardt	2001	Hospitals	—	—	—	—	✓	
Gastmans et al.	2006	Hospitals, Nursing Homes	Belgium	298	—	—	✓	
Gastmans et al.	2006	Hospitals, Nursing Homes	Belgium	298	—	—	✓	
Gastmans et al.	2006	Institutional Policies	Belgium	298	—	—	✓	✓
Goy et al.	2006	Clergy	USA	50	—	—		✓
Grassi et al.	1999	Doctors	Italy	148	36.9	—	✓	✓
Kaldijian et al.	2004	Doctors	USA	677	51	—	✓	✓
Kolodziejczyk	2020	Students	Papua New Guinea	88	—	53.4%	✓	✓

Kübler et al.	2011	Doctors	Poland	217	46	56.2%	✓	✓
Lemiengre et al.	2008	Hospitals	Belgium	71	—	—	✓	
MacLean et al.	2003	Patients	USA	542	52.3	56%		✓
Mortier et al.	2000	Doctors	Belgium	269	—	—	✓	✓
Nagi & Lazerine	1982	Clergy	USA	275	—	—	✓	✓
O'Neill et al.	2003	General Public	England	956	—	—	✓	✓
Pai et al.	2021	Doctors	USA	142	—	38.7%	✓	✓
Schioldborg	1999	Students	Norway	588	—	—	✓	✓
Tanida	2000	Religious Corporations	Japan	58	—	—	✓	
Vander Ryk et al.	1999	Students	—	51	19.9	64.7%		✓
Van Wijmen et al.	2010	General Public	Netherlands	1379	52.1*	55.8%	✓	✓
Wise	1996	General Public	England, Scotland, Wales	3500	—	—	✓	
Zimbleman	2000	Hospitals	—	—	—	—		
Total: 27 Studies				665	42.5	56.5%	22	17

* The articles checked under Euthanasia used the word MAiD

life-supporting treatment and allows for a natural death. Results found that 90% of clergies were in support of death occurring from passive voluntary euthanasia, whereas 85% of clergies were against doctors playing a role in active voluntary euthanasia, revealing the general unacceptability of PAS by clergies.[13]

The other study involving religious leaders by Goy and colleagues (2006) examined the views of hospice chaplains ($n = 50$) on PAS, and found that religious and ethical beliefs were commonly reported as reasons that influence views on PAS.[14] Among the participants, 94% identified as Christian, and 6% as Jewish and Hindu. Results indicated diverse perspectives on PAS; most hospice chaplains reported that they would not consider euthanasia ($n = 28$); 12 indicated that they would consider it, whereas 10 were unsure of their stance.[14] Hospice chaplains who stated that they would not consider euthanasia reported that only a higher spiritual being (God) is able to take a person's life. Those who favoured euthanasia/PAS cited respect for a person's self-determination as their reason for support.[14]

There is a wide variety of opinions about acceptance of euthanasia and assisted suicide among physicians globally. The varying opinions are often influenced by several factors, including religion, conflicting ethical views about euthanasia and PAS being inconsistent with the doctor's primary role of preserving life, and uncertainty about patients' mental and cognitive abilities in making the right judgement at the end of their life.[15]

Research is clear about the prominent role of the doctor and their personal values and beliefs in end-of-life decisions, although the patients and their families/caregivers ultimately make the decisions.[16] Research conducted in southern Denmark involving physicians ($n = 1485$) revealed more than 70% of physicians opposed the election of euthanasia and PAS, and fewer were opposed to sedation into unconsciousness. Opposition to these procedures was influenced by both religious and non-religious reasons, with religious reasons being statistically significant.[16] Physicians' attitudes towards euthanasia and sedation into unconsciousness in dying patients were significantly influenced by gender, age, and religiosity. Physicians who were more religious were more likely to be opposed to euthanasia, and females identified as more religious. This meant that objecting to euthanasia and identifying as female also influenced the likelihood of opposition to euthanasia, in comparison to men (odds ratio (OR) 2.38, 95% confidence interval (CI) 1.56–3.70).[16]

With religion being an overarching theme in connection with the likelihood of not accepting euthanasia and PAS, it is important to assess how much professed religious affiliations can influence these attitudes. In 2000, Mortier et al.[17] studied physicians in the city of Hasselt, Belgium who signed death certificates in 1996. Each physician was given one survey per death certificate they signed to investigate how the end-of-life decisions were made by them. Catholic physicians preferred to treat pain before exploring other end-of-life decisions.[17]

Baume et al. (1995) examined the relationship between physicians' religious affiliation and attitude towards end-of-life decisions.[18] They surveyed a total of 2000 physicians, with 1238 indicating their religious affiliation.[18] Results found that other than those who identified as agnostic/atheist or Jewish, there was no significant likelihood of physicians being sympathetic to the idea of active voluntary euthanasia or PAS. Those who identified as Catholic were the most likely to oppose these methods.[18] Further, three other studies also indicated similar trends. Bülow et al. (2012) found that religious respondents generally favoured prolongation of life and were more likely to be opposed to euthanasia or PAS.[19] In the same vein, family members and patients with stronger religious ties also were more likely to try ways of treatment to prolong and save life before considering euthanasia or physician-assisted death. Questionnaires that included self-disclosure of whether individuals would consider themselves religious or very religious were completed in six different European countries.[19] The total sample size was 1899, of which 304 were physicians. Physicians who identified as Christian and 'very religious' indicated greater opposition to euthanasia and PAS than those who were 'religious'.[19]

Further research revealed that attitudes towards euthanasia and PAS are influenced by both religion and location. For example, a more localized study investigating attitudes of Italian doctors found that doctors strongly want to consider patients' quality of life and pain management in the decision to actively participate in euthanasia or PAS.[20] This study surveyed 148 physicians in Ferra, Italy, of whom only 17.9% reported that they would endorse using those methods.[20] The rest of participants opposed those methods, with consideration to withholding lifesaving treatments.[20] Religion was again the most important determining factor influencing these attitudes.[20,21] In Poland, the results of a national survey conducted by Kübler et al. (2011) demonstrated only 5% of 217 physician participants in Polish intensive care units (ICUs) reported administering drugs until death ensued.[21] The majority (94%) reported that they had practised withholding therapy, and 75% reported withdrawing therapy completely.

Research and discussion on euthanasia and PAS can be highly nuanced with different perspectives generated if investigations are aimed at examining the differences in attitudes of support towards terminal sedation versus PAS.[22] Compared to attitudes of doctors outside the United States, a significant number (78%) of participants in the United States stated that if their terminally ill patient has intractable pain despite treatment, they would consider it ethically appropriate to provide terminal sedation. Terminal sedation was preferred over PAS, with only 38% of physicians reporting it to be ethically appropriate in very specific circumstances.[22] Participants agreeing more with terminal sedation versus PAS also indicated more frequent attendance to religious services.

Bülow and colleagues (2012) studied the perception of nurses and found that both religion and region were important factors that affected attitudes towards euthanasia.[19] End-of-life decisions and respect for patient autonomy of religious participants versus those only affiliated to that religion was evaluated through structured questionnaires. These questionnaires were completed by 304 physicians, 386 nurses, 248 patients, and 330 family members across ICUs of hospitals in six European countries.[19] The study found that individuals with only a religious affiliation were more likely to choose active euthanasia compared to participants who were religious who were often in favour of prolonging life. Most doctors and nurses expressed respect for the decision to refuse lifesaving treatment in competent patients, although nurses in southern European countries chose euthanasia more likely than their northern colleagues.

Davidson and colleagues (2022) sought to understand the values and perspectives of nurses towards medical aid in dying through a cross-sectional electronic survey sent to the American Nurses Association. Of 2043 respondents, 51.4% identified as Christian. Overall, most nurses (87%) shared that they would care for patients considering medical aid in dying, whereas 67% would be there to support the final act.[23] Non-Christian nurses had a higher OR in caring for patients in the final act of medical aid in dying (OR 0.34, 95% CI 0.28–0.41) and were more willing to care for a patient contemplating medical aid in dying (OR 0.40, 95% CI 0.30–0.52; p <0.001), compared to Christian nurses.[23] Christian nurses were also less likely to support the idea of medical aid in dying using an advance directive, compared to non-Christian nurses (OR 0.44, 95% CI 0.37–0.52; p <0.001).[23] Numerous multiple logistic regression analyses found that Christianity predicted not supporting medical aid in dying and Christian nurses were not willing to engage in caring for patients receiving medical aid in dying compared to those who identified as spiritual.

Another study by Davidson and colleagues (2022) conducted using a cross-sectional electronic survey collecting responses from 1213 nurses (80% self-identifying as white with a graduate degree, and 50.1% self-identifying as Christian) identified four themes: honouring patient autonomy without judgement; honouring with limitations; honouring not until the nurses felt certain goals had been met or specific activities had happened; and adamantly against.[24] Nurses identifying as spiritual were more inclined to promote medical aid in dying compared to nurses who were religious.

Gastmans et al. (2006) focused on Flemish Catholic hospitals and nursing homes to investigate whether they have a set of written ethics policies on euthanasia and whether the nurse's role in the process is identified and described in those policies. The study used a cross-sectional questionnaire that was mailed to 298 hospitals and nursing homes (81% were returned from hospitals, and 62% from nursing homes).[25] Of the completed questionnaires, 79% of hospitals and 30% of nursing homes had developed written ethics policies on euthanasia. Of those institutions that had these policies, 87% of hospitals and 77% of nursing homes identified the role of nurses in the action of euthanasia, with a majority reporting nurses' objections to euthanasia.[25]

Vander Ryk et al. (1999) studied 51 college students (33 female, 18 males; mean age of 19.9 years), with 78% of individuals identifying as Christian.[26] Results indicated that there was no consistent anti- or pro-death attitude among students and those who identified as Christians were not in favour of assisted suicide.[26] Similarly, a preliminary study among Norwegian students, with 38% identifying as Christian, supported euthanasia compared to 70% of those from other faiths and 65% of those without a specific faith.[27] A follow-up study one year later with the same students from the disciplines of law, medicine, and psychology revealed 39% of students who identified as Christian supported assisted suicide and even fewer (30%) supported active euthanasia for those with terminal diseases.[28] Another study conducted in Papua New Guinea asked students attending a Christian university about euthanasia, passive euthanasia, and PAS. Analysis using the chi-squared test identified that 66.6% of students did not know or knew very little about euthanasia.[18] There were also significant differences in student perceptions regarding euthanasia based on knowledge of first- and fourth-year students.[29]

Studies in Belgium, the United Kingdom, Germany, Italy, Japan, the Netherlands, Switzerland, Taiwan, and the United States on euthanasia and PAS indicate some interesting trends. In Belgium, where Christianity is the dominant ideological tradition, laws on euthanasia have been enacted since 2002.[30,31] In 2006, Gastmans et al. (2006) studied 298 Catholic hospitals and nursing homes in Belgium that had written policies regarding euthanasia, to understand the prevalence, approval, and dissemination of these policies.[30] Results showed that the reason these policies exist is because of high approval (80–83%) of euthanasia among the population. Gastmans et al.[30] highlighted Zimbelman's (2000) and Engelhardt's (2001) work, emphasizing that Catholic health care institutions are being influenced by rising social trends.[32] Another study by Gastmans et al. (2006) reported euthanasia being performed in Catholic institutions even if policies or laws exist to govern the practice.[31] The researchers recognize that there is only a minority of hospitals that prohibit euthanasia because it conflicts with Christian values.[31] Two years after the previous study, 81 hospitals were contacted to participate in a follow-up research study. Hospitals with euthanasia policies ($n = 42$) shared their documents, which were analysed.[33] Of the hospitals that responded, 69% were Catholic. When comparing Catholic to neutral hospitals, more Catholic hospitals (72%) included a position on euthanasia than neutral hospitals (28%).[33]

Researchers investigating PAS and family-assisted suicide in the United Kingdom looked at the role of technology in keeping individuals alive for longer. O'Neil et al. (2003) reflected on Wise (1996) conducting community planning research,[35] with 62% of Christian respondents, and found that 82% of community members believe doctors should have the ability to make end-of-life decisions based on patients' requests.[34] Another study conducted in the Netherlands surveying 1621 individuals, with 86% response rate, found that 60% of those who identified under the Christian umbrella (Roman Catholic or Protestant) could imagine themselves asking to end their lives depending on the circumstance.[36] Finally, a study looking at four religious groups in Japan[37] reached out to 58 Christian-specific organizations, with a response rate of 81%. Results found that among Christians, Protestant, compared to Catholic, organizations, were more favourable to doctors acting on voluntary passive euthanasia.[36] Further, Christian organizations were less in favour of voluntary active euthanasia and non-voluntary active euthanasia than Buddhist organizations.[37]

Hinduism

Hinduism is an ancient Indian religion, and Hindus form the third largest religious group globally, with over 1.2 billion individuals.[38] The majority of the world's Hindu population live in India where euthanasia and PAS are illegal. Hindu religious beliefs significantly impact end-of-life decisions made by followers,[39,40] whose attitudes vary about the practice of euthanasia and PAS.[41] This section summarizes the literature on euthanasia and PAS among doctors and students who identify as Hindu.

Hinduism and euthanasia and PAS research

A total of six research studies were found on Hinduism and euthanasia and PAS (See Table 20.3). A cross-sectional study in a hospital in South India was conducted to understand doctors' ($n = 213$) attitudes towards euthanasia in a hospital setting. This study found that the majority of the doctors (69%) supported euthanasia; 30% were against, and 1% were uncertain about their stance.[42] Relief from pain and suffering was cited as the main reason for supporting euthanasia.[42] No significant differences were found between age and gender in the doctors' perspectives on euthanasia.[42] Conversely, another study that examined doctors' perspectives on PAS ($n = 1144$) found that 69% of doctors did not agree with PAS.[39] In this study, however, only 54 doctors (5%) identified as being Hindu.[39] This study found that being Asian, affiliated with the Hindu religion, and years of experience in caring for terminally ill patients were all variables that played a role in being against PAS.[39] Bivariate analysis was conducted to examine the association between religious affiliation and PAS, and 74% of doctors affiliated with the Hindu religion objected to PAS.[39] A third study used a cross-sectional design to gather doctors' attitudes towards euthanasia.[43] Two hundred and twenty doctors were surveyed; 46.8% justified the use of euthanasia, with supporting claims of relieving patients from pain and suffering; 41% indicated that euthanasia should be legalized, and 39% said they would practise euthanasia if legalized.[43]

Bhat (2020) examined attitudes towards euthanasia and PAS in a sample ($n = 89$) of clinical postgraduate students, senior residents, assistant professors, associate professors, and professors of clinical departments.[44] Results indicated that 83% of participants stated that religion guides their beliefs about end-of-life care, with the majority against euthanasia and PAS.[44] Kamble and colleagues (2012) examined the acceptability of PAS among Indian university students ($n = 293$) in 36 medical scenarios. Among the students, the majority ($n = 281$) identified as Hindu and their views about PAS were divided into three clusters: unacceptable ($n = 79$), depending ($n = 120$), and acceptable ($n = 82$).[45] This study revealed that if a patient was old and asked for assistance in dying, students were more likely to deem PAS as acceptable.[45] Additionally, Pomfret and colleagues (2018) assessed the influence of religion on medical students' attitudes towards euthanasia and PAS.[40] A total of 400 medical students participated in the study, and 16.5% identified as Hindu. Hindu medical students were significantly more likely to disagree with actions that suggested hastening death than those from other religious groups.[40] Also, the study also found that students reported their religious beliefs guide their views on euthanasia and PAS.[40] In this study, medical students were asked to rate their views in medical scenarios that dealt with end-of-life issues. Results found that gender and being older did not influence their views about euthanasia and PAS.[40] However, the length of their academic journey did have an influence. Medical students who were further along in their academic journey (finalists and graduate-entry) were more likely to favour euthanasia and PAS.[40]

Research studies focusing on perspectives on euthanasia and PAS among doctors and Hindus are limited. Findings demonstrate mixed views about the practice of euthanasia and PAS. These mixed views resulted in differences in practising and supporting the legalization of euthanasia and PAS. While the practice of euthanasia and PAS is forbidden in Hinduism,[46] doctors and students strongly consider age, the severity of the medical condition, and patient

Table 20.3 Hinduism: Euthanasia and Physician Assisted Suicide

Author	Year	Population	Country	N	Age (years)	Female (%)	Euthanasia	PAS
Bhat	2020	Students	India	89	38	—	✓	✓
Curlin et al.	2008	Doctors	USA	144	49	26%	✓	✓
Kamath et al.	2011	Doctors	India	213	30	30.9%	✓	✓
Kamble et al.	2012	Students	India	293	23	62.1%		✓
Pomfret et al.	2018	Students	UK	400	22.7	59.8%	✓	✓
Subba et al.	2016	Doctors	India	220	37.9	66%	✓	
Total: 6 Articles				Avg.: 226.5 Range: 89-400	Avg.: 33.4	Avg.: 49%	Total: 5	Total: 5

wishes when supporting euthanasia and PAS. Future research is needed to investigate the influences of socio-demographic variables on views of euthanasia and PAS among doctors and students in other health care majors.

Islam

Islam is the second largest religion globally by population and has over 1.8 billion followers.[47] Euthanasia in Islam is considered illegal, and religious beliefs have a strong stance against euthanasia.[47] However, views on euthanasia and PAS vary among medical professionals, including doctors, nurses, and medical students who frequently see patients requesting aid in terminating their life.[48,49,50,51,52,53] This section provides some of the perspectives on, and attitudes towards, euthanasia and PAS among doctors, medical, and nursing students who identify as Muslim.

Islam and euthanasia and PAS research

A total of 13 empirical articles were found that explored euthanasia and PAS in relation to Islam (See Table 20.4). Understanding doctors' perspectives on euthanasia and PAS is critically important, as they are often asked to perform medical acts that aid patients in dying. Rathor and colleagues (2014) conducted a study exploring attitudes among doctors ($n = 195$) and patients who are terminally ill ($n = 727$) towards euthanasia.[50] In this study, there were 133 (68.2%) doctors and 347 (47.7%) patients who identified as Muslim.[50] Most doctors in this study cared for patients who were terminally ill, and 30 doctors (15%) were asked for assistance in dying by patients.[50] Results indicated that a fewer number of doctors ($n = 136$) and a larger number of patients ($n = 439$) were not in support of euthanasia. Further, among the doctors, 133 identified their religion as Islam and most ($n = 112$) were not in support of euthanasia, compared to those ($n = 19$) who were in support. A small number ($n = 2$) were unsure of their stance on euthanasia.[50]

Ahmed et al. (2001) investigated the attitudes of junior and senior Sudanese doctors towards euthanasia and medical aid in dying.[49] They surveyed 382 doctors (130 male and 118 female) through anonymous questionnaires in two main hospitals located in Khartoum, Sudan.[49] The researchers found that 92% identified as Muslim and 8% as Christian. The study highlighted that 85% of doctors in this area were opposed to both euthanasia and medical aid in dying.[49] Only 15% expressed that these options should be considered under very particular situations, with none being willing to perform the act of euthanasia themselves. The three reasons for opposition fell under the umbrella of religious beliefs, inconsistency with the doctor's role in preserving life, and fear of not adhering to prescribed requirements. The questions in the surveys were scored on a three-point scale—agree, neutral, or disagree—that inquired about the doctors' attitudes and opinions on assisted suicide, legalizing euthanasia, their willingness to be part of the process, and what limitations/restrictions they feel should be put in place if it were legal.[54]

Qidwai and colleagues (2001) examined perspectives on PAS from a convenience sample of patients ($n = 420$) who presented to family physicians in a hospital setting, and found 9% acceptability towards PAS in their sample.[51] Those who advocated for PAS were more likely to be female, older, married, and educated. Further, their support for PAS superseded their religious beliefs and gave more importance to the severity of the medical condition rather than to their religious beliefs.[51] This study revealed that a large number of patients ($n = 347$) identified their religion as Islam, most of whom ($n = 244$) did not support euthanasia compared to patients ($n = 96$) who supported euthanasia. There were no significant differences reported for demographic variables such as education, marital, or occupational status on patients' perspectives on euthanasia.[50] Patients reported religious beliefs as a reason for not supporting euthanasia over the severity of their medical condition.[50] Overall, doctors and patients did not support euthanasia and PAS, regardless of the type of medical conditions and the status of legalization of euthanasia ($p < 0.001$).

Table 20.4 Islam: Euthanasia and Physician Assisted Suicide

Author	Year	Population	Country	N	Age (years)	Female (%)	Euthanasia	PAS
Aghababaei	2013	Students	Iran	300	22.6	66%	✓	
Ahmed & Kheir	2006	Students	Sudan	141	25*	46.8%	✓	
Ahmed et al.	2001	Doctors	Sudan	248	38	48%	✓	✓
Ahmed et al.	2010	Students	Kuwait	330	21	66.7%		✓
Cavlak et al.	2007	Physio-therapists, Students	Turkey	494	35*	69.0%	✓	
Hosseinzadeh & Rafiei	2019	Students	Iran	382	62.6	61.5%	✓	
Naseh & Heidari	2017	Students	Iran	120	23.5*	65.8%	✓	
Naseh et al.	2015	Nurses	Iran	190	33.3	91.1%	✓	
Ozcelik et al.	2014	Students	Turkey	383	21.3	96.9%	✓	
Rathor et al.	2014	Doctors, Patients	Malaysia	922	48.6	48.2%	✓	
Qidwai et al.	2001	Patients	Pakistan	420	29.5*	11.2%	✓	
Tadros et al.	2011	Psychiatrists	Egypt	160	38*	29.4%		✓
Yildirim	2020	Students	Turkey	382	23.5*	63.6%	✓	
Total: 13 Articles				Avg.: 344 Range: 120-922	Avg.: 32.5	Avg.: 58.8%	Total: 11	Total: 3

* Mean calculated from data in article

Tadros and colleagues (2011) explored how Egyptian psychiatrists (*n* = 160, *n* = 134 identified as Muslim) viewed PAS. This study indicated that 50% of the participants allow their religious beliefs to strongly guide their medical practice and 12.5% indicated a weak relationship between their religious belief and their medical practice.[55] Ahmed and colleagues (2001) examined attitudes among doctors (*n* = 248) working at Khartoum's main hospitals, where all doctors identify as Muslim and were unwilling to perform euthanasia, towards euthanasia and assisted death.[56] Ninety per cent of doctors reported religious beliefs for not practising euthanasia.[56] Most doctors in this sample (*n* = 228) identified as being Muslim; almost half were male (*n* = 130), and most were familiar with the concepts of euthanasia and assisted suicide (*n* = 223). About 85% of the doctors felt that euthanasia and assisted suicide were not ethically justified, whereas 15% thought they could be justified.[56]

Studies conducted involving medical and nursing students regarding euthanasia and PAS reveal interesting insights. One study that examined the University of Khartoum's final-year medical students' ($n = 141$) attitudes towards euthanasia found that all participants identified as Muslim and that most ($n = 131$) were familiar with euthanasia but had received no formal instruction about euthanasia.[48] In addition, this study found that most medical students ($n = 108$) disagreed with euthanasia and believed it should not be legalized.[48] Those students who supported euthanasia ($n = 33$) believed that it should be legalized and indicated respecting a person's wish and autonomy to die in dignity as reasons for their support. Study participants further stated that protocols should be in place if euthanasia were legalized.[48] Most of the medical students who identified as strongly religious did not agree with euthanasia (83/87), compared to those who identified as moderately religious (25/54).[48] More female medical students (17/61) than male students (16/80) supported the legalization of euthanasia and reported that should euthanasia be legalized, they ($n = 18$) would perform it.[48]

Similarly, Cavlak and colleagues (2007) in a cross-sectional study investigated the influence of physiotherapy education on knowledge and attitudes towards euthanasia. A number of physiotherapists (PTs) ($n = 311$) and physiotherapy students (PS) ($n = 183$) participated in this study. Findings indicated that PTs ($n = 152$) were more accepting of euthanasia than PS ($n = 70$).[49] Additionally, more PTs ($n = 136$) than PS ($n = 54$) supported the legalization of euthanasia.[49] In this study, gender and age did not affect acceptance of euthanasia ($p > 0.05$), whereas religion influenced attitudes towards euthanasia. Most of the study participants defined euthanasia as permitting death ($n = 164$), identified as Muslim ($n = 478$), were women ($n = 341$), supported euthanasia ($n = 222$), and were in favour of euthanasia becoming legalized ($n = 190$).[49]

Ahmed and colleagues (2010) examined Kuwaiti university students' ($n = 330$) acceptability of PAS in 36 scenarios, including medical cases in which patients who identified as female asked for a life-ending procedure such as PAS and euthanasia. Findings were categorized into five groups, including never acceptable ($n = 142$), not very acceptable ($n = 76$), depending on patient age ($n = 54$), depending on the type of suffering ($n = 17$), and depending on patient request ($n = 35$). This study found that students were more accepting of PAS for characteristics such as an individual's request, the type of suffering, and older age, and there were no significant gender differences.[54] Aghababaei's (2013) study examined the relationship between euthanasia and religion among students ($n = 300$)

by asking about their views on euthanasia with use of the Euthanasia Attitude Scale and Religious Orientation Scale-Revised. Their study found no relationship between gender and attitudes towards euthanasia and 66.3% of participants indicated that euthanasia is morally unacceptable.[57]

Naseh and Heidari's (2017) study examined the attitudes of Muslim nursing students ($n = 120$) by using the Euthanasia Attitude Scale, and found that students had a negative view towards euthanasia.[52] This study found a significant correlation between students' gender, age, religious beliefs, and attitudes towards euthanasia.[52] Mean scores of male and female nursing students' attitudes towards euthanasia were reported in four categories, including ethical considerations (male 3.32 ± 0.84, female 2.79 ± 0.95; $p = 0.01$), practical considerations (male 2.54 ± 0.82, female 2.31 ± 0.84; $p = 0.16$), treasuring life (male 2.94 ± 0.44, female $2.89 \pm 0,43$; $p = 0.50$), and naturalist beliefs (male 2.54 ± 0.72, female 2.70 ± 0.88; $p = 0.01$).[58] Similarly, Ozcelik and colleagues (2014) examined the attitudes of undergraduate nursing students ($n = 383$) at a university in Turkey towards euthanasia. In this study, 32.4% of nursing students did not favour euthanasia.[58] Additionally, age was significantly related to nursing students being against euthanasia, the idea that euthanasia is unethical, and euthanasia could be abused.[58]

Muslim nurses ($n = 190$)—17 males and 173 females—from two hospitals (Kashani and Hajar, Iran) were surveyed about their attitudes towards euthanasia by using a cross-sectional study design.[53] Results indicated that nurses had the most negative mean score in the practical consideration domain and the most positive mean score in the treasuring life domain.[53] Nurses viewed euthanasia as unfavourable, and there was no significant difference in the nurses' attitudes towards euthanasia according to their age, marital status, years of experience, and gender.[53]

A cross-sectional study examined undergraduate nursing students' ($n = 382$) views on euthanasia.[59] This study clustered nursing students into two educational categories: freshman and sophomore students ($n = 188$); and third-year and senior students ($n = 194$).[59] Most freshman and sophomore students reported not agreeing with active euthanasia ($n = 136$), whereas a minority said they do agree ($n = 52$). Conversely, findings from third-year and senior students indicated that most did not agree with active euthanasia ($n = 111$), whereas a smaller number of participants did ($n = 83$).[59] Yildirim (2020) conducted a descriptive study examining the knowledge, opinions, and behaviours of senior nursing students ($n = 300$; 57 male and 243 female) in Turkey.[60] This study found that most nursing students were unsure ($n = 127$) of euthanasia being legal and some answered yes ($n = 107$) to legalizing euthanasia, whereas the rest reported not being in favour of legalization.[60]

While Islam holds a strong foundational belief about preserving life, research among doctors and medical and nursing students on euthanasia and PAS remains mixed. Most doctors who identified as Muslim did not support euthanasia or PAS, and religion played a crucial role in guiding their perspectives and attitudes.[50,51,55] While religious beliefs were the most cited reason for being opposed to euthanasia and PAS, there were differences in results for medical and nursing students supporting or not supporting euthanasia and PAS. Those students who were in favour of euthanasia and PAS considered patients' wishes and autonomy as the main reasons for their support. Further exploration is needed to understand the range of perspectives on, and attitudes towards, euthanasia and PAS among Muslim doctors and medical and nursing students, and the influence of demographic variables on these attitudes.

Judaism

Judaism believes that one's life is the possession of God and death is God's will.[61] The Jewish tradition considers the preservation of human life in high regard and prohibits any form of destruction to the human body or shortening of life.[61] With the significant advancement of medical technology and as human beings have more end-of-life options to consider, attitudes towards euthanasia and PAS have continued to evolve. PAS and euthanasia have received some attention in the medical and ethical literature. This section reports on research on Jewish perspectives on PAS and euthanasia.

Judaism and euthanasia and PAS research

Among the searches conducted on Judaism and euthanasia or PAS, there were 11 empirical articles identified for synthesis (See Table 20.5). One research study in the United States investigating the attitudes of students ($n = 210$, age 18–65 years) in psychology classes at Los Angeles State College towards euthanasia and PAS found that euthanasia received the most support from atheist–agnostics ($n = 35$), followed by Jewish students ($n = 25$).[62] No significant differences were identified in attitudes towards euthanasia between Jewish individuals and those from other religious groups.

Three studies exploring public opinion about euthanasia and PAS were identified: two in the United States and one in Israel. One study was conducted involving respondents aged 18 years and above ($n = 8384$) to understand American public attitudes towards euthanasia and the role of the physician.[63] This study indicated that respondents with no religion ($n = 628$) were most accepting of active euthanasia, followed by Jewish respondents ($n = 177$). Similarly, Ostheimer and Moore (1981) compared attitudes towards euthanasia among participants with Jewish ($n = 32$), Catholic ($n = 343$), Protestant ($n = 933$), and non-religious affiliations ($n = 85$), and found similar results. However, no significant difference in attitudes towards euthanasia was identified between Jewish individuals and respondents with no religion.[64] Further, Ostheimer and Moore combined non-religion individuals and Jewish individuals into a new group, and identified a significant difference in attitudes towards euthanasia between Protestants and this new group. The third study from Israel surveyed public opinion in Israel about end-of-life decisions among 515 participants aged 18 years and older. Results found that nearly half of the participants were supportive of physician-assisted death.[65] Further, 90% of ultra-orthodox and over half of religious participants opposed physician-assisted death.[65] Non-Jewish individuals were more likely to oppose physician-assisted death than Jewish individuals.

Only one study in the United States conducted with patients was identified. Silveira et al. (2000) performed a cross-sectional study of 728 outpatients in Oregon, surveying patients' knowledge about end-of-life care.[66] This study found that Jewish individuals ($n = 15$) had a higher score of knowledge related to end-of-life issues (e.g. PAS, euthanasia); however, this knowledge was not related to religion.

Four studies were identified that were conducted with health professionals, including two studies in Israel, one in multiple countries, and one in the United States. A sample of 443 Jewish physicians (mean age of 41.2 years) at four Israeli hospitals were studied.[67] Results found that very religious physicians were much less likely to agree with euthanasia of terminally ill patients than moderately religious and secular physicians.[67] Another study surveying oncology ($n = 71$, age 23–62 years) and non-oncology ($n = 52$, age 21–66 years) nurses at a teaching hospital in Israel, where the majority of nurses were Jewish, indicated favourable attitudes of nurses towards physician-assisted dying and its legalization.[68] Compared with non-oncology nurses, oncology nurses were significantly less likely to support PAS and less likely to favour its legalization.

A study conducted in multiple countries including physicians ($n = 304$), nurses ($n = 386$), family members ($n = 330$), and patients ($n = 248$) revealed that fewer Jewish professionals (67%) than Protestant (84%) and Catholic (73%) professionals would follow a competent patient's wish to reject treatment that may be lifesaving.[19] More Jewish professionals (66%) than Protestant (35%) and Catholic (53%) professionals would act against a patient's wish, even if it might be lifesaving.[19] Fewer Jewish (62%) than Protestant (88%) and Catholic (84%) professionals would try and convince a competent patient not to receive therapy that the professionals considered futile.[19]

Table 20.5 Judaism: Euthanasia and Physician Assisted Suicide

Author	Year	Population	Country	N	Age (years)	Female (%)	Euthanasia	PAS
Bodas et al.	2020	General Public	Israel	515	18+	50.1%	✓	
Bülow et al.	2012	Doctors, Nurses	Sweden, Netherlands, UK, Czech Republic, Israel, Portugal	1268	37.6	-		✓
Caddell & Newton	1995	General Public	USA	8384	44.8	56.0%	✓	
Kaldjian et al.	2002	Doctors	USA	677	51	20%		✓
Kalish	1963	Students	USA	210	28*	34.0%	✓	
Leichtentritt & Rettig	1999	Families	Israel	12	48*	83.3%	✓	
Musgrave et al.	2001	Nurses	Israel	123	38.7	95.0%		✓
Ostheimer & Moore	1981	General Public	USA	1398	18+	54.4%	✓	
Silveira et al.	2000	Patients	USA	728	46	65.0%		✓
Sonnenblick et al.	1993	Families	Israel	108	56	43.5%	✓	
Wenger & Carmel	2004	Doctors	Israel	443	41.2	29.7%	✓	
Total: 11 Articles				**Avg.:1260.5 Range: 12-8384**	**Avg.: 38.8**	**Avg.: 53.1%**	**Total: 7**	**Total: 4**

* Mean calculated from data in article.

Another study from the United States conducted with 677 respondents (mean age of 51 years) found that 28% of physicians supported legalizing PAS.[69] In this study, physicians with Jewish affiliation (45%) or no affiliation (38%) were more likely to favour legalizing PAS than those with Catholic (14%) or other Christian affiliations (19%) ($p < 0.001$).

Two studies from Israel were identified to survey offspring's decisions for their chronically or terminally ill older parents. One study of 108 offspring of 48 terminally ill older patients at Shaare-Zedek Medical Center in Israel, who were mostly Jewish, indicated that a small number ($n = 7$) of offspring requested active euthanasia.[70] Further, the nature of the relationship with their parents and the degree of religious observance significantly affected their decisions around euthanasia.[70] Another study interviewed 12 Israeli adult children (10 daughters and two sons), and indicated that over half favoured passive euthanasia for their parents when their relationship was distant and almost all opposed passive euthanasia for their parents when their relationship was close.[71] In addition, four participants favoured passive euthanasia for themselves and their partners.[71]

Current research exploring Judaism and PAS and euthanasia is limited. Studies predominantly come from the United States and Israel, which may influence the findings. While there is a lack of research exploring the reasons, overall Jewish individuals tended to be more likely to accept physician-assisted death and euthanasia than other religious groups. Also, a certain number of professionals in the health care field were found to be supportive of legalizing PAS.[67,68] In addition, the degree of religiosity was found to have an influence on individual opinions regarding PAS and euthanasia.[67,70] Further research with a focus on older adults in Jewish communities and professionals is warranted to understand more fully the relationship between Judaism and PAS and euthanasia.

Summarizing euthanasia and PAS across religions

In total, 67 studies were included in the review; 10 articles were included for substantiative context but did not include data and were not included in Tables 20.1 to 20.5. Of the 57 studies included in Tables 20.1 to 20.5, 8 (14%) were published since 2020, 17 (30%) between 2010 and 2019, 21 (37%) between 2000 and 2009, 8 (14%) between 1990 and 1999, and 3 (5%) before 1990. This rising number of publications across the decades may reflect an increased awareness informing greater research on the relationship between religion and euthanasia and PAS. Similarly, this trend may highlight a shift in how suicide, euthanasia, and PAS are perceived. This trend was not identified in all religions.

For example, studies focusing on Christianity, Hinduism, and Islam have been more recent, as compared to research on Buddhism and Judaism.

Sample characteristics varied across the studies. However, all participants were adults, with a study average age ranging from 18 to 71 years. Future research may be warranted to examine attitudes and beliefs by age. In 39 (68%) studies, gender percentages were presented or calculated from available data; 18 (32%) studies did not provide gender demographics. The percentage of female participants was slightly higher than males and ranged from 49% in studies focusing on Hinduism to 58.8% in studies focusing on Islam. Data on race and ethnicity were largely not available. It is recommended that future studies collect, and report on, sample demographics to further delineate attitudes.

Research in this area tended to investigate certain populations. The most investigated population was medical professionals (e.g. doctors, nurses) with 26 (46%) studies, followed by students with 15 (26%) studies, then followed by the general population with 6 (11%) studies, clergies with 5 (9%) studies, patients with 3 (5%) studies, and families with 2 (4%) studies. A large focus remains on medical professionals, with fewer studies investigating patients and family perceptions. Future research may want to explore a more diverse and reflective populations within their communities.

The geographical location of the research studies tended to reflect the dominant religion of the region. All studies focusing on Buddhism were conducted in Japan, Singapore, and China. Studies investigating Christianity were prevalent in the United States, the United Kingdom, and Europe. Research on Hinduism was predominantly in India. Studies examining Islam were predominantly in countries in the Middle East and North Africa (MENA). Finally, research on Judaism was mainly centred in the United States and Israel. Future research may want to explore the influence of religion on minority religious populations and heterogeneous religious communities.

Euthanasia and PAS remain controversial issues, despite growing legalization in parts of the world. Attitudes and practices around euthanasia and PAS are affected by a variety of social, religious, and legal factors, with religion being a fundamental influencing factor on how individuals view and navigate these complex concepts. Suicide, euthanasia, and PAS fall on a continuum, with large areas of overlap that need to be examined carefully. Research around religion and euthanasia is limited, mixed, and inconsistent, providing no clear picture of the effects of religious beliefs, thoughts, and practices on these issues. A deeper, more nuanced, and accurate understanding of the intersection of religion and euthanasia and PAS is warranted to advance the science on suicide prevention and intervention.

Among the dominant world religions, levels of tolerance and acceptance of suicide and, by extension, euthanasia vary, with certain faiths being more tolerant than others. Further, every dominant world religion is practised within a cultural context; hence, the influence of religion and culture on a phenomenon like euthanasia needs to be investigated carefully. Further, religious groups are not monolithic; there are large variations in beliefs, attitudes, and cultural practices within ethnic groups and geographical regions.

Research on Buddhist affiliation, beliefs, and practices on euthanasia and PAS is very limited. Further, research is almost absent from some countries in Asia that have most of their population identifying as Buddhist. Future research needs to focus on investigating attitudes, beliefs, and views of citizens of those countries on euthanasia and PAS. Further, demographic factors, including age, gender, race, and ethnicity, within Buddhist populations and their association with influences on views around euthanasia need to be investigated to determine an accurate understanding of the influence of religious affiliation and practice on euthanasia and PAS. Understanding the process of moving towards legalizing euthanasia in Buddhist-majority countries needs to be carefully examined to discern the influence of Buddhism on policy and practice of regulating euthanasia and PAS.

Research on the influence of Christian affiliation, beliefs, and practice has begun to emerge in the last few years, with some research focused on the different denominations within the Christian faith. Most research within Christianity has been conducted in Europe and North America where it is the dominant faith, with little attention to Christian populations in Asia and Africa. Further, the majority of research studies are focused on examining attitudes towards, and perspectives on, euthanasia and PAS among medical doctors, nurses, and students, given their prominent role in end-of-life care decisions. In the United States and other countries around the world, medical social workers play an important role in supporting patients and their families during end-of-life care. However, research has yet to examine the perspectives on, and attitudes towards, these issues among medical social workers. Continued research on how decisions of euthanasia and PAS impact the medical community, patients and their families, and the community at large is warranted. Research reveals that in countries where euthanasia and PAS are widely accepted, and even legal, institutional policies on euthanasia in hospitals, medical centres, and nursing homes are vague and inconsistent around issues of implementation. Research needs to examine the impact of these policies on staff and patients within these institutions, with an aim to clarify and provide consistency in understanding and implementation.

Within Hinduism, there is significant diversity among believers in thought and practice. Future research needs to investigate the influence of socio-demographic variables on attitudes towards euthanasia and PAS, particularly among physicians and medical students who affiliate with Hinduism. Cultural practices within Hinduism that influence perspectives on euthanasia and PAS need to be studied among those who identify as Hindu.

Of all the major world religions, Islam has the most prohibitive stance on suicide based on the Quran and the teachings of the Prophet. Muslims, however, are a very diverse group of people, located in every region of the world, who exhibit a variety of views on issues like euthanasia and PAS. These views might be influenced by the level of education, marital or occupational status, geographical location, religiosity, and sociocultural–political influences of the local context. Careful examination of demographic variables and cultural influences, in addition to religious identification, affiliation, and practice, on Muslims' views on the concept and practice of euthanasia and PAS is needed to determine an accurate and deeper understanding. Current research on this is mixed and indeterminate. Much of the research on Islam and euthanasia is focused on investigating perspectives of the medical community on the issue. Little research exists on determining the reasons for Muslim medical doctors and nurses opposing practices of euthanasia and PAS. Further, more attention in research needs to be paid to Muslim patients' and their families' attitudes towards acceptability of euthanasia and PAS in practice.

Research on Judaism and euthanasia and PAS is very limited, with much of the focus on investigating attitudes and perspectives of the medical community and patients on the issue. Research is lacking in understanding perspectives of older adults and terminally ill patients on this issue. Future research needs to explore the impact of the degree of religiosity on attitudes towards euthanasia and PAS. With increasing acceptance of euthanasia and PAS among Jewish populations, both health care professionals and policymakers need to pay attention to how patients understand euthanasia and PAS and the influence of this on end-of-life care.

References

1. **Annadurai K, Danasekaran R, Mani G.** Euthanasia: right to die with dignity. Journal of Family Medicine and Primary Care. 2014;**3**(4):477–8.
2. **Emanuel EJ, Onwuteaka-Philipsen BD, Urwin JW, Cohen J.** Attitudes and practices of euthanasia and physician-assisted suicide in the United States, Canada, and Europe. JAMA. 2016;**316**(1):79–90.

3. **McLachlan HV.** The ethics of killing and letting die: active and passive euthanasia. Journal of Medical Ethics. 2008;**34**(8):636–8.
4. **Draper B, Peisah C, Snowdon J, Brodaty H.** Early dementia diagnosis and the risk of suicide and euthanasia. Alzheimer's and Dementia. 2010;**6**(1):75–82.
5. **Banović B, Turanjanin V.** Euthanasia: murder or not: a comparative approach. Iranian Journal of Public Health. 2014;**43**(10):1316.
6. **Grove G, Lovell M, Best M.** Perspectives of major world religions regarding euthanasia and assisted suicide: a comparative analysis. Journal of Religion and Health. 2022;**61**(6):4758–82.
7. **Alonzo D, Gearing RE.** Suicide across Buddhism, American Indian–Alaskan Native, and African traditional religions, atheism and agnosticism: an updated systematic review. Journal of Religion and Health. 2021;**60**(4):2527–46.
8. **Yang H, Xiao S, Dong Q, Yang D.** Study of attitude towards suicide in lawyers, Buddhists, and medical staff members. Chinese Mental Health Journal. 1999;**13**(4):252–4.
9. **Low JA, Ng WC, Yap KB, Chan KM.** End-of-life issues—preferences and choices of a group of elderly Chinese subjects attending a day care centre in Singapore. Annals of the Academy of Medicine of Singapore. 2000;**29**(1):50–6.
10. **Tanida N.** The view of religions toward euthanasia and extraordinary treatments in Japan. Journal of Religion and Health. 2000;**39**(4):339–54.
11. **Balboni MJ, Sullivan A, Smith PT**, et al. The views of clergy regarding ethical controversies in care at the end of life. Journal of Pain and Symptom Management. 2018;**55**(1):65–74.
12. **MacLean CD, Susi B, Phifer N**, et al. Patient preference for physician discussion and practice of spirituality: results from a multicenter patient survey. Journal of General Internal Medicine. 2003;**18**(1):38–43.
13. **Nagi MH, Lazerine NG.** Death education and attitudes toward euthanasia and terminal illness. Death Education. 1982;**6**(1):1–5.
14. **Goy ER, Carlson B, Simopoulos N, Jackson A, Ganzini L.** Determinants of Oregon hospice chaplains' views on physician-assisted suicide. Journal of Palliative Care. 2006;**22**(2):83–90.
15. **Pai S, Andrews T, Turner A, Merchant A, Shapiro M.** Factors that influence end-of-life decision making amongst attending physicians. American Journal of Hospice and Palliative Medicine. 2022;**39**(10):1174–81.
16. **Van Randwijk CB, Opsahl T, Assing Hvidt E, Bjerrum L, Kørup AK, Hvidt NC.** Association between Danish physicians' religiosity and spirituality and their attitudes toward end-of-life procedures. Journal of Religion and Health. 2020;**59**(5):2654–63.
17. **Mortier F, Deliens L, Bilsen J, Cosyns M, Ingels K, Vander Stichele R.** End-of-life decisions of physicians in the city of Hasselt (Flanders, Belgium). Bioethics. 2000;**14**(3):254–67.
18. **Baume P, O'Malley E, Bauman A.** Professed religious affiliation and the practice of euthanasia. Journal of Medical Ethics. 1995;**21**(1):49–54.
19. **Bülow HH, Sprung CL, Baras M**, et al. Are religion and religiosity important to end-of-life decisions and patient autonomy in the ICU? The Ethicatt study. Intensive Care Medicine. 2012;**38**(7):1126–33.

20. **Grassi L, Agostini M, Magnani K.** Attitudes of Italian doctors to euthanasia and assisted suicide for terminally ill patients. The Lancet. 1999;**354**(9193):1876–7.
21. **Kübler A, Adamik B, Lipinska-Gediga M, Kedziora J, Strozecki L.** End-of-life attitudes of intensive care physicians in Poland: results of a national survey. Intensive Care Medicine. 2011;**37**(8):1290–6.
22. **Kaldjian LC, Jekel JF, Bernene JL, Rosenthal GE, Vaughan-Sarrazin M, Duffy TP.** Internists' attitudes towards terminal sedation in end of life care. Journal of Medical Ethics. 2004;**30**(5):499–503.
23. **Davidson JE, Bojorquez G, Upvall M,** et al. Nurses' values and perspectives on medical aid in dying: a survey of nurses in the United States. Journal of Hospice and Palliative Nursing. 2022;**24**(1):5–14.
24. **Davidson JE, Stokes L, DeWolf Bosek MS,** et al. Nurses' values on medical aid in dying: a qualitative analysis. Nursing Ethics. 2022:;**29(3):636–50.**
25. **Gastmans C, Lemiengre J, de Casterlé BD.** Role of nurses in institutional ethics policies on euthanasia. Journal of Advanced Nursing. 2006;**54**(1):53–61.
26. **Vander Ryk AL, O'Neill MJ, Lester D.** Attitudes toward abortion, capital punishment, and assisted suicide. Psychological Reports. 1999;**85**(3):904.
27. **Schioldborg P.** Students' attitudes to active euthanasia. Tidsskrift for den Norske Laegeforening. 1999;**119**(17):2515–19.
28. **Schioldborg P**. Students' attitudes toward active euthanasia, assisted suicide and proposed amendments to the penal code. Tidsskrift for den Norske Laegeforening. 2000;**120**(19):2283–8.
29. **Kolodziejczyk I, Kuzma J.** Knowledge and attitudes towards abortion and euthanasia among health students in Papua New Guinea. Advances in Medical Education and Practice. 2020;**11**:977.
30. **Gastmans C, Lemiengre J, de Casterlé BD.** Development and communication of written ethics policies on euthanasia in Catholic hospitals and nursing homes in Belgium (Flanders). Patient Education and Counseling. 2006;**63**(1–2):188–95.
31. **Gastmans C, Lemiengre J, van der Wal G, Schotsmans P, de Casterlé BD.** Prevalence and content of written ethics policies on euthanasia in Catholic healthcare institutions in Belgium (Flanders). Health Policy. 2006;**76**(2):169–78.
32. **Zimbelman J.** A blessing in disguise? Empowering Catholic health care institutions in the current health care environment. Christian Bioethics. 2000;**6**(3):281–94.
33. **Lemiengre J, de Casterle BD, Denier Y, Schotsmans P, Gastmans C.** How do hospitals deal with euthanasia requests in Flanders (Belgium)?: a content analysis of policy documents. Patient Education and Counseling. 2008;**71**(2):293–301.
34. **O'Neill C, Feenan D, Hughes C, McAlister DA.** Physician and family assisted suicide: results from a study of public attitudes in Britain. Social Science and Medicine. 2003;**57**(4):721–31.
35. **Wise J.** Public supports euthanasia for most desperate cases. BMJ. 1996;**313**(7070):1423.
36. **Van Wijmen MP, Rurup ML, Pasman HR, Kaspers PJ, Onwuteaka-Philipsen BD.** Advance directives in the Netherlands: an empirical contribution to the exploration of a cross-cultural perspective on advance directives. Bioethics. 2010;**24**(3):118–26.
37. **Tanida N.** The view of religions toward euthanasia and extraordinary treatments in Japan. Journal of Religion and Health. 2000;**39**(4):339–54.

38. **WorldAtlas.** The major religions in India. Available from: https://www.worldatlas.com/articles/major-religions-in-modern-india.html
39. **Curlin FA, Nwodim C, Vance JL, Chin MH, Lantos JD.** To die, to sleep: US physicians' religious and other objections to physician-assisted suicide, terminal sedation, and withdrawal of life support. American Journal of Hospice and Palliative Medicine. 2008;**25**(2):112–20.
40. **Pomfret S, Mufti S, Seale C.** Medical students and end-of-life decisions: the influence of religion. Future Healthcare Journal. 2018;**5**(1):25.
41. **Kanniyakonil S.** New developments in India concerning the policy of passive euthanasia. Developing World Bioethics. 2018;**18**(2):190–7.
42. **Kamath S, Bhate P, Mathew G, Sashidharan S, Daniel AB.** Attitudes toward euthanasia among doctors in a tertiary care hospital in South India: a cross-sectional study. Indian Journal of Palliative Care. 2011;**17**(3):197.
43. **Subba SH, Khullar V, Latafat Y, Chawla K, Nirmal A, Chaudhary T.** Doctors' attitude towards euthanasia: a cross-sectional study experience. Journal of the Association of Physicians of India. 2016;**64**(6):44–7.
44. **Bhat S.** Doctors' perception of assisted death: the effect of career stage. Biomedical Research Journal. 2020;7(2):55.
45. **Kamble SV, Sorum PC, Mullet** E. Young Indians' views of the acceptability of physician-assisted suicide. International Perspectives in Psychology. 2012;**1**(3):165–76.
46. **Madadin M, Al Sahwan HS, Altarouti KK, Altarouti SA, Al Eswaikt ZS, Menezes RG.** The Islamic perspective on physician-assisted suicide and euthanasia. Medicine, Science and the Law. 2020;**60**(4):278–86.
47. **Ali H, Hashmi HS, Wasim MH.** Islamic teachings and WHO guidelines for COVID-19 pandemic: do the conflictions exist? EasyChair; 2020:1–6.
48. **Ahmed AM, Kheir MM.** Attitudes towards euthanasia among final-year Khartoum University medical students. Eastern Mediterranean Health Journal. 2006;**12**(3–4):391–7.
49. **Cavlak U, Aslan UB, Gurso S, Yagci N, Yeldan I.** Attitudes of physiotherapists and physiotherapy students toward euthanasia: a comparative study. Advances in Therapy. 2007;**24**(1):135–45.
50. **Rathor MY, Rani MF, Shahar MA,** et al. Attitudes toward euthanasia and related issues among physicians and patients in a multi-cultural society of Malaysia. Journal of Family Medicine and Primary Care. 2014;**3**(3):230.
51. **Qidwai W, Qureshi H, Ali SS, Alam M, Azani SI.** Physician-assisted suicide perceptions among patients presenting to family physicians at a teaching hospital in Karachi, Pakistan. Journal of Pakistan Medical Association. 2001;**51**:233.
52. **Naseh L, Heidari M.** The attitudes of nursing students to euthanasia. Indian Journal of Medical Ethics. 2017;**2**(1):20–4.
53. **Naseh L, Hossein R, Mohammad H.** Nurses' attitudes towards euthanasia: a cross-sectional study in Iran. International Journal of Palliative Nursing. 2015;**21**(1):43–8.
54. **Ahmed RA, Sorum PC, Mullet E.** Young Kuwaitis' views of the acceptability of physician-assisted suicide. Journal of Medical Ethics.2010;**36**(11):671–6.
55. **Tadros G, Rakhawy MY, Khoweiled A, El-Houssini AM, Khan F.** Perception of physician-assisted suicide among Egyptian psychiatrists: cultural perspective. The Psychiatrist. 2011;**35**(1):15–18.

56. **Ahmed A, Kheir MM, Abdel Rahman A, Ahmed NH, Abdalla ME.** Attitudes towards euthanasia and assisted suicide among Sudanese doctors. Eastern Mediterranean Health Journal. 2001;7(3):551–5.
57. **Aghababaei N.** The euthanasia-religion nexus: exploring religious orientation and euthanasia attitude measures in a Muslim context. Omega (Westport). 2013;**66**(4):333–41.
58. **Ozcelik H, Tekir O, Samancioglu S, Fadiloglu C, Ozkara E.** Nursing students' approaches toward euthanasia. Omega (Westport). 2014;**69**(1):93–103.
59. **Hosseinzadeh K, Rafiei H.** Nursing student attitudes toward euthanasia: a cross-sectional study. Nursing Ethics. 2019;**26**(2):496–503.
60. **Yildirim JG.** Knowledge, opinions and behaviors of senior nursing students in Turkey regarding euthanasia and factors in Islam affecting these. Journal of Religion and Health. 2020;**59**(1):399–415.
61. **Baeke G, Wils JP, Broeckaert B.** 'There is a time to be born and a time to die' (Ecclesiastes 3: 2a): Jewish perspectives on euthanasia. Journal of Religion and Health. 2011;**50**(4):778–95.
62. **Kalish RA.** Some variables in death attitudes. Journal of Social Psychology. 1963;**59**(1):137–45.
63. **Caddell DP, Newton RR.** Euthanasia: American attitudes toward the physician's role. Social Science and Medicine. 1995;**40**(12):1671–81.
64. **Ostheimer JM, Moore Jr CL.** 'The correlates of attitudes toward euthanasia' revisited. Social Biology. 1981;**28**(1–2):145–9.
65. **Bodas M, Velan B, Kaplan G, Ziv A, Rubin C, Peleg K.** Assisted life termination and truth telling to terminally ill patients: a cross-sectional study of public opinions in Israel. Israel Journal of Health Policy Research. 2020;**9**(1):1–10.
66. **Silveira MJ, DiPiero A, Gerrity MS, Feudtner C.** Patients' knowledge of options at the end of life: ignorance in the face of death. JAMA. 2000;**284**(19):2483–8.
67. **Wenger NS, Carmel S.** Physicians' religiosity and end-of-life care attitudes and behaviors. Mount Sinai Journal of Medicine. 2004;**71**(5):335–43.
68. **Musgrave CF, Margalith I, Goldsmidt L.** Israeli oncology and nononcology nurses' attitudes toward physician-assisted dying: a comparison study. Oncology Nursing Forum. 2001;**28**(1):50–7
69. **Kaldjian LC, Jekel JF, Bernene JL, Rosenthal GE, Vaughan-Sarrazin M, Duffy TP.** Should disagreement about physician-assisted suicide discourage professional societies from engaging in public debate? A survey of 677 Connecticut internists. Connecticut Medicine. 2002;**66**(10):603–9.
70. **Sonnenblick M, Friedlander Y, Steinberg A.** Dissociation between the wishes of terminally ill parents and decisions by their offspring. Journal of the American Geriatrics Society. 1993;**41**(6):599–604.
71. **Leichtentritt RD, Rettig KD.** My parent's dignified death is different from mine: moral problem solving about euthanasia. Journal of Social and Personal Relationships. 1999;**16**(3):385–406.

Chapter 21

Suicide during the global COVID-19 pandemic

Danuta Wasserman, Miriam Iosue, and Vladimir Carli

Introduction

Throughout human history, infectious epidemics have repeatedly threatened populations and societies. The largest recorded epidemic was the '*Black Death*' that spread throughout Europe, North Africa, and the Near East in the mid-fourteenth century. The '*Spanish flu*' (1918–20) affected over a quarter of the global population and it was the first pandemic. With improvement in living conditions and health care resources, communicable diseases now play a secondary role among the leading causes of death, especially in high-income countries.[1] Recent epidemics, such as those of Ebola haemorrhagic fever in Africa and severe acute respiratory syndrome (SARS) in China, raised concerns about their possible spread across the globe. Nevertheless, they never reached the extent of a pandemic. Therefore, initially, it was difficult to imagine that COVID-19 would result in such catastrophic outcomes.

The first cases of a novel '*viral pneumonia*' were reported in December 2019 in Wuhan, China. The virus was then identified and named '*severe acute respiratory syndrome coronavirus 2*' (SARS-CoV-2), whereas the associated disease was called coronavirus disease 2019 (COVID-19). The number of confirmed cases started to increase, as well as the number of deaths. New cases were soon identified outside of China, with increasing concern from national and international authorities. The situation rapidly escalated to the point that, in March 2020, the World Health Organization (WHO) declared COVID-19 a pandemic. As of September 2021, the global number of confirmed cases reached more than 223,000,000, with more than 4,600,000 deaths, imposing a huge burden on health care systems worldwide. Furthermore, a number of containment measures have been put in place to reduce the spread of the disease, with different levels of restriction adopted across countries. Stay-at-home orders were issued in several countries, along with travel ban and restrictions, closures of schools and other public places, cancellation of public events, quarantine and isolation measures, and physical distance enforcement.[2,3] The health, socio-economic, and environmental implications of these global changes are multiple and difficult to be estimated,[4,5] and altogether pose a severe burden on global mental health and consequent suicide risk. Indeed, even if increased anxiety, stress, sleep disturbances, sadness, and feelings of helplessness may represent a normal response to crises, the global proportion of the COVID-19 pandemic and its long-term socio-economic impact may cause excessive stress on vulnerable individuals.

The prevalence of depression, anxiety, and stress among the general population during the pandemic has been calculated to be 17–34%, 15–32%, and 25–36%, respectively.[6,7,8,9,10,11] The estimated prevalence of post-traumatic stress disorder (PTSD) symptoms was 15–27%,[6,9,10] and insomnia and sleep disturbances have been reported in up to 40% of subjects.[6,8,10] Being female, being younger than 35 years old, having a lower socio-economic status, living in a rural area, being at higher risk of contracting the virus, and reporting higher media exposure during the pandemic seem to increase the risk of poor mental health, whereas social/family support and physical activity seem to play a protective role.[12] Furthermore, children, adolescents, and the elderly are considered particularly vulnerable groups in the general population.[13,14,15,16]

Nevertheless, preliminary findings from a living systematic review and meta-analysis did not show an increase in depressive and anxiety symptoms in the general population when comparing data collected during the COVID-19 pandemic and data from the preceding year.[17]

Health care workers and COVID-19 patients are considered particularly vulnerable populations. As expected, the prevalence of psychological distress (17–41%) is considerably higher among health care workers. Furthermore, depression (14–31%), anxiety (16–30%), PTSD symptoms (13–31%), and sleep disorders (37–47%) are also commonly reported.[6,8,10,11,18] Health care workers, females, nurses, and frontline professionals reported the worst mental health outcomes.[11,19]

Since the beginning of the COVID-19 pandemic, national and international agencies, associations, and experts have expressed concerns about global mental health and advocated for timely interventions that could mitigate its aftermath.[20,21,22,23] This threat is particularly serious for low- and middle-income countries (LMICs) where poverty, socio-cconomic inequalities, unemployment, violence, low educational levels, and limited availability of health and mental health services were already widespread before the pandemic.[24] Furthermore, considering the huge socio-economic impact of the COVID-19 pandemic, an increase in suicidal thoughts and behaviour has been predicted, with effects culminating after the immediate crisis has been resolved.[25,26,27,28]

This chapter aims to explore previous knowledge about suicide and epidemics, and summarizes current findings on the impact of COVID-19 on suicidality around the world.

Suicide and previous epidemics and outbreaks

The 1918 influenza pandemic was reported to increase suicide rates in the United States.[29] When adjusting for influenza mortality rate, increased social distancing resulted in significantly increased suicide rates, whereas the influenza mortality rate did not significantly predict suicide rates in 43 large cities in the United States.[30]

SARS is a viral respiratory disease that spread mainly in China in 2003 and affected more than 8000 individuals, with a mortality rate of about 11%.[31] In 2003, a significant increase in suicide rates among the elderly was reported in Hong Kong. The suicide rates in this population remained high, even in 2004. This was in contrast with a previous downward trend.[32,33] Fears about contracting the disease and of becoming a burden to the family were reported among suicidal older adults, who also had fears of separation.[34] Analysing data from an emergency department (ED) in Taiwan, a non-significant increase in admissions due to suicide attempt by drug overdose was found during the peak of the SARS epidemic, compared to the pre-epidemic stage.[35] This was in contrast with an overall decrease in patient attendances during the same period.

Between 2014 and 2016, the largest Ebola outbreak to date spread in West Africa, with more than 28,500 cases and 11,000 deaths. Guinea, Liberia, and Sierra Leone were the countries most affected.

Secor et al.[36] assessed 1495 adult survivors in these countries approximately two years after the end of the epidemic. The prevalence of depressive symptoms ranged between 13% (Guinea) and 22% (Sierra Leone). Furthermore, suicidal ideation was reported in 10–19% of the sample. Depressive symptomatology was also found to positively correlate with perceived stigma against the disease.

Besides stressful socio-economic consequences of large epidemics, other potential links between respiratory viral infections and suicide also have been hypothesized. For example, seropositivity for influenza B virus was reported to be significantly associated with a history of suicide attempts.[37] When analysing weekly suicide mortality and influenza-like illness rates in South Korea, a significant positive association was found, but only since 2009 when the H1N1 flu pandemic began to spread.[38] Furthermore, an increased neutrophil-to-lymphocyte ratio (NLR) has been proposed as a biomarker for suicidal behaviour in major depression and bipolar patients.[39,40,41]

Few studies have investigated the link between infectious epidemics and suicide. However, in their systematic review, Zortea et al.[42] concluded that the findings support this association, despite large methodological limitations.

Prevalence and trend of suicidality in different countries and world regions during the COVID-19 pandemic

According to the WHO, only 60 of its 194 Member States have good-quality mortality registration data. Even in countries with good mortality statistics, suicides can be misclassified as accidents, homicides, or death of unknown causes. This largely influences the quality of data on suicide rates, especially when estimations are conducted for relatively short time periods such as during the COVID-19 pandemic.

Pirkis et al.[43] retrieved data on suicide deaths during the COVID-19 pandemic from 21 high- and upper middle-income countries. The number of suicides remained largely unchanged or declined in the early months of the pandemic when compared to expectations based on the pre-pandemic period. On the contrary, a meta-analysis of 54 studies suggested that the event rate of suicidal ideation (10.81%) and suicide attempts (4.68%) increased during the pandemic.[44]

Preliminary conclusions of a living systematic review described evidence of a fall in hospital presentations for suicidal behaviour during the pandemic.[45] The evidence for an increase in suicide rates was not consistent.

It is important to consider that suicide rates largely vary across different countries and even across different regions within the same country, making it difficult to draw general conclusions from local data. For this reason, studies on suicidal thoughts and behaviour during the COVID-19 pandemic and changes in suicide rates are presented below, grouped according to four WHO regions. No relevant studies were identified from the Eastern Mediterranean and African regions.

Region of the Americas

The majority of studies in this region have been conducted in the United States. Only one study analysed suicide rates in a country of South America,[46] and two studies evaluated suicidal ideation and suicide attempts among Canadians.[47,48]

Suicide rates

Mitchell and Li[49] calculated a 20% decrease in the age-adjusted suicide rate during the stay-at-home period in Connecticut, United States (9.4/100,000 person-years), compared to the corresponding period in 2019 (11.7/100,000 person-years). Nevertheless, when considering only non-white residents, the age-adjusted suicide rate rose from 7.4/100,000 person-years to 12/100,000 person-years. Similarly, Bray et al.[50] described different trends for black and white people during the peak of the pandemic in Maryland, United States. Between March and May 2020, suicide mortality rates halved among white people but doubled among black people. Possible explanations proposed for the disparity in suicide trends between ethnicities are increased socio-economic impact of COVID-19 on minority groups and reduced access to mental health services for these populations. Faust et al.[51] calculated that the incident rate of suicide deaths among people aged 10 years and older during the stay-at-home period in Massachusetts remained stable when compared to the corresponding period in 2019 (0.67 vs 0.80 per 100,000 person-months), and did not deviate from projected expectations using data since 2015. No differences were found in the distribution of suicides by age and sex.

In Peru, the overall suicide rates declined during the pandemic, even if different trends were described for men and women.[46] Among men, after the initial decline, suicide rates began to increase again during the course of the pandemic.

Suicidal ideation and suicide attempts

Ontiveros et al.[52] examined suicidal poisoning cases reported to the California Poison Control System between January 2018 and May 2020. During the COVID-19 pandemic, the number of suicidal poisonings per month significantly decreased in all age groups, with the exception of people aged 70 years or older. The number of deaths by suicidal poisoning also significantly decreased.

An analysis of medical records in the University of Michigan Health System since October 2015 showed that during the first seven months of the COVID-19 pandemic, there were almost 40% fewer ED visits for suicide attempts and intentional self-harm than expected.[53] Being male, being 18–65 years of age, and having a history of three or more ED visits for suicide-related behaviour were significant risk factors for ED visits for the same reason during the pandemic. Married (vs unmarried) individuals and Asians (vs Caucasians) showed a significantly decreased risk of ED visits for suicide attempts.

Similarly, in a large healthcare delivery system in California, a significantly lower number of youths aged 5–17 years required suicide-related ED visits between March and May 2020, compared to the corresponding period in 2019.[54]

The trend subsequently returned to pre-pandemic levels. Nevertheless, female youths presented with significantly higher suicide-related ED visits during summer and autumn 2020, compared to the corresponding periods in 2019.

Using data from the Centers for Disease Control and Prevention (CDC) on ED visits, Yard et al.[55] calculated that, during spring 2020, the mean number of weekly ED visits for suspected suicide attempts decreased by 26.45% among adolescents aged 12–17 years, and by 16.80% among youths aged 18–25 years. During summer 2020 and winter 2021, the mean number of weekly ED visits for suspected suicide attempts among adolescents increased by 22.33% and 39.13%, respectively, and this was mostly due to visits by adolescent girls (+ 26.16% during spring 2020, and +50.55% during winter 2021). In the same study periods, the mean number of weekly ED visits for suspected suicide attempts remained more stable for older youths (−5.60% and +1.68%, respectively). These findings seem to indicate that adolescent females experienced more severe distress as a result of the pandemic. In 2020, two large paediatric hospitals in Montreal, Canada registered a significant 9.9% decrease in the number of ED visits for suicidal ideation, compared to the previous two years.[47]

In the early phase of the pandemic, through an online survey, 15% of a large sample of residents in the United States were categorized as being at high risk of suicidality.[56] Being black, Native American, Hispanic, or unmarried or having families with children, as well as being young and having physical symptoms or depressive symptomatology and food insecurity, positively correlates with higher levels of suicidality. On the other hand, social and psychological resources, such as strong social ties and religion, were significantly negatively correlated with suicidality.

In June 2020, Czeisler et al.[57] conducted web-based surveys involving a representative sample of adults in the United States. In this study, 10.7% of the sample reported having seriously considered suicide during the past month, which was almost twice as high as the percentage registered in 2018. Males and youths aged 18–24 years reported suicidal ideation more frequently than females and other age groups, respectively. Suicidal ideation was more common among Hispanic respondents than among white and Asian respondents. Employed respondents, especially essential workers, showed higher suicidal ideation than those who were unemployed. Finally, suicidal ideation was particularly prevalent among unpaid caregivers (30.7%). These groups also reported more often other mental health problems such as anxiety and depressive symptoms, trauma- and stress-related symptoms, and initiation of, or increase in, substance use.

Among a sample of military veterans, past-year suicidal ideation significantly decreased during the COVID-19 pandemic compared to pre-pandemic assessments.[58] However, veterans affected by COVID-19 and those who reported an increase in alcohol consumption or in loneliness were at increased risk of new-onset suicidal ideation during the pandemic.

Hill et al.[59] compared the results of a youth suicide risk screening at an ED in Texas. A higher rate of suicidal ideation was found in March and July 2020, compared to the corresponding period in 2019. Higher rates of recent suicide attempts were registered in February, March, April, and July 2020, compared to the corresponding months in 2019. The months with higher suicide-related behaviour overlapped with those with higher COVID-19 impact and community responses, indicating that youths were severely affected by stress due to the pandemic.

Suicidal ideation was reported by 18.04% of a sample of college students recruited during the initial peak of the COVID-19 pandemic in Texas, United States.[60] Furthermore, 48.14% showed moderate-to-severe depression; 38.48% presented with mild-to-severe anxiety, and 71.26% reported increased stress/anxiety levels due to the pandemic.

In a sample of Canadian adolescents, 44% reported experiencing suicidal ideation since the beginning of the pandemic.[48]

European region

Several studies were conducted in Europe and found somewhat contrasting results.

Suicide rates

Appleby et al.[61] did not find significant changes in suicide rates in England when comparing data from April through to October 2020 to the months preceding the pandemic and to the corresponding period in 2019. Similarly, no significant changes in suicide trends were reported in Leipzig, Germany[62] or in Norway in the first months of the pandemic.[63,64]

Suicidal ideation and suicide attempts

Reviewing electronic health records from general practices, Carr et al.[65] estimated that, between April and May 2020, the incidence of reported self-harm episodes decreased by 37.6% in England and by 24.5% in North Ireland, Scotland, and Wales. Similar decreases were shown also in the diagnoses of depression and anxiety disorders and in the prescriptions for antidepressants. The decrease in incidence of self-harm episodes was higher among women, patients younger than 45 years, and those belonging to deprived communities.

A significant reduction in suicide-related ED visits was reported in a large general hospital in Madrid, Spain after the beginning of the pandemic.[66]

In the United Kingdom (UK), the number of ED visits for self-harm in Oxford and Derby during the early stage of the pandemic considerably dropped compared to the preceding months (−13.5%) and the corresponding period in 2019 (−18%).[67] The reduction was observed in all age groups but was greater among females. Furthermore, self-poisoning episodes decreased more than self-injury ones. These results are somewhat in contrast with the significant increase in the total number of suicide-related ED visits reported in the first months of the pandemic, compared to the corresponding period in 2019, in a trauma centre in Birmingham.[68] In a hospital in Manchester, the absolute number of ED admissions due to deliberate self-harm remained stable when comparing March to May 2020 to the corresponding periods in 2019 and 2018.[69] Nevertheless, the proportion of admissions due to self-harm in 2020 was significantly higher than that reported in previous years (2.08% in 2020 vs 1.19% in 2018 and 1.44% in 2019).

Compared to 2018–2019, during the first months of the pandemic, there were no significant differences in the weekly rate of presentations to the ED for suicidal ideation or self-harm in a large hospital in Dublin, Ireland.[70] This was registered despite a significant 21% reduction in the weekly rate of overall psychiatric presentations. Referrals to psychiatry for self-harm decreased by 8.5% in another Irish University Hospital.[71] Nevertheless, during the pandemic, suicide attempts showed a higher degree of lethality and more often involved individuals with substance use.

Data from one of the most hit areas in Italy showed that the proportion of ED psychiatric consultations due to suicidality was higher in the first months of the pandemic than in the corresponding months in 2019 (17.2% vs 13%).[72] In a multicentre Italian study considering a longer study period, psychiatric admissions due to suicidality significantly increased in the post-lockdown phase compared to the corresponding periods in 2018 and 2019.[73] Moreover, data from nine different Italian hospitals showed that psychiatric consultations for suicidal ideation decreased by 3.4% during the lockdown period, but then rose again in the post-lockdown phase, along with an increase in consultations for suicide attempts.[74]

A French study exploring hospital admissions in children and adolescents reported a 50% decrease in the incidence of admissions for suicidal behaviour in this population during the lockdown period.[75]

Zalsman et al.[76] analysed suicide-related chats on an Internet-based crisis hotline in Israel. Compared to the corresponding period in 2019, the absolute number of suicide-related chats increased by 35% during the pandemic and followed the curve of COVID-19 cases and consequent restrictive measures, with an increase in March and then a decline between the end of April and June. A

30-fold increase in the percentage of suicide-related chats involving adults aged 50 years and over was also reported. Furthermore, the number of suicide-related chats resulting in urgent police intervention significantly increased during the lockdown period (April to May 2020) compared to the previous year.

Findings from the COVID-19 Social Study in the UK showed that, in the first month of lockdown, suicidal ideation was present in 18% of the sample, whereas 5% reported self-harm behaviours.[77] A lower prevalence was shown in a smaller survey (8.2–9.8% for suicidal ideation and 0.1–0.7% for past-week suicide attempts).[78]

The two-week prevalence of suicide attempt reported in a sample of Irish adults during spring and summer 2020 was 1–1.4%.[79]

In an online survey conducted in Norway and mostly answered by women, 3.6% of the sample reported past-month suicidal thoughts and 0.2% reported past-month suicide attempt.[80] In a repeated cross-sectional evaluation among Norwegian adults, past-month suicidal ideation did not vary between pre-pandemic (3.2%) and pandemic (3.2–4.2%) periods.[64] In this study, besides commonly recognized risk factors, such as previous suicide attempts or alcohol use, being at risk of complications if infected and having economic concerns related to the pandemic significantly increased the risk of suicidal ideation. COVID-19-related health and economic concerns also influenced the likelihood of reporting suicidal ideation in the Czech Republic where the prevalence of suicidal thoughts and behaviour tripled during the pandemic compared to previous evaluations (11.88% vs 3.88%, respectively).[81]

During the lockdown period in Greece, past-month suicidal ideation was reported by 5.2% of the sample.[82] Positive feelings towards lockdown measures, friendships, and faith in a supreme being seemed to act as protective factors. Furthermore, suicidal ideation was more often reported by those interviewed at the end of the study period than at the beginning. Another survey among Greek adults found that the vast majority did not experience any change in suicidal thoughts during the lockdown period, whereas 10.4% reported an increase and 4.2% reported a decrease.[83]

Western Pacific region

Studies conducted in this region were mostly conducted Japan, China, Australia, and New Zealand. In particular, Japan presented the most comprehensive analysis of suicide rates.

Suicide rates

Leske et al.[84] analysed data from the Queensland Suicide Register in Australia and described no differences in monthly rates of suspected suicide between the pandemic period and pre-pandemic data since 2015 (14.07/100,000 vs 14.85/100,000, respectively).

Injury mortality data from Guangdong province in China showed that suicide rates significantly decreased by more than 18% between January and June 2020, compared to the corresponding period in 2019.[85] Nevertheless, suicide rates in the 10- to 14-year age group significantly increased by 139% in the same period, and a non-significant increase was registered in the 70- to 79-year age group. A 6.9% decrease in the number of suicides between January and August 2020 was registered in South Korea, corresponding to a 10% decrease among males and a 1.4% decrease among women.[86]

Several analyses have been conducted in Japan to assess changes in suicide rates. Tanaka and Okamoto[87] examined monthly suicide rates since November 2016. They reported a 14% decrease in suicide rates between February and June 2020, and a 16% increase between July and October 2020. During the second wave of the pandemic, women (+37%) and adolescents (+49%) registered the largest increases in suicide rates. These results were confirmed by prior findings of an excess of suicide deaths among women in the summer of 2020[88] and another study extending the observations until December 2020.[89] Sakamoto et al.[90] also described a different pattern of suicide rates among men and women during the pandemic in Japan. Compared to the previous four years, suicide rates during the pandemic increased in October and November among men and from July to November among women. The largest relative increases were found among men and women aged 30 years or younger and among women aged 30–49 years. Furthermore, among occupation categories, students and homemakers showed the largest increase in suicide rates.[91]

Considering Japanese adolescents, no significant changes in suicide rates were reported during the period of school closure,[92] as the very high increase in the second wave mostly corresponded to the period after the end of school closure.[87]

Suicidal ideation and attempts

In a hospital in Sydney, Australia, no significant change in the number of trauma admissions due to self-harm was registered from March to April 2020 compared to the corresponding period in the past four years.[93] In contrast, a 26% decrease in the number of ED presentations due to suicidality and self-harm was reported in Western Australia North Metropolitan Health Services between January and May 2020 compared to the corresponding period in 2019.[94] A significant fourfold reduction in self-harming incidents was reported in six Youth Justice Centres in Australia, which was probably attributable to the timely and integrated response to the pandemic put in place in the Youth Justice System.[95]

Considering the proportion of mental health presentations due to self-harm in a hospital in New Zealand, a significant 3.5% increase was registered during lockdown compared with the pre-lockdown period.[96]

In an online survey of adult New Zealanders, 6% of the sample reported suicidal ideation during the lockdown period, with 2.1% reporting suicide planning and 2.1% reporting suicide attempts.[97] Nevertheless, 83% of those experiencing suicidal ideation during the lockdown period reported having experienced such thoughts also in the preceding 12 months.

In a large survey of Chinese adults, more than 16% of the sample showed at least some degree of suicidal ideation at the beginning of the pandemic.[98] Among COVID-19-related factors, being a confirmed or suspected COVID-19 case, living in the most severely affected region, experience of quarantine, unemployment, being a frontline worker, perceiving higher psychological stress, and having greater difficulty in accessing information on psychological interventions significantly increased the risk of suicidal ideation. Conversely, paying more attention to information about the pandemic, having a better understanding of COVID-19-related knowledge, and having greater access to knowledge about psychological interventions were significantly associated with a lower risk of suicidal ideation. A prevalence of 6.47% of suicidal ideation was reported among Chinese hospital staff.[99] The significant risk factors were a need for current psychological intervention, infection of family members or relatives, poor self-rated health status, poor marital relationships, depression and anxiety symptoms, and higher perceived stress. Furthermore, 2% of a sample of university students in Wuhan, China reported suicidal ideation.[100] Among other factors, high stress and alcohol use during the pandemic increased the risk of suicidality in this population.

South East Asia region

Few studies assessing suicidality during the COVID-19 pandemic were conducted in this region.

Suicide rates

An analysis of suicide cases registered in autopsies conducted in New Delhi, India, reported a significant 42% reduction of suicide deaths during the lockdown period compared to the corresponding period in 2019.[101] Moreover, an increase of suicide in the post-lockdown period, compared to the lockdown period, was also described.

Suicidal ideation and suicide attempts

Using data from a hospital in Sri Lanka, Knipe et al.[102] estimated a significant 32% reduction in presentations for self-poisoning during the pandemic period compared to the pre-pandemic period. In contrast, in a Nepalese hospital, the proportion of ED visits due to suicide and self-harm during the lockdown period was 44% and 72% higher than during the corresponding period in 2019 and the months preceding the lockdown period, respectively.[103]

Pathare et al.[104] analysed online news media reports of suicide and suicidal behaviour. During the lockdown period in India, there was a 67.7% increase in these reports compared to the corresponding period in 2019. Suicide cases reported during the pandemic significantly more often involved males, people aged 31–50 years, and married and employed individuals. Concerning suicide methods, hanging was reported significantly more often, whereas cases of poisoning and jumping in front of a train decreased. However, similar changes in socio-demographic characteristics of suicides were not found in Bangladesh.[105]

Different online surveys were conducted in Bangladesh. The largest survey showed a 5% prevalence of COVID-19-related suicidal ideation in the general population during the early phase of the pandemic.[106] A higher prevalence was reported among university students (12.8%)[107] and in a sample recruited in July 2020 (19%).[108] In this survey, COVID-19-related factors associated with increased suicidality included living in high-hit areas, having economic loss due to the pandemic, having relatives or acquaintances die from COVID-19, and being afraid of COVID-19 infection.

Mental health and suicidality among migrants and indigenous people during the COVID-19 pandemic

During the last decade, large-scale displacement was triggered by conflicts (e.g. Syria, Congo), natural disasters (e.g. India, the Philippines), and economic and political instability (e.g. Venezuela). According to the World Migration Report 2020,[109] there are more than 272 million international migrants, accounting for 3.5% of the world population, of whom nearly two-thirds are labour migrants and almost 26 million are refugees. Before, during, and after migration, migrants may face several adverse experiences (e.g. persecution, violence, separation from family, social isolation, unemployment) that place them at a higher risk of developing mental disorders. Furthermore, migrants, especially those who are undocumented, encounter barriers in accessing mental health care due to a lack of knowledge of the health care system in the host country, language difficulties, cultural expectations and beliefs, and a lack of trust in professionals and authorities.[110] Indeed, immigration status is a social determinant of health,[111] and the COVID-19 pandemic exacerbated existing social and health inequalities.[112] A limited number of studies were conducted during the COVID-19 pandemic on migrants' mental health, none of which assessed suicidality.

In a small survey of Indian migrant workers, the authors reported worsening mental health since the beginning of the pandemic.[113] In particular, the prevalence of anxiety and depression symptoms was found to be twice that of the general population during the lockdown period. Further, 47.2% of a sample of immigrants in South Korea showed severe anxiety symptoms.[114] Economic difficulties, such as job loss due to COVID-19, significantly increased the risk of higher levels of anxiety in this sample. More than 20,500 refugees and migrants participated in an online global survey between April and November 2020.[115] A deterioration of mental health status was reported, as indicated by increased depression, anxiety, loneliness, irritability, and hopelessness. Worse mental health outcomes were shown, particularly among women and those with difficulties in fulfilling basic needs (i.e. food, work, and housing). Ethiopian migrant returnees in the context of COVID-19 showed a high prevalence of depression (55%), anxiety (49%), and stress (36%),[116] whereas better outcomes were reported among Indonesian migrant returnees (10% depression, 10% anxiety, 2% stress).[117] Finally, Canadian clinicians caring for refugees and migrants described an increase in the demand for mental health support.[118] Difficulties in delivering psychotherapy through digital channels, such as technological barriers and privacy concerns, were also reported.

There are more than 5 million indigenous people in the United States, and more than 2 million in Canada.[119] Indigenous people represent 8.3% of the population in Latin America, and 3.3% of the population in Australia. Compared to the general population, higher suicide rates have been registered among indigenous people such as the Aboriginal people in Australia, Māori in New Zealand, and Native Americans in the United States and Canada.[120] Like migrants, indigenous people are exposed to increased socio-economic hardships and discrimination due to the pandemic crisis and their mental health needs may be neglected.[119] An in-person survey was conducted at the beginning of 2021 among the indigenous people in Bangladesh.[121] The prevalence rates of depression, anxiety, and stress were 49%, 47%, and 37%, respectively. In an online survey among Australian residents, being Aboriginal or Torres Strait Islander significantly increased the risk of experiencing anxiety and stress symptoms during the pandemic.[122] Similar results were reported for indigenous people in Canada.[123] Furthermore, in a national survey conducted by the Canadian Mental Health Association between March and September 2020, 10% of the sample exhibited suicidal ideation during the pandemic (compared to 2.5% in 2019), whereas the prevalence of suicidal thoughts among indigenous people was 20%.[124] Finally, news reports described suicide clusters among indigenous communities in the United States and Canada, with social isolation due to the COVID-19 pandemic probably as an important proximal risk factor.[125,126]

Conclusion

The majority of studies on suicidality during the COVID-19 pandemic have been conducted in high- and middle-income countries. Research on this topic is particularly lacking in South American, African, and East Mediterranean regions.

A preliminary analysis in 21 countries and findings from the United States described no changes or a decline in suicide rates during the first wave of the pandemic.[43,49,50,51] Similar results were reported also in studies from Europe, Peru, China, and South Korea by using national registries and extending their observations to September or October 2020.[46,61,62,63,64,85,86] However, this stabilization or decline was not consistently observed in different subgroups. For example, in the United States, suicide rates decreased among whites but increased among non-white residents.[49,50] In Guangdong, China, despite an overall reduction in suicide mortality, suicide rates significantly increased among youths aged 10–14 years.[85]

Japan has the highest quality of data on suicide rates during the COVID-19 pandemic. Study results showed a decrease in suicide rates in the first phase of the pandemic, followed by a statistically significant increase starting in July 2020 and mostly driven by a surge in female suicides.[87,88,89,91] A similar trend was reported also in Bangladesh by using data from autopsy records.[101] Furthermore, these findings are in line with what is described, in the context of natural disasters and other epidemics, as the 'honeymoon' phase, characterized by a strong sense of belonging to the community, which is followed by a phase of 'disillusionment', characterized by increased distress and loss of hope.[32,89,127]

Concerning hospital presentations and psychiatric consultations due to suicidality, a decline in the number of visits has been described in the United States,[53] Canada,[47] the UK,[67] Spain,[66] Ireland,[70,71] France,[75] and Australia.[94] Nevertheless, an increase in suicide-related visits by female youths has been described starting from summer 2020 in the United States.[54,55] When looking at the proportion of suicide-related visits compared to all visits during the pandemic, a rise was found in New Zealand,[96] the UK,[69] and Italy.[72] Furthermore, an increase was reported in suicide-related visits during the pandemic in Birmingham, UK,[68] as well as in psychiatric admissions due to suicidality in Italy in the post-lockdown period.[73]

Assessment of suicidal thoughts and behaviour during the pandemic was mostly conducted via online cross-sectional surveys by using different psychometric tools (e.g. Patient Health Questionnaire, Suicide Behaviors Questionnaire-Revised) and different time frames, making it difficult to compare the results. Three studies were based on repeated cross-sectional surveys and found either an increase in suicidality[59,81] or no significant differences[64] between the pandemic and the comparison period.

Migrants and indigenous people are considered vulnerable groups for mental health problems and suicidality. Even though studies examining the COVID-19 mental health impact on these populations received less attention, exacerbation of already existing social and health inequalities places them at increased risk.

Commonly recognized risk factors for suicidality, such as unemployment, depressive and anxiety symptoms, loneliness, interpersonal violence, and conflicts, were exacerbated during the COVID-19 pandemic. Furthermore, restrictive measures to contain the infection augmented barriers to accessing health and mental health care services.[25,26] In addition, other specific COVID-related suicide risk factors have been identified such as living in highly infected areas, having health and economic concerns, being infected or having experienced quarantine, having relatives who have been infected, bereavement due to COVID-19, higher perceived psychological stress, increased alcohol consumption, and difficulties in accessing information concerning mental health interventions.[58,80,81,98,99,100,108] Conversely, better knowledge and understanding of the disease, positive feelings towards lockdown measures, greater access to information concerning mental health interventions, friendships, and faith in a supreme being have been described as protective factors against suicidality during the pandemic.[82,98]

Since the beginning of the pandemic, there were concerns about its huge impact on global mental health. Therefore, national and international institutions and organizations disseminated general recommendations to increase psychological well-being, and health and mental health services tried to rapidly adjust.[128] Digital interventions played a pivotal role in mitigating the psychological impact of the pandemic and demonstrated to be safe, effective, and well accepted by users.[129] Besides this, evidence-based suicide preventive strategies also need to be adapted. In particular, universal interventions, such as active labour market policies and social protection, should be strengthened, and specific interventions for newly identified vulnerable groups, such as COVID-19 patients and frontline responders, should be developed.[26] More rigorous research designs and methods are also needed.[21] Finally, efforts should be made to overcome the research and treatment gap in mental health that affect low- and middle-income countries and rural communities.[130,131]

References

1. **World Health Organization** (2020). The top 10 causes of death. Available from: https://www.who.int/news-room/fact-sheets/detail/the-top-10-causes-of-death
2. **Wasserman D, van der Gaag R, Wise J.** The term 'physical distancing' is recommended rather than 'social distancing' during the COVID-19 pandemic for reducing feelings of rejection among people with mental health problems. European Psychiatry. 2020;**63**(1):e52.

3. **Wasserman D, van der Gaag R, Wise J.** Terms 'physical distancing' and 'emotional closeness' should be used and not 'social distancing' when defeating the Covid-19 pandemic. Science. 2020;**367**:1282.
4. **Sarkodie SA, Owusu PA.** Global assessment of environment, health and economic impact of the novel coronavirus (COVID-19). Environment, Development and Sustainability. 2021;**23**:5005–15.
5. **El Keshky MES, Basyouni SS, Al Sabban AM.** Getting through COVID-19: the pandemic's impact on the psychology of sustainability, quality of life, and the global economy—a systematic review. Frontiers in Psychology. 2020;**11**:3188.
6. **Krishnamoorthy Y, Nagarajan R, Saya GK, Menon V.** Prevalence of psychological morbidities among general population, healthcare workers and COVID-19 patients amidst the COVID-19 pandemic: a systematic review and meta-analysis. Psychiatry Research. 2020;**293**:113382.
7. **Salari N, Hosseinian-Far A, Jalali R**, et al. Prevalence of stress, anxiety, depression among the general population during the COVID-19 pandemic: a systematic review and meta-analysis. Globalization and Health. 2020;**16**(57):1–11.
8. **Wu T, Jia X, Shi H**, et al. Prevalence of mental health problems during the COVID-19 pandemic: a systematic review and meta-analysis. Journal of Affective Disorders. 2021;**281**:91–8.
9. **Cooke JE, Eirich R, Racine N, Madigan S.** Prevalence of posttraumatic and general psychological stress during COVID-19: a rapid review and meta-analysis. Psychiatry Research. 2020;**292**:113347.
10. **Cénat JM, Blais-Rochette C, Kokou-Kpolou CK**, et al. Prevalence of symptoms of depression, anxiety, insomnia, posttraumatic stress disorder, and psychological distress among populations affected by the COVID-19 pandemic: a systematic review and meta-analysis. Psychiatry Research. 2021;**295**:113599.
11. **Luo M, Guo L, Yu M, Jiang W, Wang H.** The psychological and mental impact of coronavirus disease 2019 (COVID-19) on medical staff and general public: a systematic review and meta-analysis. Psychiatry Research. 2020;**291**:113190.
12. **Wang Y, Kala MP, Jafar TH.** Factors associated with psychological distress during the coronavirus disease 2019 (COVID-19) pandemic on the predominantly general population: a systematic review and meta-analysis. PLoS One. 2020;**15**(12):e0244630.
13. **Nearchou F, Flinn C, Niland R, Subramaniam SS, Hennessy E.** Exploring the impact of COVID-19 on mental health outcomes in children and adolescents: a systematic review. International Journal of Environmental Research and Public Health. 2020;**17**(22):8479.
14. **Meherali S, Punjani N, Louie-Poon S**, et al. Mental health of children and adolescents amidst COVID-19 and past pandemics: a rapid systematic review. International Journal of Environmental Research and Public Health. 2021;**18**(7):3432.
15. **Sepúlveda-Loyola W, Rodríguez-Sánchez I, Pérez-Rodríguez P**, et al. Impact of social isolation due to COVID-19 on health in older people: mental and physical effects and recommendations. Journal of Nutrition, Health and Aging. 2020;**24**(9):938–47.
16. **Jones EAK, Mitra AK, Bhuiyan AR.** Impact of COVID-19 on mental health in adolescents: a systematic review. International Journal of Environmental Research and Public Health. 2021;**18**(5):2470.

17. **Sun Y, Wu Y, Bonardi O**, et al. Comparison of mental health symptoms prior to and during COVID-19: evidence from a living systematic review and meta-analysis. medRxiv. 2021:2021.05.10.21256920.
18. **Marvaldi M, Mallet J, Dubertret C, Moro MR, Guessoum SB.** Anxiety, depression, trauma-related, and sleep disorders among healthcare workers during the COVID-19 pandemic: a systematic review and meta-analysis. Neuroscience and Biobehavioral Reviews. 2021;**126**:252–64.
19. **Pappa S, Ntella V, Giannakas T, Giannakoulis VG, Papoutsi E, Katsaounou P.** Prevalence of depression, anxiety, and insomnia among healthcare workers during the COVID-19 pandemic: a systematic review and meta-analysis. Brain, Behavior, and Immunity. 2020;**88**:901–7.
20. **Fiorillo A, Gorwood P.** The consequences of the COVID-19 pandemic on mental health and implications for clinical practice. European Psychiatry. 2020;**63**(1):e32.
21. **Holmes EA, O'Connor RC, Perry VH**, et al. Multidisciplinary research priorities for the COVID-19 pandemic: a call for action for mental health science. The Lancet Psychiatry. 2020;7(6):547–60.
22. **United Nations** (2020). Policy brief: COVID-19 and the need for action on mental health 2020. Available from: https://unsdg.un.org/resources/policy-brief-covid-19-and-need-action-mental-health
23. **Adhanom Ghebreyesus T.** Addressing mental health needs: an integral part of COVID-19 response. World Psychiatry. 2020;**19**(2):129–30.
24. **Kola L, Kohrt BA, Hanlon C**, et al. COVID-19 mental health impact and responses in low-income and middle-income countries: reimagining global mental health. The Lancet Psychiatry. 2021;**8**(6):535–50.
25. **Gunnell D, Appleby L, Arensman E**, et al. Suicide risk and prevention during the COVID-19 pandemic. The Lancet Psychiatry. 2020;7(6):468–71.
26. **Wasserman D, Iosue M, Wuestefeld A, Carli V.** Adaptation of evidence-based suicide prevention strategies during and after the COVID-19 pandemic. World Psychiatry. 2020;**19**(3):294–306.
27. **Zalsman G, Stanley B, Szanto K, Clarke DE, Carli V, Mehlum L.** Suicide in the time of COVID-19: review and Recommendations. Archives of Suicide Research. 2020;**24**(4):477–82.
28. **Sarchiapone M, Lopez-Castroman J, Gramaglia C**, et al. Increased risk for mental disorders and suicide during the COVID-19 pandemic. Position statement of the Section on Suicidology and Suicide Prevention of the European Psychiatric Association. Global Psychiatry. 2021;**4**(1):4–19.
29. **Wasserman IM.** The impact of epidemic, war, prohibition and media on suicide: United States, 1910–1920. Suicide and Life-Threatening Behavior. 1992;**22**(2):240–54.
30. **Stack S, Rockett IRH.** Social distancing predicts suicide rates: analysis of the 1918 flu pandemic in 43 large cities, research note. Suicide and Life-Threatening Behavior. 2021;51(5):833–5.
31. **Chan-Yeung M, Xu R-H.** SARS: epidemiology. Respirology. 2003;**8**(s1):S9–14.
32. **Chan SMS, Chiu FKH, Lam CWL, Leung PYV, Conwell Y.** Elderly suicide and the 2003 SARS epidemic in Hong Kong. International Journal of Geriatric Psychiatry. 2006;**21**(2):113–18.

33. **Cheung YT, Chau PH, Yip PSF.** A revisit on older adults suicides and severe acute respiratory syndrome (SARS) epidemic in Hong Kong. International Journal of Geriatric Psychiatry. 2008;**23**(12):1231–8.
34. **Yip PS, Cheung YT, Chau PH, Law YW.** The impact of epidemic outbreak: the case of severe acute respiratory syndrome (SARS) and suicide among older adults in Hong Kong. Crisis. 2010;**31**(2):86–92.
35. **Huang C-C, Yen DH-T, Huang H-H**, et al. Impact of severe acute respiratory syndrome (SARS) outbreaks on the use of emergency department medical resources. Journal of the Chinese Medical Association. 2005;**68**(6):254–9.
36. **Secor A, Macauley R, Stan L**, et al. Mental health among Ebola survivors in Liberia, Sierra Leone and Guinea: results from a cross-sectional study. BMJ Open. 2020;**10**(5):e035217.
37. **Okusaga O, Yolken RH, Langenberg P**, et al. Association of seropositivity for influenza and coronaviruses with history of mood disorders and suicide attempts. Journal of Affective Disorders. 2011;**130**(1–2):220–5.
38. **Jung SJ, Lim S-S, Yoon J-H.** Fluctuations in influenza-like illness epidemics and suicide mortality: a time-series regression of 13-year mortality data in South Korea. PLoS One. 2021;**16**(2):e0244596.
39. **Ivkovic M, Pantovic-Stefanovic M, Dunjic-Kostic B**, et al. Neutrophil-to-lymphocyte ratio predicting suicide risk in euthymic patients with bipolar disorder: moderatory effect of family history. Comprehensive Psychiatry. 2016;**66**:87–95.
40. **Ekinci O, Ekinci A.** The connections among suicidal behavior, lipid profile and low-grade inflammation in patients with major depressive disorder: a specific relationship with the neutrophil-to-lymphocyte ratio. Nordic Journal of Psychiatry. 2017;**71**(8):574–80.
41. **Velasco A, Rodriguez-Revuelta J, Olie E**, et al. Neutrophil-to-lymphocyte ratio: a potential new peripheral biomarker of suicidal behavior. European Psychiatry. 2020;**63**(1):e14.
42. **Zortea TC, Brenna CTA, Joyce M**, et al. The impact of infectious disease-related public health emergencies on suicide, suicidal behavior, and suicidal thoughts. Crisis. 2020:1–14.
43. **Pirkis J, John A, Shin S**, et al. Suicide trends in the early months of the COVID-19 pandemic: an interrupted time-series analysis of preliminary data from 21 countries. The Lancet Psychiatry. 2021;**8**(7):579–88.
44. **Dubé JP, Smith MM, Sherry SB, Hewitt PL, Stewart SH.** Suicide behaviors during the COVID-19 pandemic: a meta-analysis of 54 studies. Psychiatry Research. 2021;**301**:113998.
45. **John A, Eyles E, Webb RT**, et al. The impact of the COVID-19 pandemic on self-harm and suicidal behaviour: update of living systematic review. F1000Research. 2021;**9**:1097.
46. **Calderon-Anyosa RJC, Kaufman JS.** Impact of COVID-19 lockdown policy on homicide, suicide, and motor vehicle deaths in Peru. Preventive Medicine. 2021;**143**:106331.
47. **Chadi N, Spinoso-Di Piano C, Osmanlliu E, Gravel J, Drouin O.** Mental health-related emergency department visits in adolescents before and during the COVID-19 pandemic: a multicentric retrospective study. Journal of Adolescent Health. 2021;69(5):847–50.

48. **Turner BJ, Robillard CL, Ames ME, Craig SG.** Prevalence and correlates of suicidal ideation and deliberate self-harm in Canadian adolescents during the coronavirus disease 2019 pandemic. Canadian Journal of Psychiatry. 2022;**67**(5):403–6.
49. **Mitchell TO, Li L.** State-level data on suicide mortality during COVID-19 quarantine: early evidence of a disproportionate impact on racial minorities. Psychiatry Research. 2021;**295**:113629.
50. **Bray MJC, Daneshvari NO, Radhakrishnan I,** et al. Racial differences in statewide suicide mortality trends in Maryland during the coronavirus disease 2019 (COVID-19) pandemic. JAMA Psychiatry. 2021;**78**(4):444.
51. **Faust JS, Shah SB, Du C, Li S-X, Lin Z, Krumholz HM.** Suicide deaths during the COVID-19 stay-at-home advisory in Massachusetts, March to May 2020. JAMA Network Open. 2021;**4**(1):e2034273.
52. **Ontiveros ST, Levine MD, Cantrell FL, Thomas C, Minns AB.** Despair in the time of COVID: a look at suicidal ingestions reported to the California Poison Control System during the pandemic. Academic Emergency Medicine. 2021;**28**(3):300–5.
53. **Bergmans RS, Larson PS.** Suicide attempt and intentional self-harm during the earlier phase of the COVID-19 pandemic in Washtenaw County, Michigan. Journal of Epidemiology and Community Health. 2021;**75**:963–9.
54. **Ridout KK, Alavi M, Ridout SJ,** et al. Emergency department encounters among youth with suicidal thoughts or behaviors during the COVID-19 pandemic. JAMA Psychiatry. 2021;78(12):1319–28.
55. **Yard E.** Emergency department visits for suspected suicide attempts among persons aged 12–25 years before and during the COVID-19 pandemic—United States, January 2019–May 2021. MMWR Morbidity and Mortality Weekly Report. 2021;**70**(24):888–94.
56. **Fitzpatrick KM, Harris C, Drawve G.** How bad is it? Suicidality in the middle of the COVID-19 pandemic. Suicide and Life-Threatening Behavior. 2020;**50**(6):1241–9.
57. **Czeisler MÉ, Lane RI, Petrosky E,** et al. Mental health, substance use, and suicidal ideation during the COVID-19 pandemic—United States, June 24–30, 2020. MMWR Morbidity and Mortality Weekly Report. 2020;**69**(32):1049–57.
58. **Nichter B, Hill ML, Na PJ,** et al. Prevalence and trends in suicidal behavior among US military veterans during the COVID-19 pandemic. JAMA Psychiatry. 2021;78(11):1218–27.
59. **Hill RM, Rufino K, Kurian S, Saxena J, Saxena K, Williams L.** Suicide ideation and attempts in a pediatric emergency department before and during COVID-19. Pediatrics. 2021;**147**(3):e2020029280.
60. **Wang X, Hegde S, Son C, Keller B, Smith A, Sasangohar F.** Investigating mental health of US college students during the COVID-19 pandemic: cross-sectional survey study. Journal of Medical Internet Research. 2020;**22**(9):e22817.
61. **Appleby L, Richards N, Ibrahim S, Turnbull P, Rodway C, Kapur N.** Suicide in England in the COVID-19 pandemic: early observational data from real time surveillance. The Lancet Regional Health—Europe. 2021;**4**:100110.
62. **Radeloff D, Papsdorf R, Uhlig K, Vasilache A, Putnam K, Von Klitzing K.** Trends in suicide rates during the COVID-19 pandemic restrictions in a major German city. Epidemiology and Psychiatric Sciences. 2021;**30**:1–19.

63. **Qin P, Mehlum L.** National observation of death by suicide in the first 3 months under COVID-19 pandemic. Acta Psychiatrica Scandinavica. 2021;**143**(1):92–3.
64. **Knudsen AKS, Stene-Larsen K, Gustavson K,** et al. Prevalence of mental disorders, suicidal ideation and suicides in the general population before and during the COVID-19 pandemic in Norway: a population-based repeated cross-sectional analysis. The Lancet Regional Health—Europe. 2021;**4**:100071.
65. **Carr MJ, Steeg S, Webb RT,** et al. Effects of the COVID-19 pandemic on primary care-recorded mental illness and self-harm episodes in the UK: a population-based cohort study. The Lancet Public Health. 2021;**6**(2):e124–35.
66. **Hernández-Calle D, Martínez-Alés G, Mediavilla R, Aguirre P, Rodríguez-Vega B, Bravo-Ortiz MF.** Trends in psychiatric emergency department visits due to suicidal ideation and suicide attempts during the COVID-19 pandemic in Madrid, Spain. Journal of Clinical Psychiatry. 2020;**81**(5):21721.
67. **Hawton K, Casey D, Bale E,** et al. Self-harm during the early period of the COVID-19 pandemic in England: comparative trend analysis of hospital presentations. Journal of Affective Disorders. 2021;**282**:991–5.
68. **Henry N, Parthiban S, Farroha A.** The effect of COVID-19 lockdown on the incidence of deliberate self-harm injuries presenting to the emergency room. International Journal of Psychiatry in Medicine. 2021;**56**(4):266–77.
69. **Shields C, Bernard J, Mirza OI, Reeves D, Wells A, Heagerty A.** Covid-19, lockdown and self-isolation: evaluation of deliberate self-harm admissions. Frontiers in Psychiatry. 2021;**12**:662885.
70. **McAndrew J, O'Leary J, Cotter D,** et al. Impact of initial COVID-19 restrictions on psychiatry presentations to the emergency department of a large academic teaching hospital. Irish Journal of Psychological Medicine. 2021;**38**(2):108–15.
71. **McIntyre A, Tong K, Mcmahon E, Doherty AM.** COVID-19 and its effect on emergency presentations to a tertiary hospital with self-harm in Ireland. Irish Journal of Psychological Medicine. 2021;**38**(2):116–22.
72. **Gesi C, Grasso F, Dragogna F,** et al. How did COVID-19 affect suicidality? Data from a multicentric study in Lombardy. Journal of Clinical Medicine. 2021;**10**(11):2410.
73. **Boldrini T, Girardi P, Clerici M,** et al. Consequences of the COVID-19 pandemic on admissions to general hospital psychiatric wards in Italy: reduced psychiatric hospitalizations and increased suicidality. Progress in Neuro-Psychopharmacology and Biological Psychiatry. 2021;**110**:110304.
74. **Balestrieri M, Rucci P, Amendola D,** et al. Emergency psychiatric consultations during and after the COVID-19 lockdown in Italy. A multicentre study. Frontiers in Psychiatry. 2021;**12**:697058.
75. **Mourouvaye M, Bottemanne H, Bonny G,** et al. Association between suicide behaviours in children and adolescents and the COVID-19 lockdown in Paris, France: a retrospective observational study. Archives of Disease in Childhood. 2021;**106**(9):918–19.
76. **Zalsman G, Levy Y, Sommerfeld E,** et al. Suicide-related calls to a national crisis chat hotline service during the COVID-19 pandemic and lockdown. Journal of Psychiatric Research. 2021;**139**:193–6.
77. **Iob E, Steptoe A, Fancourt D.** Abuse, self-harm and suicidal ideation in the UK during the COVID-19 pandemic. British Journal of Psychiatry. 2020;**217**(4):543–6.

78. **O'Connor RC, Wetherall K, Cleare S**, et al. Mental health and well-being during the COVID-19 pandemic: longitudinal analyses of adults in the UK COVID-19 Mental Health & Wellbeing study. British Journal of Psychiatry. 2021;**218**(6):326–33.
79. **Hyland P, Rochford S, Munnelly A**, et al. Predicting risk along the suicidality continuum: a longitudinal, nationally representative study of the Irish population during the COVID-19 pandemic. Suicide and Life-Threatening Behavior. 2022;**52**(1):83–98.
80. **Bonsaksen T, Skogstad L, Heir T, Ekeberg Ø, Schou-Bredal I, Grimholt TK.** Suicide thoughts and attempts in the Norwegian general population during the early stage of the COVID-19 outbreak. International Journal of Environmental Research and Public Health. 2021;**18**(8):4102.
81. **Winkler P, Formanek T, Mlada K**, et al. Increase in prevalence of current mental disorders in the context of COVID-19: analysis of repeated nationwide cross-sectional surveys. Epidemiology and Psychiatric Sciences. 2020;**29**:1–17.
82. **Papadopoulou A, Efstathiou V, Yotsidi V**, et al. Suicidal ideation during COVID-19 lockdown in Greece: prevalence in the community, risk and protective factors. Psychiatry Research. 2021;**297**:113713.
83. **Fountoulakis KN, Apostolidou MK, Atsiova MB**, et al. Self-reported changes in anxiety, depression and suicidality during the COVID-19 lockdown in Greece. Journal of Affective Disorders. 2021;**279**:624–9.
84. **Leske S, Kõlves K, Crompton D, Arensman E, De Leo D.** Real-time suicide mortality data from police reports in Queensland, Australia, during the COVID-19 pandemic: an interrupted time-series analysis. The Lancet Psychiatry. 2021;**8**(1):58–63.
85. **Zheng X-Y, Tang S-L, Ma S-L**, et al. Trends of injury mortality during the COVID-19 period in Guangdong, China: a population-based retrospective analysis. BMJ Open. 2021;**11**(6):e045317.
86. **Kim AM.** The short-term impact of the COVID-19 outbreak on suicides in Korea. Psychiatry Research. 2021;**295**:113632.
87. **Tanaka T, Okamoto S.** Increase in suicide following an initial decline during the COVID-19 pandemic in Japan. Nature Human Behaviour. 2021;**5**(2):229–38.
88. **Nomura S, Kawashima T, Yoneoka D**, et al. Trends in suicide in Japan by gender during the COVID-19 pandemic, up to September 2020. Psychiatry Research. 2021;**295**:113622.
89. **Osaki Y, Otsuki H, Imamoto A**, et al. Suicide rates during social crises: changes in the suicide rate in Japan after the Great East Japan earthquake and during the COVID-19 pandemic. Journal of Psychiatric Research. 2021;**140**:39–44.
90. **Sakamoto H, Ishikane M, Ghaznavi C, Ueda P.** Assessment of suicide in Japan during the COVID-19 pandemic vs previous years. JAMA Network Open. 2021;**4**(2):e2037378.
91. **Ueda M, Nordström R, Matsubayashi T.** Suicide and mental health during the COVID-19 pandemic in Japan. Journal of Public Health. 2022;44(3):541–8.
92. **Isumi A, Doi S, Yamaoka Y, Takahashi K, Fujiwara T.** Do suicide rates in children and adolescents change during school closure in Japan? The acute effect of the first wave of COVID-19 pandemic on child and adolescent mental health. Child Abuse and Neglect. 2020;**110**:104680.

93. **Jacob S, Mwagiru D, Thakur I, Moghadam A, Oh T, Hsu J.** Impact of societal restrictions and lockdown on trauma admissions during the COVID-19 pandemic: a single-centre cross-sectional observational study. ANZ Journal of Surgery. 2020;**90**(11):2227–31.
94. **Dragovic M, Pascu V, Hall T, Ingram J, Waters F.** Emergency department mental health presentations before and during the COVID-19 outbreak in Western Australia. Australasian Psychiatry. 2020;**28**(6):627–31.
95. **Kasinathan J, Haysom L, Andriotis H,** et al. Keeping COVID out: a collaborative approach to COVID-19 is associated with a significant reduction in self-harm in young people in custody. Australasian Psychiatry. 2021;**29**(4):412–6.
96. **Joyce LR, Richardson SK, McCombie A, Hamilton GJ, Ardagh MW.** Mental health presentations to Christchurch Hospital Emergency Department during COVID-19 lockdown. Emergency Medicine Australasia. 2021;**33**(2):324–30.
97. **Every-Palmer S, Jenkins M, Gendall P,** et al. Psychological distress, anxiety, family violence, suicidality, and wellbeing in New Zealand during the COVID-19 lockdown: a cross-sectional study. PLoS One. 2020;**15**(11):e0241658.
98. **Shi L, Que J-Y, Lu Z-A,** et al. Prevalence and correlates of suicidal ideation among the general population in China during the COVID-19 pandemic. European Psychiatry. 2021;**64**(1):1–29.
99. **Xu X, Wang W, Chen J,** et al. Suicidal and self-harm ideation among Chinese hospital staff during the COVID-19 pandemic: prevalence and correlates. Psychiatry Research. 2021;**296**:113654.
100. **Xu Y, Su S, Jiang Z,** et al. Prevalence and risk factors of mental health symptoms and suicidal behavior among university students in Wuhan, China during the COVID-19 pandemic. Frontiers in Psychiatry. 2021;**12**:695017.
101. **Behera C, Gupta SK, Singh S, Balhara YPS.** Trends in deaths attributable to suicide during COVID-19 pandemic and its association with alcohol use and mental disorders: findings from autopsies conducted in two districts of India. Asian Journal of Psychiatry. 2021;**58**:102597.
102. **Knipe D, Silva T, Aroos A,** et al. Hospital presentations for self-poisoning during COVID-19 in Sri Lanka: an interrupted time-series analysis. The Lancet Psychiatry. 2021;8(10):892–900.
103. **Shrestha R, Siwakoti S, Singh S, Shrestha AP.** Impact of the COVID-19 pandemic on suicide and self-harm among patients presenting to the emergency department of a teaching hospital in Nepal. PLoS One. 2021;**16**(4):e0250706.
104. **Pathare S, Vijayakumar L, Fernandes TN,** et al. Analysis of news media reports of suicides and attempted suicides during the COVID-19 lockdown in India. International Journal of Mental Health Systems. 2020;**14**(88):1–9.
105. **Kar SK, Menon V, Arafat SMY,** et al. Impact of COVID-19 pandemic related lockdown on suicide: analysis of newspaper reports during pre-lockdown and lockdown period in Bangladesh and India. Asian Journal of Psychiatry. 2021;**60**:102649.
106. **Mamun MA, Sakib N, Gozal D,** et al. The COVID-19 pandemic and serious psychological consequences in Bangladesh: a population-based nationwide study. Journal of Affective Disorders. 2021;**279**:462–72.

107. **Tasnim R, Islam MS, Sujan MSH, Sikder MT, Potenza MN.** Suicidal ideation among Bangladeshi university students early during the COVID-19 pandemic: prevalence estimates and correlates. Children and Youth Services Review. 2020;**119**:105703.
108. **Rahman ME, Zubayer AA, Al Mazid Bhuiyan MR, Jobe MC, Ahsan Khan MK.** Suicidal behaviors and suicide risk among Bangladeshi people during the COVID-19 pandemic: an online cross-sectional survey. Heliyon. 2021;**7**(2):e05937.
109. **International Organization for Migration.** *World Migration Report 2020*. Geneva: International Organization for Migration; 2019.
110. **Priebe S, Giacco D, El-Nagib R.** *Public Health Aspects of Mental Health among Migrants and Refugees: A Review of the Evidence on Mental Health Care for Refugees, Asylum Seekers and Irregular Migrants in the WHO European Region*. Copenhagen: World Health Organization, Regional Office for Europe; 2016.
111. **Castañeda H, Holmes SM, Madrigal DS, Young ME, Beyeler N, Quesada J.** Immigration as a social determinant of health. Annual Review of Public Health. 2015;**36**:375–92.
112. **Bambra C, Riordan R, Ford J, Matthews F.** The COVID-19 pandemic and health inequalities. Journal of Epidemiology and Community Health. 2020;**74**:964–8.
113. **Kumar K, Mehra A, Sahoo S, Nehra R, Grover S.** The psychological impact of COVID-19 pandemic and lockdown on the migrant workers: a cross-sectional survey. Asian Journal of Psychiatry. 2020;**53**:102252.
114. **Acharya SR, Moon DH, Chun JH, Shin YC.** COVID-19 and mental health: anxiety disorders among immigrants due to COVID-19 outbreak in South Korea. International Journal of Psychiatry in Medicine. 2022;**57**(4):323–37.
115. **Spiritus-Beerden E, Verelst A, Devlieger I,** et al. Mental health of refugees and migrants during the COVID-19 pandemic: the role of experienced discrimination and daily stressors. International Journal of Environmental Research and Public Health. 2021;**18**(12):6354.
116. **Habtamu K, Desie Y, Asnake M, Lera EG, Mequanint T.** Psychological distress among Ethiopian migrant returnees who were in quarantine in the context of COVID-19: institution-based cross-sectional study. BMC Psychiatry. 2021;**21**(1):424.
117. **Harjana NPA, Januraga PP, Indrayathi PA, Gesesew HA, Ward PR.** Prevalence of depression, anxiety, and stress among repatriated Indonesian migrant workers during the COVID-19 pandemic. Frontiers in Public Health. 2021;**9**:630295.
118. **Benjamen J, Girard V, Jamani S,** et al. Access to refugee and migrant mental health care services during the first six months of the COVID-19 pandemic: a Canadian refugee clinician survey. International Journal of Environmental Research and Public Health. 2021;**18**(10):5266.
119. **Júnior JG, Moreira MM, Pinheiro WR,** et al. The mental health of those whose rights have been taken away: an essay on the mental health of indigenous peoples in the face of the 2019 coronavirus (2019-nCoV) outbreak. Psychiatry Research. 2020;**289**:113094.
120. **Clifford AC, Doran CM, Tsey K.** A systematic review of suicide prevention interventions targeting indigenous peoples in Australia, United States, Canada and New Zealand. BMC Public Health. 2013;**13**(1):463.
121. **Faruk MO, Ching U, Chowdhury KUA.** Mental health and well-being of indigenous people during the COVID-19 pandemic in Bangladesh. Heliyon. 2021;**7**(7):e07582.

122. **Newby JM, O'Moore K, Tang S, Christensen H, Faasse K.** Acute mental health responses during the COVID-19 pandemic in Australia. PLoS One. 2020;**15**(7):e0236562.
123. **Lawal MA, Shalaby R, Chima C**, et al. COVID-19 pandemic: stress, anxiety, and depression levels highest amongst indigenous peoples in Alberta. Behavioral Sciences. 2021;**11**(9):115.
124. **Canadian Mental Health Association** (2020). Despair and suicidal feelings deepen as pandemic wears on. Available from: https://cmha.ca/despair-and-suicidal-feelings-deepen-as-pandemic-wears-on/
125. **Reardon S** (2020). Health officials fear COVID-19 pandemic-related suicide spike among indigenous youth. Available from: https://time.com/5921715/indigenous-youth-suicide-covid-19/
126. **Olivia S** (2021). 'We don't want any more tears': First Nations urge Ottawa to boost mental health. Available from: https://www.cbc.ca/news/politics/indigenous-mental-health-resources-federal-budget-2021-1.5989070
127. **Kõlves K, Kõlves KE, De Leo D.** Natural disasters and suicidal behaviours: a systematic literature review. Journal of Affective Disorders. 2013;**146**(1):1–14.
128. **Clemente-Suárez VJ, Navarro-Jiménez E, Jimenez M**, et al. Impact of COVID-19 pandemic in public mental health: an extensive narrative review. Sustainability. 2021;**13**(6):3221.
129. **Rauschenberg C, Schick A, Hirjak D**, et al. Evidence synthesis of digital interventions to mitigate the negative impact of the COVID-19 pandemic on public mental health: rapid meta-review. Journal of Medical Internet Research. 2021;**23**(3):e23365.
130. **Kohn R, Saxena S, Levav I, Saraceno B.** The treatment gap in mental health care. Bulletin of the World Health Organization. 2004;**82**(11):858–66.
131. **Monteith LL, Holliday R, Brown TL, Brenner LA, Mohatt NV.** Preventing suicide in rural communities during the COVID-19 pandemic. Journal of Rural Health. 2021;**37**(1):179–84.

Part 5

Prevention concepts and programs

Chapter 22

National strategies and plans for the prevention of suicide

José Manoel Bertolote

Introduction

Suicide is a phenomenon that has been a companion to mankind since its dawn. In fact, in most, if not all, ancient texts dealing with cosmology, one can find references to what is now referred to as suicide. Nevertheless, a common word to designate it, at least in Europe, appeared only in the mid-seventeenth century.

In 1643, Thomas Browne published, in Latin, *Religio Medici*[1] (*The Religion of a Doctor*), and when discussing the moral implications of Cato's death, he coined in Greek the neologism *autofonos* (murder of oneself). Given the wide acclaim of that book, both in England and elsewhere, in 1645, it was published in an English translation, however while retaining its now famous Latin title,[2] in which *autofonos* was translated to *suicide*; thereafter, suicide was a staple word translated into many other languages.

Before Browne's book, many other ancient texts had dealt with this concept (e.g. *Gilgamesh*, *Mahabharata*, the *Ancient Testament*, old texts from Assyria, Babylon, and Egypt, not to mention the classic Greek literature), in which suicide was always taking place among heroes, philosophers, and members of the nobility. No reports of suicide in commoners are found in those texts, to a large extent because commoners were not frequent characters therein.

However, in Europe at least, from the Middle Ages onwards, suicide lost its aura of nobility and started to be reported in growing numbers in people of all classes.[3] It increased so much that the World Health Organization (WHO) estimated that about 877,000 cases of deaths from suicide took place in 2002 worldwide, of which 549,000 were males and 328,000 were females.[4] By 2021, that estimation had decreased to 700,000 deaths per year worldwide;[5] it is assumed that the observed reduction was due to effective measures adopted and implemented in some countries.

Although there are references to initiatives aimed at the prevention of suicide since the beginning of the twentieth century, these bloomed among private humanitarian, philanthropic, or religious agencies such as the Save-a-Life League in New York and the Salvation Army in London.[5] Only by the end of the twentieth century, intergovernmental organizations, such as the United Nations (UN) and the WHO, got involved in the matter.

Role of international governmental organizations: the UN and the WHO

In 1996, the UN published a seminal document jointly produced by the WHO and the Economic and Social Council (ECOSOC) of the UN on *Suicide Prevention: Guidelines for the Formulation and Implementation of National Strategies*.[6] In this document, suicide was recognized as a major 'social and economic problem affecting several nations'.

The document was the product of a meeting organized in 1993 by the UN and the WHO, held in Calgary and Banff, Canada, with participants and observers from 13 countries (Australia, Canada, China, Estonia, Finland, India, Hungary, Japan, the Netherlands, Nigeria, Sweden, United States, and United Arab Emirates). It was the first time that such respected and authoritative international agencies as the UN and the WHO declared, based on the best evidence available at the time, that suicide was indeed a major public health problem that deserved not only sanitary, but also political, attention.[8]

Already in 1986, the 39th World Health Assembly (WHA) had adopted Resolution WHA39.25 on *Prevention of Mental, Neurological and Psychosocial Disorders*,[8] giving a mandate to the WHO Secretariat to develop programmes related to this extremely broad topic. However, no specific disorders were mentioned in this Resolution, and it was evident that not all mental, neurological, and psychosocial disorders could be prevented, which left the WHO Secretariat with the thorny question of deciding where to begin.

Given the worrisome numbers of deaths by suicide and the WHA Resolution, in 1989, the WHO selected suicide as one of the psychosocial disorders that needed to be addressed. Following a series of working groups to examine the existing evidence on effective interventions to reduce the impact of suicide, in 1998, a technical publication was published that included suicide as one example of a psychosocial disorder that could be prevented.[9]

While complying with Resolution WHA39.25, and considering that *all* mental, neurological, and psychosocial disorders could *not* be prevented, this technical publication opted to give but a few examples of such conditions for which some form of prevention was known at the time—among them, suicide.

The five specific interventions identified to be effective for the prevention of suicide were:

- Treatment of mental disorders;
- Gun control;
- Gas detoxification;
- Control of toxic substances;
- Responsible media reporting.

Of these, as only treatment of mental disorders was clearly and directly health-related, another novel strategy had to be identified.

Countries with a suicide prevention strategy

In 2013, the WHO, together with the International Association for Suicide Prevention (IASP), conducted a survey of 157 countries which had IASP associated members to identify how many, and which, of the countries had national strategies for prevention of suicide. Responses were obtained from 90 countries (57%); however, when considering the number of WHO Member States, the global coverage was nearly only 30%.[10]

Suicide was perceived as a significant public health problem in 55 countries (61%, but equivalent to 28% of WHO Member States); however, only 35 (39%) of responding countries (18% of WHO Member States) had a national standalone strategy or action plan for prevention of suicide. Another 22 (24%) countries (11% of WHO Member States) had some suicide prevention activities integrated into their general or mental health programme (e.g. India, Russian Federation, Spain, Uganda, Vanuatu), or had suicide prevention programmes available at a regional level only (e.g. Belgium) or for specific populations (e.g. Croatia, Italy).

Table 22.1 shows the distribution of these countries, according to WHO Regional Offices. It is worth nothing that all countries included in Table 22.1 developed their strategy or action plan after the publication of the 1996 UN document mentioned previously. This might help us to hope that there are more countries that are WHO Member States with formal suicide prevention strategies than the 29% identified in the WHO-IASP survey.[1]

In 55 (61%) of the responding countries, suicide was perceived to be a significant public health concern. Within the different WHO regions, this varied from 20 (77%) responding countries in the European Region to two (29%) in the South East Asia Region.

[1] This might well be the case, as at least Brazil and Finland, to the author's knowledge, have national strategies for prevention of suicide and were not among respondents to the WHO-IASP survey.

Table 22.1 Countries with a national stand-alone suicide prevention strategy or action plan, or other type of activity related to prevention of suicidal behaviours[11]

	National stand-alone suicide prevention strategy or action plan	Other, non specific actions
WHO region	**Country**	
Africa	Namibia	Chad
		Mozambique
		Uganda
Americas	Argentina	Canada
	Chile	Ecuador
	Costa Rica	El Salvador
	Cuba	
	Dominican Republic	
	Nicaragua	
	Panama	
	Suriname	
	United States	
	Uruguay	
Eastern Mediterranean	Afghanistan	
	Iran	
Europe	Austria	Belgium
	Belarus	Croatia
	Bulgaria	Germany
	France	Italy
	Israel	Monaco
	Lithuania	Romania
	Luxembourg	Russian Federation
	Netherlands	Slovakia
	Norway	Spain
	Portugal	Turkey
	Sweden	
	Switzerland	
	Germany	
	United Kingdom	
	Uzbekistan	

Table 22.1 Continued

	National stand-alone suicide prevention strategy or action plan	Other, non specific actions
WHO region	**Country**	
South East Asia	Buthan	India
	Sri Lanka	
	Thailand	
Western Pacific	Australia	Cook Islands
	Fiji	Marshall Islands
	Japan	Philippines
	Korea	Timor-Leste
	Malaysia	Vanuatu
	New Zealand	

In 28 (31%) of the responding countries, a comprehensive national strategy or action plan was adopted by the government (see Table 22.2). In the vast majority of countries, this has developed since 2000. Of all the countries in the world, only 38 have a national suicide prevention strategy, according to the WHO report from 2018, which is perhaps not enough.[11]

Possible reasons why not more countries have a strategy for prevention of suicide

Surely there is no single and simple answer to that big question. Nevertheless, several hypotheses can be raised.

Complexity of the nature of the task

As one can see from Table 22.1, the majority of countries with a suicide prevention strategy are high-income countries (HICs). Although they represent about 18% of the world population, they have 24% of world's suicides. In HICs, deaths from other non-natural causes are relatively less common than in low- and middle-income countries (LMICs), which thus increases the prominence of deaths from suicide. On the other hand, in most LMICs, deaths due to accidents and homicides are more frequent than deaths from suicide, particularly among young people, which therefore prioritizes the former group over deaths from suicide.

However, perhaps a major obstacle to governments putting in place a strategy for prevention of suicide lies in the complexity of the strategy itself. According to the 1996 UN document,[7] the aim of such a national strategy would be 'to

Table 22.2 Typical components of national strategies

Component	Goals and objectives
Surveillance	Increases the quality and timeliness of national data collection on suicide and suicide attempts. Supports the establishment of an integrated data collection system which serves to identify vulnerable groups, individuals, and situations
Means restriction	Reduces the availability, accessibility, and attractiveness of the means of suicide (e.g. pesticides, firearms, high places). Reduces toxicity/lethality of available means
Media	Promote implementation of media guidelines to support responsible media reporting of suicide in print, broadcasting, and social media
Access to services	Promotes increased access to comprehensive services for those vulnerable to suicidal behaviours. Removes barriers to care
Training and education	Maintain comprehensive training programmes for identified gatekeepers (e.g. health workers, educators, police). Improve the competencies of mental health and primary care providers in the recognition and treatment of vulnerable persons
Treatment	Improves the quality of clinical care and evidence-based clinical interventions, especially for individuals who present to hospital following a suicide attempt. Improves research and evaluation of effective interventions
Crisis intervention	Ensures that communities have the capacity to respond to crises with appropriate interventions and that individuals in a crisis situation have access to emergency mental health care, including through telephone helplines or the Internet
Postvention	Improves response to, and caring for, those affected by suicide and suicide attempts. Provides support to persons affected by suicide attempts
Awareness	Establishes public information campaigns to support the understanding that suicides are preventable. Increases public and professional access to information on all aspects of preventing suicidal behaviour
Stigma reduction	Promotes the use of mental health services, and services for prevention of substance abuse and suicide. Reduces discrimination against people using these services
Oversight and coordination	Establish institutions or agencies to promote and coordinate research, training, and service delivery in respect of suicidal behaviours. Strengthen the health and social system response to suicidal behaviours

promote, coordinate and support culturally appropriate intersectorial programmes for the prevention of suicidal behaviour at the national, regional and local levels'. It goes on to identifying the types of activities and approaches that could support the achievement of national strategy goals:

1. Developing a nation-specific conceptual framework for implementing, monitoring, and evaluating suicide intervention programmes that address the specifics of the problem and fit the unique characteristics of the country;
2. Adopting a standard taxonomy for suicidal behaviour;
3. Promoting early identification, assessment, treatment, and referral of persons at risk of suicidal behaviour for appropriate health care;
4. Increasing public and professional access to information about all aspects of preventing suicidal behaviour;
5. Promoting and/or supporting the establishment of an integrated data collection system which serves to identify at-risk groups, individuals, situations, and settings associated with life-threatening behaviour;
6. Promoting public awareness with regard to issues of mental well-being, suicidal behaviour, the consequences of stress, and effective crisis management;
7. Developing or maintaining a comprehensive training programme for identified gatekeepers (e.g. police, educators, clergy, primary health care providers, mental health professionals);
8. Where indicated, adopting culture-appropriate protocols for public reporting of suicidal events;
9. Promoting greater access to comprehensive services for those at risk of, or affected by, the full range of suicidal behaviours;
10. Providing supporting and rehabilitation services to persons affected by suicidal behaviour: those at risk of, or who have attempted, suicide, their family, friends, colleagues, and other relations;
11. Reducing the availability, accessibility, and attractiveness of the means for suicidal behaviour;
12. Identifying and/or establishing institutions or agencies to promote and coordinate research, training, and service delivery with respect to suicidal behaviour;
13. Developing or modifying relevant legislation and administrative regulations to facilitate the implementation of national objectives.[7]

This is a very comprehensive list of activities, to which, from today's perspective, one can hardly add anything further, except perhaps mentioning the importance of addressing also the role of protective factors against—in addition to risk factors for—suicidal behaviours.[12]

Also, according to the 1996 UN document,[7] the mandate of this person/agency/organization, in addition to formulating a national strategy, includes also the development, implementation, and coordination of activities leading to the prevention of suicide, by means of:

1. Surveillance, to monitor the problem;
2. Basic research, to identify risk factors;
3. Programme development, to develop intervention programmes and services; and
4. Evaluation research, to develop means to test the effectiveness of interventions.

Further to the 1996 UN document, and in line with the 39th WHA, in 1999, the WHO established a specific Suicide Prevention (SUPRE) programme, which aimed at producing—within its limitations of financial and personnel resources, but with the invaluable support from experts from around the world, relevant non-governmental organizations, and WHO Collaborating Centres—technical resources that address each of the above-listed activities.

Aiming to assist WHO Member States in adopting and implementing their national suicide prevention strategies and programmes, the WHO Department of Mental Health produced a series of technical documents and resources, improved the analysis of national suicide mortality data, periodically updated information on risk factors—and initiated systematic information gathering of protective factors—and developed a multisite intervention research programme aimed at identifying effective means to reduce suicidal behaviours in people who have already attempted suicide.[13] Additionally effort, a recent WHO technical document[14] updated and elaborated on the typical components of national strategies, as indicated in Table 22.2.

Of major importance is the advice from the 1996 UN document that governments should provide 'the coordinating body with the executive, financial and technical resources that will enable it to carry out its formulation and implementation responsibilities effectively and efficiently'.[7]

Effectiveness and cost-effectiveness of suicide prevention programmes

Platt et al.[15] aptly remarked that the paucity of published studies or reports on the effectiveness and cost-effectiveness of national strategies for the prevention of suicide could be a problem in this respect.

One of the reasons for such paucity could be the same complexity and diversity of components of most national strategies for the prevention of suicide mentioned earlier.[16]

Most studies have focused on one or few of these components, thus compromising whichever overall conclusion on this topic. Nevertheless, there are several robust studies on the effectiveness of those national strategies, but less so on their cost-effectiveness.

For instance, Zalsman et al.,[17] in their review of 1797 studies, including 23 systematic reviews, 12 meta-analyses, 40 randomized controlled trials (RCTs), 67 cohort trials, and 22 ecological or population-based investigations, concluded that 'no single strategy clearly stands above the others' and that 'the paucity of RCTs is a major limitation in the evaluation of preventive interventions'. They also rated the strength of evidence of the reviewed strategies by using the Oxford criteria,[19] which is summarized in Table 22.3.

One example of the complexity mentioned here is given by measurement of the component Helpline support. Its strength varies from very high for people attempting suicide in an RCT[20] to low in a cohort study of crisis line callers,[21] and to very low in another study of crisis line callers.[22]

By using a different approach—a segmented regression analysis of interrupted time series data, Lewitzka et al.[23] analysed outcomes in four countries which launched a national suicide prevention strategy in the late 1990s (Australia, Finland, Norway, and Sweden), compared to four control countries without such strategies (Austria, Canada, Denmark, and Switzerland) over 30 years (from 22 years before the launch of the national suicide prevention strategy to six years after its launch). Their main conclusion was that 'the implementation of a national strategy is an effective tool to reduce suicide rates'; however, it correlated with sex and age. More specifically, the reduction was significant for males of all ages, except those aged 65 years and older for whom there was also a reduction, albeit non-significant. The same effect was observed for females.

A different picture emerges with respect to studies on the cost-effectiveness of national strategies for prevention of suicide. As noted by McDaid and Kennelly,[24] one of the difficulties associated with these studies derives from the fact that in order to conduct them, both the specific cost of each type of specific interventions (not to mention the complexity of combined community-based interventions)[25] and the direct and indirect costs of suicide must be obtained.

One of the few—now classic—examples of evaluation of the cost-effectiveness of a suicide prevention strategy is the study reported in 2003 by Zaloshnja et al.[26] Despite its limitations (focused primarily on indigenous young people from a New Mexico jurisdictions), it showed cost savings of US$1.7 million, with

Table 22.3 Strength of evidence for some components of suicide prevention strategies

Component of suicide prevention strategies	Strength of evidence
Brief intervention in emergency room and follow-up contact	Very high
Restricting access to lethal means	High
Restricting access to hotspots for suicide by jumping	High
School-based awareness programme	High*
Anti-suicidal effects of clozapine and lithium	High
Treatments of depression	High
Screening in primary care and education of physicians	Insufficient evidence
General public education	Insufficient evidence
Media guidelines	Insufficient evidence
Gatekeeper training	Insufficient evidence
Internet and helpline support	Insufficient evidence

* For suicidal ideation and suicide attempts only.

highly cost-effective benefits of 43 times greater than costs incurred. The programmes evaluated included community education programmes, peer training of young people, postvention, and suicide risk screening.

Given the complexity of components of national strategies for prevention of suicide, what can be found more frequently is evaluation of single components of strategies, such as case-control economic evaluation of a specific brief therapy for individuals who attempted suicide conducted in Switzerland[26] or of the use of a particular class of antidepressant medication for people with depression conducted in the United States.[27]

Both studies used quite distinct methodologies. The Swiss case-control study found that psychiatric hospital costs and total health care costs were lower, albeit not significantly, in the brief intervention group, whereas general hospital costs were significantly lower in the brief intervention group, as compared to the control group. The US study found that the cost per statistical life saved from increasing the use of a particular class of antidepressant was around US$20,000.

At any rate, studies like these do not address the full complexity of evaluating the cost-effectiveness of a complete national strategy for prevention of suicide. However, in McDaid and Kennelly's words:[23] 'The limited evidence available to date would suggest that investment in effective interventions is likely to be hghly cost-effective compared with other uses of public resources.'

Locus of responsibility

A critical issue for the adoption and implementation of a national strategy for prevention of suicide is the identification of the person/agency/organization that will champion it—that is, that will be entrusted with the responsibility of transforming its objectives into reality.

More often that not, the locus of responsibility for suicide prevention in the government structure falls upon the health (or, more precisely, the mental health) sector—after all, WHO's correspondents are usually ministries of health. However, according to the WHO, the list of stakeholders relevant to the development of national prevention strategies include quite diversified sectors and disciplines, well beyond the health sector, as shown in Figure 22.1.[28]

It is clear from the range of stakeholders indicated in Figure 22.1 that it is not an easy task to identify where, in the specific administration of each country, management of suicide prevention programmes should be placed. So much so that in a few countries, this function has been given to civil society agencies and/or organizations directly interested in suicide prevention.[29] Furthermore, in some countries with a federal, decentralized political organization, the adopted strategy or action does not cover the whole country, but one or more regions (state, province, land, canton, etc.) that are more particularly affected by, or interested in, suicidal behaviours.

The diversification mentioned earlier could well be another hypothesis to explain why more countries are reluctant to adopt a national strategy or plan to prevent suicide, despite acknowledging the importance of the problem.

Conclusion

It should be clear by now that the 1996 UN document on guidelines for the formulation and implementation of national strategies for prevention of suicide[7] (or rather the 1993 Calgary–Banff UN-WHO meeting from which the document originated) was a turning point in the history of global prevention of suicide. Despite documented reports on suicide since the beginning of history, and the worrisome rise in the number of suicides since the Middle Ages in Europe, there was no known concerted action at national level until the publication of the 1996 UN document, and more specifically after 2000, when the WHO established SUPRE and the publication of several technical documents on the same topic.[15] These two actions combined served as a wake-up call to governments concerned with avoidable losses of so many lives to suicide.

Yet, there are still many countries with very high suicide-related mortality incidence and rates that have not yet taken any effective measures to change this sad situation. The amount of WHO technical documents and the availability

Health

Social

Welfare

Education

Employment

Legislation

Agriculture

Transport

Law enforcement

Defense

Private sector

Parliamentarians

Health/Mental health professionals

Nongovernmental organizations

Professional associations

Media

Researchers

Communities and volunteers

Vulnerable groups

Survivors and families

Traditional healers

Spiritual and religious leaders

Figure 22.1 Disciplines and sectors relevant to the development of a national prevention strategies.[29]

of technical assistance from both WHO staff and its network of experts from around the world leave no room for excuses for inaction.

Admittedly, we—especially in LMICs—are far from the utopian idea that governments should be ruled by wisdom and knowledge (which might be true in very few of HICs only). In most instances, immediate interests and strategies determine the course of action of governments, however democratic they might be.

At any rate, hundreds of thousands of lives continue to be unnecessarily lost every year, no matter the amount of culturally appropriate frameworks, guidelines, and technical information there might be. They lay around waiting for articulated advocacy from societies and a grain of political will from governments.

References

1. **Browne T.** Religio Medici. 1643. Available from: https://books.google.com/books
2. **Browne T.** *Religio Medici*. Cambridge: Cambridge University Press; 2008.
3. **Minois G.** *Histoire du suicide*. Paris: Fayard; 1995.
4. **Bertolote JM, Fleischmann A.** A global perspective of the magnitude of suicide mortality. In: **Wasserman D, Wasserman C**, editors. *Oxford Textbook of Suicidology and Suicide Prevention*. Oxford: Oxford University Press; 2009. pp. 91–8.
5. **World Health Organization** (2023). Suicide. Available from: https://www.who.int/news-room/fact-sheets/detail/suicide
6. **United Nations**. *Suicide Prevention: Guidelines for the Formulation and Implementation of National Strategies*. New York, NY: United Nations; 1996.
7. **Bertolote JM.** Suicide prevention: at what level does it work? *World Psychiatry*. 2004;**3**(3):147–51.
8. **United Nations**. *Suicide Prevention: Guidelines for the Formulation and Implementation of National Strategies*. New York, NY: United Nations; 1996.
9. **Bertolote JM.** Prevention of suicidal behaviors. In: **Nock MK**, editor. *Oxford Handbook of Suicide and Self-Injury*. Oxford: Oxford University Press; 2014. pp. 355–65.
10. **World Health Assembly, 39** (1986). Prevention of mental, neurological and psychosocial disorders. Geneva: World Health Organization. Available from: https://apps.who.int/iris/handle/10665/163186
11. **World Health Organization** (1998). Primary prevention of mental, neurological and psychosocial disorders. Geneva: World Health Organization. Available from: https://apps.who.int/iris/handle/10665/42043
12. **World Health Organization**. *National Suicide Prevention Strategies: Progress, Examples and Indicators*. Geneva: World Health Organization; 2018.
13. **Bertolote JM.** Primary prevention of mental disorders. In: **Gelder MG, Andreasen N, Lopez-Ibor JJ, Geddes J**, editors. *New Oxford Textbook of Psychiatry*, Volume **2**. Oxford: Oxford University Press; 2012. pp. 1446–51.
14. **Fleischmann A, Bertolote JM, De Leo D, Wasserman D.** Instruments used in the SUPRE-MISS: the WHO multisite intervention study on suicidal behaviours. In: **Wassermam D, Wasserman C**, editors. *Oxford Textbook of Suicidology and Suicide Prevention*. Oxford: Oxford University Press; 2009. pp 313–18.
15. **World Health Organization**. *Preventing Suicide: A Global Imperative*. Geneva: World Health Organization; 2014.
16. **Platt S, Arensman E, Rezaeian M.** National suicide prevention strategies: progress and challenges. Crisis. 2019;**40**:75–82.
17. **Turecki G.** Preventing suicide: where are we? The Lancet Psychiatry. 2016;**3**:597–8.
18. **Zalsman G, Hawton K, Wasserman D**, et al. Suicide prevention strategies revisited: 10-year systematic review. The Lancet Psychiatry. 2016;**3**:646–59.

19. **Oxford Centre for Evidence-Based Medicine** (2009). Levels of evidence. Available from: http://www.cebm.net/oxford-centre-evidence-based-medicine-levels-evidence-march-2009/
20. **Marasinghe RB, Edirippulige S, Kavanagh D, Smith A, Jiffry MT.** Effect of mobile phone-based psychotherapy in suicide prevention: a randomized controlled trial in Sri Lanka. Journal of Telemedicine and Telecare. 2012;**18**:151–5.
21. **Gould MS, Munfakh JL, Kleinman M, Lake AM.** National suicide prevention lifeline: enhancing mental health care for suicidal individuals and other people in crisis. Suicide and Life-Threatening Behavior. 2012;**42**:22–35.
22. **Mishara BL, Chagnon F, Daigle M,** et al. Which helper behaviors and intervention styles are related to better short-term outcomes in telephone crisis intervention? Results from a silent monitoring study of calls to the U.S. 1-800-SUICIDE Network. Suicide and Life-Threatening Behavior. 2007;**37**:308–21.
23. **Lewitzka U, Sauer C, Bauer M, Felber W.** Are national suicide prevention programs effective? A comparison of 4 verum and 4 control countries over 30 years. BMC Psychiatry. 2019;**19**:158–68.
24. **McDaid D, Kennelly B.** An economic perspective on suicide across the five continents. In: **Wasserman D, Wasserman C**, editors. *Oxford Textbook on Suicidology and Suicide Prevention*. Oxford: Oxford University Press; 2009. pp. 359–67.
25. **Beautrais A.** National strategies for the reduction and prevention of suicide. Crisis. 2005;**26**:1–3.
26. **Zaloshnja E, Miller TR, Galbraith MS,** et al. Reducing injuries among Native Americans: five cost–outcome analyses. Accident Analysis and Prevention. 2003;**35**:631–9.
27. **Park AL, Gysin-Maillart A, Müller TJ, Exadaktylos A, Michel K.** Cost-effectiveness of a brief structured intervention program aimed at preventing repeat suicide attempts among those who previously attempted suicide: a secondary analysis of the ASSIP randomized clinical trial. JAMA Network Open. 2018;**1**(6):e183680.
28. **Ludwig J, Marcotte K** (2007). Anti-depressants and suicide. National Bureau of Economic Research Working Paper No. 12906. Available from: https://www.nber.org/system/files/working_papers/w12906/w12906.pdf
29. **World Health Organization**. *Public Health Action for the Prevention of Suicide: A Framework*. Geneva: World Health Organization; 2012.

Chapter 23

Mass media and suicide in low- and middle-income countries: Learnings from India

Gregory Armstrong and Lakshmi Vijayakumar

Introduction

Responsible media reporting of suicides has been identified as a promising and potentially effective population-level suicide prevention intervention.[1,2] While further research on the impact of media-based interventions is needed, the focus on media portrayals of suicide is based on evidence around copycat suicides, dissemination of suicide methods and behaviours, and the imperative to deliver tailored suicide prevention messaging in media content.[3,4,5,6] There are also important concerns based on observations that media can present simplistic monocausal explanations for suicide and can selectively present 'newsworthy' stories that do not reflect the broader array of suicide events in the population, thus impacting the public's knowledge and beliefs about suicide.[7] Empirical research has also observed that the way in which media reports about suicide are worded and framed can influence the public's knowledge, beliefs, and attitudes about suicide.[8,9,10]

Consequently, the World Health Organization (WHO) has prescribed guidelines for responsible media reporting of suicide.[11] However, implementation of the guidelines has been varied, with minimal take-up in low-resource settings where care and nuance are required to ensure successful local implementation.

Media research gap in low- and middle-income countries and why it matters

Despite a majority of suicides occurring in low- and middle-income countries (LMICs), suicide research is predominantly undertaken in high-income countries (HICs), which is not surprising, given the wide global disparity in resources to devote to research. A scientometric analysis of suicide research published between 1990 and 2018 observed that approximately 60% of suicide studies were published by 10 countries, all HICs, and almost a third of outputs were published by the United States; further, the analysis observed that India produced 1.5% of suicide research, yet it accounts for over a quarter of global suicides.[12,13] The same gap applies to research specifically focused on media and suicide. For example, a recent meta-analysis on the association between media reports of suicides and subsequent suicides in the population did manage to incorporate findings from a diverse range of countries, yet it was exclusively based on findings from high-income settings;[14] the authors were clearly not at fault—they were simply drawing on the available high-quality evidence. While there is an extensive history of media and suicide research in countries like the United States, Australia, Canada, Japan, and Austria, media and suicide research is in its infancy in most LMIC settings where contemporary studies primarily focus on performing formative content analysis research (i.e. how does media report on suicide in our country?) that was undertaken several years ago in many HICs. It is a game of catch-up on limited resources, impeded by the limited availability of reliable suicide data in LMICs.

Why is this research gap important? Given that the drivers of suicide vary across nations,[15] and across regions within nations, the implementation of suicide prevention strategies will also need to vary and such strategies benefit from quality local evidence. It is unlikely this point needs to be further laboured in a book such as this, but this is not just an issue of low resources. Local culture plays an important role in suicidal phenomena, with culture contributing significantly to the occurrence, patterns, and responses to suicidal behaviour in a society.[15] Culture also influences the way in which suicide is understood and represented. From historical representations of suicide in Kabuki theatre in Japan to narratives around suicide in ancient Hindu texts in India, various forms of media and cultural and religious texts have long represented suicide in a variety of ways across cultures. This diversity is not simply a cause for anthropological curiosity; it is as much about contemporary representations as it is about historical representations and sometimes the connection between the two. The way in which contemporary mass media represents suicide across settings, and the way in which suicide stories/narratives are produced and consumed, remains integral, rather than incidental, to localized approaches to the development and implementation of media-based suicide prevention guidelines and interventions.

Some learnings from India

South East Asia accounts for approximately 40% of suicide deaths globally and is the frontline for delivering on the aspirational Sustainable Development Goal (SDG) of a one-third reduction in suicide rate by 2030. Suicide rates in

India are among the highest in the world. The most recent suicide rate estimates ranged between 18 and 21 deaths per 100,000 population (cf. 11 per 100,000 globally), resulting in an estimated 230,000–250,000 suicide deaths annually, which equate to approximately 28% of global suicides (cf. approximately 17% of the world population).[12,13] Under-reporting of suicide is ubiquitous in official suicide statistics,[16] and suicide rates and methods vary substantially across regions.[17,18,19] A public health approach to suicide prevention is gaining momentum in India, with calls for the development of national-, state-, and community-level suicide prevention plans and strategies.[20] As an indication of this momentum, the first national suicide prevention strategy is in the final stages of development and the Press Council of India has adopted the WHO guidelines for media reporting of suicide.

In response to the above-mentioned gap in suicide and media research, we have undertaken multidisciplinary research on suicide and media in the middle-income country of India. Below we present some of the learnings from our research that may assist others in thinking through this issue in other LMICs. While our research in this area is still evolving and growing, the learnings discussed below are based on our content analysis of media reports,[21] epidemiological analyses,[22,23] and qualitative interviews with media professionals.[24,25] All methodological queries can be referred to these source articles.

Suicide as clickbait in a competitive mass media market

Before embarking on engagement with mass media on the issue of suicide reporting, it is important to get an understanding of the mass media marketplace and how it may be impacting on suicide reporting. The mass media market in India has observed exponential growth and diversification in the number of mass media outlets since the market was privatised in the late 1990s.[26] While other countries have observed a decline in print media, India has maintained steady annual growth in terms of publications and income.[27] Competition is fierce to attract lucrative advertising revenue, with global commercial interests in the huge number of potential consumers in India and the rapidly expanding middle class aspiring to a 'Western' lifestyle.[28] As in many countries, this has seen a rapid expansion of a 24/7 breaking news culture. In alignment with this, suicide reporting is intertwined with commercial competitiveness in India, with media professionals articulating that 'deaths make news' and that suicide stories are frequently 'clickbait', drawing in readers with sensationalized content.[24] The 24/7 breaking news culture can result in a high level of competition for exclusive and detailed updates in relation to suicides of high interest to the audience, creating drama and giving the suicide a high profile. Media reports occur before post-mortems have been concluded, with emphasis on the speed of breaking news rather than on accuracy.

The media market is also deeply influenced by the diversity of cultures and languages in India, with strong audience demand for a wide array of local/regional news channels catering to diverse languages and tastes.[26] In connection with this, our research observed that suicide stories in the Indian media are overwhelmingly about incidents that are geographically local to the readership base of the publication, rather than about incidents from elsewhere in the country or the world.[22] For example, over 80% of suicide stories in major newspapers in Tamil Nadu are about suicides in Tamil Nadu. This is important and speaks to the way in which suicide news is being produced at a very local level. It may also have implications for concerns around imitation suicide if audiences more closely identify with suicidal people from their local area and cultural and linguistic background.

Assessing the quality of media reporting against international guidelines

An essential early step in the process of engaging on the issue of media and suicide is to gain a thorough understanding as to whether the mass media are covering suicide news in alignment with international guidelines.[11] Our content analysis study of approximately 1600 suicide reports in Southern India found that, on average, newspapers were reporting one suicide incident per day, providing a daily diet of suicide news to their readers.[21] These suicide reports were typically short, explicit in their detail of suicide methods, repetitive, and simplistic. Compared to the WHO suicide reporting guidelines, it was clear that a high proportion of these media reports carried content that was potentially harmful. Key concerns were the high proportions of articles reporting detail that may create risks related to imitation suicides, as well as information that simplifies the reasons for suicide. For example, it was common for articles to report: the suicide method (93%); specific detail around the suicide method (43%); information on public locations where suicide incidents had taken place (8%) that could become the next location for a suicide cluster; and simplistic single-cause explanations for suicide (53%) that impede suicide literacy as well as provide audience members with a model for how people in their community respond to issues in their life such as unemployment and marital breakdown. The high frequency of suicide articles and harmful reporting characteristics that we observed is generally consistent with concerns that adherence to guidelines is particularly low in Asia where suicide deaths are highly newsworthy events.[29,30,31,32]

The suicide-related articles we examined did little to educate the public about the issue of suicide, consolidating findings from a small prior study of newspapers in the city of Bangalore.[33] Very few articles contained expert opinions from health professionals, research findings, suicide statistics, or information about suicide prevention programmes, all of which are useful ways to educate the public about the issue of suicide and to inform that help is available for those in crisis. Very few articles reported in a way that served to dispel the myths that there is nothing you can do to prevent suicide and that there are no preceding warning signs. This is an unfortunate missed opportunity, considering that a recent household survey in a major South Indian city found that over 50% of people believe in the myth that 'suicide happens without warning'.[34] Similarly, few articles recognized the link between poor mental health and drug/alcohol abuse with suicidality, both of which are major risk factors for suicide.[35,36,37,38,39,40] and something that is a challenge to address in India where mental health literacy is low and stigmatizing attitudes are prominent.[41,42,43]

We have subsequently collaborated on the development of a scorecard tool for assessing the quality of suicide reports in the Indian media,[44] the results of which are providing an ongoing and publicly available update on media performance according to international guidelines. We have collaborated on content analysis work from the neighbouring countries of Bangladesh and Sri Lanka,[45,46] which has also observed similar challenges in the current approach to media reporting, indicating some potential value in regional collaborative networks to develop common solutions to common problems.

Impact of colonial legacies of suicide criminality on media reporting

In many countries, including India, it is relevant to reflect on the impact of colonial legacies with regard to attitudes and policies related to suicide, and on how this may impact media reporting. It is critical to note that until early 2017, 'attempt to commit suicide' was a crime under the Indian Penal Code, as formulated by the British Raj[47] and as has been the case in many former British colonies. Consistent with this, it is often crime journalists who report on suicide incidents in India, and they have a relationship with the police that provides the information on these incidents.[24] Given this, it is unlikely such reports will contain broader helpful suicide prevention information. The recent decriminalization of suicide may prove to be an important and timely catalyst, shifting suicide out of the criminal realm and into the health sphere. Responsible media reporting of suicide by health and social, rather than by crime, journalists will be an important component of shifting suicide out of the criminal realm and into the health sphere.

Our qualitative interviews with media professionals in India observed that reporters on the crime beat and the police are playing dominant roles in the production of suicide news in India, with the police being a key stakeholder in improving reporting practices.[24] The crime reporter approach to suicide news was described as being largely incident-based, following a simple format for writing a news story, answering 'who, what, why, where and when',[48] with information and photos provided readily by police officers via WhatsApp groups and other media. The police are frequently both the unofficial and the official sources of information on suicides and they share personal and sensitive information on those who have died by suicide with crime reporters who have no knowledge or training in responsible approaches to covering suicide news.

It is important to appreciate the disconnect between the policy approach to suicide prevention and the current practices of the police and crime reporters. The national approach of decriminalization of suicide has seen moves away from criminality and towards a public health framework. Yet, it is still 'business as usual' in terms of crime coverage of suicide news, and there appears to be a *street-level bureaucracy* phenomenon at play. The street-level bureaucracy theory[49,50] seeks to explain the working practices of people delivering services on the frontline and how they may differ from public policy. Addressing this disconnect will need to be an important aspect of initiatives targeting media reporting of suicide in India, and addressing attitudes and literacy related to suicide among the police and media professionals will be key.

Culture and the newsworthiness of suicide

Culture is intertwined with decisions made by media professionals as to which suicides on which they report and which aspects of the incident may be emphasized. Our study revealed that the perceived newsworthiness of a suicide event in India was, in part, influenced by the profile of the suicidal person,[22,24] which is largely unsurprising and accords with practice elsewhere in the world.[51,52,53] We identified substantial disparities between the characteristics of suicides in the population and those in the Indian media.[22] Suicides involving females, those aged under 30 years, and separated or widowed males and unmarried females were significantly over-reported relative to their occurrence in the broader population. Students and persons working in the agricultural sector were also over-reported.

The focus on suicides of younger persons aged under 30 years is largely consistent with research elsewhere, including from Australia,[54] Austria,[55] and

China.[30] However, over-representation of female suicides in media coverage appears to be in stark contrast to what has been observed elsewhere. In India, the female suicide rate is among the highest in the world, and is nearly three times higher than the rate expected globally for countries at similar levels on the Socio-Demographic Index.[13] This well-documented fact about suicide in India could possibly permeate the minds of media professionals, who may then give greater emphasis to the plight of females who take their lives. Notwithstanding this, it is also likely that there are some other reasons why media professionals decide that suicides of females are more newsworthy. Based on our conversations with media professionals, female suicides are perceived to generate a greater empathic response among readers of newspapers in India.[24] Stories of suicides of females may also align with paternalistic narratives about the risks to women in Indian society and the family's and collective responsibility to protect them.[56]

Our observation of under-reporting of suicides of married males and females is also noteworthy to conversations around culture. Marriage and family are at the core of the social fabric in India,[57] and the family is the main source of welfare protection. We speculate that risks associated with being outside of the institution of marriage may be emphasized by media professionals through their selection of suicide stories pertaining to people whose marriage has been lost or who are yet to enter marriage. Through this under-reporting of suicides of married people, these media reports may actually be giving an incorrect signal to the population with regard to any suicide prevention protection that may be gained from being married. While marriage is typically understood to protect against suicide (particularly for men), based on findings from studies in Western settings,[58] this is not the case in India. Research undertaken in India has yielded mixed findings regarding the relationship between marital status and suicide for both men and women, suggesting that either marriage is not a protective factor against suicide or the risk of suicide is indeed higher among those who are married.[59,60] This epidemiological reality regarding marriage and suicide may conflict with narratives in India that locate 'the family' as the main source of social protection.

Our finding that suicides of students and people engaged in the agricultural sector were significantly over-represented is not surprising, given that both occupational groups are of significant interest to the public discourse and narratives around suicide in India.[17,61] Our qualitative research indicated that media professionals are well aware that reports on such deaths would resonate strongly with readers.[24] Student suicides are a major and topical policy issue in India, frequently located within discussions around the fierce competition for student places, the accompanying intensity of exam pressure, and the prominent media coverage of exam results with photos of top-scoring students.[62] Reporting on this issue will likely be of great interest to parents, who may carry a level of fear around suicide happening to their own children. Farmer suicides are highly politicized in India and have been the subject of numerous government commissions and policy dialogues. This has been largely with a focus on issues around the high levels of indebtedness among farmers, a decline in secure institutional credit, water scarcity and climate change, trade liberalization, and vulnerability to 'crop failure'.[63] Farmer suicides have been described as 'public deaths' due to the sensational coverage of these by mass media.[64] This issue has even been the subject of a popular fictional Hindi film *Peepli Live*, a 2010 satirical comedy that explores farmer suicides and the media frenzy that can ensue.

Beyond specific population groups of interest, other sociocultural issues also play a major role in determining the newsworthiness of suicide events in India. Suicide articles in India are replete with important cultural narratives, such as stories of bringing shame on family, dowry disputes, and young lovers unable to wed due to caste, religion, or other issues. Media professionals reported to us that compelling social narratives that are based in cultural mores are believed to stimulate greater audience interest in a suicide.[24] Furthermore, the capacity to link a suicide event with the detrimental impact of social/policy issues allowed a suicide report to generate controversy and apportioning of blame, again believed to stimulate audience interest. For some media professionals, this was linked with beliefs in India that some suicide events are a form of protest and martyrdom related to larger social issues, informed by major historical events where high-profile protest suicides have taken place. The concept of suicide as protest or martyrdom is a phenomenon that has also appeared in the academic literature on suicide in India, especially in reference to suicide by self-immolation.[65,66] In connection with this, media professionals see themselves as playing an important advocacy role in using suicides as a catalyst for raising awareness about social issues. A similar finding was observed in Hong Kong,[52] leading the authors to assert that suicide is perceived to be the result of social problems in many Asian societies. In one sense, this resonates with the push for taking a broad public health approach to suicide prevention that equally emphasizes the role of major social issues and policies rather than solely focusing on individual-level pathologized distress.[67] In another sense, such a predilection may lead to an oversimplification of suicide, including overlooking the important role of individual-level suicide risk factors like mental illness and drug and alcohol issues. Importantly, it is worth considering the extent to which reporting on suicide from such a framework may risk justifying the suicidal behaviour, inadvertently modelling suicide as an acceptable option in the face of intractable social ills. It may also model suicidal behaviour as a way to gain public notoriety via media coverage and to seek public retribution against people or institutions.

Media and imitation suicide: the need for local evidence

Imitation suicides are a prime concern in relation to media reporting of suicide, with research highlighting the potential for media reporting to impact population suicide rates in both harmful and protective ways.[3,14] The majority of evidence comes from outside India in HICs, although our recent study in India has captured the large and concerning impact of a reported high-profile celebrity suicide on suicide-related Internet search behaviours in the population.[23] Several media professionals to whom we spoke acknowledge the possibility that their reporting may have negatively influenced vulnerable people in the population, leading to imitation suicides. Several participants even provided anecdotal accounts of specific instances that they perceived to be imitation suicide events stemming from media reporting such as high-profile reports of metro suicides in Delhi; this phenomenon around media coverage of metro suicides has also been observed in Austria, where the introduction of media guidelines was associated with a decline in metro suicides.[68] This raises a query as to what is preventing action from taking place. A repeated point made by reporters was that they had little power or autonomy in the process of deciding how suicide-related news is covered, indicating a strong need for engagement at editorial and higher levels of media organizations, with evidence and locally accepted guidelines in hand.

Furthermore, a minority of media professionals dismissed or minimized concerns around imitation suicides, and others raised legitimate queries as to whether the harmful effects of graphic suicide scenes in fictional media were likely to be of greater concern than those presented in non-fictional media. What is clear is that there is a real need for strong local evidence of imitation suicidal behaviour in the population after media reports. International evidence is helpful, but alone it is not sufficient to easily convince all media professionals and owners in India of the need to adjust reporting styles to reduce the risk of imitation suicides.

While there has been this predominant focus on preventing imitation suicide, recent trends in the media and suicide research field have highlighted the potential protective effects on the population from media reporting that covers stories of people coping and surviving periods of suicidality. In our analyses of newspapers reports in India, such media reports were almost non-existent. It is a space with great potential for making a positive contribution in India and other LMICs, and further research is required to understand the dynamics of how this phenomenon might work across cultural settings.

Mass media and the suicide prevention ecosystem

Another key aspect to media guidance is for media reports to provide information on suicide helplines and any other relevant supports/programmes. Despite sounding simple and common sense, this recommendation is not without its complications. In India, media professionals with whom we spoke frequently expressed hesitance to publish contact details for suicide helplines or any other helplines/services on a regular basis.[25] A wide range of state and national helplines are available across India, from the long-standing Chennai-based SNEHA suicide prevention helpline to government helplines, to the recently launched nationwide KIRAN mental health helpline, and the quality and systems surrounding each inevitably vary. Media professionals raise legitimate doubts around how the helpline model works, alongside a lack of trust in the quality of the services, some of which are run by non-governmental organizations who may not have undertaken rigorous evaluations of their programme. The issue of quality is paramount in the minds of media professionals, who are concerned about promoting a helpline that may end up causing harm or providing a sub-par service to audience members who may be distressed. This is compounded by a media culture that does not encourage repeating the same helpline or advisory, due to concerns that it starts to become like an advertisement or a promotion for a particular organization or service.

We should not too quickly dismiss what are genuine concerns from media professionals around the programme theory and efficacy of helplines. To address any misunderstandings, suicide prevention experts should seek to provide media professionals with a clear rationale for the helpline model and an explanation as to how they operate, perhaps including on-site tours, with clear examples given of the processes involved and accounts from people with lived experience of using helplines for support during a suicide crisis. Local research evidence on the effectiveness of helplines[69] may also help to provide confidence to media professionals in giving helpline information to the public.

There is also a larger issue at play, with the need to understand how the different pieces of the suicide prevention puzzle come together. Media can provide details of helplines and create demand for these services, but if the helplines themselves are not well resourced or poorly functioning, and people have negative or harmful experiences, this can be counterproductive. It is also a function of demand and supply where media coverage of suicide prevention services may create demand that exceeds the supply capacity of such services. The recommendation to provide this information is simple to give, but support and guidance may be required around its implementation.

Melding mental health and social perspectives on suicide

It is clear that a public health framework around suicide reporting is emerging in India, with health reporters starting to tackle stories on the trends and causes of suicide, including the role of poor mental health and approaches to preventing suicide. However, our content analysis work observed that it was uncommon for mental health to be identified as an issue in suicide reports in the media.[21] In qualitative interviews, we found that media professionals held concerns that it is not possible to simply replicate the mental health discourse used in 'the West'.[24] Important concerns were raised that it may not be appropriate for Indian media to start promoting mental illness framings and treatments for suicide, when in many cases, it may be understandable (rather than pathological) human distress in the face of serious social issues such as deeply entrenched and intergenerational poverty, gender inequality, caste discrimination, and the socio-political-environmental challenges in the agricultural sector. Suicidal behaviour may also strongly intersect with culture, which is typically not a feature of discourses around mental health and suicide.

This emerging public health discourse around suicide in India needs to be able to equally incorporate the cultural and socio-economic drivers of suicide in India, as well as conversations around mental health. Kleinman's theory of social suffering has some relevance to this discussion.[70] Kleinman uses the term *social suffering*: (1) to emphasize that health problems are at times caused by socio-economic, cultural, and political forces such as the link between depression and poverty; and (2) to break down the distinction between health and social problems, and to frame ill-health as demanding both health and social responses. This perspective may be helpful in shaping nuanced framings of suicide in India in mass media reports.

Conclusion

We have sought to share some learnings from our research into mass media and suicide in India, in the hope that it may be of relevance to other LMICs attempting to address this same issue. Future research is needed that engages with fictional media, social media, and other forms of online media. It is evident that mass media-based suicide prevention interventions need to be developed, with a solid foundation in culture and the local context. Distribution of international guidelines may be insufficient on its own. It is also worth reflecting that WHO guidelines, while based on a considerable amount of international evidence and input from people across several countries, have nonetheless been written for a global, rather than for a local, audience. Being an international standard, they have necessarily been developed in somewhat of a culture and context vacuum, so that they are of broader utility. However, our research has highlighted how suicide reporting in India is intimately intertwined with sociocultural frameworks. Our current paper also reveals a range of attitudes and systematic reporting issues, such as reluctance to consistently report details of helplines (or other 'health advisories'), that need to be addressed through national guidelines adapted for the Indian context. Our findings indicate a clear need for guidelines that are situated in the Indian context and that have a strong basis in high-quality research evidence, with a priority for integrating research evidence and reporting examples from within India and the South Asia region. Most core recommendations (e.g. avoiding to give details of suicide methods) would be largely unchanged, but they would be positioned and communicated within an understanding of the Indian sociocultural and media practice context.

References

1. **Zalsman G, Hawton K, Wasserman D,** et al. Suicide prevention strategies revisited: 10-year systematic review. The Lancet Psychiatry. 2016;**3**(7):646–59.
2. **Turecki G, Brent DA.** Suicide and suicidal behaviour. The Lancet. 2016;**387**(10024):1227–39.
3. **Niederkrotenthaler T, Voracek M, Herberth A,** et al. Role of media reports in completed and prevented suicide: Werther v. Papageno effects. British Journal of Psychiatry. 2010;**197**(3):234–43.
4. **Cheng Q, Chen F, Yip PS.** Media effects on suicide methods: a case study on Hong Kong 1998–2005. PLoS One. 2017;**12**(4):e0175580.
5. **Niederkrotenthaler T, Fu KW, Yip PS,** et al. Changes in suicide rates following media reports on celebrity suicide: a meta-analysis. Journal of Epidemiology and Community Health. 2012;**66**(11):1037–42.
6. **Chen YY, Chen F, Yip PS.** The impact of media reporting of suicide on actual suicides in Taiwan, 2002–05. Journal of Epidemiology and Community Health. 2011;**65**(10):934–40.
7. **Niederkrotenthaler T, Stack S.** *Media and Suicide: International Perspectives on Research, Theory, and Policy*. New York, NY: Taylor & Francis; 2017.
8. **Till B, Arendt F, Scherr S, Niederkrotenthaler T.** Effect of educative suicide prevention news articles featuring experts with vs without personal experience of suicidal ideation. Journal of Clinical Psychiatry. 2018;**80**(1):17m11975.
9. **Till B, Wild TA, Arendt F, Scherr S, Niederkrotenthaler T.** Associations of tabloid newspaper use with endorsement of suicide myths, suicide-related knowledge, and stigmatizing attitudes toward suicidal individuals. Crisis. 2018;**39**(6):428–37.

10. **Arendt F, Scherr S, Niederkrotenthaler T, Till B.** The role of language in suicide reporting: investigating the influence of problematic suicide referents. Social Science and Medicine. 2018;**208**:165–71.
11. **World Health Organization, International Association for Suicide Prevention.** *Preventing Suicide: A Resource for Media Professionals, Update 2017.* Geneva: World Health Organization; 2017.
12. **World Health Organization.** *Preventing Suicide: A Global Imperative.* Geneva: World Health Organization; 2014.
13. **India State-Level Disease Burden Initiative Suicide Collaborators.** Gender differentials and state variations in suicide deaths in India: the Global Burden of Disease Study 1990–2016. The Lancet Public Health. 2018;**3**(10):e478–89.
14. **Niederkrotenthaler T, Braun M, Pirkis J**, et al. Association between suicide reporting in the media and suicide: systematic review and meta-analysis. BMJ. 2020;**368**:m575.
15. **Naghavi M; Global Burden of Disease Self-Harm Collaborators.** Global, regional, and national burden of suicide mortality 1990 to 2016: systematic analysis for the Global Burden of Disease Study 2016. BMJ. 2019;**364**:l94.
16. **Arya V, Page A, Armstrong G, Kumar A, Dandona R.** Estimating patterns in the under-reporting of suicide deaths in India: comparison of administrative data and Global Burden of Disease Study estimates, 2005–2015. Journal of Epidemiology and Community Health. 2021;75(6):550–5.
17. **Arya V, Page A, River J, Armstrong G, Mayer P.** Trends and socio-economic determinants of suicide in India: 2001–2013. Social Psychiatry and Psychiatric Epidemiology. 2018;**53**(3):269–78.
18. **Arya V, Page A, Dandona R, Vijayakumar L, Mayer P, Armstrong G.** The geographic heterogeneity of suicide rates in India by religion, caste, tribe, and other backward classes. Crisis. 2019;**40**(5):370–4.
19. **Arya V, Page A, Gunnell D**, et al. Suicide by hanging is a priority for suicide prevention: method specific suicide in India (2001–2014). Journal of Affective Disorders. 2019;**257**:1–9.
20. **Armstrong G, Vijayakumar L.** Suicide in India: a complex public health tragedy in need of a plan. The Lancet Public Health. 2018;3(10):e459–e460.
21. **Armstrong G, Vijayakumar L, Niederkrotenthaler T**, et al. Assessing the quality of media reporting of suicide news in India against World Health Organization guidelines: a content analysis study of nine major newspapers in Tamil Nadu. Australian and New Zealand Journal of Psychiatry. 2018;**52**(9):856–63.
22. **Armstrong G, Vijayakumar L, Pirkis J**, et al. Mass media representation of suicide in a high suicide state in India: an epidemiological comparison with suicide deaths in the population. BMJ Open. 2019;**9**(7):e030836.
23. **Armstrong G, Haregu T, Arya V**, et al. Suicide-related Internet search queries in India following media reports of a celebrity suicide: an interrupted time series analysis. World Psychiatry. 2021;**20**(1):143–4.
24. **Armstrong G, Vijayakumar L, Cherian AV, Krishnaswamy K.** 'It's a battle for eyeballs and suicide is clickbait': the media experience of suicide reporting in India. PLoS One. 2020;**15**(9): e0239280.
25. **Armstrong G, Vijayakumar L, Cherian A, Krishnaswamy K, Pathare S.** Indian media professionals' perspectives regarding the role of media in suicide prevention and receptiveness to media guidelines: a qualitative study. BMJ Open. 2021;**11**:e047166.

26. **Rao U.** *News as Culture: Journalistic Practices and the Remaking of Indian Leadership Traditions*. New York, NY: Berghahn Books; 2010.
27. **The Economist** (2016). Why India's newspaper business is booming.
28. **Thussu DK.** Privatizing the airwaves: the impact of globalization on broadcasting in India. Media, Culture and Society. 1999;**21**:125–31.
29. **Beautrais A, Hendin H, Yip P**, et al. Improving portrayal of suicide in the media in Asia. In: **Hendin H, Phillips M, Vijayakumar L**, et al., editors. *Suicide and Suicide Prevention in Asia*. Geneva: World Health Organization; 2008. pp. 39–49.
30. **Fu KW, Chan YY, Yip PS.** Newspaper reporting of suicides in Hong Kong, Taiwan and Guangzhou: compliance with WHO media guidelines and epidemiological comparisons. Journal of Epidemiology and Community Health. 2011;**65**(10):928–33.
31. **Ju Ji N, Young Lee W, Seok Noh M, Yip PS.** The impact of indiscriminate media coverage of a celebrity suicide on a society with a high suicide rate: epidemiological findings on copycat suicides from South Korea. Journal of Affective Disorders. 2014;**156**:56–61.
32. **Fu KW, Yip PS.** Estimating the risk for suicide following the suicide deaths of 3 Asian entertainment celebrities: a meta-analytic approach. Journal of Clinical Psychiatry. 2009;**70**(6):869–78.
33. **Chandra PS, Doraiswamy P, Padmanabh A, Philip M.** Do newspaper reports of suicides comply with standard suicide reporting guidelines? A study from Bangalore, India. International Journal of Social Psychiatry. 2014;**60**(7):687–94.
34. **Poreddi V, Thimmaiah R, Ramu R**, et al. Gender differences related to attitudes toward suicide and suicidal behavior. Community Mental Health Journal. 2016;**52**(2):228–32.
35. **Cavanagh JT, Carson AJ, Sharpe M, Lawrie SM.** Psychological autopsy studies of suicide: a systematic review. Psychological Medicine. 2003;**33**(3):395–405.
36. **Armstrong G, Jorm AF, Samson L, Joubert L, Singh S, Kermode M.** Suicidal ideation and attempts among men who inject drugs in Delhi, India: psychological and social risk factors. Social Psychiatry and Psychiatric Epidemiology. 2014;**49**(9):1367–77.
37. **Hawton K, van Heeringen K.** Suicide. The Lancet. 2009;**373**(9672):1372–81.
38. **Nock MK, Borges G, Bromet EJ**, et al. Cross-national prevalence and risk factors for suicidal ideation, plans and attempts. British Journal of Psychiatry. 2008;**192**(2):98–105.
39. **Borges G, Bagge CL, Cherpitel CJ, Conner KR, Orozco R, Rossow I.** A meta-analysis of acute use of alcohol and the risk of suicide attempt. Psychological Medicine. 2017;**47**(5):949–57.
40. **Cottler LB, Campbell W, Krishna VA, Cunningham-Williams RM, Abdallah AB.** Predictors of high rates of suicidal ideation among drug users. Journal of Nervous Mental Disorders. 2005;**193**(7):431–7.
41. **Shidhaye R, Kermode M.** Stigma and discrimination as a barrier to mental health service utilization in India. International health. 2013;**5**(1):6–8.
42. **Armstrong G, Kermode M, Raja S, Suja S, Chandra P, Jorm AF.** A mental health training program for community health workers in India: impact on knowledge and attitudes. International Journal of Mental Health Systems. 2011;**5**(1):17.
43. **Hofmann-Broussard C, Armstrong G, Boschen MJ, Somasundaram KV.** A mental health training program for community health workers in India: impact on recognition of mental disorders, stigmatizing attitudes and confidence. International Journal of Culture and Mental Health. 2017;**10**(1):62–74.

44. **Vijayakumar L, Shastri M, Fernandes T**, et al. Application of a scorecard tool for assessing and engaging media on responsible reporting of suicide-related news in India. International Journal of Environmental Research and Public Health. 2021;**18**:6206.
45. **Arafat SMY, Khan MM, Niederkrotenthaler T, Ueda M, Armstrong G.** Assessing the quality of media reporting of suicide deaths in Bangladesh against World Health Organization guidelines. Crisis. 2020;**41**:47–53.
46. **Sorensen JB, Pearson M, Armstrong G**, et al. A qualitative analysis of self-harm and suicide in Sri Lankan printed newspapers. Crisis. 2020;**42**:56–63.
47. **Ranjan R, Kumar S, Pattanayak RD, Dhawan A, Sagar R.** (De-) criminalization of attempted suicide in India: a review. Industrial Psychiatry Journal. 2014;**23**(1):4–9.
48. **Richardson J.** *Analysing Newspapers: An Approach from Critical Discourse Analysis*. London: United Kingdom: Palgrave Macmillan; 2007.
49. **Cooper MJ, Sornalingam S, O'Donnell C.** Street-level bureaucracy: an underused theoretical model for general practice? British Journal of General Practice. 2015;**65**(636):376–7.
50. **Lipsky M.** *Street-Level Bureacracy: Dilemmas of the Individual in Public Services*, 2nd edition. New York, NY: Russell Sage Foundation; 2010.
51. **Collings SC, Kemp CG.** Death knocks, professional practice, and the public good: the media experience of suicide reporting in New Zealand. Social Science and Medicine. 2010;**71**(2):244–8.
52. **Cheng Q, Fu KW, Caine E, Yip PS.** Why do we report suicides and how can we facilitate suicide prevention efforts? Perspectives of Hong Kong media professionals. Crisis. 2014;**35**(2):74–81.
53. **Jamieson P, Jamieson KH, Romer D.** The responsible reporting of suicide in print journalism. American Behavioral Scientist. 2003;**46**(12):1643–60.
54. **Machlin A, Pirkis J, Spittal MJ.** Which suicides are reported in the media—and what makes them 'newsworthy'? Crisis. 2013;**34**(5):305–13.
55. **Niederkrotenthaler T, Till B, Herberth A**, et al. The gap between suicide characteristics in the print media and in the population. European Journal of Public Health. 2009;**19**(4):361–4.
56. **Chanana K.** Hinduism and female sexuality: social control and education of girls in India. Sociological Bulletin. 2001;**50**(1):37–63.
57. **Mullatti L.** Families in India: beliefs and realities. Journal of Comparative Family Studies. 1995;**26**:11–25.
58. **Kposowa AJ.** Marital status and suicide in the National Longitudinal Mortality Study. Journal of Epidemiology and Community Health. 2000;**54**(4):254–61.
59. **Latha KS, Bhat SM, D'Souza P.** Suicide attempters in a general hospital unit in India: their socio-demographic and clinical profile—emphasis on cross-cultural aspects. Acta Psychiatrica Scandinavica. 1996;**94**(1):26–30.
60. **Srivastava MK, Sahoo RN, Ghotekar LH**, et al. Risk factors associated with attempted suicide: a case control study. Indian Journal of Psychiatry. 2004;**46**(1):33–8.
61. **Bhola P, Manjula M, Rajappa V, Phillip M.** Predictors of non-suicidal and suicidal self-injurious behaviours, among adolescents and young adults in urban India. Asian Journal of Psychiatry. 2017;**29**:123–8.
62. **Mary RA, Marslin G, Franklin G, Sheeba CJ.** Test anxiety levels of board exam going students in Tamil Nadu, India. BioMed Research International. 2014;**2014**:578323.

63. **Kennedy J, King L.** The political economy of farmers' suicides in India: indebted cash-crop farmers with marginal landholdings explain state-level variation in suicide rates. Global Health. 2014;**10**:16.
64. **Munster D.** Farmers' suicides as public death: politics, agency and statistics in a suicide-prone district (South India). Modern Asian Studies. 2015;**49**(5):1580–605.
65. **Singh SP, Santosh PJ, Avasthi A, Kulhara P.** A psychosocial study of 'self-immolation' in India. Acta Psychiatrica Scandinavica. 1998;**97**(1):71–5.
66. **Dey A.** Women as martyrs: mass suicides at Thoa Khalsa during the partition of India. Spanish Journal of India Studies. 2016;**3**:7–17.
67. **Caine ED.** Forging an agenda for suicide prevention in the United States. American Journal of Public Health. 2013;**103**(5):822–9.
68. **Niederkrotenthaler T, Sonneck G.** Assessing the impact of media guidelines for reporting on suicides in Austria: interrupted time series analysis. Australian and New Zealand Journal of Psychiatry. 2007;**41**(5):419–28.
69. **Hoffberg AS, Stearns-Yoder KA, Brenner LA.** The effectiveness of crisis line services: a systematic review. Frontiers in Public Health. 2019;**7**:399.
70. **Kleinman A.** Four social theories for global health. The Lancet. 2010;**375**(9725):1518–19.

Chapter 24

Ethnic aspects in pharmacological treatment of suicidality

Eva Döring-Brandl

Introduction

Over 700,000 people die from suicide every year, making suicide the cause of death for 1.3% of the population.[1] Although there are regional differences in suicide rates, suicides occur worldwide across all cultures and age groups. Especially in individuals with psychiatric disorders, suicidality is a serious concern. Psychiatric disorders are among the main risk factors for suicidality.[2] It has been estimated that approximately 90% of suicides occur in individuals with mental disorders.[3] While most suicide attempts and suicides are conducted by patients with depression, other psychiatric disorders such as bipolar disorder, schizophrenia or substance use disorders are known also to lead to an increased suicide risk.

A higher risk of suicidal behaviour and death from suicide has been shown for several groups of migrants and ethnic minorities. In particular, women of non-European background are at increased risk. Language barriers, separation from family, and several other social factors, such as loss of status or lack in knowledge of health care systems and possibilities of obtaining support, may contribute to this increased risk.[4]

Suicidal ideations and suicide attempts are serious issues in psychiatric treatment and usually require fast interventions, independent of the underlying disorder causing the suicidality. Besides psychotherapeutic strategies, medication is often part of the treatment for suicidal patients. However, many psychopharmacological approaches are used for treatment of suicidal patients without sufficient efficacy or evidence of benefit. For some types of medication used in acute treatment of suicidal patients with different types of psychiatric disorders, ethnic factors that may influence metabolism, tolerability, or efficacy of the medication should be considered. While it is well established that there are ethnic differences in pharmacokinetic and pharmacodynamic factors influencing treatment response to some medications, these factors are often not considered sufficiently in clinical practice. This chapter reviews ethnic aspects of medication commonly used in treatment of suicidal behaviour.

Antidepressants

Depression is the most common psychiatric disorders in individuals dying from suicide.[5] Suicidal behaviour is a key symptom of depressive episodes and very often plays an important role in treatment of depression patients. Acute, as well as chronic, suicidality may occur and requires consideration throughout psychiatric treatment.

Depression is commonly treated with antidepressants. The prescription rates of these types of medication have been rising dramatically over the past few decades. It is often assumed by psychiatrists, as well as by affected individuals, that antidepressants not only alleviate the severity of depression itself, but also are effective against suicidal ideations or suicide attempts. A large number of studies have investigated the impact of antidepressants on suicidality. Several large meta-analyses have been published, each incorporating up to almost 100,000 patients (e.g. Khan et al.,[6] Fergusson et al.,[7] and Stone et al.).[8] These have shown that antidepressants are not superior in preventing suicide, compared to placebo. Since it may be argued that the anti-suicide effect of antidepressants may begin only after a longer treatment duration, a more recent meta-analysis has investigated the effect of treatment of at least 12 weeks' duration on suicidality. This study even reported a higher suicide risk in patients taking antidepressants, compared to the placebo group.[9] An increased suicide risk in patients younger than 25 years taking an antidepressant has been reported in another meta-analysis, whereas this increased risk was not observed in patients older than 25 years.[8] Although antidepressants do not seem to reduce the risk of dying by suicide, they have been shown to reduce suicidal ideations, in particular in elderly subjects,[8,10] which might be rather caused by the effect against depression and less by a generally anti-suicidal effect. Current clinical practice guidelines do not contain convergent recommendations regarding antidepressants and suicidality.[11]

Despite these limitations, antidepressants are commonly used in psychiatric treatment of suicidal patients with depression. It has been shown that prescription patterns to ethnic minority patients differ from those to ethnic majorities. For example, the box warning regarding the increased risk of suicidal ideations has been shown to be followed less by health care providers caring for ethnic minority children and adolescents.[12] In elderly individuals with depression, differences in symptom presentation and prescription patterns of antidepressant medication with generally lower prescription rates have been described.[13] Treatment adherence to antidepressants in ethnic minority patients has been shown to be lower. This may be caused by various factors, including language barriers, differences in attitude towards treatment, and insufficient consideration of specific cultural factors.[14] Another reason may be a lack of understanding of biological differences between ethnic groups that can lead to poor antidepressant efficacy or tolerability. One important example are the ethnic differences in frequency of genetic variants influencing the cytochrome (CYP) P450 system. Most antidepressants are metabolized by one or more CYP enzymes. Genetic variants can affect the activity and inducibility of almost all known CYP enzymes, leading to clinical phenotypes with regular (extensive metabolizer (EM)), slightly lower (intermediate metabolizer (IM)), lacking (poor metabolizer (PM)), or increased (ultrarapid metabolizer, UM) enzyme activity. There are large differences in the frequency of these phenotypes across ethnic groups. For example, up to 40% of individuals from North Africa have a UM status for CYP2D6, as compared to under 5% of the European population.[15] CYP2D6 is one of the key CYP enzymes for most antidepressants (e.g. paroxetine, fluoxetine, amitriptyline, venlafaxine) and antipsychotics (e.g. aripiprazole, haloperidol, risperidone). Increased metabolism of substrates leads to lower plasma levels and potentially worse treatment response.[16] Another relevant CYP enzyme for medication used in psychiatric treatment is CYP2C19, which metabolizes escitalopram, citalopram, and sertraline, among others. Approximately 25% of individuals from East Asia have a PM status for CYP2C19, leading to increased plasma levels and a higher risk of side effects from medication. This may be the reason for the higher risk of medication adverse effects in East Asian individuals and has led to recommendations for lower starting doses of medication in patients of Asian descent.[15] While a broad use of CYP genotyping in psychiatric practice is not recommended to date, consideration of ethnic differences in CYP variation potentially underlying poor treatment outcome may be helpful in individual cases.

Besides these pharmacokinetic variants, genetic variation influencing pharmacodynamics (i.e. the action of a medication on tissues, receptors, etc.) is also known to differ across ethnic groups. Although the clinical relevance of most pharmacodynamic variants influencing antidepressant response and/or side effects is yet to be fully determined,[17,18] several pharmacodynamic variants have repeatedly been shown to have different, or even opposite, effects. One well-examined example is the 5-HTTLPR polymorphism in the promoter region of the serotonin transporter gene. The serotonin transporter is one of the main targets of antidepressants, and therefore of specific pharmacogenetic interest. The 5-HTTLPR polymorphism can lead to a long ('l') or short ('s') variant of the promoter region. In individuals of European ancestry, the l-allele has repeatedly been shown to be associated with better antidepressant response, whereas in Asians, better response in s-allele carriers has been observed.[19] The 5-HTTLPR polymorphism has also been associated with suicidality with opposite effects across ethnicities. While in Europeans, the s-allele has been found to be associated with a lower suicide risk, it has been found to be associated with an increased risk in all other examined ethnicities.[20] Due to contradictory research findings and low effect size of the polymorphism, 5-HTTLPR genotyping is not part of clinical practice to date but serves as an important example of ethnic differences in pharmacodynamic variation.

Mood stabilizers

It has been estimated that up to 50% of bipolar patients will attempt to die by suicide at least once, and up to 19% of individuals with bipolar disorder complete suicide.[21] Therefore, suicidality is a serious concern in treatment of patients with bipolar disorder. While there is good evidence for an anti-suicidal effect of lithium, other mood stabilizers have shown much weaker or no effects on suicide risk. However, since they are commonly used in treatment of bipolar patients, they are also discussed within this section.

Valproate

While valproate is only approved for treatment of acute mania in patients with bipolar disorder, it is commonly used also as maintenance treatment. In addition, valproate is used in clinical practice for treatment of various other symptoms and psychiatric disorders. Although it has not been shown to be superior to lithium in treatment of acute mania, valproate is commonly used for treatment of manic episodes where it has been shown repeatedly to be effective.[22] Limited evidence also supports an effect on depressive episodes in bipolar patients. Valproate has been shown to have some efficacy in prevention of new disease episodes, although it also has not been demonstrated to be superior to lithium maintenance treatment.[23] A recent meta-analysis has investigated the effect of valproate on suicidality in bipolar patients. Here, no reduction in suicide risk could be demonstrated,[24] showing that valproate does not have an anti-suicidal effect.

Valproate is mainly metabolized by several hepatic pathways, including CYP2A6, CYP2B6, and CYP2C9. Mitochondrial beta-oxidation and microsomal glucuronide conjugation also participate in its metabolism. Regarding pharmacodynamics, effects on *N*-methyl-*D*-aspartate receptors and gamma-aminobutyric acid signalling, and alterations in monoamine levels, as well as epigenetic effects, have been described.[23] A variety of pharmacokinetic, as well as pharmacodynamic, candidate genes for valproate response have been examined during the past years.[25] However, to the best of the author's knowledge, there are no studies focusing on ethnic differences in these variants in the context of treatment of suicidal bipolar patients. With the additional lack of evidence for an anti-suicidal effect of valproate, current knowledge does not allow any specific recommendations for patients from different ethnicities in this context.

Lithium

Lithium is the only medication used for treatment of affective disorders with a proven anti-suicidal effect. Meta-analyses have shown that lithium treatment lowers the suicide risk in patients with unipolar depression or bipolar disorder, compared to the general population.[26,27,28] Large population-based register studies have confirmed the anti-suicidal effect of lithium. While in a large Danish study, the suicide risk in individuals receiving lithium prescriptions in general was higher than in the general population, regular intake (defined as two or more lithium prescriptions) significantly lowered the suicide rate, as compared to irregular or short-term intake of lithium.[29] Another large register study from the United Kingdom found a significantly reduced suicide rate in bipolar patients receiving lithium, compared to patients receiving valproate or atypical antipsychotics.[30] In summary, there is extensive evidence for the anti-suicidal effect of lithium from both large randomized controlled trials and population-based register studies.

Regarding ethnicity and lithium treatment, there are only limited data available. In general, patients of African or Afro-Caribbean ancestry seem to be misdiagnosed with other disorders than bipolar disorder more often than patients of other ethnicities, leading to an underrepresentation in clinical and genomic studies, as well as in clinical treatment settings.[31,32] Therefore, insufficient treatment of this ethnic group with lithium and other mood stabilizers in general can be assumed. A recent randomized controlled trial reported better response to low-dose lithium in African–American individuals with bipolar depression, as compared to non-Hispanic subjects of European ancestry.[33]

Lithium undergoes renal elimination, making cytochrome variants irrelevant for its elimination. One study from the 1980s reported slightly faster distribution and elimination in subjects of European origin, as compared to those of Afro-Caribbean origin.[34] However, this difference was not statistically significant.

With the exact biological mechanism of action of lithium not yet fully understood, no genetic variants with clinically relevant impact on treatment response or side effects have been identified to date. However, a number of candidate genes for lithium response have been identified. Recent genome-wide association studies have identified a number of loci of potential interest; however, further studies are required for confirmation of these findings and for an assessment of their clinical relevance.[16] A recent large study examining the association of a polygenic score for major depression with lithium response in bipolar patients reported a similar trend in the effect of the polygenic score on lithium response in European and Asian subjects; however, the association was only significant in the European, but not the Asian, subsample.[35]

Carbamazepine

There are only sparse data available on the effect of carbamazepine on suicidality. Data from Taiwan indicate a reduced risk of completed suicide in bipolar patients treated with carbamazepine, valproate, or lithium, with similar effects of the medications.[36] A retrospective chart review in veterans with bipolar disorder found similar rates of non-lethal suicidal behaviour during treatment with lithium, valproate, or carbamazepine.[37] However, a recent review of the literature reported a higher rate of suicide attempts in bipolar patients receiving carbamazepine versus those treated with valproate or lithium.[38]

While the effect of carbamazepine on suicidality needs further assessment, it is the medication used in psychiatric treatment with the clearest evidence for a major impact of patients' ethnicity on tolerability. A massively increased risk of development of Stevens–Johnson syndrome (SJS) or toxic epidermal necrolysis (TEN)—both rare, but dangerous, side effects of carbamazepine—in Asians, especially in Han Chinese patients, has been observed. This elevated risk is linked with the higher prevalence of risk alleles for SJS and TEN in genes encoding the human leucocyte antigen (HLA) system in individuals of Asian origin. In particular, the HLA-B*1502 allele has been associated with a massively increased risk of SJS and TEN, with an odds ratio of 2504.[39] The HLA-B*1511 allele also has been associated with an increased risk, whereas the HLA-A*2402 allele seems to be protective.[40]

The high risk of SJS/TEN in carriers of HLA-B*1502 has led to the incorporation in box warnings from the Food and Drug Administration (FDA) of the recommendation for genotyping prior to treatment initiation with carbamazepine in at-risk populations.[41]

Antipsychotics

Schizophrenia patients are at increased risk of death by suicide. However, there are only limited data on the impact of antipsychotic medication on suicidality. The only antipsychotic with some indication for an anti-suicidal effect is clozapine. One randomized controlled trial found significantly fewer suicide attempts in patients taking clozapine, compared to those treated with olanzapine; however, there was no significant difference in completed suicides.[42] A register-based study from Finland found a reduced suicide rate in patients receiving clozapine, whereas there was no reduction in those receiving haloperidol, thioridazine, olanzapine, perphenazine, risperidone, or quetiapine.[43] However, while a recent meta-analysis reported reduced long-term mortality in schizophrenia patients taking clozapine, no significant difference in death by suicide between clozapine and other antipsychotics could be found.[44]

Ethnic differences in response to, and tolerability of, antipsychotics have been reported—however, not in terms of suicidality, but rather in general response to treatment. Treatment-resistant schizophrenia seems to be more common in individuals of European origin, as compared to other ethnicities.[45] Patients of Asian origin seem to respond to lower doses of medication, which might be caused by pharmacokinetic variation. While a review from 1999 assumed that most differences in antipsychotic response in African–American subjects may rather be caused by different prescription practices of treating clinicians,[46] a recent quasi-systematic review identified a number of pharmacodynamics variants, mainly including variants in the dopamine D1 and D4 receptors, that influence antipsychotic response and tolerability in African–Americans, but not in Europeans.[47] While no clinical recommendations can be derived from these pharmacogenetic findings to date, they underline the necessity for consideration of ethnicity in pharmacogenetic studies, as well as in clinical treatment settings.

Regarding pharmacokinetic influences on antipsychotic response, the above-mentioned higher frequency of CYP2D6 UM status in North African subjects can lead to faster metabolism of antipsychotics metabolized by CYP2D6. This can result in lower plasma levels and 'pseudo-refractoriness' to the medication.[15] A polymorphism in CYP3A43, rs472660, is significantly more common in African–Americans, compared to Europeans, and has been linked with faster olanzapine clearance and poorer response;[48] however, this finding requires further investigation.

Benzodiazepines

Benzodiazepines are commonly used in acute treatment of suicidal patients, especially as a combination treatment with antidepressants. A combination of antidepressants and benzodiazepines in the first four weeks of depression treatment was shown in a meta-analysis to have better efficacy than antidepressant monotherapy with regard to the antidepressant effect; however, anti-suicidal effects were not assessed in the study.[49] In a case-control study, suicide victims had received benzodiazepine prescriptions significantly more often than the control group,[50] which may either indicate that individuals with a high suicide risk receive prescriptions more often or that benzodiazepines themselves increase the suicide risk. A literature review found indications of an increased suicide risk in individuals receiving benzodiazepine prescriptions, which might be caused by increased aggression, impulsivity, or withdrawal symptoms.[51] These data indicate that benzodiazepines generally should be prescribed with caution and suicidality needs to be regularly assessed.

Regarding ethnic aspects of benzodiazepine treatment, similarly to other types of psychotropic medication, differences in prescription patterns have been observed. A recent study showed a much higher likelihood for subjects of European ancestry to have benzodiazepine dependence and to receive prescriptions, as compared to African–American, Asian, or Hispanic subjects.[12]

In terms of pharmacokinetics, the higher frequency of poor metabolizers for CYP2C19 from East Asia should be considered when diazepam is prescribed. The slower metabolism could lead to an increased risk of initial oversedation. Therefore, a lower starting dosage in patients of Asian origin has been recommended.[52]

Conclusion

In summary, while a number of medications are used for treatment of suicidal patients with various psychiatric disorders, there is only limited evidence for an anti-suicidal effect of psychopharmacological medication. The only drug with a substantial indication for a reduction in suicidality to date is lithium. However, other medications have their place in treatment of disorders underlying suicidal behaviour (e.g. affective or psychotic disorders). For a number of psychiatric medications, ethnic differences in pharmacokinetics and pharmacodynamics have been demonstrated. To date, only few of these have been shown to be of high clinical relevance. Among these, the higher risk of SJS/TEN in East Asians receiving carbamazepine is associated with genetic variation, which carries the best evidence for genetic testing prior to treatment onset. Nonetheless, knowledge and consideration of ethnic variation in the frequency of slow or fast CYP metabolizers in clinical practice have been shown to be helpful in reducing treatment resistance or adverse events.

With the generally limited evidence for anti-suicidal efficacy of current psychotropic substances, novel pharmacological treatment approaches are warranted. Ketamine, for example, has been shown to have beneficial fast effects on depression symptoms and suicidal ideations;[53] however, further assessment of anti-suicidal effects of this substance is needed.

References

1. **World Health Organization**. 2023. Available from: https://www.who.int/news-room/fact-sheets/detail/suicide
2. **Carrasco-Barrios MT, Huertas P, Martin P**, et al. Determinants of suicidality in the European general population: a systematic review and meta-analysis. International Journal of Environmental Research and Public Health. 2020;**17**(11):4115.
3. **Bradvik L.** Suicide risk and mental disorders. International Journal of Environmental Research and Public Health. 2018;**15**(9):2028.
4. **Forte A, Trobia F, Gualtieri F**, et al. Suicide risk among immigrants and ethnic minorities: a literature overview. International Journal of Environmental Research and Public Health. 2018;**15**(7):1438.
5. **Hawton K, Casanas ICC, Haw C, Saunders K.** Risk factors for suicide in individuals with depression: a systematic review. Journal of Affective Disorders. 2013;**147**(1–3):17–28.
6. **Khan A, Khan S, Kolts R, Brown WA.** Suicide rates in clinical trials of SSRIs, other antidepressants, and placebo: analysis of FDA reports. American Journal of Psychiatry. 2003;**160**(4):790–2.
7. **Fergusson D, Doucette S, Glass KC**, et al. Association between suicide attempts and selective serotonin reuptake inhibitors: systematic review of randomised controlled trials. BMJ. 2005;**330**(7488):396.
8. **Stone M, Laughren T, Jones ML**, et al. Risk of suicidality in clinical trials of antidepressants in adults: analysis of proprietary data submitted to US Food and Drug Administration. BMJ. 2009;**339**:b2880.
9. **Braun C, Bschor T, Franklin J, Baethge C.** Suicides and suicide attempts during long-term treatment with antidepressants: a meta-analysis of 29 placebo-controlled studies including 6,934 patients with major depressive disorder. Psychotherapy and Psychosomatics. 2016;**85**(3):171–9.
10. **Gibbons RD, Brown CH, Hur K, Davis J, Mann JJ.** Suicidal thoughts and behavior with antidepressant treatment: reanalysis of the randomized placebo-controlled studies of fluoxetine and venlafaxine. Archives of General Psychiatry. 2012;**69**(6):580–7.
11. **Gabriel FC, de Melo DO, Fraguas R, Leite-Santos NC, Mantovani da Silva RA, Ribeiro E.** Pharmacological treatment of depression: a systematic review comparing clinical practice guideline recommendations. PLoS One. 2020;**15**(4):e0231700.
12. **Cook B, Creedon T, Wang Y**, et al. Examining racial/ethnic differences in patterns of benzodiazepine prescription and misuse. Drug and Alcohol Dependence. 2018;**187**:29–34.
13. **Mansour R, Tsamakis K, Rizos E**, et al. Late-life depression in people from ethnic minority backgrounds: differences in presentation and management. Journal of Affective Disorders. 2020;**264**:340–7.
14. **Brandl EJ, Dietrich N, Mell N**, et al. Attitudes towards psychopharmacology and psychotherapy in psychiatric patients with and without migration background. BMC Psychiatry. 2020;**20**(1):176.

15. **Brandl EJ, Eckermann G.** [Ethnische Aspekte in der Psychopharmakologie]. In: **Graef-Calliess I, Schouler-Ocak M,** editors. [*Migration und Transkulturalität-Neue Aufgaben in Psychiatrie und Psychotherapie*]. Schattauer, Stuttgart; 2017. pp. 345–57.
16. **Muller DJ, Brandl EJ, Degenhardt F,** et al. [Pharmacogenetics in psychiatry: state of the art]. Der Nervenarzt. 2018;**89**(3):290–9.
17. **Gvozdic K, Brandl EJ, Taylor DL, Muller DJ.** Genetics and personalized medicine in antidepressant treatment. Current Pharmaceutical Design. 2012;**18**(36):5853–78.
18. **Lett TA, Walter H, Brandl EJ.** Pharmacogenetics and imaging—pharmacogenetics of antidepressant response: towards translational strategies. CNS Drugs. 2016;**30**(12):1169–89.
19. **Porcelli S, Fabbri C, Serretti A.** Meta-analysis of serotonin transporter gene promoter polymorphism (5-HTTLPR) association with antidepressant efficacy. European Neuropsychopharmacology. 2012;**22**(4):239–58.
20. **Schild AH, Nader IW, Pietschnig J, Voracek M.** Ethnicity moderates the association between 5-HTTLPR and national suicide rates. Archives of Suicide Research. 2014;**18**(1):1–13.
21. **Latalova K, Kamaradova D, Prasko J.** Suicide in bipolar disorder: a review. Psychiatria Danubina. 2014;**26**(2):108–14.
22. **Baldessarini RJ, Tondo L, Vazquez GH.** Pharmacological treatment of adult bipolar disorder. Molecular Psychiatry. 2019;**24**(2):198–217.
23. **Schäfer M, Brandl EJ.** Mood stabilizers: valproate. In: **Riederer P, Laux G, Mulsant B, Le W, Nagatsu T,** editors. *NeuroPsychopharmacotherapy*. Springer, Cham; 2022. pp. 1549–57.
24. **Chen TY, Kamali M, Chu CS,** et al. Divalproex and its effect on suicide risk in bipolar disorder: a systematic review and meta-analysis of multinational observational studies. Journal of Affective Disorders. 2019;**245**:812–18.
25. **Ghodke-Puranik Y, Thorn CF, Lamba JK,** et al. Valproic acid pathway: pharmacokinetics and pharmacodynamics. Pharmacogenetics and Genomics. 2013;**23**(4):236–41.
26. **Tondo L, Hennen J, Baldessarini RJ.** Lower suicide risk with long-term lithium treatment in major affective illness: a meta-analysis. Acta Psychiatrica Scandinavica. 2001;**104**(3):163–72.
27. **Guzzetta F, Tondo L, Centorrino F, Baldessarini RJ.** Lithium treatment reduces suicide risk in recurrent major depressive disorder. Journal of Clinical Psychiatry. 2007;**68**(3):380–3.
28. **Cipriani A, Hawton K, Stockton S, Geddes JR.** Lithium in the prevention of suicide in mood disorders: updated systematic review and meta-analysis. BMJ. 2013;**346**:f3646.
29. **Kessing LV, Sondergard L, Kvist K, Andersen PK.** Suicide risk in patients treated with lithium. Archives of General Psychiatry. 2005;**62**(8):860–6.
30. **Hayes JF, Pitman A, Marston L,** et al. Self-harm, unintentional injury, and suicide in bipolar disorder during maintenance mood stabilizer treatment: a UK population-based electronic health records study. JAMA Psychiatry. 2016;**73**(6):630–7.
31. **Akinhanmi MO, Biernacka JM, Strakowski SM,** et al. Racial disparities in bipolar disorder treatment and research: a call to action. Bipolar Disorders. 2018;**20**(6):506–14.
32. **Kirov G, Murray RM.** Ethnic differences in the presentation of bipolar affective disorder. European Psychiatry. 1999;**14**(4):199–204.

33. **Gonzalez Arnold J, Salcedo S, Ketter TA**, et al. An exploratory study of responses to low-dose lithium in African Americans and Hispanics. Journal of Affective Disorders. 2015;**178**:224–8.
34. **Shelley RK.** Are there ethnic differences in lithium pharmacokinetics and side-effects? International Clinical Psychopharmacology. 1987;**2**(4):337–42.
35. **Amare AT, Schubert KO, Hou L**, et al. Association of polygenic score for major depression with response to lithium in patients with bipolar disorder. Molecular Psychiatry. 2021 Jun; 26(6):2457–70.
36. **Tsai CJ, Cheng C, Chou PH**, et al. The rapid suicide protection of mood stabilizers on patients with bipolar disorder: a nationwide observational cohort study in Taiwan. Journal of Affective Disorders. 2016;**196**:71–7.
37. **Yerevanian BI, Koek RJ, Mintz J.** Bipolar pharmacotherapy and suicidal behavior. Part I: lithium, divalproex and carbamazepine. Journal of Affective Disorders. 2007;**103**(1-3):5–11.
38. **Caley CF, Perriello E, Golden J.** Antiepileptic drugs and suicide-related outcomes in bipolar disorder: a descriptive review of published data. Mental Health Clinician. 2018;**8**(3):138–47.
39. **Ferrell PB, Jr, McLeod HL.** Carbamazepine, HLA-B*1502 and risk of Stevens–Johnson syndrome and toxic epidermal necrolysis: US FDA recommendations. Pharmacogenomics. 2008;**9**(10):1543–6.
40. **Grover S, Kukreti R.** HLA alleles and hypersensitivity to carbamazepine: an updated systematic review with meta-analysis. Pharmacogenetics and Genomics. 2014;**24**(2):94–112.
41. **Food and Drug Administration** (2009). Tegretol®. Available from: https://www.accessdata.fda.gov/drugsatfda_docs/label/2009/016608s101,018281s048lbl.pdf
42. **Meltzer HY, Alphs L, Green AI**, et al. Clozapine treatment for suicidality in schizophrenia: International Suicide Prevention Trial (InterSePT). Archives of General Psychiatry. 2003;**60**(1):82–91.
43. **Tiihonen J, Lonnqvist J, Wahlbeck K**, et al. 11-year follow-up of mortality in patients with schizophrenia: a population-based cohort study (FIN11 study). The Lancet. 2009;**374**(9690):620–7.
44. **Vermeulen JM, van Rooijen G, van de Kerkhof MPJ, Sutterland AL, Correll CU, de Haan L.** Clozapine and long-term mortality risk in patients with schizophrenia: a systematic review and meta-analysis of studies lasting 1.1–12.5 years. Schizophrenia Bulletin. 2019;**45**(2):315–29.
45. **Teo C, Borlido C, Kennedy JL, De Luca V.** The role of ethnicity in treatment refractory schizophrenia. Comprehensive Psychiatry. 2013;**54**(2):167–72.
46. **Frackiewicz EJ, Sramek JJ, Herrera JM, Kurtz NM, Cutler NR.** Ethnicity and antipsychotic response. Annals of Pharmacotherapy. 1997;**31**(11):1360–9.
47. **Jerome RN, Pulley JM, Sathe NA**, et al. Exploring biologic predictors response disparities to atypical antipsychotics among blacks: a quasi-systematic review. Ethnicity and Disease. 2020;**30**(Suppl 1):229–40.
48. **Bigos KL, Bies RR, Pollock BG, Lowy JJ, Zhang F, Weinberger DR.** Genetic variation in CYP3A43 explains racial difference in olanzapine clearance. Molecular Psychiatry. 2011;**16**(6):620–5.

49. **Ogawa Y, Takeshima N, Hayasaka Y**, et al. Antidepressants plus benzodiazepines for adults with major depression. Cochrane Database of Systematic Reviews. 2019;**6**:CD001026.
50. **Cato V, Hollandare F, Nordenskjold A, Sellin T.** Association between benzodiazepines and suicide risk: a matched case-control study. BMC Psychiatry. 2019;**19**(1):317.
51. **Dodds TJ.** Prescribed benzodiazepines and suicide risk: a review of the literature. Primary Care Companion for CNS Disorders. 2017;**19**(2):22746.
52. **Chen JP, Barron C, Lin KM, Chung H.** Prescribing medication for Asians with mental disorders. Western Journal of Medicine. 2002;**176**(4):271–5.
53. **Wilkinson ST, Ballard ED, Bloch MH**, et al. The effect of a single dose of intravenous ketamine on suicidal ideation: a systematic review and individual participant data meta-analysis. American Journal of Psychiatry. 2018;**175**(2):150–8.

Index

For the benefit of digital users, indexed terms that span two pages (e.g., 52–53) may, on occasion, appear on only one of those pages.

Tables and figures are indicated by an italic *t* and *f* following the page/paragraph number